HANDBOOK OF OBESITY TREATMENT

Edited by
Thomas A. Wadden
Albert J. Stunkard

THE GUILFORD PRESS
New York   London

© 2002 The Guilford Press
A Division of Guilford Publications, Inc.
72 Spring Street, New York, NY 10012
www.guilford.com

Printed in the United States of America

This book is printed on acid-free paper.

Last digit is print number: 9   8   7   6   5   4

Library of Congress Cataloging-in-Publication Data

Handbook of obesity treatment / edited by Thomas A. Wadden, Albert J. Stunkard.
     p. cm.
     Updated ed. The 2nd ed. was previously published as: Obesity : theory and therapy.
     Includes bibliographical references and index.
     ISBN 1-57230-722-6 (hc.)   ISBN 1-59385-094-8 (pbk.)
     1. Obesity.   I. Wadden, Thomas A.   II. Stunkard, Albert J., 1922–   III. Obesity.

RC628 .O32 2001
616.3′98—dc21   2001040507

For David, Michael, and Steven
and for Elana
with deepest love and affection

About the Editors

Thomas A. Wadden, PhD, is Professor of Psychology at the University of Pennsylvania School of Medicine, where he also is Director of the Weight and Eating Disorders Program. He received his AB from Brown University and his doctorate in clinical psychology from the University of North Carolina at Chapel Hill. Dr. Wadden has published over 150 scientific papers and is the coeditor of two books. He has investigated the treatment of obesity by several methods, including behavior modification, very-low-calorie diets, exercise, pharmacotherapy, and surgery. He serves on the National Task Force for the Prevention and Treatment of Obesity and on the Council of the North American Association for the Study of Obesity.

Albert J. Stunkard, MD, is Professor of Psychiatry at the University of Pennsylvania School of Medicine where, in 1957, he founded the Obesity Research Group (now the Weight and Eating Disorders Program). He received his BS from Yale University and his MD from Columbia University. Dr. Stunkard is the author of nearly 400 publications, primarily in the field of obesity, and his research has been supported for 40 years by the National Institutes of Health. He is a member of the Institute of Medicine and serves on the editorial boards of seven journals in the fields of nutrition and behavioral medicine.

Contributors

Drew A. Anderson, PhD, Department of Psychology, State University of New York at Albany, Albany, NY

Louis J. Aronne, MD, Department of Medicine, Weill College of Cornell University, New York, NY

Richard L. Atkinson, MD, Department of Medicine and Nutritional Sciences and Beers–Murphy Clinical Nutrition Center, University of Wisconsin, Madison, WI

Joaquin Barnoya, MD, Department of Nutrition, Harvard School of Public Health, Boston, MA

Robert I. Berkowitz, MD, Department of Psychiatry, University of Pennsylvania School of Medicine, Philadelphia, PA

Steven N. Blair, PED, The Cooper Institute, Dallas, TX

George A. Bray, MD, Pennington Biomedical Research Center, Louisiana State University, Baton Rouge, LA

Kelly D. Brownell, PhD, Department of Psychology, Yale University, New Haven, CT

Streamson C. Chua, Jr., MD, PhD, Division of Molecular Genetics, Department of Pediatrics, Naomi Berrie Diabetes Center, Columbia University College of Physicians and Surgeons, New York, NY

Graham A. Colditz, MD, DrPH, Department of Medicine, Channing Laboratory, Brigham and Women's Hospital and Harvard Medical School, Boston, MA

Zafra Cooper, DPhil, DipClinPsych, Department of Psychiatry, Oxford University, Oxford, England

Joyce A. Corsica, PhD, Department of Clinical and Health Psychology, University of Florida, Gainesville, FL

Eric J. De Maria, MD, Department of Surgery, Medical College of Virginia at Virginia Commonwealth University, Richmond, VA

Johanna Dwyer, DSc, RD, Jean Mayer Human Nutrition Center on Aging and Tufts University Schools of Medicine and Nutrition, Boston, MA; Frances Stern Nutrition Center, New England Medical Center, Boston, MA

Leonard H. Epstein, PhD, Department of Pediatrics, State University of New York at Buffalo, Buffalo, NY

Christopher G. Fairburn, DM, FRCPsych, Department of Psychiatry, Oxford University, Oxford, England

Alison E. Field, ScD, Department of Medicine, Channing Laboratory, Brigham and Women's Hospital and Harvard Medical School, Boston, MA

Gary D. Foster, PhD, Department of Psychiatry, University of Pennsylvania School of Medicine, Philadelphia, PA

Gary S. Goldfield, PhD, Department of Psychology, State University of New York at Buffalo, Buffalo, NY

Edward W. Gregg, PhD, Division of Diabetes Translation, National Center for Chronic Disease Prevention and Health Promotion, Centers for Disease Control and Prevention, Atlanta, GA

Katherine Battle Horgen, PhD, Department of Psychology, Yale University, New Haven, CT

Robert W. Jeffery, PhD, Division of Epidemiology, University of Minnesota, Minneapolis, MN

Carol Johnson, MA, Largely Positive, Incorporated, Milwaukee, WI

John M. Kellum, MD, Department of Surgery, Medical College of Virginia at Virginia Commonwealth University, Richmond, VA

Shiriki K. Kumanyika, PhD, MPH, RD, Center for Clinical Epidemiology and Biostatistics, University of Pennsylvania School of Medicine, Philadelphia, PA

Rifat Latifi, MD, Department of Surgery, Medical College of Virginia at Virginia Commonwealth University, Richmond, VA

Elizabeth A. Leermakers, PhD, The Cooper Institute, Dallas, TX

Rudolph L. Leibel, MD, Division of Molecular Genetics, Department of Pediatrics, Naomi Berrie Diabetes Center, Columbia University College of Physicians and Surgeons, New York, NY

Brian G. McGuckin, EdM, Department of Psychiatry, University of Pennsylvania School of Medicine, Philadelphia, PA

Kathleen Melanson, PhD, RD, LD, Department of Nutrition and Food Sciences, University of Rhode Island, Kingston, RI

Suzette Osei, MD, PhD, Department of Medicine, University of Pennsylvania School of Medicine, Philadelphia, PA

Michael G. Perri, PhD, Department of Clinical and Health Psychology, University of Florida, Gainesville, FL

Suzanne Phelan, PhD, Weight Control and Diabetes Research Center, Miriam Hospital, and Department of Psychiatry and Human Behavior, Brown University Medical School, Providence, RI.

R. Arlen Price, PhD, Center for Neurobiology and Behavior, University of Pennsylvania, Philadelphia, PA

Eric Ravussin, PhD, Pennington Biomedical Research Institute, Baton Rouge, LA

Hollie A. Raynor, MS, RD, Department of Psychology, State University of New York at Buffalo, Buffalo, NY

David B. Sarwer, PhD, Departments of Psychiatry and Surgery and The Edwin and Fannie Gray Hall Center for Human Appearance, University of Pennsylvania School of Medicine, Philadelphia, PA

Kathryn H. Schmitz, PhD, MPH, Division of Epidemiology, University of Minnesota, Minneapolis, MN

Albert J. Stunkard, MD, Department of Psychiatry, University of Pennsylvania School of Medicine, Philadelphia, PA

Harvey J. Sugerman, MD, Department of Surgery, Medical College of Virginia at Virginia Commonwealth University, Richmond, VA

P. A. Tataranni, MD, National Institute of Diabetes and Digestive and Kidney Diseases, National Institutes of Health, Tucson, AZ

J. Kevin Thompson, PhD, Department of Psychology, University of South Florida, Tampa, FL

Thomas A. Wadden, PhD, Department of Psychiatry, University of Pennsylvania School of Medicine, Philadelphia, PA

Shirley S. Wang, Department of Psychology, Yale University, New Haven, CT

David F. Williamson, PhD, Division of Diabetes Translation, National Center for Chronic Disease Prevention and Health Promotion, Centers for Disease Control and Prevention, Atlanta, GA

Rena R. Wing, PhD, Weight Control and Diabetes Research Center, Miriam Hospital, and Department of Psychiatry and Human Behavior, Brown University Medical School, Providence, RI

Leslie G. Womble, PhD, Department of Psychiatry, University of Pennsylvania School of Medicine, Philadelphia, PA

Preface

The past decade has witnessed unprecedented interest in the topic of obesity. The discovery in 1994 of the *ob/ob* gene and its protein product, leptin, will long remain a watershed mark in the history of obesity research, revealing as it did key mechanisms of body weight regulation. This discovery came at an opportune time, for other research completed the same year revealed that the United States was experiencing an epidemic of obesity. Fully 55% of adults were found to be either overweight or obese. Data from 1999 found that the prevalence had increased to 61%, placing overweight/obesity among our nation's most pressing public health problems. Regrettably, this problem is shared with growing numbers of developed nations—a fact that has led the World Health Organization to declare obesity a "global epidemic."

This volume seeks to improve the treatment of obesity by providing practitioners with a thorough review of its assessment and of therapies available to manage it. Particular attention is paid to identifying the most appropriate intervention for a given individual. The book also seeks to illuminate the causes of the obesity epidemic, with the ultimate goal of identifying innovative strategies to prevent the development of this disorder in both children and adults.

PLAN OF THE BOOK

This volume is divided into six parts. We hope that all will be of interest to the reader; however, researchers probably will be drawn particularly to the first two parts, and practitioners to the latter four. The parts are as follows:

- *Part I. Prevalence, Consequences, and Etiology of Obesity.* The opening chapter by Field and colleagues chronicles the growth of the nation's obesity epidemic and the very significant health and economic burden that it imposes. The three chapters that follow describe basic mechanisms of body weight regulation and the remarkable advances in this field in the past decade. As Chua and Liebel reveal in Chapter 2, our understanding of the neural and hormonal factors that regulate appetite has progressed well beyond leptin. Tataranni and Ravussin provide a more general overview in Chapter 3 of the regulation of energy intake and expenditure, as well as of body composition. Price, in Chapter 4, discusses advances in the genetics of obesity; he makes it clear that most cases of human obesity are likely to involve the interaction of multiple genes, which have yet to be identified. Only a handful of obese individuals, for example, suffer from a defect in the *ob/ob* gene. In Chapter 5, Horgen and Brownell argue convincingly that the obesity epidemic is the product of a "toxic environment" that explicitly encourages the consumption of super-sized portions, while implicitly discouraging physical activity. Stunkard concludes this part in Chapter 6 by discussing two groups who appear to be most adversely affected by this environment: those who suffer from binge-eating disorder, and those with the newly defined night-eating syndrome.

• *Part II. Health Consequences of Weight Reduction.* Before the assessment and treatment of obesity are considered, the two chapters in this part evaluate the health consequences of weight loss. This is an important issue, given recent concerns that weight loss, as well as cycles of weight loss and regain, may be associated with an increased risk of health complications. Gregg and Williamson, however, conclude in Chapter 7 that intentional weight loss (as contrasted to unintentional loss) appears to be associated with decreased risks of morbidity and mortality. Wadden and colleagues similarly conclude in Chapter 8 that weight reduction is associated with improvements in mood and quality of life, and that dieting (i.e., caloric restriction) in obese adults is not associated with the development of eating disorders. Thus obese adults should not be dissuaded from attempting to lose weight because of fears about adverse health consequences.

• *Part III. Assessment of the Obese Adult.* Obesity is easily diagnosed, usually by sight alone. In Chapter 9, however, Atkinson provides a thorough description of the history and physical examination that should be conducted on overweight or obese individuals. This assessment is critical for identifying health complications of obesity, and thus the medical need for weight reduction. Wadden and Phelan discuss the behavioral evaluation of the obese individual in Chapter 10; this includes assessing eating and activity habits, psychosocial status, and readiness for weight loss. This assessment is aided by the patient's completion of a questionnaire that is included as an appendix to the chapter.

• *Part IV. Treatment of Adult Obesity.* An expert panel convened in 1998 by the National Heart, Lung, and Blood Institute completed an exhaustive review of the safety and efficacy of treatments for obesity. The contributions in this part of the book build upon this foundation. Wadden and Osei present an algorithm in Chapter 11 that will assist health care providers in selecting an appropriate therapy, based on the patient's body mass index (BMI) and risk of health complications. As a rule, patients with a BMI < 30 kg/m^2 are most appropriately treated by a program of diet, exercise, and behavior modification. In Chapter 12, Melanson and Dwyer discuss the characteristics of a well-balanced reducing diet, in addition to identifying the potential liabilities of several "best-selling" approaches. Exercise is a critical component of long-term weight control, as reiterated by Blair and Leermakers in Chapter 13. These authors, however, highlight new findings that exercise is important for improving cardiovascular health, independently of its effects on body weight, and that health benefits can be obtained with relatively modest levels of physical activity. In Chapter 14, on behavioral weight control, Wing reviews the efficacy of a comprehensive program that combines diet, exercise, and behavior modification. She also describes efforts over the past decade to improve both the induction and maintenance of weight loss; promising methods include the use of social support and the long-term provision of meal replacement products.

Patients with a BMI ≥ 30 kg/m^2 are usually at greater risk of weight-related health complications and often have failed to reduce their weight with the interventions previously described. These individuals are candidates for pharmacological therapy, as described in Chapter 15 by Bray, who thoroughly reviews the medications that are currently available and those that may come to market in future years. Patients with a BMI ≥ 40 kg/m^2 who do not achieve a satisfactory outcome with behavioral or pharmacological approaches are eligible for bariatric surgery, which is described by Latifi and colleagues in Chapter 16. Surgical intervention is clearly associated with greater iatrogenic risks than the aforementioned therapies but is also associated with the best long-term results. The central challenge for all obesity therapies, that of maintaining weight loss, is discussed by Perri and Corsica in Chapter 17.

• *Part V. Treatment of Adult Obesity: Additional Approaches and Resources.* The interventions described in Part IV have been extensively evaluated, and their safety and efficacy have been described. Overweight and obese individuals, however, are treated by a variety of other approaches. In some cases, they do not have access to the aforementioned therapies; in other cases, patients may seek therapies that address psychosocial issues, in addition to their weight. Part V thus highlights other treatments available.

Primary care physicians can play an important role in the management of obesity, either by providing treatment directly or by referring patients to an appropriate program. In Chapter 18, Aronne describes the barriers that physicians frequently encounter in treating obesity, and provides suggestions for overcoming them. For practitioners unable to provide diet and exercise counseling in the office, referral to a self-help or commercial program may be considered. Womble and colleagues review criteria proposed by the Federal Trade Commission for evaluating commercial programs, and describe the treatment components of several popular approaches, in Chapter 19.

The five chapters that follow examine methods of adapting treatment to patients' individual needs, as well as addressing concerns beyond weight reduction. In Chapter 20, Kumanyika reviews findings that African Americans lose significantly less weight than whites when treated by a behavioral intervention. She explores cultural factors that may influence outcome, and proposes innovative ways to improve treatment in minority group members. Complaints of body image dissatisfaction are pervasive among overweight and obese individuals and are a new focus of behavioral treatment, as described by Sarwer and Thompson in Chapter 21. Cooper and Fairburn argue even more strongly in Chapter 22 that the failure to achieve their desired body image is what causes patients to regain lost weight. These authors propose adding a more intensive cognitive component to behavioral weight control therapy, to address body image dissatisfaction and unrealistic weight loss expectations. In Chapter 23, Johnson discusses the importance of improving not only body image but feelings of self-worth. She provides physicians with practical suggestions for improving their care of overweight patients, and encourages obese individuals to confront the weight-related prejudice and discrimination that can rob them of self-esteem. Efforts to improve body image and self-esteem in obese individuals have frequently been combined with programs that discourage participants from dieting (i.e., restricting calorie intake), in favor of eating in response to the body's natural hunger and satiety cues. In Chapter 24, Foster and McGuckin review the effects of these nondieting approaches on body weight, psychological functioning, and physical health.

• *Part VI. Childhood Obesity and Obesity Prevention.* This volume focuses principally on the treatment of adult obesity. This is consistent with the exceptionally high prevalence of overweight and obesity in U.S. men and women. Although researchers and practitioners must continue to search for more effective treatments for adult obesity, such efforts alone will not be adequate to halt and ultimately reverse the epidemic of obesity. More effective methods are needed to manage obesity in children and adolescents, in order to spare them the health complications that will beset them in adulthood. Of even more pressing concern, however, is the need to prevent the development of obesity in both children and adults. These issues are the topics of the volume's final three chapters.

The prevention and treatment of obesity in children require the identification of risk factors for this condition, which are reviewed by Berkowitz and Stunkard in Chapter 25. One of the review's principal conclusions is that children who become obese do not have low resting energy requirements, contrary to a recent hypothesis. In Chapter 26, Goldfield and colleagues describe behavioral interventions for obese children. The finding that children remain significantly less overweight fully 10 years after receiving treatment stands in sharp contrast to the results of treatment with adults and makes a strong argument for early intervention. Schmitz and Jeffery, in Chapter 27, tackle the challenge of preventing obesity; they review the results of school, workplace, and community interventions. Although some promising findings are reported, the chapter makes clear that efforts in this area must be increased many times over if we are to reverse the epidemic of obesity.

ACKNOWLEDGMENTS

We are grateful to have received contributions from an outstanding group of investigators, who are the world's experts in their areas of study. We are fortunate to count many of them among our closest friends and colleagues. All have our deepest thanks and appreciation.

Jim Nageotte, senior editor at The Guilford Press, provided invaluable counsel on all aspects of the book, from framing the big picture to addressing the smallest details. We thank him, as we do Laura Specht Patchkofsky and Marie Sprayberry (whose editorial expertise and superb copy editing, respectively, contributed to the uniformly high quality of all the chapters). We also thank Seymour Weingarten, editor-in-chief at The Guilford Press, for making this work possible.

This book would not have been completed without the superb editorial assistance of Shirley Wang, our unit's former research coordinator, who is now pursing her doctorate in clinical psychology. She, with the able assistance of Rebecca Rothman, read multiple drafts of chapters, tracked down missing references and figures, and maintained exceptionally good humor throughout the production of the book. We also thank Jane Seagrave and John Kennedy for their generous assistance with these efforts.

Our research on obesity has been supported for many years by the National Institutes of Health, to which we are grateful. Preparation of the individual chapters that we contributed was supported in part by Grant Nos. DK-56114 and DK-56124 (to Thomas A. Wadden) and by Grant Nos. DK-56735 and MH-56251 (to Albert J. Stunkard).

And finally, we thank our wives for their love, support, and understanding. They ultimately have contributed to this volume, as they do to all significant events in our lives.

THOMAS A. WADDEN
ALBERT J. STUNKARD

Contents

PART I. PREVALENCE, CONSEQUENCES, AND ETIOLOGY OF OBESITY

1. Epidemiology and Health and Economic Consequences of Obesity   3
   Alison E. Field, Joaquin Barnoya, and Graham A. Colditz

2. Body Weight Regulation: Neural, Endocrine, and Autocrine Mechanisms   19
   Streamson C. Chua, Jr., and Rudolph L. Leibel

3. Energy Metabolism and Obesity   42
   P. A. Tataranni and Eric Ravussin

4. Genetics and Common Obesities: Background, Current Status, Strategies,   73
   and Future Prospects
   R. Arlen Price

5. Confronting the Toxic Environment: Environmental Public Health Actions   95
   in a World Crisis
   Katherine Battle Horgen and Kelly D. Brownell

6. Binge-Eating Disorder and Night-Eating Syndrome   107
   Albert J. Stunkard

PART II. HEALTH CONSEQUENCES OF WEIGHT REDUCTION

7. The Relationship of Intentional Weight Loss to Disease Incidence and Mortality   125
   Edward W. Gregg and David F. Williamson

8. Psychosocial Consequences of Obesity and Weight Loss   144
   *Thomas A. Wadden, Leslie G. Womble, Albert J. Stunkard, and
   Drew A. Anderson*

PART III. ASSESSMENT OF THE OBESE ADULT

9. Medical Evaluation of the Obese Patient   173
   Richard L. Atkinson

10. Behavioral Assessment of the Obese Patient   186
Thomas A. Wadden and Suzanne Phelan

PART IV. TREATMENT OF ADULT OBESITY

11. The Treatment of Obesity: An Overview   229
Thomas A. Wadden and Suzette Osei

12. Popular Diets for Treatment of Overweight and Obesity   249
Kathleen Melanson and Johanna Dwyer

13. Exercise and Weight Management   283
Steven N. Blair and Elizabeth A. Leermakers

14. Behavioral Weight Control   301
Rena R. Wing

15. Drug Treatment of Obesity   317
George A. Bray

16. Surgical Treatment of Obesity   339
Rifat Latifi, John M. Kellum, Eric J. De Maria, and Harvey J. Sugerman

17. Improving the Maintenance of Weight Lost in Behavioral Treatment of Obesity   357
Michael G. Perri and Joyce A. Corsica

PART V. TREATMENT OF ADULT OBESITY:
ADDITIONAL APPROACHES AND RESOURCES

18. Treatment of Obesity in the Primary Care Setting   383
Louis J. Aronne

19. Commercial and Self-Help Weight Loss Programs   395
Leslie G. Womble, Shirley S. Wang, and Thomas A. Wadden

20. Obesity Treatment in Minorities   416
Shiriki K. Kumanyika

21. Obesity and Body Image Disturbance   447
David B. Sarwer and J. Kevin Thompson

22. Cognitive-Behavioral Treatment of Obesity   465
Zafra Cooper and Christopher G. Fairburn

23. Obesity, Weight Management, and Self-Esteem   480
Carol Johnson

24. Nondieting Approaches: Principles, Practices, and Evidence   494
Gary D. Foster and Brian G. McGuckin

PART VI. CHILDHOOD OBESITY AND OBESITY PREVENTION

25. Development of Childhood Obesity   515
    Robert I. Berkowitz and Albert J. Stunkard

26. Treatment of Pediatric Obesity   532
    Gary S. Goldfield, Hollie A. Raynor, and Leonard H. Epstein

27. Prevention of Obesity   556
    Kathryn H. Schmitz and Robert W. Jeffery

Author Index   595

Subject Index   617

PART I

PREVALENCE, CONSEQUENCES, AND ETIOLOGY OF OBESITY

1

Epidemiology and Health and Economic Consequences of Obesity

ALISON E. FIELD
JOAQUIN BARNOYA
GRAHAM A. COLDITZ

Obesity is a serious public health problem in the United States. The prevalence of obesity has increased sharply among children and adults over the past three decades. According to the third National Health and Nutrition Examination Survey (NHANES III), 32% of adults in the United States are overweight, and an additional 22.5% are obese (Flegal, Caroll, Kuczmarski, & Johnson, 1998). The prevalences are much higher among African Americans and Hispanics. Approximately 67% of adult African American and Hispanic women are overweight or obese, compared with 46% of non-Hispanic white women. Obesity is also a public health problem in other developed and affluent countries and is now spreading to less affluent countries, such as Mexico, Brazil, and Cuba (Popkin, 1994).

Although the terms "overweight" and "obesity" are used almost interchangeably in the scientific and lay literature, the two concepts are not identical. "Overweight" refers to weighing more than a standard level for height and age; "obesity" refers to excessive body fat. Overweight individuals may have excessive stores of body fat; however, highly active people who have substantial muscle mass may weigh slightly more than the standard for their height despite low body fat. Thus people may be overweight but not over-fat. Obesity has traditionally been classified based on body fat stores, but now is frequently defined as weighing substantially more than a standard level for age and height. The assumption has been that individuals who weigh much more than the standard for their height are very likely to have excessive body fat stores. This approach to categorizing people works quite well, since it is rare for an athlete to have sufficient muscle mass to be misclassified as obese. In clinical practice, it is obvious that a highly fit individual does not have excessive body fat; thus misclassification is only a potential problem in nonclinical settings.

Obesity and higher relative weights in adults are risk factors for cardiovascular disease (CVD) (Manson et al., 1990; Rexrode et al., 1997), certain cancers (Huang et al., 1997; Shoff & Newcomb, 1998; Tornberg & Carstensen, 1994), diabetes (Colditz et al., 1990), and mortality (Manson et al., 1995; Willett, Dietz, & Colditz, 1999). Excessive weight also exacerbates many other chronic diseases, such as hypertension (Witteman et al., 1990), osteoarthritis (Carman, Sowers, Hawthorne, & Weissfeld, 1994; Davis, Ettinger, Neuhaus, & Hauck, 1988), gallstones (Maclure et al., 1989), dyslipidemia, and musculoskeletal problems (Beirman & Hirsch, 1981; Mann, 1974; VanItallie, 1979). In addition to the physical health problems related to obesity, there are numerous psychological and psychosocial effects (Fine et al., 1999). Because psychological and psychosocial factors ultimately influence health and general well-being, the social impact of obesity is far-reaching.

DEFINITIONS, PREVALENCE, AND AGE-RELATED CHANGES

Definitions of Overweight and Obesity

Body mass index (BMI), a formula that combines weight and height, is commonly used in epidemiological studies assessing the relationship between weight and disease. In addition, the public health recommendations on body weight are based on BMI, which is computed as weight (in kilograms) divided by height (in meters) squared. The advantage of using BMI instead of weight in pounds or kilograms is that it accounts for height—an essential piece of information when one is evaluating weight. For example, a woman who weighs 145 pounds is overweight if she is 5 feet 4 inches tall, but a healthy weight if she is 5 feet 8 inches tall. The World Health Organization (1998) and the National Heart, Lung, and Blood Institue (NHLBI, 1998) have classified BMI as follows: <18.5 kg/m^2 is underweight; 18.5–24.9 kg/m^2 is the healthy weight range; 25–29.9 kg/m^2 is overweight; and ≥30 kg/m^2 is obese. As can be seen in Figure 1.1, a woman, who at 5 feet 4 inches and 145 pounds is considered overweight would be considered obese if she weighed 180 pounds.

Prevalence of Overweight and Obesity

Currently, approximately 60 million U.S. adults are overweight (Flegal et al., 1998; National Center for Health Statistics, 1996), and the prevalence of both overweight and obesity has been increasing (Kuczmarski, Flegal, Campbell, & Johnson, 1994). The age-adjusted prevalence of obesity increased by 8% from 1980 to 1994 (Flegal et al., 1998). More than 50% of U.S. adults over 20 years old exceed the healthy weight ranges (i.e., BMI > 25 kg/m^2): 59.3% of men and 49.6% of women, or 54.4% of the total U.S. population. In addition, 24.9% of women and 19.9% of men, or overall 25.4% of adults, are obese (BMI > 30 kg/m^2).

Body Weight and Age

Body weight and body composition are a function of genetics, health status, basal metabolic factors, dietary intake, physical activity, race, and hormonal factors. The onset (i.e., childhood, adolescence, or adulthood) and duration of obesity, as well as weight change, may have an important impact on health. Changes over time in basal metabolic factors, hormones, dietary intake, and physical activity result in changes in body weight and composition. Although BMI does an adequate job of classifying young- and middle-aged people in terms of body weight, it is less accurate among elderly individuals. Old age is frequently accompanied by a decline in lean body mass and changes in the distribution of body fat. Therefore, when body weight and risk of disease are being assessed among elderly persons, both BMI and waist circumference should be used.

WL	100	105	110	115	120	125	130	135	140	145	150	155	160	165	170	175	180
HL																	
5'0"	20	21	21	22	23	24	25	26	27	28	29	30	31	32	33	34	35
5'1"	19	20	21	22	23	24	25	26	26	27	28	29	30	31	31	33	34
5'2"	18	19	20	21	22	23	24	25	26	27	27	28	29	30	31	32	33
5'3"	18	19	19	20	21	22	23	24	25	26	27	27	28	29	30	31	32
5'4"	17	18	19	20	21	21	22	23	24	25	26	27	27	28	29	30	31
5'5"	17	17	18	19	20	21	22	22	23	24	25	26	27	27	28	29	30
5'6"	16	17	18	19	19	20	21	22	23	23	24	25	26	27	27	28	29
5'7"	16	16	17	18	19	20	20	21	22	23	23	24	25	26	27	27	28
5'8"	15	16	17	17	18	19	20	21	21	22	23	24	24	25	26	27	27
5'9"	15	16	16	17	18	18	19	20	21	21	22	23	24	24	25	26	27
5'10"	14	15	16	17	17	18	19	19	20	21	22	22	23	24	24	25	26
5'11"	14	15	15	16	17	17	18	19	20	20	21	22	22	23	24	24	25
6'0"	14	14	15	16	16	17	18	18	19	20	20	21	22	22	23	24	24
6'1"	14	14	15	15	16	16	17	18	18	19	20	20	21	22	22	23	24
6'2"	14	13	14	15	15	16	17	17	18	19	19	20	21	21	22	22	23
6'3"	12	13	14	14	14	16	16	17	17	18	19	19	20	21	21	22	22
6'4"	12	13	13	14	14	15	16	16	17	18	18	19	19	20	21	21	22

☐ (18.5–24.9) = NORMAL WEIGHT
▨ (25–29.9) = OVERWEIGHT
▪ (≥30) = OBESE
▢ (≤18.5) = UNDERWEIGHT

FIGURE 1.1. BMI chart.

CONSEQUENCES OF OVERWEIGHT

Mortality

Excessive weight increases the risk of death, particularly death due to CVD. Although there has been debate about whether the relationship between weight and risk of death is linear or J-shaped, the results have consistently shown that adults with BMI over 30 kg/m² are at increased risk of death (Manson et al., 1995; Stevens et al., 1998). Among 45- to 75-year-old men and women in the American Cancer Society's Cancer Prevention Study I, the risk of death increased linearly with BMI among those who had never smoked. The risk was particularly pronounced for death from CVD and among men (Stevens et al., 1998). Among 115,195 women in the Nurses' Health Study, Manson and colleagues (1995) observed that the risk of death over 16 years of follow-up rose steadily with BMI (see Figure 1.2). Although there was evidence of a J-shaped curve in the age-adjusted analysis, there was no evidence of an increased risk of death among the leanest women in the group who had never smoked.

Although mortality is a clearly defined outcome, the results of mortality analyses can

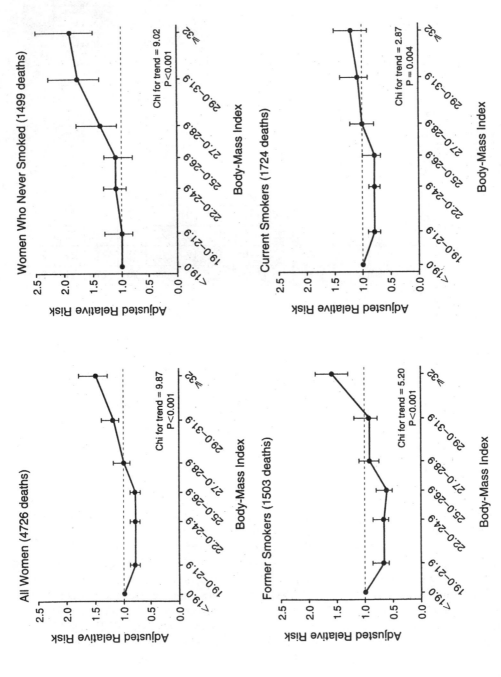

FIGURE 1.2. Relative risk of death from all causes, 1976 through 1992, according to body mass index, for all women, women who never smoked, former smokers, and current smokers. All relative risks have been adjusted for age in 5-year categories. For the total cohort and for current smokers, relative risks have been additionally adjusted for the intensity of smoking (1 to 14, 15 to 24, or ≥ 25 cigarettes per day). The bars represent 95% confidence intervals. In all cases, the reference category is the women with a body mass index below 19.0. From Manson et al. (1995). Copyright 1995 by Massachusetts Medical Society. Reprinted by permission.

be difficult to interpret. Except for diseases that are almost always fatal regardless of treatment, mortality is a function of incidence of disease, stage of illness at diagnosis, and the effectiveness of treatment. Many forms of CVD are treatable by either pharmacotherapy or intervention (i.e., angioplasty or surgery). Thus the relationship between excess weight and death from CVD does not necessarily translate to the same relationship with the development of CVD.

Morbidity

Cardiovascular Disease

CVD is the leading cause of death in the United States, accounting for 45.2% of all deaths. Approximately 58 million persons in the United States have one or more types of CVD ("Missed Opportunities in Preventive Counseling," 1998), including coronary heart disease (CHD), stroke, and hypertension.

Heart Disease. Young and middle-aged men and women who are overweight or obese are more likely than their leaner peers to develop heart disease (see Figure 1.3). Rimm and colleagues (1995) followed 29,122 U.S. men who were 40 to 75 years of age. They observed that among the men under 65 years of age, the risk of developing CHD increased with increasing category of BMI. Men who were overweight were almost twice as likely as those with a BMI below 23 kg/m^2 to develop CHD (relative risk [RR] = 1.7, 95% confidence interval [CI] = 1.1–2.7), whereas men with a BMI of at least 33 kg/m^2 were three times more likely to develop CHD (RR = 3.4, 95% CI = 1.7–7.1) during the 3 years of follow-up.

CHD is less common among women than men, particularly before menopause. Nevertheless, associations between excessive weight and CHD have been observed in adult women. Harris, Ballard-Barbasch, Madans, Makue, and Feldman (1993) observed that

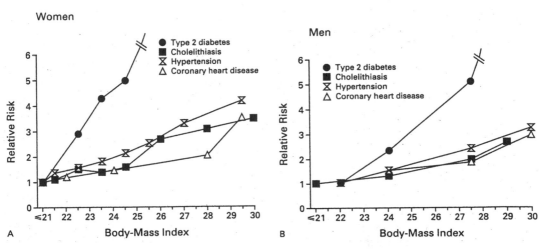

FIGURE 1.3. Relation between body mass index up to 30 and the relative risk of Type 2 diabetes, hypertension, coronary heart disease, and cholelithiasis. Panel A shows these relations for women in the Nurses' Health Study, initially 30 to 55 years of age, who were followed for up to 18 years. Panel B shows the same relations for men in the Health Professionals Follow-Up Study, initially 40 to 65 years of age, who were followed for up to 10 years. From Willett, Dietz, and Colditz (1999). Copyright 1999 by Massachusetts Medical Society. Reprinted by permission.

among 1,259 white women in NHANES I, those who were overweight (BMI > 29 kg/m²) and had fairly stable weights had a threefold increased risk (RR = 2.7, 95% CI = 1.7–4.4) of developing CHD. In addition, independent of overall adiposity (as measured by BMI), women with a large waist circumference (38 inches) or waist-to-hip ratio (WHR ≥ 0.88) were approximately three times more likely than their peers to develop CHD over an 8-year period (Rexrode et al., 1998). Overweight women are also at increased risk of ischemic stroke. Among 116,759 women aged 30 to 55 years in the Nurses' Health Study, women with BMI over 29 kg/m² were approximately twice as likely as women with BMI under 21 kg/m² to have an ischemic stroke during 16 years of follow-up (Rexrode et al., 1997).

Not only are obese adults more likely to develop CHD, but they are also more likely to die from it. During 12 years of follow-up of 48,287 Dutch men and women aged 30 to 54 , Seidell, Verschuren, van Leer, and Kromhout (1996) observed that men and women who were obese (i.e., BMI ≥ 30 kg/m²) were three times more likely than their nonoverweight peers (BMI < 25 kg/m²) to die from CHD. Moreover, the authors estimated that 20%–30% of the CHD mortality could be attributed to being overweight. Excessive weight earlier in life is also predictive of CHD mortality. Must, Jacques, Dallal, Bajema, and Dietz (1992) followed 508 adolescents who participated in the Harvard Growth Study of 1922 to 1935. The adolescents who were overweight were twice as likely as their lean peers to die from CHD during adulthood (RR = 2.3, 95% CI = 1.4–4.1).

There are several mechanisms through which obesity and weight gain might increase the risk of CHD. Hyperlipidemia is one mechanism. BMI is correlated with triglyceride levels, as well as high-density lipoprotein (HDL) levels. Low HDL levels are more predictive than high total cholesterol of developing heart disease. Thus obesity increases risk of heart disease in part by increasing total triglycerides and making the ratio of HDL to low-density lipoprotein (LDL) less favorable (Bray, 1996).

Hypertension. Approximately 25% of adult Americans have high blood pressure. From 1986 to 1996, the death rate from high blood pressure increased 6.8% (American Heart Association, 2000). Although high blood pressure (i.e., hypertension) is a highly treatable condition, if left untreated its consequences are severe. Hypertension is a strong predictor of more severe CVD. The combination of obesity and hypertension is associated with an increased risk of cardiac failure due to thickening of the ventricular wall and increased heart volume (Alpert & Hashimi, 1993).

Both weight (Ascherio et al., 1992; Folsom, Prineas, Kaye, & Soler, 1989; Witteman et al., 1989) and weight gain (Field et al., 1999; Yong, Kuller, Rutan, & Bunker, 1993) are positively associated with the development of hypertension. Among both men and women, there is a linear relation between body weight and blood pressure. Witteman and colleagues (1989) observed that women with a BMI between 26 and 28 kg/m² were approximately three times more likely then women with a BMI under 23 kg/m² (RR = 2.8) to develop hypertension over a 4-year period, and women with a BMI of 32 kg/m² or more were almost six times more likely to develop hypertension.

Blood pressure is very sensitive to weight change. A maintained weight loss of 10%–15% can result in a sustained lowering of blood pressure, as well as improving other CHD risk factors (Wing & Jeffrey, 1995). Thus weight loss is recommended to patients with mildly elevated blood pressure or risk factors for developing CVD. Huang and colleagues (1998) observed that among 82,473 women in the Nurses' Health Study, those who lost at least 10 kg and were able to maintain the loss for at least 2 years were 45% less likely to develop hypertension (RR = 0.6, 95% CI = 0.4–0.7) than their peers who were weight-stable. By contrast, women who gained 10–19.9 kg were twice as likely (RR = 2.2, 95% CI = 2.0–2.4) to develop hypertension. There are several mechanisms through which obesity causes hypertension. Hyperinsulinemia, which is common among overweight and obese individuals, can cause activation of the sympathetic nervous system as well as sodium retention, both of which increase the risk of developing hypertension (Mikhail, Golub, & Tuck, 1999).

Diabetes

The incidence of Type 2 diabetes mellitus has risen steadily over the past 30 years. Diabetes is a prevalent and serious disease, affecting approximately 14 million people in the United States (National Institute of Diabetes and Digestive and Kidney Diseases [NIDDK], 2000b). People with diabetes are at substantially elevated risk for blindness, kidney disease, heart disease, stroke, and death. Diabetes is the seventh leading cause of death in the United States (NIDDK, 2000b)

Type 2 diabetes is characterized by peripheral insulin resistance, impaired regulation of hepatic glucose production, and low β-cell function. Excessive weight increases the risk of Type 2 diabetes through insulin resistance (Mahler & Adler, 1999). Not only are overweight men and women at substantially increased risk for developing Type 2 diabetes (Chan, Rimm, Colditz, Stampfer, & Willett, 1994; Lundgren, Bengtsson, Blohme, Lapidus, & Sjöström, 1988), but adults at the upper end of the "healthy weight range" (i.e., BMI of 20–24.9 kg/m^2) are also at risk because of the strong linear relation between BMI and risk. In addition, even after adjustment for weight, weight gain has been observed to be strongly associated with the risk of developing diabetes (Colditz, Willett, Rotnitsky, & Manson, 1995; Holbrook, Barrett-Connor, & Wingard, 1989). Colditz and colleagues (1995) observed that among 114,281 female nurses 30 to 55 years of age, even a modest weight gain (5–7.9 kg) since age 18 was associated with a 90% increase in risk of diabetes (RR = 1.9; 95% CI = 1.5–2.3). Moreover, similar results were observed in a parallel study among men (Chan et al., 1994).

Independent of weight, location of adiposity has an important role in the development of Type 2 diabetes. Carey and colleagues (1997) observed that women with a large waist circumference (36.2 inches) were more than five times as likely as their peers with small waists (26.2 inches) to develop Type 2 diabetes, regardless of their overall adiposity (measured by BMI). Moreover, among 15,432 women, Hartz, Rupley, Kalkhoff, and Rimm (1983) found that the prevalence of diabetes within each weight stratum (nonobese, moderately obese, and severely obese) increased with WHR. Among the nonobese women, the risk increased in a gradual linear fashion. Among the severely obese women, the risk increased sharply from approximately 6% for those with a WHR under 0.72 to 16.5% among women with a WHR over 0.81. Similar associations have been seen in men. Ohlson and colleagues (1985) observed that BMI and WHR were significant independent predictors of developing diabetes over a 13.5-year follow-up of 792 Swedish men. Approximately 15% of the men in the highest tertile of both WHR and BMI developed diabetes, compared with only 0.5% of the men in the lowest tertile of both factors.

Cancers

Excessive weight is associated with the development of numerous types of cancer, including breast (among postmenopausal women), endometrial, gastric, and colon. The racial differences in the prevalence of excessive weight may partially explain the elevated rate of certain cancers among African Americans. Obesity is thought to increase risk of developing cancer primarily through its effect on hormones. However, certain cancers (e.g., renal cell carcinoma) are related to obesity through other, not well-understood mechanisms.

Among premenopausal women, those who are overweight are less likely to develop breast cancer (Peacock, White, Daling, Voigt, & Malone, 1999). The decrease in risk may be due to a higher prevalence of menstrual irregularities and their associated low estrogen levels in overweight women. The relation is quite different in postmenopausal women, among whom obesity is associated with an increased risk of developing breast cancer. Adipose tissue is the primary source of estrogen among postmenopausal women who do not use hormone replacement therapy. Therefore, it is not surprising that the obesity-related increase in risk is restricted to women who do not use hormone replacement therapy (Huang et al., 1997). Breast cancer is more common among post- than premenopausal women; therefore, it is it fair to say that obesity promotes more breast cancers than it prevents. In addition, among women diagnosed with breast cancer, obesity is associated with a higher mortality rate (Kyogoku et al., 1990).

Overweight women are more likely than their leaner peers to develop endometrial cancer (Shoff & Newcomb, 1998), which is the most common gynecological cancer in the United States and the fourth most common cancer overall in women. The increase in risk is strongest in older women (Tornberg & Carstensen, 1994). Although the data are quite limited, the results from primarily case–control studies suggest that the risk of ovarian cancer increases with relative weight (Farrow, Weiss, Lyon, & Daling, 1989).

In addition to increasing the risk of developing hormone-related cancers, obesity is associated with the development of other types of cancer, such as esophageal, stomach, and colon cancer. Obesity has a known relationship with gastroesophageal reflux, a risk factor for esophogeal adenocarcinoma (Vaughn, Davis, Fristal, & Thomas, 1995). Obese adults are up to 16 times as likely as lean adults to develop this type of cancer (Lagergren, Bergstrom, & Nyren, 1999). The increasing prevalence of obesity, coupled with the strength of the association between obesity and adenocarcinoma of the gastric cardia, may explain why the incidence of the tumor has been increasing dramatically in the recent past (Vaughn et al., 1995). Colon cancer is the third most common cancer in the United States. Among the 13,420 men and women in the NHANES I follow-up study, the risk of colon cancer associated with excess weight was similar in men and women (Ford, 1999). Although other researchers have observed an increase in risk associated with weight only among men (Giovannucci et al., 1995; Le Marchang, Wilkens, Kolonel, Hankin, & Lyu, 1997), the more recent data show an elevated risk in women (Martinez et al., 1997).

Gallstones

Gallstones are a fairly common, often quite painful condition and are most common among overweight adults. Gallstones are believed to form when the bile contains too much cholesterol or bilirubin or not enough bile salts, or when the gallbladder does not empty properly. Stones can range in size, and many of them are asymptomatic; however, if the stones lodge in any of the ducts that carry bile from the liver, problems can arise. The trapped bile in the ducts can lead to inflammation in the gallbladder, the ducts themselves, or the liver. If prolonged, the blockages can have severe consequences affecting the gallbladder, liver, or pancreas.

Gallstones that are symptomatic can be very painful. The most common course of treatment is laparoscopic surgery to remove the gallbladder (i.e., laparoscopic cholecystectomy). Although gallstones do form in lean adults, the relationship among weight, weight change, and gallstone formation is very strong. Moreover, women are more likely than men to develop gallstones. Among 16,884 adults in NHANES III, the prevalence of gallbladder disease significantly increased with weight status (Must et al., 1999). The relationship was stronger among women than men, and stronger in those less than 55 years of age. Compared with women in the healthy weight range, overweight women were twice as likely to report gallbladder disease (odds ratio [OR] = 1.9, 95% CI = 1.3–3.0), and women with a BMI of 40 kg/m^2 or over were more than five times as likely to report the diagnosis (OR = 5.2, 95% CI = 2.9–8.8). The association between body weight and gallbladder disease also has been observed prospectively. Over an 8-year period, 2,122 cases of symptomatic gallstones were diagnosed among the 90,302 women in the Nurses' Health Study (Stampfer, Maclure, Colditz, Manson, & Willett, 1992). The risk of developing symptomatic gallstones (that were not removed) and the risk of having a cholecystectomy increased linearly with BMI. Women with a BMI between 25 and 26 kg/m^2 were approximately 60% more likely than women with a BMI under 24 kg/m^2 to have a cholecystectomy or develop symptomatic gallstones (RR = 1.6, 95% CI = 1.4–1.9), whereas women with a BMI of 30–34.9 kg/m^2 were more than three times as likely to develop gallstones (RR = 3.5, 95% CI = 3.1–4.0).

The most likely mechanism through which obesity increases the risk of developing gallstones is the reduction in the amount of bile salts in bile, which results in more cholesterol. In addition, obesity is associated with decreased gallbladder emptying (NIDDK, 2000a).

Osteoarthritis

Approximately 16 million people in the United States have osteoarthritis (Arthritis Foundation, 2000), a disease that causes the breakdown of cartilage in joints. The hips, knees, and spine are the most common sites of osteoarthritis. As a result of the degeneration of the cartilage, bones that were previously cushioned by cartilage rub together and cause considerable pain. Although the condition has not been as well studied as other chronic diseases, such as CHD and cancer, it does appear that overweight adults are more than twice as likely as their leaner peers to develop osteoarthritis in the hip (Cooper et al., 1998). In addition, excessive weight is associated with the development and course of osteoarthritis of the knee (Cicuttini, Baker, & Spector, 1996; Hart & Spector, 1993; Manninen, Riihimaki, Heliovaara, & Makela, 1996). Excessive weight causes additional strain on the joints and can lead to their degradation.

Benign Prostatic Hyperplasia

Prostate enlargement is common among men. Benign prostatic hyperplasia (BPH) rarely causes symptoms among young men; however, more than 50% of men in their 60s and an estimated 90% in their 70s and 80s have some symptoms of BPH (Patient Information Resource, 2000). Surgical treatment (i.e., prostatectomy) is very common. An estimated 350,000 operations are preformed annually in the United States (Patient Information Resource, 2000). Among 25,892 men in the Health Professionals' Follow-Up Study, independent of age, smoking, and BMI, men with a large waist circumference (≥43 inches vs. <35 inches) were more than twice as likely (OR = 2.4, 95% CI = 1.4–4.0) to develop BPH and have a prostatectomy (Giovannucci et al., 1994). Centrally located adiposity may increase the risk of developing BPH by increasing the estrogen-to-androgen ratio and sympathetic nervous activity.

Mental Health and Lifestyle Outcomes

Despite the rapid increase in the prevalence of overweight, there are considerable social consequences of being overweight in a Westernized society that values thinness and fitness. Obese women are less likely to be hired, more likely to have their performance rated negatively, and less likely to be promoted (Larkin & Pines, 1979; Roe & Eichwort, 1976). Moreover, among both normal and overweight women, weight gain is associated with poorer well-being (Rumpel, Ingram, Harris, & Madans, 1994). Among approximately 1,000 adults in a weight gain prevention program, 22% of the women and 17% of the men reported that they had been mistreated because of their weight (Falkner et al., 1999). The prevalence increased across quartiles of BMI, from 5.7% among the leanest quartile to 42.5% among the heaviest participants. Gortmaker, Must, Perrin, Sobol, and Dietz (1993) followed a sample of 16- to 24-year-old people over 8 years. They observed that women who were overweight were approximately 20% and overweight men 11% less likely to marry. In addition to the adverse social consequences, overweight individuals are less likely than their leaner peers to be promoted at work (Wadden & Stunkard, 1985). Sonne-Holm and Sorensen (1986) observed that among 3,267 men in Copenhagen at each level of education attainment, the attained level of social class was significantly lower for obese men.

Obesity has an impact on many aspects of quality of life. The association between quality of life and body weight has been assessed among women in the Nurses' Health Study. In both cross-sectional (Coakley et al., 1998) and prospective (Fine et al., 1999) analyses using the Medical Outcome Study 36-Item Short-Form Health Survey to measure health-related quality of life, there was a linear association between increasing BMI and decreases in physical functioning and vitality. Moreover, weight change over a 4-year period was associated with changes in quality of life. Women who gained more than 20 pounds over the 4 years had significant decreases in physical functioning, whereas weight losses were associated with increases in functioning and vitality.

ECONOMIC COSTS OF OBESITY

Disease burden is commonly measured by mortality; however, it is an inadequate measure because it does not account for the morbidity associated with chronic conditions, nor does it capture the impact of lifestyle on health-related quality of life. Economic measures, on the other hand, can summarize this broad range of health effects and account for both nonfatal and fatal conditions. Thus they may provide a more comprehensive summary of the public health impact of such conditions as obesity.

Economic costs can be compartmentalized into direct and indirect costs. The direct costs of illness include the costs of diagnosis and treatment related to any disease (hospital stay, nursing home, medications, physician visits). Indirect costs include the value of lost productivity, including wages lost by people unable to work because of disease and wages forgone due to premature mortality.

In the United States, the direct cost of obesity has been estimated to be $70 billion, or 7% of health care expenditures. In other countries, the costs range from 2% in France (Levy, Levy, Le Pen, & Basdevant, 1995) and Australia (Segal, Carter, & Zimmet, 1994) to 4% of the national health care costs in the Netherlands (Seidell, 1995). The indirect costs of early retirement and increased risk of disability pensions are not insignificant. Among adult women in Sweden, obese subjects were 1.5 to 1.9 times more likely to take sick leave, and 12% of obese women had disability pensions attributable to obesity (Narbro, Jonsson, Larsson, Wedel, & Sjöström, 1996). Overall, approximately 10% of sick leave and disability pensions for women may be related to obesity and obesity-related conditions.

Colditz (1999) estimated that the indirect costs attributable to obesity in the United States amounted to at least $48 billion in 1995. However, Colditz noted that because there are adverse health effects associated with overweight below a BMI of 30 (NHLBI, 1998; U.S. Department of Agriculture and U.S. Department of Health and Human Services,

1995), his estimate is the lower bound of the health care cost, since substantial additional costs are incurred among those who are overweight (i.e., a BMI of 25–29.9 kg/m^2) but not obese.

Gorsky, Pamuk, Williamson, Shaffer, and Koplan (1996) simulated three hypothetical cohorts to estimate the costs of health care according to level of obesity over a 25-year period, discounting future costs at 3% per year. They estimated that an additional $16 billion will be spent over the next 25 years in treating adverse health effects of obesity in middle-aged women. Using an incidence-based approach to cost of illness, Thompson, Edelsberg, Colditz, Bird, and Oster (1999) estimated the excess costs of health services according to level of obesity. Using a conservative approach that did not include any future weight gain, and starting with NHANES III population estimates for BMI, cholesterol, hypertension, and diabetes, they estimated the lifetime future costs per person as comparable to those for smoking.

The health care costs that have been estimated to date are underestimations of the true costs, since they do not consider the impact of reduced physical functioning (Coakley et al., 1998; Fontaine, Cheskin, & Barofsky, 1996), the increased risk of infertility among young women (Rich-Edwards et al., 1994), or the increased risk of asthma, all of which are directly associated with increasing adiposity. The costs associated with infertility and asthma treatment are substantial and should be included in future analyses of the costs of obesity.

CONCLUSION

Obesity is a serious public health problem in the United States and other developed countries, and is becoming a problem in developing countries as well. The prevalence of obesity in both children and adults in the United States, as well as in other Westernized countries, is rising rapidly, so that we can expect the rates of CVD, diabetes, certain cancers, gallbladder disease, and osteoarthritis to rise over the next several decades.

Despite the health risks of obesity and the societal pressures to be thin, most adult Americans are steadily gaining weight. With rare exceptions, obesity is a preventable disease. Prevention of the development of obesity needs to be made a public health priority. In addition, doctors should counsel their patients on the importance of maintaining a healthy weight and help their overweight patients lose weight and maintain the loss. Physical activity is important for maintaining weight losses, as well as preventing excessive weight gain. In addition, the deleterious health effects of excessive weight are at least partially alleviated by being fit (Blair & Brodney, 1999). Thus it is essential that children and adults be encouraged to be active, regardless of their weight.

The benefits of weight loss are substantial in terms of reducing the risk of diabetes and hypertension. Although many people may be unable to lose and maintain a sufficient amount of weight for them to be happy with their weight and shape, even a modest 10% sustained weight loss can have tremendous benefits for their physical health. Although treatments for CVD and cancer have improved, prevention should be the goal. If the development of obesity could be prevented, a substantial proportion of the burden of CVD, cancer, and gallbladder disease could be avoided.

REFERENCES

Alpert, M. A., & Hashimi, M. W. (1993). Obesity and the heart. *American Journal of Medical Science, 306,* 117–123.

American Heart Association. (2000). *High blood pressure*. [Online]. Available: http://www.american-heart.org/statistics/06hghbld.html [2000, January 27].

Arthritis Foundation. (2000). *Osteoarthritis* [Online]. Available: http://www.arthritis.org/offices/al/about/osteoarthritis.asp [2000, January 27].

Ascherio, A., Rimm, E. B., Giovannucci, E. L., Colditz, G. A., Rosner, B., Willett, W. C., Sacks, F., & Stampfer, M. J. (1992). A prospective study of nutritional factors and hypertension among US men. *Circulation, 86*, 1475–1484.

Beirman, E. L., & Hirsch, J. (1981). Obesity. In R. H. Williams (Ed.), *Textbook of endocrinology* (pp. 906–921). Philadelphia: W.B. Saunders.

Blair, S. N., & Brodney, S. (1999). Effects of physical inactivity and obesity on morbidity and mortality: Current evidence and research issues. *Medical Science in Sports and Exercise, 31*(Suppl.), 646–662.

Bray, G. A. (1996). Health hazards of obesity. *Endocrinology and Metabolism Clinics of North America, 25*, 907–919.

Carey, V. J., Walters, E. E., Colditz, G. A., Solomon, C. G., Willett, W. C., Rosner, B. A., Speizer, F. E., & Manson, J. E. (1997). Body fat distribution and risk of non-insulin-dependent diabetes mellitus in women: The Nurses' Health Study. *American Journal of Epidemiology, 145*, 614–619.

Carman, W. J., Sowers, M., Hawthorne, V. M., & Weissfeld, L. A. (1994). Obesity as a risk factor for osteoarthritis of the hand and wrist: A prospective study. *American Journal of Epidemiology, 139*, 119–129.

Chan, J. M., Rimm, E. B., Colditz, G. A., Stampfer, M. J., & Willett, W. C. (1994). Obesity, fat distribution, and weight gain as a risk factor for clinical diabetes in men. *Diabetes Care, 17*, 961–969.

Cicuttini, F. M., Baker, J. R., & Spector, T. D. (1996). The association of obesity with osteoarthritis of the hand and knee in women: A twin study. *Journal of Rheumatology, 23*, 1221–1226.

Coakley, E. H., Kawachi, I., Manson, J. E., Speizer, F. E., Willett, W. C., & Colditz, G. A. (1998). Lower levels of physical function are associated with higher body mass index among middle-aged and older women. *International Journal of Obesity, 22*, 958–965.

Colditz, G. A. (1999). Economic costs of obesity and inactivity. *Medical Science in Sports and Exercise, 31*(Suppl. 11), S663–S667

Colditz, G. A., Willett, W. C., Rotnitsky, A., & Manson, J. E. (1995). Weight gain as a risk factor for clinical diabetes mellitus in women. *Annals of Internal Medicine, 122*, 481–486.

Colditz, G. A., Willett, W. C., Stampfer, M. J., Manson, J. E., Arkey, R. A., Hennekens, C. H., & Speizer, F. E. (1990). Weight as a risk factor for clinical diabetes in women. *American Journal of Epidemiology, 132*, 501–513.

Cooper, C., Inskip, H., Croft, P., Campbell, L., Smith, G., McLaren, M., & Coggon, D. (1998). Individual risk factors for hip osteoarthritis: Obesity, hip injury, and physical activity. *American Journal of Epidemiology, 147*, 516–522.

Davis, M. A., Ettinger, W. H., Neuhaus, J. M., & Hauck, W. W. (1988). Sex differences in osteoarthritis of the knee: The role of obesity. *American Journal of Epidemiology, 127*, 1019–1030.

Falkner, N. H., French, S. A., Jeffery, R. W., Neumark-Sztainer, D., Sherwood, N. E., & Morton, N. (1999). Mistreatment due to weight: Prevalence and sources of perceived mistreatment in women and men. *Obesity Research, 7*, 572–576.

Farrow, D. C., Weiss, N. S., Lyon, J. L., & Daling, J. R. (1989). Association of obesity and ovarian cancer in a case–control study. *American Journal of Epidemiology, 129*, 1300–1304.

Field, A. E., Byers, T., Hunter, D. J., Laird, N. M., Manson, J. E., Williamson, D. F., & Willett, W. C. (1999). Weight cycling, weight gain, and risk of hypertension in women. *American Journal of Epidemiology, 150*, 573–579.

Fine, J. T., Colditz, G. A., Coakley, E. H., Moseley, G., Manson, J. E., Willett, W. C., & Kawachi, I. (1999). A prospective study of weight change and health-related quality of life in women. *Journal of the American Medical Association, 282*, 2136–2142.

Flegal, K. M., Caroll, M. D., Kuczmarski, R. J., & Johnson, C. L. (1998). Overweight and obesity in the United States: Prevalence and trends, 1960–1994. *International Journal of Obesity, 22*, 39–47.

Folsom, A. R., Prineas, R. J., Kaye, S. A., & Soler, J. T. (1989). Body fat distribution and self-reported prevalence of hypertension, heart attack, and heart disease in older women. *International Journal of Epidemiology, 18,* 361–367.

Fontaine, K., Cheskin, L., & Barofsky, I. (1996). Health-related quality of life in obese persons seeking treatment. *Journal of Family Practice, 43,* 265–270.

Ford, E. S. (1999). Body mass index and colon cancer in a national sample of adult US men and women. *American Journal of Epidemiology, 15,* 390–398.

Giovannucci, E., Ascherio, A., Rimm, E. B., Colditz, G. A., Stampfer, M. J., & Willett, W. C. (1995). Physical activity, obesity, and risk for colon cancer and adenoma in men. *Annals of Internal Medicine, 122,* 327–334.

Giovannucci, E., Rimm, E. B., Chute, C. G., Kawachi, I., Colditz, G. A., Stampfer, M. J., & Willett, W. C. (1994). Obesity and benign prostatic hyperplasia. *American Journal of Epidemiology, 140,* 989–1002.

Gorsky, R., Pamuk, E., Williamson, D. F., Shaffer, P., & Koplan, J. (1996). The 25-year health care costs of women who remain overweight after 40 years of age. *American Journal of Preventative Medicine, 12,* 388–394.

Gortmaker, S. L., Must, A., Perrin, J. M., Sobol, A. M., & Dietz, W. H. (1993). Social and economic consequences of overweight in adolescence and young adulthood. *New England Journal of Medicine, 329,* 1008–1012.

Harris, T. B., Ballard-Barbasch, R., Madans, J., Makue, D. M., & Feldman, J. J. (1993). Overweight, weight loss, and risk of coronary heart disease in older women: The NHANES I Epidemiologic Follow-Up Study. *American Journal of Epidemiology, 137,* 1318–1327.

Hart, D. J., & Spector, T. D. (1993). The relationship of obesity, fat distribution and osteoarthritis in women in the general population: The Chingford Study. *Journal of Rheumatology, 20,* 331–335.

Hartz, A. J., Rupley, D. C., Kalkhoff, R. D., & Rimm, A. A. (1983). Relationship of obesity to diabetes: Influence of obesity level and body fat distribution. *Prevention Medicine, 12,* 351–357.

Holbrook, T. L., Barrett-Conner, E., & Wingard, D. L. (1989). The association of lifetime weight and weight control patterns with diabetes among men and women in an adult community. *International Journal of Obesity, 13,* 723–729.

Huang, Z., Hankinson, S. E., Colditz, G. A., Stampfer, M. J., Hunter, D. J., Manson, J. E., Hennekens, C. H., Rosner, B., Speizer, F. E., & Willett, W. C. (1997). Dual effects of weight and weight gain on breast cancer risk. *Journal of the American Medical Association, 278,* 1407–1411.

Huang, Z., Willett, W. C., Manson, J. E., Rosner, B., Stampfer, M. J., Speizer, F. E., & Colditz, G. A. (1998). Body weight, weight change, and risk for hypertension in women. *Annals of Internal Medicine, 128,* 81–88.

Kuczmarski, R. J., Flegal, K. M., Campbell, S. M., & Johnson, C. L. (1994). Increasing prevalence of overweight among US adults: The National Health and Nutrition Examination Surveys, 1960 to 1991. *Journal of the American Medical Association, 272,* 205–211.

Kyogoku, S., Hirohata, T., Takeshita, S., Nomura, Y., Shigematsu, T., & Horie, A. (1990). Survival of breast-cancer patients and body size indicators. *International Journal of Cancer, 46,* 824–831.

Lagergren, J., Bergstrom, R., & Nyren, O. (1999). Association between body mass and adenocarcinoma of the esophagus and gastric cardia. *Annals of Internal Medicine, 130,* 883–890.

Larkin, J., & Pines, H. (1979). No fat person need apply. *Sociology of Work and Occupations, 6,* 312–327.

Le Marchand, L., Wilkens, L. R., Kolonel, L. N., Hankin, J. H., & Lyu, L. C. (1997). Associations of sedentary lifestyle, obesity, smoking, alcohol use, and diabetes with the risk of colorectal cancer. *Cancer Research, 57,* 4787–4794.

Levy, E., Levy, P., Le Pen, C., & Basdevant, A. (1995). Economic cost of obesity: The French situation. *International Journal of Obesity, 19,* 788–792.

Lundgren, H., Bengtsson, C., Blohme, G., Lapidus, L., & Sjöström, L. (1988). Adiposity and adipose tissue distribution in relation to incidence of diabetes in women: Results from a prospective population study in Gothenburg, Sweden. *International Journal of Obesity, 13,* 413–423.

Maclure, K. M., Hayes, K. C., Colditz, G. A., Stampfer, M. J., Speizer, F. E., & Willett, W. C. (1989).

F. E., Rosner, B., & Hennekens, C. H. (1990). Moderate alcohol consumption and increased risk of systemic hypertension. *American Journal of Cardiology, 65,* 633–637.

Witteman, J. C. M., Willett, W. C., Stampfer, M. J., Colditz, G. A., Sacks, F. M., Speizer, F. E., Rosner, B., & Hennekens, C. H. (1989). A prospective study of nutritional factors and hypertension among US women. *Circulation, 80,* 1320–1327.

World Health Organization. (1998). *Obesity: Preventing and managing the global epidemic. Report of a WHO Consultation on Obesity, Geneva, June 3–5, 1997* (Publication No. WHO/NUT/NCD/98.1). Geneva: Author.

Yong, L. C., Kuller, L. H., Rutan, G., & Bunker, C. (1993). Longitudinal study of blood pressure: Changes and determinants from adolescents to middle age. The Dormont High School follow-up study, 1957–1963 to 1989–1990. *American Journal of Epidemiology, 138,* 973–983.

2

Body Weight Regulation: Neural, Endocrine, and Autocrine Mechanisms

STREAMSON C. CHUA, JR.
RUDOLPH L. LEIBEL

The biology of body weight regulation is complex and operates through effects on energy intake, energy expenditure, and caloric partitioning (i.e., the chemical composition of somatic energy stores). Body weight is maintained in a steady state by a balance between caloric intake and energy expenditure. Alterations of intake or expenditure are usually accompanied by compensatory changes in the other components of energy balance, tending thereby to maintain relative constancy of body weight and composition.

The absolute caloric requirements for an organism are dependent on actual metabolic mass rather than absolute body mass. This is because some body compartments are less metabolically active, such as adipose tissue and bone, which are primarily composed of inert triglyceride and minerals, respectively. Furthermore, the various tissues have different qualitative and quantitative fuel requirements (Gallagher et al., 1998). Rates of fuel consumption per unit mass are higher in brain and heart than, for example, in skeletal muscle at rest. Thus body composition and the metabolic mass of specific organs are important factors in energy balance.

IS BODY WEIGHT REGULATED?

Experiments on animals (Hervey, 1988) and humans (Sims et al., 1973) suggest that absolute body weight is regulated (Leibel, Rosenbaum, & Hirsch, 1995). Weight loss induced by caloric restriction is countered by increased food intake and weight regain when food is presented *ad libitum*. This phenomenon is also seen in growing organisms and is part of the biological response to deprivation-induced growth failure, termed catch-up growth. However, there are limits to "catch-up growth." Severe long-term caloric restriction of developing organisms causes permanent, though not equivalent, stunting in all compartments of somatic mass (Hughes, 1982; Widdowson & McCance, 1975). Thus early environmental factors can exert powerful influences on adult body weight.

Body weight gain can be induced by overfeeding and presenting highly palatable diets that induce hyperphagia (Levin, Dunn-Meynell, Balkan, & Keesey, 1997; Levin & Keesey, 1998). Upon cessation of the overfeeding or the palatable diet, body weight loss occurs as a result of diminished intake or increased energy expenditure until the premanipulation weight is attained. However, long-term effects can be induced by early overnutrition of rodents during the preweaning phase of development (Johnson, Stern, Greenwood, Zucker, & Hirsch, 1973), leading to permanent excess adiposity in the adult rat and associated metabolic changes, such as mild insulin insensitivity (You, Gotz, Rohde, & Dorner, 1990).

Dramatic alterations in body mass can be achieved by mechanical or chemical lesions centered in the hypothalamus. Hyperphagia and obesity result from bilateral lesions of the medial hypothalamus (Hetherington & Ranson, 1940; Keesey & Hirvonen, 1997), affecting the ventromedial and arcuate nuclei. A similar syndrome of hyperphagia and obesity is observed in rodents and humans with mutations that inactivate genes whose products function as modulators of ingestive behavior and energy balance—for example, leptin, leptin receptor (LEPR), neuropeptide Y (NPY), agouti gene-related peptide (AGRP), pro-opiomelanocortin (POMC), melanocortin receptor 4 (MC4R), and corticotropin-releasing hormone (CRH) (see Table 2.1). In contrast, aphagia and severe weight loss occur as a result of bilateral lesions of the lateral hypothalamic areas (Anand & Brobeck, 1951). This hypothalamic area contains neurons that secrete orexigenic peptides: melanin-concentrating hormone (MCH) and oxexin/hypocretin.

These experimental observations indicate that body weight is regulated by a system coordinated in the central nervous system. However, tissue-specific growth also plays a role in the control of body composition (see Table 2.2). Several questions are raised by these simple observations:

1. Is the factor being regulated absolute body weight, a component of body mass, or total fuel stores? What are the signals and the sensors for the regulated factor(s)?

2. Are each of the body compartments regulated independently, or are there systems that affect multiple tissues and organs?

3. Is there a hierarchy for preservation of these body compartments?

4. Are the metabolic pathways for response to weight loss and weight gain identical?

5. What is the nature of the coupling among caloric intake, substrate partitioning, and energy expenditure? Since perfect coupling of the components of energy balance would result in the maintenance of a constant body weight and body composition, it is obvious that the coupling of the components of energy balance is imperfect.

Table 2.1. Genes Expressed in the Central Nervous System That Regulate Body Weight

Orexigenic/anabolic molecules	Anorectic/catabolic molecules
Neuropeptide Y (NPY)	Leptin receptor (LEPR)
Agouti gene-related peptide (AGRP)	Pro-opiomelanocortin (POMC)
Agouti-related transcript (ART)	Melanocortin receptor 4 (MC4R)
Melanin-concentrating hormone (MCH)	Corticotropin-releasing hormone (CRH)
Dopamine	Serotonin receptor subtype 2C (5-HT2C)
	Glucagon-like peptide 1 receptor (GLP-1R)

Table 2.2. Genes Expressed in Peripheral Tissues That Regulate Body Weight

Skeletal muscle	White adipose tissue
Myostatin (MYO)	Leptin
Callipyge	CCAAT enhancer-binding proteins—α, β, δ (CEBP-α, CEBP-β,
Ryanodine receptor 1 (RYR1)	CEBP-δ)
Myogenin	Nuclear sterol regulatory-element-binding protein 1c (SREBP-1c)
Myogenic differentiation antigen 1	High-mobility group protein isoform I-C (HMGIC)
Myogenic factor 5	Lipoprotein lipase (LPL)
Myogenic factor 4	Fatty-acid-binding protein 4, expressed in adipocytes (aP2)
	Peroxisome proliferator-activated receptor gamma (PPARG)
Brown adipose tissue	**Gut**
Uncoupling protein 1 (UCP1)	Cholecystokinin receptor A (CCK-A)
	Bombesin receptor subtype 3 (BRS-3)
	Glucagon-like peptide 1 (GLP–1)

WHAT COMPONENTS OF ENERGY BALANCE ARE REGULATED?

In early studies of the effects of precise neuroanatomical lesions within the hypothalamus, gross alterations of body mass were produced in rats. Ventromedial lesions caused hyperphagia and severe obesity. Lesions of the lateral hypothalamic area caused hypophagia and profound weight loss. These studies led to a hypothesis of dual centers in the hypothalamus that controlled body weight (Elmquist, Elias, & Saper, 1999). The ventromedial hypothalamic area was viewed as a satiety center, whereas the lateral hypothalamic area was proposed as the "eating center." Debates ensued as to whether intrinsic neurons of the two areas or neuronal axons passing through these areas were the principal mediators of the apparent regulatory roles associated with the respective anatomical regions. Molecular genetic studies, which enable the disruption of specific neurotransmitters in specific cell bodies and their connections, have indicated that both intrinsic neurons and fibers of passage are important in mediating the effects of these two types of lesions (Elmquist et al., 1999). Neuroanatomical studies of neurochemically defined neuronal populations (Elmquist et al., 1999) provide a detailed picture of the pathways that control energy balance.

REGULATION OF BODY WEIGHT BY SKELETAL MUSCLE METABOLISM

By virtue of its mass, skeletal muscle mass accounts for a substantial portion of oxidative metabolism, even at rest. Skeletal muscle mass can increase by myocyte hypertrophy resulting from mechanical loads. On the other hand, muscle mass can atrophy during unloading. Therefore, it is not surprising that several genes have been identified that directly affect muscle mass: myostatin (MYO), callipyge, and ryanodine receptor 1 (RYR1). These genes have apparent effects in multiple muscle groups and appear to alter body composition by increasing muscle mass and decreasing adipose tissue mass.

A member of the transforming growth factor family, MYO is expressed early in development within skeletal muscle precursor cells that have a probable role of inhibiting myocyte growth and/or differentiation (Lee & McPherron, 1999). Mice and cattle without MYO have increased skeletal muscle mass (Grobet et al., 1997; Kambadur, Sharma, Smith, & Bass, 1997; McPherron & Lee, 1997; Szabo et al., 1998). For MYO-knockout cattle, the increase in muscle mass appears to be at the expense of other tissues, since the absolute weights of adipose tissue and all visceral organs are diminished. Although this phenomenon of "metabolic steal" has not been observed in MYO-knockout mice, further investigations are warranted to document this finding in cattle, in light of the fact that callipyge sheep (Cockett et al., 1996; Jackson, Miller, & Green, 1997) and RYR1-mutant pigs (Fujii et al., 1991; MacLennan, 1992) have increased muscle mass and diminished fat mass. Alleles of the RYR1 gene that cause malignant hyperthermia phenotype in humans and pigs also cause increased calcium release in myocytes, leading to increased expense of mechanical force during contractions (Gallant & Lentz, 1992; Reiss et al., 1991). Thus it is possible that humans who are susceptible to malignant hyperthermia may have increased muscle mass. A phenotypic test that can identify individuals (humans and pigs) susceptible to malignant hyperthermia has been verified by correlation with genotype at the RYR1 gene. The test relies on increased contractility of muscle upon exposure to caffeine and 4-chloro-m-cresol *in vitro* (Baur et al., 2000). Unfortunately, there have been no reports regarding the effect of the RYR1 mutations on human body composition.

Developmental factors contribute to the determination of skeletal muscle mass. Numerous transcription factors—for example, myogenin, myogenic differentiation antigen 1, myogenic factor 5, and myogenic factor 4—have been identified that are necessary for normal skeletal development (Hasty et al., 1993; Nabeshima et al., 1993; Rawls et al., 1998; Rudnicki et al., 1993). Although genetic ablations of these genes cause a profound reduction of skeletal muscle, and often a complete absence of skeletal muscle, the adult phenotype cannot be observed since the knockout mice die within a few minutes of birth, presumably due to an inability to initiate respiration. In the aggregate, these experimental observations indicate that skeletal muscle produces factors that affect skeletal muscle mass as well as other tissue compartments.

EFFECTS OF BROWN ADIPOSE TISSUE ON BODY WEIGHT

The brown adipose tissue (BAT) of small mammals is responsible for producing up to 50% of the energy required to maintain a constant body weight (Himms-Hagen, 1990). The control of nonshivering thermogenesis (NST) is exerted through sympathetic nervous system input to BAT. Therefore, it is not surprising that mice with a transgene that ablates BAT become obese (Lowell et al., 1993). BAT is ablated by producing the α chain of diphtheria toxin in BAT under the control of the uncoupling protein (UCP) promoter. If these mice are reared under thermoneutral conditions, preventing BAT deterioration and production of the toxin, the obese phenotype is not manifested. This indicates that the obesity is due to the loss of BAT and the concomitant decrease in energy expenditure (Klaus, Munzberg, Truloff, & Heldmaier, 1998; Melnyk, Harper, & Himms-Hagen, 1997).

In transgenic mice, the loss of BAT is only partial and temporary, since BAT regenerates after inactivation of the toxic transgene. Surprisingly, mice with UCP1 (the major UCP of BAT) knocked out do not develop obesity or any alterations in food intake (Enerback et al., 1997). It is probable that other proteins compensate for the lack of UCP1. Two proteins, UCP2 and UCP3, appear to be homologous to UCP1. However, two lines of evidence suggest that this is unlikely. First, humans who are homozygous for a truncating mutation of UCP3 are not uniformly obese (Chung et al., 1999). Second, sequence comparisons indicate that crucial histidine residues (145 and 147), which are required for the uncoupling activity of UCP1, are not conserved in UCP2 and UCP3 (Bienengraeber, Echtay, & Klingenberg, 1998; Echtay, Bienengraeber, Winkler, & Klingenberg, 1998). It is possible that uncoupling proteins are not the sole mediators of NST. Other mitochondrial molecules that can facilitate mitochondrial uncoupling may be identified.

REGULATION OF BODY WEIGHT BY WHITE ADIPOSE TISSUE DEVELOPMENT

Development and Proliferation of White Adipose Tissue

Lipodystrophy, the phenotype associated with a lack of some or all adipose tissue depots, consists of several distinct syndromes in humans. Lamin A/C gene mutations have been implicated in some humans (Cao & Hegele, 2000; Shackleton et al., 2000; Speckman et al., 2000). The mechanism, however, whereby a ubiquitously expressed nuclear membrane protein can cause a disease specific to white adipose tissue (WAT) remains to be identified. Mouse models of lipodystrophy have been generated by the expression of dominant negative proteins that inhibit the activities of transcription factors necessary for the differentiation of white adipocytes. One of these synthetic constructs, A-ZIP/F-1, encodes (1) a leucine zipper-dimerizing domain that forms heterodimers with CCAAT enhancer-binding proteins (CEBPs) and JUNs; and (2) an acidic amphipathic helix that replaces the basic DNA-binding domain (McKnight, 1998). The heterodimers containing A-ZIP/F-1 are stable and devoid of DNA-binding and transcription-enhancing activities.

The second synthetic construct, nuclear sterol regulatory-element-binding protein 1c (SREBP-1c), lacks the Golgi membrane attachment domain and is constitutively targeted to the nucleus (Shimomura et al., 1998). Nuclear SREBP-1c is a transcription factor that binds sterol regulatory elements. Mice expressing these transgenes have greatly diminished WAT and BAT, visceromegaly, hyperinsulinemia, and hyperglycemia. Lipodystrophic humans and rodents demonstrate increased metabolic rate, severe insulin resistance, and glucose intolerance as a result of the lack of WAT. Although many of the manifestations of lipodystrophy, such as hyperphagia and altered insulin sensitivity, can be attributed to the lack of leptin secretion, the increased metabolic rate of lipodystrophy is not the result of leptin deficiency (see below). Thus WAT apparently produces a factor that regulates metabolic rate, or the loss of WAT alters metabolic pathways in such a way as to favor a catabolic state.

CEBPs are a family of transcription factors necessary for the differentiation of preadipocytes to adipocytes. The CEBP-α form is expressed mainly in adipocytes. Mice with a homozygous knockout of the CEBP-α gene are nearly devoid of WAT and BAT (Wang et al., 1995). Most of the mice are born alive but die within a few hours of birth. Mice with combined mutations of the CEBP-β and CEBP-δ isoforms have a similar phenotype of reduced adipose tissue mass and increased neonatal mortality (Tanaka, Yoshida, Kishimoto, & Akira, 1997).

Variant alleles of the peroxisome proliferator-activated receptor gamma (PPARG) have been associated with obesity and/or diabetes (Barroso et al., 1999; Deeb et al., 1998). The PPARG peptide forms a heterodimer with the retinoid X receptor (Kliewer, Umesono, Noonan, Heyman, & Evans, 1992) that binds prostaglandin J2 and the synthetic thiazolidinediones (Forman et al., 1995; Lehmann et al., 1995; Nagy, Tontonoz, Alvarez, Chen, & Evans, 1998). Due to the insulin-sensitizing activity of thiazolidinediones and the association of activating mutations of PPARG with diabetes and obesity, it is assumed that PPARG is an important mediator of lipid accumulation in adipocytes. Mice with a homozygous deletion of PPARG die during embryonic development (Barak et al., 1999; Miles, Barak, He, Evans, & Olefsky, 2000). However, mice with reduced PPARG activity, by virtue of hemizygosity for a knockout allele of PPARG, are protected from diet-induced obesity. On a high-fat diet, the PPARG hemizygotes had less adipose tissue mass than wild-type mice, although the adipocytes were larger.

Adipocytes differentiate from a precursor cell, probably from a fibroblast/mesenchymal lineage. The high-mobility group protein isoform I-C (HMGIC) gene is induced in adipose tissue by feeding mice a high-fat diet (Anand & Chada, 2000), suggesting that it may

a partial compensation of fatty acid binding by overexpression of keratinocyte lipid-binding protein (Coe, Simpson, & Bernlohr, 1999). It is possible that the failure of aP2-knockout mice to develop insulin resistance on a high-fat diet is due to an alteration of the composition of circulating fatty acids (indirectly by alterations in fatty acid metabolism due to the aP2 deficiency). Although there are only minor differences between normal and knockout mice in total plasma free fatty acids, as well as fatty acid composition, β-adrenergic stimulation *in vivo* causes significant changes in fatty acid composition.

Deficiencies in either of two lipolytic enzymes, lipoprotein lipase (LPL) and hormone-sensitive lipase (LIPE), cause hyperlipidemia and increased mortality. Mice that do not have LIPE (Osuga et al., 2000) are superficially normal, although the males are sterile. Without LIPE, mice have a normal amount of WAT, although adipocyte size is enlarged twofold. The BAT mass of LIPE-deficient mice is increased fivefold. Mice and humans without LPL suffer early mortality due to hyperchylomicronemia. The LPL-knockout mice can be rescued by a transgene expressing LPL in skeletal muscle only (Weinstock et al., 1995, 1997). The LPL-knockout mice appear to have fewer adipose tissue stores. However, numerous human cases of partial and complete LPL deficiency have been reported, and no clear association to obesity has been observed.

REGULATION OF BODY WEIGHT BY THE HYPOTHALAMUS

Mediation of Leptin's Actions by LEPR

The LEPR is a member of the cytokine receptor superfamily and has a single transmembrane region (Tartaglia et al., 1995). The LEPR forms a homodimer, and each monomer is capable of binding one leptin molecule (Devos et al., 1997). There are binding sites for Janus kinase (JAK) and signal transducer and activator of transcription (STAT) proteins, which are intracellular signal transducers of leptin (Baumann et al., 1996; Ghilardi et al., 1996; Vaisse et al., 1996). The LEPR gene encodes numerous isoforms (some of which are species-specific) with identical leptin-binding sites but different carboxyl termini due to splicing of alternative 3′ terminal exons. There is a soluble receptor (LEPR-E) that does not contain a transmembrane domain and is highly expressed in the mouse placenta, leading to hyperleptinemia (Gavrilova, Barr, Marcus-Samuels, & Reitman, 1997) during pregnancy (i.e., up to a 100-fold increase in circulating leptin concentrations). However, this isoform accumulates in the blood only up to twofold during gestation in humans (Henson, Swan, & O'Neil, 1998) and rats (Kawai et al., 1997), suggesting that leptin's role during gestation may not be universal.

The human LEPR gene has lost the polyadenylation signal in the 3′ terminal exon for the LEPR-E form, indicating that soluble human LEPR is produced by cleavage of membrane bound LEPR isoforms (Chua et al., 1997). There are several membrane-bound isoforms—LEPR-A, LEPR-B, LEPR-C, LEPR-D, and LEPR-F—all of which contain the identical JAK docking site. However, only LEPR-B bears a STAT docking motif. Moreover, loss of the LEPR-B isoform in the *Lepr^{db}* mouse is sufficient to produce an obesity–diabetes syndrome that is identical to complete LEPR deficiency and leptin deficiency (Brown, Chua, Liu, Andrews, & Vandenbergh, 2000; Chen et al., 1996; Chua, Chung, et al., 1996; Chua, White, et al., 1996; Lee et al., 1996, 1997; Liu, Leibel, & Chua, 1998; Wu-Peng et al., 1997). Therefore, the genetic evidence indicates that leptin signals relevant to the obesity–diabetes phenotype are mediated by the LEPR-B isoform only, and that the JAK and STAT proteins, rather than JAK proteins alone, initiate the intracellular signaling cascade. Other actions of leptin, such as stimulation of angiogenesis (Sierra-Honigmann et al.,

1998) and immune responses (Lord et al., 1998), remain to be more fully explored in terms of signal transduction.

Rodents with defective LEPR genes exhibit an obesity–diabetes syndrome that is identical to the syndrome caused by leptin deficiency (Argiles, 1989; Aubert, Herzog, Camus, Guenet, & Lemonnier, 1985; Brown et al., 2000; Hummel, Dickie, & Coleman, 1966; Koletsky, 1973; Leiter, Coleman, Eisenstein, & Strack, 1980). This includes (1) early-onset obesity associated with hyperphagia, decreased NST, and preferential fat deposition; (2) neuroendocrine disturbances at the hypothalamic level; and (3) Type 2 diabetes associated with insulin resistance and defective insulin secretion. Humans with LEPR deficiency (Clement et al., 1998) have hyperphagic obesity and neuroendocrine disturbances similar to those of LEPR-deficient rodents (but without insulin resistance or diabetes). Although LEPR is expressed in many tissues with pleiotropic effects, its main site of action relevant to energy balance lies in the hypothalamus. This influence is supported by several lines of evidence:

1. Disruption of the STAT-signaling competent LEPR-B isoform, as observed in the Lepr^{db} mouse, is sufficient to produce the obesity–diabetes syndrome of complete LEPR deficiency in the Lepr^{dbPas} mouse and the Lepr^{faf} rat.

2. LEPR-B constitutes a major fraction of LEPR (up to 40%) expressed in the hypothalamus, whereas LEPR-B constitutes ~1% of LEPR in almost every tissue except lymph nodes (Ghilardi et al., 1996).

3. Delivery of leptin to the brain, in doses too small to detect in the circulation, mimics the effects of physiological doses of leptin delivered to the periphery (Campfield, Smith, Guisez, Devos, & Burn, 1995; Halaas et al., 1995; Pelleymounter et al., 1995).

4. Leptin administration causes the activation of the STAT-signaling pathway in the hypothalamus (Vaisse et al., 1996)—an effect that is not observed in peripheral tissues—and produces major alterations in the expression of neuropeptide genes, such as NPY and POMC (Baskin, Hahn, & Schwartz, 1999).

LEPR is expressed within many neuronal cell types that are important in regulating ingestion, and the neuropeptide genes expressed within these neuronal types are modulated by leptin. Within the arcuate nucleus, NPY/AGRP neurons (Broberger, Johansen, Johansson, Schalling, & Hokfelt, 1998; Hahn, Breininger, Baskin, & Schwartz, 1998; Wilson et al., 1999) and POMC/cocaine- and amphetamine-regulated transcript (CART) neurons (Ahima et al., 1999; Elias et al., 1999; Korner, Chua, Williams, Leibel, & Wardlaw, 1999) express LEPR. The transcriptional activities of these neuropeptide genes appear to be regulated in part by leptin. Interestingly, the orexigenic peptides NPY and AGRP are coexpressed within the same neurons, while the anorectic peptides POMC and CART are coexpressed. Within the lateral hypothalamus, both MCH neurons and hypocretin/orexin neurons are regulated by leptin (Elias et al., 1998). Similarly, within the paraventricular nucleus, CRH (Schwartz, Seeley, Campfield, Burn, & Baskin, 1996) and thyrotropin-releasing hormone (TRH) (Legradi, Emerson, Ahima, Flier, & Lechan, 1997) neurons are sensitive to leptin. Physiological states associated with diminished circulating leptin concentrations, such as food restriction, are correlated with increased expression of the orexigenic peptides (NPY, AGRP, hypocretin/orexin, and MCH) and diminished expression of the anorectic neuropeptides (POMC, CART, and CRH). Diminished leptin concentrations are associated with decreased TRH messenger RNA (mRNA). Leptin administration during food restriction prevents many of these fasting-associated changes of gene expression, indicating that the primary role of leptin may be to regulate the physiological response to diminished availability of calories and/or diminished triglyceride stores.

ingestive drive is reduced even after L-dopa treatment (Szczypka et al., 1999). Similarly, loss of dopaminergic transmission by lateral hypothalamic lesions, or by chemicals that disrupt dopaminergic neurons, might induce a movement disorder rather than a specific effect on appetitive behavior. Many of the genes encoding the large family of dopamine receptors have been genetically ablated. Mice with a knockout of individual dopamine receptors do not manifest hypophagia or hypodipsia: D_1 (Xu et al., 1994), D_2 (Baik et al., 1995; Maldonado et al., 1997), D_3 (Xu et al., 1997), and the dopamine transporter (Jones et al., 1999). Therefore, it remains to be conclusively shown that loss of dopaminergic activity and transmission has a specific effect on ingestive behavior, independent of its effects on motor control.

Serotonergic Pathways

Serotonin has been implicated in body weight regulation (Simansky, 1996). Furthermore, weight gain during treatment with antidepressants that interfere with serotonin's activity has been widely observed (Vickers, Clifton, Dourish, & Tecott, 1999). Tricyclic antidepressants enhance the sensitivity of postsynaptic receptors (Chaput, de Montigny, & Blier, 1991), whereas selective serotonin reuptake inhibitors, such as sibutramine, antagonize the negative feedback effect of serotonin on presynaptic receptors. Due to the large number of serotonin receptors, the receptors responsible for the effects of serotonin on ingestive behavior have been difficult to identify with pharmacological agents. Molecular genetic ablation of one receptor subtype, serotonin receptor subtype 2C (5-HT_{2C}), results in obese mice that are prone to seizures (Tecott, Logue, Wehner, & Kauer, 1998). The obesity is produced primarily by hyperphagia, since pair-feeding mutant mice with wild-type mice results in mutant mice with normal body weights and normal body composition. Thus pharmacological agents that do not interfere with the 5-HT_{2C} receptor might have minimal effects on body weight gain. Conversely, agents that selectively activate 5-HT_{2C} may be efficacious compounds for appetite suppression and weight loss.

REGULATION BY THE GUT

The gut is able to sense the presence of ingested calories and to generate signals leading to meal termination (Smith & Romsos, 1984). Therefore, it is not surprising that the release of endogenous gut factors can modulate meal size. Molecular genetic data analysis has identified two receptors that mediate satiety signals: the A receptor for cholecystokinin (CCK-A) (Moran & Schwartz, 1994) and the bombesin receptor subtype 3 (BRS-3) (Fathi et al., 1996). A rat model of obesity, the Otsuka Long–Evans Tokushima Fatty (OLETF) rat, is characterized by obesity associated with large meals and resistance to the satiating effects of CCK-A (Moran, Katz, Plata-Salaman, & Schwartz, 1998). These rats have an inactivating mutation within the CCK-A receptor gene (Funakoshi et al., 1995; Moran et al., 1998). The phenotype of delayed satiety is commensurate with the postulated function of the CCK-A receptor. However, other associated genetic alterations in the OLETF rat strain may interact with the CCK-A receptor mutation to produce obesity, since inactivating mutations of the CCK-A receptor in humans and mice (Kopin et al., 1999) are not associated with obesity.

Genetic ablation of the BRS-3 gene produces hyperphagic mice (Ohki-Hamazaki et al., 1997) that do not display any other alterations in other components of energy homeostasis. Pair-feeding of the mutant mice, compared to normal controls, completely normalizes the body composition of the BRS-3-deficient mice. However, the endogenous ligand for the

BRS-3 molecule remains to be identified, as mice with genetic ablations of the mammalian homologues of bombesin-like ligands and receptors—gastrin (Friis-Hansen et al., 1998), gastrin receptor (Wang & Dockray, 1999), gastrin-releasing peptide receptor (Hampton et al., 1998), and neuromedin B receptor (Ohki-Hamazaki et al., 1999)—do not develop obesity.

The glucagon gene encodes glucagon and a splice variant, glucagon-like peptide 1 (GLP-1). A receptor for GLP-1 (GLP-1R) has been identified in the hypothalamus. Treatment with GLP-1 inhibits feeding, while exendin, a long-acting inverse agonist of GLP-1R, stimulates feeding (Larsen, Tang-Christensen, & Jessop, 1997; Turton et al., 1996). Despite these observations, mice with a targeted knockout of GLP-1R do not exhibit obesity or hyperphagia, even when fed a high-fat diet (Scrocchi et al., 1996). The GLP-1R-knockout mice do exhibit glucose intolerance with a glucose challenge, and *in vitro* testing supports the requirement of GLP-1 and GLP-1R for the stimulation of insulin release from beta cells exposed to glucose.

SUMMARY

The range of molecules and cell types committed to the regulation of energy homeostasis is large and still only partly known. From a physiological perspective, this plethora of agents and pathways clearly reflects the critical nature of this process for organismic survival and ability to reproduce, and for the diverse systems that participate in a coordinated way to determine body energy stores (e.g., ingestive behavior, nutrient partitioning, energy expenditure). The rodent mutations with the most striking impact on body fatness (e.g., *ob* and *db*) have effects on all three of these compartments. Genetic alterations affecting single compartments generally produce less striking phenotypic effects. The redundancy of the pathways, and the ability of one "limb" of control to compensate for changes in another (e.g., decline in energy expenditure with decreased metabolic fuel flux), provide a caution to those endeavoring to interrupt these pathways for therapeutic purposes. Better understanding of the full panoply of molecules and pathways, however, should ultimately permit very specific manipulations of energy intake and expenditure without substantial counterresponses by the organism.

REFERENCES

Ahima, R. S., Kelly, J., Elmquist, J. K., & Flier, J. S. (1999). Distinct physiologic and neuronal responses to decreased leptin and mild hyperleptinemia. *Endocrinology, 140*(11), 4923–4931.

Ahima, R. S., Prabakaran, D., Mantzoros, C., Qu, D., Lowell, B., Maratos-Flier, E., & Flier, J. S. (1996). Role of leptin in the neuroendocrine response to fasting. *Nature, 382*(6588), 250–252.

Anand, A., & Chada, K. (2000). In vivo modulation of HMGIC reduces obesity. *Nature Genetics, 24*(4), 377–380.

Anand, B. K., & Brobeck, J. R. (1951). Hypothalamic control of food intake in rats and cats. *Yale Journal of Biology and Medicine, 24*.

Argiles, J. M. (1989). The obese Zucker rat: A choice for fat metabolism 1968–1988. Twenty years of research on the insights of the Zucker mutation. *Progress in Lipid Research, 28*(1), 53–66.

Aubert, R., Herzog, J., Camus, M. C., Guenet, J. L., & Lemonnier, D. (1985). Description of a new model of genetic obesity: The *dbPas* mouse. *Journal of Nutrition, 115*(3), 327–333.

Baik, J. H., Picetti, R., Saiardi, A., Thiriet, G., Dierich, A., Depaulis, A., Le Meur, M., & Borrelli, E. (1995). Parkinsonian-like locomotor impairment in mice lacking dopamine D2 receptors. *Nature, 377*(6548), 424–428.

Elmquist, J. K., Elias, C. F., & Saper, C. B. (1999). From lesions to leptin: hypothalamic control of food intake and body weight. *Neuron, 22*(2), 221–232.

Enerback, S., Jacobsson, A., Simpson, E. M., Guerra, C., Yamashita, H., Harper, M. E., & Kozak, L. P. (1997). Mice lacking mitochondrial uncoupling protein are cold-sensitive but not obese. *Nature, 387*(6628), 90–94.

Erickson, J. C., Hollopeter, G., & Palmiter, R. D. (1996). Attenuation of the obesity syndrome of *ob/ob* mice by the loss of neuropeptide Y. *Science, 274*(5293), 1704–1707.

Fathi, Z., Way, J. W., Corjay, M. H., Viallet, J., Sausville, E. A., & Battey, J. F. (1996). Bombesin receptor structure and expression in human lung carcinoma cell lines. *Journal of Cellular Biochemistry, 24*(Suppl.), 237–246.

Flier, J. S. (1998). Clinical review 94: What's in a name? In search of leptin's physiologic role. *Journal of Clinical Endocrinology and Metabolism, 83*(5), 1407–1413.

Forman, B. M., Tontonoz, P., Chen, J., Brun, R. P., Spiegelman, B. M., & Evans, R. M. (1995). 15-Deoxy-delta 12, 14-prostaglandin J2 is a ligand for the adipocyte determination factor PPAR gamma. *Cell, 83*(5), 803–812.

Frederich, R. C., Lollmann, B., Hamann, A., Napolitano-Rosen, A., Kahn, B. B., Lowell, B. B., & Flier, J. S. (1995). Expression of *ob* mRNA and its encoded protein in rodents: Impact of nutrition and obesity. *Journal of Clinical Investigation, 96*(3), 1658–1663.

Friis-Hansen, L., Sundler, F., Li, Y., Gillespie, P. J., Saunders, T. L., Greenson, J. K., Owyang, C., Rehfeld, J. F., & Samuelson, L. C. (1998). Impaired gastric acid secretion in gastrin-deficient mice. *American Journal of Physiology, 274*(3, Pt. 1), G561–G568.

Fujii, J., Otsu, K., Zorzato, F., de Leon, S., Khanna, V. K., Weiler, J. E., O'Brien, P. J., & MacLennan, D. H. (1991). Identification of a mutation in porcine ryanodine receptor associated with malignant hyperthermia. *Science, 253*(5018), 448–451.

Funakoshi, A., Miyasaka, K., Shinozaki, H., Masuda, M., Kawanami, T., Takata, Y., & Kono, A. (1995). An animal model of congenital defect of gene expression of cholecystokinin (CCK)-A receptor. *Biochemical and Biophysical Research Communications, 210*(3), 787–796.

Gallagher, D., Belmonte, D., Deurenberg, P., Wang, Z., Krasnow, N., Pi-Sunyer, F. X., & Heymsfield, S. B. (1998). Organ-tissue mass measurement allows modeling of REE and metabolically active tissue mass. *American Journal of Physiology, 275*(2, Pt. 1), E249–E258.

Gallant, E. M., & Lentz, L. R. (1992). Excitation–contraction coupling in pigs heterozygous for malignant hyperthermia. *American Journal of Physiology, 262*(2, Pt. 1), C422–C426.

Gavrilova, O., Barr, V., Marcus-Samuels, B., & Reitman, M. (1997). Hyperleptinemia of pregnancy associated with the appearance of a circulating form of the leptin receptor. *Journal of Biological Chemistry, 272*(48), 30546–30551.

Ghilardi, N., Ziegler, S., Wiestner, A., Stoffel, R., Heim, M. H., & Skoda, R. C. (1996). Defective STAT signaling by the leptin receptor in diabetic mice. *Proceedings of the National Academy of Sciences USA, 93*(13), 6231–6235.

Grobet, L., Martin, L. J., Poncelet, D., Pirottin, D., Brouwers, B., Riquet, J., Schoeberlein, A., Dunner, S., Menissier, F., Massabanda, J., Fries, R., Hanset, R., & Georges, M. (1997). A deletion in the bovine myostatin gene causes the double-muscled phenotype in cattle. *Nature Genetics, 17*(1), 71–74.

Hahn, T. M., Breininger, J. F., Baskin, D. G., & Schwartz, M. W. (1998). Coexpression of AGRP and NPY in fasting-activated hypothalamic neurons. *Nature Neuroscience, 1*(4), 271–272.

Halaas, J. L., Boozer, C., Blair-West, J., Fidahusein, N., Denton, D. A., & Friedman, J. M. (1997). Physiological response to long-term peripheral and central leptin infusion in lean and obese mice. *Proceedings of the National Academy of Sciences USA, 94*(16), 8878–8883.

Halaas, J. L., Gajiwala, K. S., Maffei, M., Cohen, S. L., Chait, B. T., Rabinowitz, D., Lallone, R. L., Burley, S. K., & Friedman, J. M. (1995). Weight-reducing effects of the plasma protein encoded by the obese gene. *Science, 269*(5223), 543–546.

Hampton, L. L., Ladenheim, E. E., Akeson, M., Way, J. M., Weber, H. C., Sutliff, V. E., Jensen, R. T., Wine, L. J., Arnheiter, H., & Battey, J. F. (1998). Loss of bombesin-induced feeding suppression in gastrin-releasing peptide receptor-deficient mice. *Proceedings of the National Academy of Sciences USA, 95*(6), 3188–3192.

Hasty, P., Bradley, A., Morris, J. H., Edmondson, D. G., Venuti, J. M., Olson, E. N., & Klein, W. H. (1993). Muscle deficiency and neonatal death in mice with a targeted mutation in the myogenin gene. *Nature, 364*(6437), 501–506.

Henson, M. C., Swan, K. F., & O'Neil, J. S. (1998). Expression of placental leptin and leptin receptor transcripts in early pregnancy and at term. *Obstetrics and Gynecology, 92*(6), 1020–1028.

Hervey, G. R. (1988). Physiological factors involved in long-term control of food intake. *International Journal for Vitamin and Nutrition Research, 58*(4), 477–490.

Hetherington, A. W., & Ranson, S. W. (1940). Hypothalamic lesions and adiposity in the rat. *Anatomical Record, 78,* 149–172.

Heymsfield, S. B., Greenberg, A. S., Fujioka, K., Dixon, R. M., Kushner, R., Hunt, T., Lubina, J. A., Patane, J., Self, B., Hunt, P., & McCamish, M. (1999). Recombinant leptin for weight loss in obese and lean adults: A randomized, controlled, dose-escalation trial. *Journal of the American Medical Association, 282*(16), 1568–1575.

Himms-Hagen, J. (1990). Brown adipose tissue thermogenesis: Interdisciplinary studies. *FASEB Journal, 4*(11), 2890–2898.

Hinney, A., Bornscheuer, A., Depenbusch, M., Mierke, B., Tolle, A., Mayer, H., Siegfried, W., Remschmidt, H., & Hebebrand, J. (1997). Absence of leptin deficiency mutation in extremely obese German children and adolescents [Letter to the editor]. *International Journal of Obesity, 21*(12), 1190.

Ho, G., & MacKenzie, R. G. (1999). Functional characterization of mutations in melanocortin–4 receptor associated with human obesity. *Journal of Biological Chemistry, 274*(50), 35816–35822.

Hotamisligil, G. S., Johnson, R. S., Distel, R. J., Ellis, R., Papaioannou, V. E., & Spiegelman, B. M. (1996). Uncoupling of obesity from insulin resistance through a targeted mutation in aP2, the adipocyte fatty acid binding protein. *Science, 274*(5291), 1377–1379.

Hughes, P. C. (1982). Morphometric studies of catch-up growth in the rat. *Progress in Clinical and Biological Research, 101,* 433–446.

Hummel, K. P., Dickie, M. M., & Coleman, D. L. (1966). Diabetes, a new mutation in the mouse. *Science, 153*(740), 1127–1128.

Huszar, D., Lynch, C. A., Fairchild-Huntress, V., Dunmore, J. H., Fang, Q., Berkemeier, L. R., Gu, W., Kesterson, R. A., Boston, B. A., Cone, R. D., Smith, F. J., Campfield, L. A., Burn, P., & Lee, F. (1997). Targeted disruption of the melanocortin-4 receptor results in obesity in mice. *Cell, 88*(1), 131–141.

Jackson, S. P., Miller, M. F., & Green, R. D. (1997). Phenotypic characterization of Rambouillet sheep expressing the callipyge gene: II. Carcass characteristics and retail yield. *Journal of Animal Science, 75*(1), 125–132.

Jhanwar-Uniyal, M., & Chua, S. C., Jr. (1993). Critical effects of aging and nutritional state on hypothalamic neuropeptide Y and galanin gene expression in lean and genetically obese Zucker rats. *Brain Research: Molecular Brain Research, 19*(3), 195–202.

Johnson, P. R., Stern, J. S., Greenwood, M. R., Zucker, L. M., & Hirsch, J. (1973). Effect of early nutrition on adipose cellularity and pancreatic insulin release in the Zucker rat. *Journal of Nutrition, 103*(5), 738–743.

Jones, S. R., Gainetdinov, R. R., Hu, X. T., Cooper, D. C., Wightman, R. M., White, F. J., & Caron, M. G. (1999). Loss of autoreceptor functions in mice lacking the dopamine transporter. *Nature Neuroscience, 2*(7), 649–655.

Kambadur, R., Sharma, M., Smith, T. P., & Bass, J. J. (1997). Mutations in myostatin (GDF8) in double-muscled Belgian blue and Piedmontese cattle. *Genome Research, 7*(9), 910–916.

Kanatani, A., Mashiko, S., Murai, N., Sugimoto, N., Ito, J., Fukuroda, T., Fukami, T., Morin, N., MacNeil, D. J., Van der Ploeg, L. H., Saga, Y., Nishimura, S., & Ihara, M. (2000). Role of the Y1 receptor in the regulation of neuropeptide Y-mediated feeding: Comparison of wild-type, Y1 receptor-deficient, and Y5 receptor-deficient mice. *Endocrinology, 141*(3), 1011–1016.

Kawai, M., Yamaguchi, M., Murakami, T., Shima, K., Murata, Y., & Kishi, K. (1997). The placenta is not the main source of leptin production in pregnant rat: Gestational profile of leptin in plasma and adipose tissues. *Biochemical and Biophysical Research Communications, 240*(3), 798–802.

(1997). Effects of gender, ethnicity, body composition, and fat distribution on serum leptin concentrations in children. *Journal of Clinical Endocrinology and Metabolism, 82*(7), 2148–2152.

Nahon, J. L. (1994). The melanin-concentrating hormone: From the peptide to the gene. *Critical Reviews in Neurobiology, 8*(4), 221–262.

Naveilhan, P., Hassani, H., Canals, J. M., Ekstrand, A. J., Larefalk, A., Chhajlani, V., Arenas, E., Gedda, K., Svensson, L., Thoren, P., & Ernfors, P. (1999). Normal feeding behavior, body weight and leptin response require the neuropeptide Y Y2 receptor. *Nature Medicine, 5*(10), 1188–1193.

Ohki-Hamazaki, H., Sakai, Y., Kamata, K., Ogura, H., Okuyama, S., Watase, K., Yamada, K., & Wada, K. (1999). Functional properties of two bombesin-like peptide receptors revealed by the analysis of mice lacking neuromedin B receptor. *Journal of Neuroscience, 19*(3), 948–954.

Ohki-Hamazaki, H., Watase, K., Yamamoto, K., Ogura, H., Yamano, M., Yamada, K., Maeno, H., Imaki, J., Kikuyama, S., Wada, E., & Wada, K. (1997). Mice lacking bombesin receptor subtype–3 develop metabolic defects and obesity. *Nature, 390*(6656), 165–169.

Ollmann, M. M., Lamoreux, M. L., Wilson, B. D., & Barsh, G. S. (1998). Interaction of agouti protein with the melanocortin 1 receptor *in vitro* and *in vivo. Genes and Development, 12*(3), 316–330.

Ollmann, M. M., Wilson, B. D., Yang, Y. K., Kerns, J. A., Chen, Y., Gantz, I., & Barsh, G. S. (1997). Antagonism of central melanocortin receptors *in vitro* and *in vivo* by agouti-related protein [published erratum appears in *Science, 281*(5383), 1615]. *Science, 278*(5335), 135–138.

Osuga, J., Ishibashi, S., Oka, T., Yagyu, H., Tozawa, R., Fujimoto, A., Shionoiri, F., Yahagi, N., Kraemer, F. B., Tsutsumi, O., & Yamada, N. (2000). Targeted disruption of hormone-sensitive lipase results in male sterility and adipocyte hypertrophy, but not in obesity. *Proceedings of the National Academy of Sciences USA, 97*(2), 787–792.

Ozata, M., Ozdemir, I. C., & Licinio, J. (1999). Human leptin deficiency caused by a missense mutation: Multiple endocrine defects, decreased sympathetic tone, and immune system dysfunction indicate new targets for leptin action, greater central than peripheral resistance to the effects of leptin, and spontaneous correction of leptin-mediated defects [published erratum appears in *Journal of Clinical Endocrinology and Metabolism, 85*(1), 416]. *Journal of Clinical Endocrinology and Metabolism, 84*(10), 3686–3695.

Pelleymounter, M. A., Cullen, M. J., Baker, M. B., Hecht, R., Winters, D., Boone, T., & Collins, F. (1995). Effects of the obese gene product on body weight regulation in *ob/ob* mice. *Science, 269*(5223), 540–543.

Qu, D., Ludwig, D. S., Gammeltoft, S., Piper, M., Pelleymounter, M. A., Cullen, M. J., Mathes, W. F., Przypek, R., Kanarek, R., & Maratos-Flier, E. (1996). A role for melanin-concentrating hormone in the central regulation of feeding behaviour. *Nature, 380*(6571), 243–247.

Rau, H., Reaves, B. J., O'Rahilly, S., & Whitehead, J. P. (1999). Truncated human leptin (delta133) associated with extreme obesity undergoes proteasomal degradation after defective intracellular transport. *Endocrinology, 140*(4), 1718–1723.

Rawls, A., Valdez, M. R., Zhang, W., Richardson, J., Klein, W. H., & Olson, E. N. (1998). Overlapping functions of the myogenic bhlh genes MRF4 and MYOD revealed in double mutant mice. *Development, 125*(13), 2349–2358.

Reiss, G. K., Desmoulin, F., Martin, C. F., Monin, G., Renou, J. P., Canioni, P., & Cozzone, P. J. (1991). *In vitro* correlation between force and energy metabolism in porcine malignant hyperthermic muscle studied by 31p NMR. *Archives of Biochemistry and Biophysics, 287*(2), 312–319.

Rosenbaum, M., & Leibel, R. L. (1999). The role of leptin in human physiology. *New England Journal of Medicine, 341*(12), 913–915.

Rosenbaum, M., Nicolson, M., Hirsch, J., Heymsfield, S. B., Gallagher, D., Chu, F., & Leibel, R. L. (1996). Effects of gender, body composition, and menopause on plasma concentrations of leptin. *Journal of Clinical Endocrinology and Metabolism, 81*(9), 3424–3427.

Rosenbaum, M., Nicolson, M., Hirsch, J., Murphy, E., Chu, F., & Leibel, R. L. (1997). Effects of weight change on plasma leptin concentrations and energy expenditure. *Journal of Clinical Endocrinology and Metabolism, 82*(11), 3647–3654.

Rudnicki, M. A., Schnegelsberg, P. N., Stead, R. H., Braun, T., Arnold, H. H., & Jaenisch, R. (1993). MYOD or MYF-5 is required for the formation of skeletal muscle. *Cell, 75*(7), 1351–1359.

Russell, C. D., Petersen, R. N., Rao, S. P., Ricci, M. R., Prasad, A., Zhang, Y., Brolin, R. E., & Fried, S. K. (1998). Leptin expression in adipose tissue from obese humans: Depot-specific regulation by insulin and dexamethasone. *American Journal of Physiology, 275*(3, Pt. 1), E507–E515.

Saito, M., & Bray, G. A. (1983). Diurnal rhythm for corticosterone in obese (*ob/ob*) diabetes (*db/db*) and gold-thioglucose-induced obesity in mice. *Endocrinology, 113*(6), 2181–2185.

Saito, Y., Nothacker, H. P., Wang, Z., Lin, S. H., Leslie, F., & Civelli, O. (1999). Molecular characterization of the melanin-concentrating-hormone receptor. *Nature, 400*(6741), 265–269.

Scarpace, P. J., Matheny, M., Pollock, B. H., & Tumer, N. (1997). Leptin increases uncoupling protein expression and energy expenditure. *American Journal of Physiology, 273*(1, Pt. 1), E226–E230.

Schwartz, M. W., Seeley, R. J., Campfield, L. A., Burn, P., & Baskin, D. G. (1996). Identification of targets of leptin action in rat hypothalamus. *Journal of Clinical Investigation, 98*(5), 1101–1106.

Scrocchi, L. A., Brown, T. J., MaClusky, N., Brubaker, P. L., Auerbach, A. B., Joyner, A. L., & Drucker, D. J. (1996). Glucose intolerance but normal satiety in mice with a null mutation in the glucagon-like peptide 1 receptor gene. *Nature Medicine, 2*(11), 1254–1258.

Shackleton, S., Lloyd, D. J., Jackson, S. N., Evans, R., Niermeijer, M. F., Singh, B. M., Schmidt, H., Brabant, G., Kumar, S., Durrington, P. N., Gregory, S., O'Rahilly, S., & Trembath, R. C. (2000). LMNA, encoding lamin A/C, is mutated in partial lipodystrophy. *Nature Genetics, 24*(2), 153–156.

Shimomura, I., Hammer, R. E., Richardson, J. A., Ikemoto, S., Bashmakov, Y., Goldstein, J. L., & Brown, M. S. (1998). Insulin resistance and diabetes mellitus in transgenic mice expressing nuclear SREBP-1c in adipose tissue: Model for congenital generalized lipodystrophy. *Genes and Development, 12*(20), 3182–3194.

Shimomura, Y., Mori, M., Sugo, T., Ishibashi, Y., Abe, M., Kurokawa, T., Onda, H., Nishimura, O., Sumino, Y., & Fujino, M. (1999). Isolation and identification of melanin-concentrating hormone as the endogenous ligand of the SLC-1 receptor. *Biochemical and Biophysical Research Communications, 261*(3), 622–626.

Shutter, J. R., Graham, M., Kinsey, A. C., Scully, S., Luthy, R., & Stark, K. L. (1997). Hypothalamic expression of ART, a novel gene related to agouti, is up-regulated in obese and diabetic mutant mice. *Genes and Development, 11*(5), 593–602.

Sierra-Honigmann, M. R., Nath, A. K., Murakami, C., Garcia-Cardena, G., Papapetropoulos, A., Sessa, W. C., Madge, L. A., Schechner, J. S., Schwabb, M. B., Polverini, P. J., & Flores-Riveros, J. R. (1998). Biological action of leptin as an angiogenic factor. *Science, 281*(5383), 1683–1686.

Simansky, K. J. (1996). Serotonergic control of the organization of feeding and satiety. *Behavioural Brain Research, 73*(1–2), 37–42.

Sims, E. A., Danforth, E., Jr., Horton, E. S., Bray, G. A., Glennon, J. A., & Salans, L. B. (1973). Endocrine and metabolic effects of experimental obesity in man. *Recent Progress in Hormone Research, 29,* 457–496.

Sivitz, W. I., Walsh, S., Morgan, D., Donohoue, P., Haynes, W., & Leibel, R. L. (1998). Plasma leptin in diabetic and insulin-treated diabetic and normal rats. *Metabolism, 47*(5), 584–591.

Smith, C. K., & Romsos, D. R. (1984). Cold acclimation of obese (*ob/ob*) mice: Effects on skeletal muscle and bone. *Metabolism, 33*(9), 858–863.

Speckman, R. A., Garg, A., Du, F., Bennett, L., Veile, R., Arioglu, E., Taylor, S. I., Lovett, M., & Bowcock, A. M. (2000). Mutational and haplotype analyses of families with familial partial lipodystrophy (Dunnigan variety) reveal recurrent missense mutations in the globular C-terminal domain of lamin A/C. *American Journal of Human Genetics, 66*(4), 1192–1198.

Stehling, O., Doring, H., Nuesslein-Hildesheim, B., Olbort, M., & Schmidt, I. (1997). Leptin does not reduce body fat content but augments cold defense abilities in thermoneutrally reared rat pups. *Pflugers Archiv: European Journal of Physiology 434*(6), 694–697.

Szabo, G., Dallmann, G., Muller, G., Patthy, L., Soller, M., & Varga, L. (1998). A deletion in the myostatin gene causes the compact (*cmpt*) hypermuscular mutation in mice. *Mammalian Genome, 9*(8), 671–672.

Szczypka, M. S., Rainey, M. A., Kim, D. S., Alaynick, W. A., Marck, B. T., Matsumoto, A. M., &

3

Energy Metabolism and Obesity

P. A. TATARANNI
ERIC RAVUSSIN

Throughout evolution, humans and animals have evolved redundant mechanisms promoting accumulation of fat during periods of feast to survive periods of famine. However, what was an asset during evolution has become a liability in the current "pathoenvironment" (Ravussin, 1995). With the recent abrupt change in environmental conditions, in which high-fat food is constantly available and in which there is little need for physical activity, obesity has reached epidemic proportions in industrialized countries and in urbanized populations around the world (World Health Organization, 1998).

In the United States in the late 1990s, one out of two adult Americans was overweight and one out of four was obese (Mokdad et al., 1999). More alarming, the prevalence of obesity is drastically increasing among children (Troiano & Flegal, 1998). The World Health Organization (1998) has identified obesity as one of the major emerging chronic diseases. Obesity increases the risk for a number of noncommunicable diseases (e.g., Type 2 diabetes, hypertension, dyslipidemias) and reduces life expectancy (Must et al., 1999). In the United States alone, the yearly cost of obesity to the public health system is estimated to be close to $100 billion. This represents between 5% and 10% of the U.S. health care budget (Wolf & Colditz, 1996).

Obesity results from a chronic imbalance between energy intake and energy expenditure. Hyperphagia, a low metabolic rate, low rates of fat oxidation, and impaired sympathetic nervous system (SNS) activity characterize animal models of obesity. Similar metabolic factors have been found to characterize humans susceptible to weight gain. Recent research has provided an unprecedented expansion of our knowledge about the molecular mechanisms that may underlie such metabolic risk factors. Perhaps the greatest impact has resulted from the cloning of genes corresponding to several mouse monogenic obesity syndromes, and the subsequent characterization of the pathways involved. Three of these genes (*ob, db,* and *A^y*) have already led to potential drugs (leptin) or drug targets (leptin receptor, melanocortin receptor 4 [MC4R], neuropeptide Y [NPY] Y1 and Y5 receptors, and others) currently in pharmaceutical development.

Over the past 15 years, we and others have focused on understanding how much of the genetic predisposition to obesity, estimated to explain as much as 70% of body mass index (BMI) variability (Stunkard, Harris, Pedersen, & McClearn, 1990), is related to energy metabolism in humans. In this chapter we review the current knowledge of the role of daily energy expenditure and its major components in the etiology of obesity.

METHODS OF MEASURING DAILY ENERGY EXPENDITURE

Several methods have been developed to measure daily energy expenditure. The most accurate methods involve continuous measurements of heat output (direct calorimetry) or gas exchange (indirect calorimetry) in subjects confined in metabolic chambers. Because confined subjects are unable to pursue habitual activities, a number of field methods have been developed to measure energy expenditure in free-living conditions, including factorial methods, heart rate monitoring, body weight clamping, and the doubly labeled water method; because the last of these has proven to be the most satisfactory, it is discussed in more detail than the others.

Direct Calorimetry

Total heat loss from the body can be assessed by direct calorimetry. This method has been extensively applied to animal studies and, in a few instances, to human studies (Benzinger & Kitzinger, 1963; Spinnler, Jequier, Favre, Dolivo, & Vannotti, 1973; Webb, 1985). The technique of direct calorimetry requires placing an individual in a small chamber in which all the heat released in the form of either dry or evaporative heat is measured. Dry heat loss represents the heat dissipated by convection and radiation, whereas evaporative heat loss is related to the evaporation of water from the lungs and skin. Direct calorimeters have been useful for validating other indirect methods, but they have become largely obsolete because they are very expensive and require the confinement of subjects in a very small room.

Indirect Calorimetry

Under normal physiological conditions, neither oxygen nor carbon dioxide is stored within the body. Therefore, an indirect method of assessing energy expenditure is to measure oxygen consumption, carbon dioxide production, and nitrogen excretion. Protein oxidation is estimated on the basis of urinary nitrogen excretion. A nonprotein respiratory quotient (nonprotein VCO_2/nonprotein VO_2) can be calculated, and the ratio between carbohydrate and lipid oxidation can be assessed (Jequier, Acheson, & Schutz, 1987). When the amount of each energy substrate oxidized (i.e., carbohydrate, fat, and protein) is known, it is possible to calculate the energy generated as a function of these oxidative processes.

Indirect calorimetry has proved useful for the study of energy expenditure and/or substrate oxidation in normal and diseased states. Early measurements were performed on individuals wearing mouthpieces or face masks, which were later replaced by ventilated hood systems. The latter systems have the advantage of being easily tolerated for several hours. During the past two decades, the indirect calorimetry method has been applied to respiratory chambers (Dauncey, Murgatroyd, & Cole, 1978; Dulloo et al., 1988; Jequier & Schutz, 1983; Mingheli, Schutz, Charbonnier, Whitehead, & Jequier, 1990; Ravussin, Lillioja, Anderson, Christin, & Bogardus, 1986; Rumpler, Seale, Conway, & Moe, 1990; Van Es et al., 1984). These are rooms large enough (12,000–40,000 liters) for a subject to live in comfortably for up to several days. The measurements from the chamber are accurate and are now used extensively to assess the determinants of daily sedentary energy expenditure in hu-

has formed the basis for the development of widely used equations to predict RMR from height and weight (Boothby & Sandiford, 1922; Cunningham, 1991; Harris & Benedict, 1919; Roza & Shizgal, 1984; Schofield, 1985). We and many others, however, have shown that at any given body size, RMR can vary as much as 20% among individuals. In our search for the possible mechanisms underlying the intersubject variability in RMR, we have explored the impact of body composition, gender, physical training, age, muscle metabolism, SNS activity, and body temperature on RMR. In a study of 130 siblings from 54 Pima Indian families, we have shown that RMR correlated best with fat-free mass (Bogardus et al., 1986). In white volunteers, we found that females had a lower RMR when compared to males (~100 kcal/day less), independent of differences in fat-free mass, fat mass, and age (Ferraro et al., 1992). This might have been due to the effect of sex hormones on metabolic rate. Whether level of physical activity and training are determinants of the RMR remains controversial (Davis et al., 1983; Donahoe, Daria, Kirschenbaum, & Keesey, 1984; Hill, Sparling, Shields, & Heller, 1987; Lennon, Nagle, Stratment, Shrago, & Dennis, 1985; Poehlman, Melby, & Bradylak, 1988; Schulz, Nyomba, Alger, Anderson, & Ravussin, 1991; Stern et al., 1980; Tremblay, Nadeau, Fournier, & Bouchard, 1988; Tremblay et al., 1986).

Cross-sectional studies of RMR indicate significant age-related declines (Boothby, Berkson, & Dunn, 1936; Shock & Yiengst, 1955; Vaughan, Zurlo, & Ravussin, 1991). Based on longitudinal data, Keys, Taylor, and Grande (1987) estimated that the decline in RMR was less than 1%–2% per decade from the second to the seventh decade of life. Subsequent work has supported Keys and colleagues' conclusion that the decrease in RMR seen in elderly people can be explained largely by decreases in fat-free mass (Calloway & Zanni, 1980; Cohn et al., 1980; Tzankoff & Norris, 1977).

Data from studies using indirect assessment of SNS activity suggest that the SNS may be involved in the regulation of RMR under eucaloric conditions (Saad et al., 1991; Schwartz, Jaeger, & Veith, 1988). Using a more direct measurement (microneurography), we found that the variability in energy expenditure was related to the variability of muscle sympathetic nerve activity (Spraul et al., 1993). Resting skeletal muscle metabolism seems also to be a significant determinant of whole-body metabolism (Kirkwood, Zurlo, Larson, & Ravussin, 1991; Zurlo, Larson, Bogardus, & Ravussin, 1990), and recent studies suggest that uncoupling protein 3 (UCP3) expression appears to underlie some of this variability (Schrauwen, Xia, Walder, Snitker, & Ravussin, 1999). Finally, we have observed that variability in RMR, after adjustments for differences in fat-free mass, fat mass, and age, was related to the variability in body temperature in males (Rising, Keys, Ravussin, & Bogardus, 1992). These results indicate that body temperature could be a marker for a high or low relative metabolic rate. It is not clear whether the heat production in the body (i.e., the metabolic rate) is regulated to maintain a given "preset" temperature, or whether the temperature is simply a reflection of the equilibrium between the heat-producing and heat-losing mechanisms that are controlled by other factors.

Fat-free mass, fat mass, age, and sex are the major determinants of RMR, explaining ~80% of its variance (Jequier & Schutz, 1983; Ravussin, Lillioja, et al., 1986). However, some of the remaining variance is explained by family membership, suggesting that RMR is at least partly genetically determined (Bogardus et al., 1986). Further support for a genetic determinant of RMR comes from studies of twins by Bouchard and colleagues (1989).

Thermic Effect of Food

The TEF (i.e., the increase in energy expenditure observed after the administration of a meal) accounts for approximately 5%–15% of the daily energy expenditure (Tataranni, Larson, Snitker, & Ravussin, 1995; Weststrate, 1993). Many factors influence TEF: meal size and composition; palatability of the food; time of the meal; and the subject's genetic background, age, physical fitness, and sensitivity to insulin. Brundin, Thorne, and Wharen (1992) have shown that TEF is also a function of the heat leakage across the abdominal wall, which is inversely related to the thickness of the abdominal adipose tissue layer. These influences, plus technical aspects such as the position of the subject and the duration of measurement, make TEF the most difficult-to-measure and the least reproducible component of daily energy expenditure (Tataranni et al., 1995; Weststrate, 1993). TEF has long been regarded as a component of daily energy expenditure that could cause significant variations in daily energy balance and therefore predispose individuals to obesity. TEF may have evolved as a mechanism for enriching protein-poor diets by disposing of the excess nonessential energy (Dulloo & Jacquet, 1999; Stock, 1999). Consequently, Stock (1999) and Dulloo and Jacquet (1999) have recently argued that large interindividual differences in TEF can only be uncovered under conditions of overfeeding with protein-depleted diets. However, given adequate protein and other essential nutrients in the diet, one can safely state that individual differences in TEF can account for only small differences in daily energy expenditure. Although a review of the published literature suggests that obesity may be associated with an impaired TEF (de Jonge & Bray, 1997), it is important to note that numerous studies have been published showing either a defect (Pittet, Chappuis, Acheson, de Techtermann, & Jequier, 1976; Ravussin et al., 1983; Schwartz, Halter, & Bierman, 1983; Schutz, Golay, Felber, & Jequier, 1984; Segal, Gutin, Nyman, & Pi-Sunyer, 1985; Thorne, Hallberg, & Wahren, 1989) or no defect in TEF in obese versus lean subjects (Blaza & Garrow, 1983; D'Alessio et al., 1988; Ravussin, Acheson, Vernet, Danforth, & Jequier, 1985; Schwartz, Ravussin, Massari, O'Connell, & Robbins, 1985; Thorne, Naslund, & Wahren, 1990; Welle & Campbell, 1983). Furthermore, in our prospective study, we found no relationship between TEF and weight change in more than 100 subjects (Tataranni et al., 1995). Decreased thermogenesis is therefore a very unlikely explanation for significant degrees of obesity.

Physical Activity

Physical activity, the most variable component of daily energy expenditure, can account for a significant amount of calories in very active people. However, sedentary adult individuals exhibit a range of physical activity that represents only 20%–30% of total energy expenditure.

Reduced physical activity as a cause of obesity is an obvious and attractive hypothesis. The energy expended in physical activity is quite variable, and the secular increase in obesity parallels the increase in sedentary lifestyles. Prentice and Jebb (1995) have presented evidence that in the United Kingdom, the prevalence of obesity has increased dramatically over the past three decades, despite a marked decrease in energy intake (Scalfi, Coltorti, & Contaldo, 1991). They resolve this paradox by hypothesizing that physical activity has decreased even more during the same period; they provide data using a proxy for activity (or inactivity), such as the numbers of hours of television viewing and the number of cars per household, both of which have increased continuously over the same period. (See Blair & Leermakers, Chapter 13, this volume, for more on exercise and weight management.)

However, until the relatively recent introduction of the doubly labeled water method for measuring energy expenditure in free-living conditions (Schoeller & Field, 1991; Schoeller & van Santen, 1982), there has been no satisfactory method by which to assess the impact of physical activity on daily energy expenditure. Schulz and Schoeller (1994) have provided data on more than 200 subjects and have observed a wide variability in total energy expenditure, and therefore in physical activity. Using the ratio between total energy expenditure and RMR as an index of the level of physical activity (Figure 3.1), they have also shown that physical activity is decreased in heavier or fatter subjects. In a review of 574 doubly labeled water measurements, Black, Coward, Cole, and Prentice (1996) compiled data to (1) establish the limits of sustainable human energy expenditure; (2) establish the average and range of habitual energy expenditure in relationship to age and sex; and (3) describe the lifestyles and activity patterns associated with different levels of physical activity. Prentice, Black, Coward, and Cole (1996) described the relationship between graded levels of obesity and free-living energy expenditure in men and women of affluent societies, and confirmed that habitual total energy expenditure is increased with obesity because of concomitant increase in fat-free mass. They also suggested that except in massive obesity, the level and cost of physical activity are quite similar at different levels of body weight and BMI.

This, however, does not exclude the possibility that an inactive lifestyle may be an important risk factor for the development of obesity. Whether a low level of physical activity is a cause or a consequence of obesity can only be tested in prospective studies. Prospective studies are providing initial evidence that even differences in nonvolitional muscle activity (i.e., fidgeting, muscle tone, maintenance of posture, etc.) may be important in determining predisposition to obesity and/or resistance to diet-induced weight gain (Levine, Eberhardt, & Jensen, 1999).

ENERGY BALANCE EQUATIONS

The balance between energy intake and energy expenditure determines energy stores. Since living organisms must obey the first law of thermodynamics, the energy balance equation has been used to predict changes in body weight when energy intake or expenditure is changed. However, the classic equation of energy balance, which states that the body energy store is equal to energy intake minus energy expenditure, has provided both insight and confusion in the understanding of energy balance in humans. Much of the confusion comes from inappropriate energy calculations using the static equation of energy balance (see below).

Equation during Weight Maintenance

$$\text{Energy Intake} = \text{Energy Expenditure}$$

This equation is self-evident and quite accurate under conditions of weight maintenance, as only limited changes in body composition are possible without changing body weight. It has been most useful in uncovering problems with reported energy intake. Most dietary intake studies show either no correlation or a negative correlation between energy intake and body weight (Lichtman et al., 1992; Romieu et al., 1988). This is in marked contrast to studies of energy expenditure, where there is a positive relationship (Figure 3.2). In addition to their greater fat mass, obese individuals have a greater fat-free mass, which is the main determinant of both RMR and 24-hour metabolic rate as measured in a respiratory chamber (Ravussin, Lillioja, et al., 1986). Studies involving free-living individuals have simultaneously measured energy expenditure via the doubly labeled water technique and energy intake via continuous recording of diet diaries (Bandini, Schoeller, Cyr, & Dietz, 1990; Mertz et al., 1991; Prentice et al., 1986). Under these careful conditions of food intake assessment, the obese subjects reported only one-half to two-thirds of their total energy intake; by contrast, lean subjects reported 80%–100% (Lichtman et al. 1992). This gap between the food that obese people perceive themselves eating and what they actually eat has been termed the

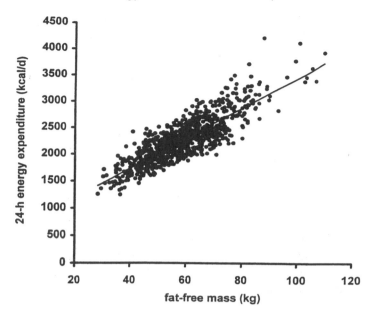

24-h energy expenditure			Total variance (SD) = 422	
		Determinant	Residual variance √ MSE	p-value
24-EE = 696	+ 18.9	FFM (kg)	224	<0.0001
(kcal/d)	+ 10.0	FM (kg)	178	<0.0001
	+ 180	male	165	<0.0001
	- 1.9	age (y)	164	<0.001
	+ 7.1	WTR (decimal)	163	<0.05
	+ 44	Pima Indian	162	<0.001

FIGURE 3.2. Relationship between 24-hour energy expenditure (24-EE) and fat-free mass (FFM) in over 900 subjects. The 24-hour energy expenditure was measured after at least 3 days on a weight-maintaining diet (50% carbohydrate, 30% fat, 20% protein) and FFM was assessed by hydrodensitometry or dual energy X-ray absorptiometry (DEXA). FFM is the major determinant of 24-hour energy expenditure, explaining a large proportion of its variance. Other determinants of 24-EE include fat mass (FM), waist-to-thigh ratio (WTR), sex, age, and race. From Weyer, Snitker, Rising, Bogardus, and Ravussin (1999). Copyright 1999 by the Nature Publishing Group. Reprinted by permission.

"eye–mouth gap" and represents a major challenge for psychologists and psychiatrists interested in obesity and food intake.

Static Energy Balance Equation

Change in Energy Stores = Energy Intake – Energy Expenditure

This is the most common equation used in discussions and calculations of energy balance. Intuitively, it seems valid; however, Alpert (1990) has elegantly demonstrated that this

Fat Balance

In marked contrast to the other nutrients, body fat stores are large, and fat intake has no influence on fat oxidation (Flatt et al., 1985; Schutz et al., 1989). As with protein, the daily fat intake represents less than 1% of the total energy stored as fat, but the fat stores contain about six times the energy of the protein stores (Bray, 1991) (Figure 3.3). These fat stores are the energy buffer for the body, and the slope of the relationship between energy balance and fat balance is determined by conditions of day-to-day small positive or negative energy balances (Abbott et al., 1988). A deficit of 200 kilocalories (kcal) of energy over 24 hours means that 200 kcal comes from the fat stores, and the same holds true for an excess of 200 kcal of energy, which ends up in the fat stores. Even in conditions of spontaneous overfeeding the entire excess fat intake is stored as body fat (Rising, Alger, et al., 1992). Ingestion of a mixed meal is followed by an increase in carbohydrate oxidation and a decrease in fat oxidation and the addition of extra fat does not alter that mix of nutrient oxidation (Flatt et al., 1985; Schutz et al., 1989). What promotes fat oxidation, if it is not dietary fat intake? The amount of total body fat exerts a small but significant effect on fat oxidation, and this promotion of fat oxidation at higher body fat levels may represent a mechanism for attenuating the rate of weight gain (Zurlo, Lillioja, et al., 1990). Energy balance is the driving force for fat oxidation (Abbott et al., 1988; Zurlo, Lillioja, et al., 1990); when it is negative (i.e., energy expenditure exceeding intake), fat oxidation increases.

In summary, when one considers energy balance in humans under physiological conditions, fat is the only nutrient that maintains a chronic imbalance between intake and oxidation, thus directly contributing to the increase in adipose tissue. The other nutrients will indirectly influence adiposity by their contribution to overall energy balance, and thus to fat balance, as emphasized by Frayn (1995). The use of the fat balance equation instead of the energy balance equation offers a new framework for understanding the pathogenesis of obesity.

Alcohol Balance

There is an inconsistent relationship between reported alcohol intake and BMI, with many studies showing a negative relationship (Colditz et al., 1991; Hellerstedt, Jeffery, & Murray, 1990). However, it has been shown that in healthy individuals the fate of ingested alcohol is oxidation and not storage (as fat), and therefore perfect alcohol balance is achieved (Shelmet et al., 1988). In the same manner as dietary carbohydrate and protein, alcohol diverts dietary fat away from oxidation and toward storage, and it inhibits lipolysis. Therefore, a chronic imbalance between alcohol intake and oxidation cannot be a direct cause of obesity, although by contributing to overall energy balance, it may indirectly influence fat balance. (For further reading on the nutrient content of foods, see Appendix 12.1 in Melanson & Dwyer, Chapter 12, this volume.)

METABOLIC RISK FACTORS FOR BODY WEIGHT GAIN IN ADULTS

An understanding of the etiology of human obesity demands longitudinal studies. Cross-sectional studies have added little to our understanding of the physiological mechanisms predisposing to weight gain (Ravussin & Swinburn, 1993). Cross-sectional studies can only provide associations, whereas longitudinal studies reveal predictors or risk factors. Several studies have examined these predictors in the Pima Indian population in Arizona. Obesity is extremely prevalent among the Pima; therefore, weight gain is very common in young adults, making this group well suited for longitudinal studies of various metabolic risk factors of weight gain (Knowler et al., 1991).

Low Metabolic Rate

Because obesity is associated with high absolute metabolic rate, both in resting conditions and over 24 hours (Ravussin, Lillioja, et al., 1986; Weyer et al., 1999), it cannot be caused by a low absolute metabolic rate, as is often proposed. Many investigators who have studied energy expenditure in humans have suggested that in the absence of a clear defect in energy expenditure in obese subjects, obesity can only be the result of excessive energy intake. However, the scatter around the regression line between metabolic rate and body size suggests that at any given body size, individuals can have a "high," "normal," or "low" relative metabolic rate. This concept is expressed graphically in Figure 3.4. From our own studies in adult nondiabetic Pima Indians, we found that a low relative metabolic rate (resting and 24-hour), adjusted for differences in fat-free mass, fat mass, age, and sex, was a risk factor for body weight gain (Ravussin et al., 1988). After 4 years of follow-up, the risk of gaining 10 kg was approximately eight times greater in subjects with the lowest RMR (lower tertile) than in those with the highest RMR (higher tertile) (Figure 3.5). According to a recent meta-analysis of published studies, formerly obese subjects have a 3%–5% lower mean relative RMR than control subjects, which is likely to contribute to the high rate of weight regain in formerly obese persons (Astrup et al., 1999).

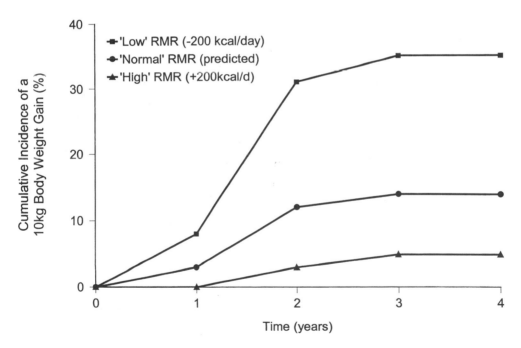

FIGURE 3.4. Cumulative incidence of a 10-kg body weight gain for a subject with a "high" relative metabolic rate (200 kcal/day above that predicted for body size and body composition), for a subject with a "normal" RMR (equal to that predicted), and for a subject with a "low" RMR (200 kcal/day below that predicted). The cumulative incidence was calculated on the basis of follow-up data obtained in 126 Pima Indians followed for an average of 3 years via a survival analysis (proportional hazard linear model). Note that subjects with a "low" RMR had approximately eight times the risk of gaining weight compared to those with a "high" RMR had.

Low SNS Activity

Studies in European Americans indicate that the activity of the SNS is related to the three major components of energy expenditure: (1) RMR (Spraul et al., 1993); (2) TEF (Schwartz et al., 1988); and (3) spontaneous physical activity (Christin, O'Connell, Bogardus, Danforth, & Ravussin, 1993). We have recently shown that SNS activity is also negatively correlated with the 24-hour respiratory quotient (Snitker, Tataranni, & Ravussin, 1998). Further indications of the possible role of SNS activity in the regulation of energy balance in humans comes from a study showing that low SNS activity was associated with a poor weight loss outcome in obese subjects treated with diet (Astrup et al., 1995). Furthermore, Pima Indians, who are prone to obesity, have low rates of muscle sympathetic nerve activity compared to weight-matched European Americans (Spraul et al., 1993). In a prospective study, we found that baseline urinary excretion rate of norepinephrine, a global index of SNS activity, was negatively correlated with body weight gain in male Pima Indians (Tataranni, Young, Bogardus, & Ravussin, 1997). Thus low SNS activity is associated with the development of obesity.

Low Plasma Concentration of Leptin

Leptin, the product of the *ob* gene, is a hormone produced by the adipose tissue that inhibits food intake and increases energy expenditure (Caro, Sinha, Kolaczynski, Zhang, & Considine, 1997). To investigate whether individuals prone to weight gain are hypoleptinemic, we measured fasting plasma leptin concentrations in two groups of weight-matched, nondiabetic Pima Indians followed for approximately 3 years, 19 of whom subsequently gained weight (average weight gain 23 kg) and 17 of whom maintained their weight within 0.5 kg. After adjustment for initial percentage of body fat, mean plasma leptin concentration was lower in those who gained weight than in those whose weight was stable (Ravussin et al., 1997). Despite the leptin resistance apparent in obesity (Caro et al., 1997), these data indicate that relatively low plasma leptin concentrations may play a role in the development of obesity in some Pima Indians. Of note, relative hypoleptinemia is not a risk factor for obesity in other populations (Lissner et al., 1999; McNeely et al., 1999).

METABOLIC RISK FACTORS FOR BODY WEIGHT GAIN IN CHILDREN

One of the most troubling aspects of the current epidemic of obesity (Mokdad et al., 1999) is the increasing prevalence of obesity and Type 2 diabetes among children. Childhood obesity is a very serious problem because tracking of overweight, albeit moderate, is observed between childhood and adulthood (Serdula et al., 1993). Furthermore, duration of obesity is an independent predictor of health outcomes (McCance et al., 1994). The risk of developing obesity seems to be especially elevated during early infancy, the adiposity rebound period during prepubertal growth, and the adolescent growth phase (Dietz, 1994).

The observation that obesity occurs more frequently in children of obese parents has led to various studies to determine how much of the genetic predisposition to obesity is related to energy metabolism. Stunkard, Berkowitz, Stallings, and Schoeller (1999) reported data on energy intake and energy expenditure in infants born to lean and overweight mothers; they concluded that excessive energy intake, rather than low energy expenditure, is the cause of obesity in infants at high risk of obesity. This is a vastly unexplored area, and more studies are needed to understand how eating behavior forms and solidifies in conjunction with the final maturation of the human brain from childhood to adulthood. In their study of 18 subjects, Roberts, Savage, Coward, Chew, and Lucas (1988) measured energy expenditure by doubly labeled water in infants at 3 months of age and divided them post hoc into overweight and normal-weight groups at age 12 months. Energy expenditure (mostly activity) was on average 20% lower in those who became overweight at 12 months than in those who did not. Similarly, Griffiths, Payne, Stunkard, Rivers, and Cox (1990) reported that low energy expenditure in 5-year-old girls was negatively correlated with BMI at adolescence. In girls, reduction in total energy expenditure as a result of a marked reduction in physical activity during prepubertal growth has recently been reported (Goran, Gower, Nagy, & Johnson, 1998). However, other studies have failed to confirm that resting energy expenditure, total energy expenditure, or activity energy expenditure measured in early childhood is inversely related to the development of obesity (Goran, Hunter, Nagy, & Johnson, 1997; Johnson et al., 1999). Despite these large inconsistencies in the literature, it seems reasonable to conclude that a sedentary lifestyle in early childhood should be discouraged, because low levels of aerobic fitness (Johnson et al., 1999), excessive TV viewing (Robinson, 1999; Salbe, Weyer, Fontvieille, & Ravussin, 1998), and limited playing time (Salbe et al., 1998) have all been associated with increased risk of weight gain.

Some studies have suggested that higher plasma insulin concentration early in life may predispose to obesity. In 5- to 10-year-old Pima Indian children, a high fasting plasma insulin concentration (probably reflecting insulin resistance) predicted overweight 7–8 years later, especially in boys (Odeleye, de Courten, Pettitt, & Ravussin, 1997). Le Stunff and Bougneres (1994) reported that a hyperisulinemic response to meals is the earliest detectable abnormality in obese children, followed by the development of fasting hyperinsulinemia and insulin resistance. Although investigators are far from reaching a consensus in this area, these results seem to indicate that hyperinsulinemia, perhaps through the antilipolytic effect of insulin, may be an early risk factor for obesity.

Despite the attractiveness of prevention strategies aimed at children, which could be based on correcting some of these early risk factors for obesity, caution should be exercised. Until we fully comprehend the interplay among variability of energy metabolism, growth, and obesity, we must be concerned about the risk of unforeseen adverse consequences, particularly in respect to interruption of normal growth pattern in early childhood and distorted body image, excessive dieting, and anorexia nervosa in adolescence.

Additional information on child obesity is provided by Berkowitz and Stunkard and by Goldfield, Raynor, and Epstein in Chapters 25 and 26 of this volume, respectively.

METABOLIC ADAPTATION

Studies in adult Pima Indians have allowed us to identify metabolic risk factors for body weight gain, such as a relatively low metabolic rate and low rate of spontaneous physical activity, a high respiratory quotient, and insulin sensitivity. We have also observed that after weight gain the original abnormal state becomes normalized, and because the change in metabolic risk factors is greater than the cross-sectional data would predict, this may be a mechanism to counteract further weight gain (Figure 3.4).

Changes in metabolic factors, which are not explained by changes in body weight and composition, are the hallmarks of metabolic adaptation. The concept of metabolic adaptation was introduced by the pioneering work of Keys and colleagues, who defined the drop in energy expenditure observed in healthy men in response to semistarvation "a useful adjustment to altered circumstances" (Keys, Brozek, Henschel, Mickelsen, & Taylor, 1950). A more recent definition of adaptation has been proposed in a report by several U.N. agencies (Food and Argriculture Organization, World Health Organization, & United Nations Uni-

stimulating hormone (α-MSH) at the hypothalamic MC4R (Gantz et al., 1993). In addition, MC4R-knockout mice exhibit an obesity phenotype similar to that observed in A^y mice (Huszar et al., 1997). α-MSH is derived from the gene known as pro-opiomelanocortin (POMC), which was found to be linked with body fat content in Mexican Americans (Comuzzie et al., 1997), suggesting a possible role for this pathway in the pathophysiology of human obesity. In addition, two individuals with mutations in the POMC gene were recently described with severe, early-onset obesity and bright red hair (Krude et al., 1998). Finally, several individuals from three different human pedigrees have been described to have a mutation of MC4R that is associated with hyperphagia and severe obesity (Hinney et al., 1999; Vaisse, Clement, Guy-Grant, & Froguel, 1998; Yeo et al., 1998).

At least three other hypothalamic peptides have been discovered recently in animal models of obesity, which may be important in energy balance. Melanin-concentrating hormone (MCH), discovered by differential display studies in *ob/ob* mice, is overexpressed in some animal models of obesity, and administration of MCH increased food intake in rats (Qu et al., 1996). A recent study suggests that MCH may act as a functional antagonist of the melanocortin pathway described above (Ludwig et al., 1998). Orexins A and B are recently described hypothalamic peptides that stimulate food consumption in rats (Sakurai et al., 1998). However, recent data suggest that orexins have more to do with arousal than with eating behavior (Lin et al., 1999). Another hypothalamic peptide known as cocaine- and amphetamine-related transcript (CART) was recently discovered by differential display studies in animal models (Douglass, McKinzie, & Couceyro, 1995). Administration of CART to rats inhibited both basal and starvation-induced feeding (Kristensen et al., 1998). Further investigation of these and other hypothalamic peptides is likely to add to our understanding of the central regulation of energy balance in humans.

Other studies in animal models have increased our knowledge of the role of certain genes in energy balance. For example, the recently discovered uncoupling proteins UCP2 and UCP3 have been suggested to play a role in energy balance in rodents, and studies are currently underway to investigate the role of these proteins in humans. Studies in our laboratory suggest that genetic variation at UCP2–UCP3 is associated with metabolic rate in Pima Indians (Schrauwen et al., 1999; Walder et al., 1998). In summary, recent studies in animal models have contributed greatly to our understanding of the regulation of energy balance. New peptides and pathways have been discovered that could potentially lead to new therapies for the treatment of human obesity.

FUTURE DIRECTIONS

Our studies on the regulation of energy expenditure in humans have provided evidence that approximately 30% of the interindividual variability of body weight can be attributable to familial traits such as daily energy expenditure (10%–15%), respiratory quotient (5%), and spontaneous physical activity (10%). With the knowledge that up to 70% of the variance in BMI is genetically determined, one has to conclude that a large proportion of the variance in BMI may be due to the effect of genes on factors not measured in our studies—that is, eating behavior and habitual physical activity in free-living conditions (Figure 3.7).

In contrast to animal models, however, it has been very difficult to study the molecular mechanisms and resulting behaviors that underlie excessive energy intake in humans. Nevertheless, the identification of severe hyperphagia in individuals with mutations of the leptin, leptin receptor, and MC4R genes leaves little doubt that energy intake is as highly regulated at the molecular levels in humans as it is in animals. Furthermore, based on the results that have emerged from the recent use of new techniques such as positron emission tomog-

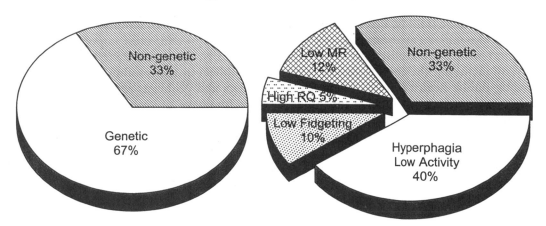

FIGURE 3.7. Studies in monozygotic twins reared apart suggest that approximately 70% of the variability in BMI is attributable to genetic factors and 30% to the environment. Based in part on results from our longitudinal studies in Pima Indians, we submit that the contribution of genetic factors controlling metabolic rate, respiratory quotient, fidgeting, daily physical activity, and hyperphagia to BMI variability can be estimated. From Ravussin and Bogardus (2000).

raphy and functional magnetic resonance imaging (fMRI), it seems likely that the level of complexity of the neuroanatomical correlates of eating behavior in humans could be much higher than it is in rodents. We have recently shown that in response to a single meal, neuronal activity increases in the prefrontal cortex and decreases in the hypothalamus, thalamus, insular cortex, orbitofrontal cortex, and hippocampal formation in the brains of healthy men (Tataranni et al., 1999). An inhibition of neuronal activity in the hypothalamic region following a meal was confirmed in a second study using fMRI (Matsuda et al., 1999). Most importantly, preliminary data suggest that brain responses to a meal may be substantially different between lean and obese subjects (Gautier et al., 2000). Such techniques applied to formerly obese subjects, as well as subjects suffering from eating disorders, may help identify the neurological pathways responsible for hyperphagia and obesity.

Past difficulties in measuring habitual physical activity in humans have largely been alleviated by the advent of the doubly labeled water technique. Thus in the near future, it should be possible to better understand the interaction between the energy expended in daily physical activities and the development of obesity in children and adults.

A greater knowledge of the physiology of obesity will ultimately come from the current efforts to isolate all the genes related to weight gain. Over the past few years, genetic linkage studies have increasingly focused on complex traits such as obesity. Genome-wide scans have been completed in Mexican Americans (Comuzzie et al., 1997), in Pima Indians (Hanson, Ehm, & Pettitt, 1998; Norman et al., 1998), in a diverse population of European and African Americans (Lee et al., 1999), in French Canadian families (Chagnon, Perusse, Weisnagel, Rankinen, & Bouchard, 2000), and in French families (Hager et al., 1998). From all these studies, major loci linked to obesity have been found on chromosomes 2, 5, 10, 11, and 20. Those areas of the genome are currently under intense investigation as they may lead to the cloning of obesity susceptibility genes.

Although many of us would like to think that obesity is a disease with multiple genetic/molecular explanations, a new paradigm may emerge from such research indicating that obesity results from "normal physiological variability within a pathoenvironment." The corollary of this is that the pathology does not lie within the individual, but within

Coleman, D. L. (1973). Effects of parabiosis of obesity with diabetes and normal mice. *Diabetologia, 9,* 294–298.

Comuzzie, A. G., Hixson, J. E., Almasy, L., Mitchell, B. D., Mahaney, M. C., Dyer, T. D., Stern, M. P., MacCluer, J. W., & Blangero, J. (1997). A major quantitative trait locus determining serum leptin levels and fat mass is located on human chromosome 2. *Nature Genetics, 15,* 273–276.

Considine, R. V., Sinha, M. K., Heiman, M. L., Kriauciunas, A., Stephens, T. W., Nyce, M. R., Ohannesian, J. P., Marco, C. C., McKee, L. J., Bauer, T. L., & Caro, J. F. (1996). Serum immunoreactive-leptin concentrations in normal-weight and obese humans. *New England Journal of Medicine, 334,* 292–295.

Coward, W. A., Prentice, A. M., Murgatroyd, P. R., et al. (1984). Measurement of CO_2 and water production rates in man using ^2H, ^{18}O-labelled H_2O: comparisons between calorimeter and isotope values. In A. J. Van Es & A. J. H. Wageningen (Eds.), *European nutrition report: Vol 5. Human energy metabolism: Physical activity and energy expenditure measurements in epidemiological research based upon direct and indirect calorimetry* (pp. 126–128). Stichting Netherlands Instituut voor de Voeding.

Cunningham, J. J. (1991). Body composition as a determinant of energy expenditure: A synthetic review and a proposed general prediction equation. *American Journal of Clinical Nutrition, 54,* 963–969.

D'Alessio, D. A., Kavle, E. C., Mozzoli, M. A., Smalley, K. J., Polansky, M., Kendrick, Z. V., Owen, L. R., Bushman, M. C., Boden, G., & Owen, O. E. (1988). Thermic effect of food in lean and obese men. *Journal of Clinical Investigation, 81,* 1781–1789.

Dauncey, Y. M. J., Murgatroyd, P. R., & Cole, T. J. (1979). A human calorimeter for the direct and indirect measurement of 24 h energy expenditure. *British Journal of Nutrition, 39,* 557–566.

Davis, J. R., Tagliaferro, A. R., Kertzer, R., Gerardo, T., Nichols, J., & Wheeler, J. (1983). Variations in dietary-induced thermogenesis and body fatness with aerobic capacity. *European Journal of Applied Physiology, 50,* 319–329.

de Jonge, L., & Bray, G. A. (1997). The thermic effect of food and obesity: A critical review. *Obesity Research, 5,* 622–631.

Dietz, W. H. (1994). Critical periods in childhood for the development of obesity. *American Journal of Clinical Nutrition, 59,* 955–959.

Donahoe, C. P., Daria, H. L., Kirschenbaum, D. S., & Keesey, R. E. (1984). Metabolic consequences of dieting and exercise in the treatment of obesity. *Journal of Consulting and Clinical Psychology, 52,* 827–886.

Douglass, J., McKinzie, A. A., & Couceyro, P. (1995). PCR differential display identifies a rat brain mRNA that is transcriptionally regulated by cocaine and amphetamine. *Journal of Neurosciences, 15,* 2471–2481.

Dulloo, A. G., Ismail, M. N., Ryall, M., Meals, G., Geissler, C. A., & Miller, D. S. (1988). A low budget easy-to-operate room respirometer for measuring daily energy expenditure in man. *American Journal of Clinical Nutrition, 48,* 1267–1274.

Dulloo, A. G., & Jacquet, J. (1999). Low-protein overfeeding: A tool to unmask susceptibility to obesity in humans. *International Journal of Obesity, 23,* 1118–1121.

Durnin, J. V. G. A. (1959). Determination of total daily energy expenditure in man by indirect calorimetry: Assessment of the accuracy of a modern technique. *British Journal of Nutrition, 13,* 41–53.

Durnin, J. V. G. A. (1978). Indirect calorimetry in man: A critique of practical problems. *Proceedings of the Nutrition Society, 37,* 5–12.

Durnin, J. V. G. A., Edholm, O. G., Miller, D. S., & Waterlow, J. (1973). How much food does man require? *Nature, 242,* 418.

Durnin, J. V. G. A., & Passemore, R. (1967). *Energy, work and leisure.* London: Heinemann.

Eckel, R. H. (1992). Insulin resistance: an adaptation for weight maintenance. *Lancet, 340,* 1452–1453.

Edholm, O. G. (1973). Energy expenditure and food intake. In M. Apfelbaum (Ed.), *Energy balance in man* (pp. 51–60). Paris: Masson.

Elliot, D. L., Goldberg, L., Kuehl, K. S., & Bennett, W. M. (1989). Sustained suppression of resting metabolic rate after massive weight loss. *International Journal of Obesity, 49,* 93–96.

Ferraro, R., Lillioja, S., Fontvieille, A. M., Rising, R., Bogardus, C., & Ravussin, E. (1992). Lower sedentary metabolic rate in women compared with men. *Journal of Clinical Investigation, 90,* 780–784.

Flatt, J. P., Ravussin, E., Acheson, K. J., & Jequier, E. (1985). Effects of dietary fat on postprandial substrate oxidation and on carbohydrate and fat balance. *Journal of Clinical Investigation, 76,* 1019–1024.

Food and Agriculture Organization, World Health Organization, & United Nations University. (1985). *Energy and protein requirements* (WHO Technical Report Series No. 724). Geneva: World Health Organization.

Frayn, K. N. (1995). Physiological regulation of macronutrient balance. *International Journal of Obesity, 19,* S4–S10.

Froidevaux, F., Schutz, Y., Christin, L., & Jequier, E. (1993). Energy expenditure in obese women before and during weight loss, after refeeding and in the weight-relapse period. *American Journal of Clinical Nutrition, 57,* 35–42.

Gantz, I., Miwa, H., Konda, Y., Shimoto, Y., Tashiro, T., Watson, S. J., Delvalle, J., & Yamada, T. (1993). Molecular cloning, expression and gene localisation of a 4th melanocortin receptor. *Journal of Biological Chemistry, 268,* 15174–15179.

Garrow, J. S. (1974). *Energy balance and obesity in man.* Amsterdam: North-Holland.

Gautier, J. F., Chen, K., Salbe, A. D., Bandy, D., Pratley, R. E., Heinman, M., Ravussin, E., Reiman, E., & Tataranni, P. A. (2000). Differential brain responses to satiation in obese and lean men. *Diabetes, 49,* 838–846.

Geissler, C. A., Dzumbira, T. M. O., & Noor, M. I. (1986). Validation of a field technique for the measurement of energy expenditure: Factorial method versus continuous respirometry. *American Journal of Clinical Nutrition, 44,* 596–602.

Goran, M. I., Gower, B. A., Nagy, T. R., & Johnson, R. K. (1998). Developmental changes in energy expenditure and physical activity in children: Evidence for a decline in physical activity in girls before puberty. *Pediatrics, 101,* 887–891.

Goran, M. I., Hunter, G., Nagy, T. R., & Johnson, R. (1997). Physical activity related energy expenditure and fat mass in young children. *International Journal of Obesity, 21,* 171–178.

Griffiths, M., Payne, P. R., Stunkard, A. J., Rivers, J. P. W., & Cox, M. (1990). Metabolic rate and physical development in children at risk of obesity. *Lancet, 336,* 76–78.

Hager, J., Dina, C., Franeke, S., Dubois, S., Houari, M., Vatin, V., Vaillant, V., Lorentz, N., Basdevant, A., Clement, K., Guy-Grand, B., & Froguel, P. (1998). A genome-wide scan for human obesity genes reveals a major susceptibility locus on chromosome 10. *Nature Genetics, 20,* 304–308.

Hanson, R. L., Ehm, M. G., & Pettitt, D. J. (1998). An autosomal genomic scan for loci linked to Type 2 diabetes mellitus and body mass index in Pima Indians. *American Journal of Human Genetics, 63,* 1130–1138.

Harris, J. A., & Benedict, F. G. (1919). *A biometric study of basal metabolism in man.* Washington, DC: Carnegie Institute.

Hellerstedt, W. L., Jeffery, R. W., & Murray, D. M. (1990). The association between alcohol intake and adiposity in the general population. *American Journal of Epidemiology, 132,* 594–611.

Heska, S., Yang, M. U., Wand, J., Burt, P., & Pi-Sunyer, F. X. (1990). Weight loss and change in resting metabolic rate. *American Journal of Clinical Nutrition, 52,* 981–986.

Heymsfield, S. B., Darby, P. C., Muhlheim, L. S., Gallagher, D., Wolper, C., & Allison, D. B. (1995). The calorie: Myth, measurement, and reality. *American Journal of Clinical Nutrition, 62,* 1034S–1041S.

Heymsfield, S. B., Greenberg, A. S., Fujioka, K., Dixon, R. M., Kushner, R., Hunt, T., Lubina, J. A., Patane, J., Self, B., Hunt, P., & McCamish, M. (1999). Recombinant leptin for weight loss in obese and lean adults: A randomized, controlled, dose escalation trial. *Journal for the American Medical Association, 282,* 1568–1575.

Hill, J. O., & Peters, J. C. (1998). Environmental contributions to the obesity epidemic. *Science, 280,* 1371–1374.

E., Mohammed, S. N., Hurst, J. A., Cheetham, C. H., Earley, A. R., Barnett, A. H., Prins, J. B., & O'Rahilly, S. (1997). Congenital leptin deficiency is associated with severe early-onset obesity in humans. *Nature, 387,* 903–908.

Must, A., Spadano, J., Coakley, E. H., Field, A. E., Colditz, G., & Dietz, W. H. (1999). The disease burden associated with overweight and obesity. *Journal of the American Medical Association, 282,* 1523–1529.

Norgan, N. G., & Durnin, J. V. G. A. (1980). The effect of 6 weeks of overfeeding on the body weight, body composition, and energy metabolism in young men. *American Journal of Clinical Nutrition, 33,* 978–988.

Norman, R., Tataranni, P. A., Pratley, R. E., Thompson, D. B., Hanson, R. L., Prochazka, M., Baier, L., Ehm, M. G., Sakul, H., Foroud, T., Garvey, W. T., Burney, D., Knowler, W. C., Bennett, P. H., Bogardus, C., & Ravussin, E. (1998). Autosomal genomic scan for loci linked to obesity and energy metabolism in Pima Indians. *American Journal of Human Genetics, 62,* 659–668.

Odeleye, O. E., de Courten, M., Pettitt, D. J., & Ravussin, E. (1997). Fasting hyperinsulinemia is a predictor of increased body weight gain and obesity in Pima Indian children. *Diabetes, 46,* 1341–1345.

Pittet, P. H., Chappuis, P. H., Acheson, K., de Techtermann, F., & Jequier, E. (1976). Thermic effect of glucose in obese subjects studied by direct and indirect calorimetry. *British Journal of Nutrition, 35,* 281–292.

Poehlman, E. T., Melby, C. L., & Bradylak, S. J. (1988). Resting metabolic rate and postprandial thermogenesis in highly trained and untrained males. *American Journal of Clinical Nutrition, 47,* 793–798.

Prentice, A. M., Black, A. E., Coward, W. A., & Cole, T. J. (1996). Energy expenditure in overweight and obese adults in affluent societies: An analysis of 319 doubly-labeled water measurements. *European Journal of Clinical Nutrition, 50,* 93–97.

Prentice, A. M., Black, A. E., Coward, W. A., Davies, H. L., Goldberg, G. R., Murgatroyd, P. R., Ashford, J., Sawyer, M., & Whitehead, R. G. (1986). High levels of energy expenditure in obese women. *British Medical Journal, 292,* 983–987.

Prentice, A. M., & Jebb, S. A. (1995). Obesity in Britain: Gluttony or sloth? *British Medical Journal, 311,* 437–439.

Qu, D., Ludwig, D. S., Gammeltoft, S., Piper, M., Pelleymounter, M. A., Cullen, M. J., Mathes, W. F., Przypek, J., Kanarek, R., & Maratos-Flier, E. (1996). A role for melanin-concentrating hormone in the central regulation of feeding behavior. *Nature, 380,* 243–247.

Ravussin, E. (1995). Obesity in Britain: Rising trend may be due to "pathoenvironment" [Letter to the editor]. *British Medical Journal, 311,* 1569.

Ravussin, E., Acheson, K. J., Vernet, O., Danforth, E., & Jequier, E. (1985). Evidence that insulin resistance is responsible for the decreased thermic effect of glucose in human obesity. *Journal of Clinical Investigation, 76,* 1268–1273.

Ravussin, E., & Bogardus, C. (2000). Energy balance and weight regulation: Genetics versus environment. *British Journal of Nutrition, 83,* 17–20.

Ravussin, E., Bogardus, C., Schwartz, R. S., Robbins, D. C., Wolfe, R. R., Horton, E. S., Danforth, E., & Sims, E. A. (1983). Thermic effect of infused glucose and insulin in man: Decreased response with increased insulin resistance in obesity and non-insulin dependent diabetes mellitus. *Journal of Clinical Investigation, 72,* 893–902.

Ravussin, E., Harper, I. T., Rising, R., & Bogardus, C. (1986). Energy expenditure by doubly labeled water: Validation in lean and obese subjects. *American Journal of Physiology, 261,* E402–E409.

Ravussin, E., Lillioja, S., Anderson, T. E., Christin, L., & Bogardus, C. (1986). Determinants of 24-hour energy expenditure in man: Methods and results using a respiratory chamber. *Journal of Clinical Investigation, 78,* 1568–1578.

Ravussin, E., Lillioja, S., Knowler, W. C., Christin, L., Freymond, D., Abbott, W. G., Boyce, V., Howard, B. V., & Bogardus, C. (1988). Reduced rate of energy expenditure as a risk factor for body weight gain. *New England Journal of Medicine, 318,* 467–472.

Ravussin, E., Pratley, R. E., Maffei, M., Wang, H., Friedman, J. M., Bennett, P. H., & Bogardus, C. (1997). Relatively low plasma leptin concentrations precede weight gain in Pima Indians. *Nature Medicine, 3,* 238–240.

Ravussin, E., & Swinburn, B. A. (1993). Metabolic predictors of obesity: Cross-sectional versus longitudinal data. *International Journal of Obesity, 17,* S28–S31.

Rising, R., Alger, S., Boyce, V., Seagle, H., Ferraro, R., Fontvieille, A. M., & Ravussin, E. (1992). Food intake measured by an automated food-selection system: Relationship to energy expenditure. *American Journal of Clinical Nutrition, 55,* 343–349.

Rising, R., Keys, A., Ravussin, E., & Bogardus, C. (1992). Concomitant inter-individual variation in body temperature and metabolic rate. *American Journal of Physiology, 263,* E730–E734.

Roberts, S. B., Coward, W. A., Schlingenseigpen, K. H., Nohria, V., & Lucas, A. (1986). Comparison of the doubly labeled water ($H_2^{18}O$) method with indirect calorimetry and a nutrient balance study for simultaneous determination of energy expenditure, water intake, and metabolized energy intake in preterm infants. *American Journal of Clinical Nutrition, 44,* 315–322.

Roberts, S. B., Savage, J., Coward, W. A., Chew, B., & Lucas, A. (1988). Energy expenditure and intake in infants born to lean and overweight mothers. *New England Journal of Medicine, 318,* 461–466.

Robinson, T. N. (1999). Reducing children's television viewing to prevent obesity: A randomized controlled trial. *Journal of the American Medical Association, 282,* 1561–1567.

Romieu, I., Willett, W. C., Stampfer, M. J., Colditz, G. A., Sampson, L., Rosner, B., Hennekens, C. H., & Speizer, F. E. (1988). Energy intake and other determinants of relative weight. *American Journal of Clinical Nutrition, 47,* 406–412.

Roza, A. M., & Shizgal, H. M. (1984). The Harris–Benedict equation reevaluated: Resting energy requirements and the body cell mass. *American Journal of Clinical Nutrition, 40,* 168–182.

Rumpler, W. V., Seale, J. L., Conway, J. M., & Moe, P. W. (1990). Repeatability of 24-h energy expenditure in humans by indirect calorimetry. *American Journal of Clinical Nutrition, 51,* 147–152.

Saad, M. F., Alger, S. A., Zurlo, F., Young, J. B., Bogardus, C., & Ravussin, E. (1991). Ethnic differences in sympathetic nervous system-mediated energy expenditure. *American Journal of Physiology, 261,* E789–E794.

Sakurai, T., Amemiya, A., Ishii, M., Matsuzaki, I., Chemelli, R. M., Tanaka, H., Williams, S. C., Richardson, J. A., Kozlowski, G. P., Wilson, S., Arch, J. R. S., Buckingham, R. E., Haynes, A. C., Carr, S. A., Annan, R. S., McNulty, D. E., Liu, W.-S., Terrett, J. A., Elshourbagy, N. A., Bergsma, D. J., & Yanagisawa, M. (1998). Orexins and orexin receptors: A family of hypothalamic neuropeptides and G protein-coupled receptors that regulate feeding behavior. *Cell, 92,* 573–585.

Salbe, A. D., Weyer, C., Fontvieille, A. M., & Ravussin, E. (1998). Low levels of physical activity and time spent viewing television at 9 years of age predict weight gain 8 years later in Pima Indian children. *International Journal of Obesity, 22*(Suppl. 4), S10.

Scalfi, L., Coltorti, A., & Contaldo, F. (1991). Postprandial thermogenesis in lean and obese subjects after meals supplemented with medium-chain and long-chain triglycerides. *American Journal of Clinical Nutrition, 53,* 1130–1133.

Schoeller, D. A., & Field, C. R. (1991). Human energy metabolism: What have we learned from the doubly labeled water method? *Annual Review of Nutrition, 11,* 355–373.

Schoeller, D. A., Ravussin, E., Schutz, Y., Acheson, K. J., Baertschi, P., & Jequier, E. (1986). Energy expenditure by doubly labeled water: Validation in humans and proposed calculation. *American Journal of Physiology, 250,* R823–R830.

Schoeller, D. A., & van Santen, E. (1982). Measurement of energy expenditure in humans by doubly labeled water method. *Journal of Appled Physiology, 53,* 955–959.

Schoeller, D. A., & Webb, P. (1984). Five-day comparison of the doubly labeled water method with respiratory gas exchange. *American Journal of Clinical Nutrition, 40,* 143–158.

Schofield, W. N. (1985). Predicting basal metabolic rate: New standards and review of previous work. *Human Nutrition: Clinical Nutrition, 39C*(Suppl. 1), 5–14.

Schrauwen, P., Xia, J., Walder, K., Snitker, S., & Ravussin, E. (1999). A novel polymorphism in the proximal UCP3 promoter region: Effect on skeletal muscle UCP3 mRNA expression and obesity in male non-diabetic Pima Indians. *International Journal of Obesity, 23,* 1242–1245.

Schulz, L. O., Nyomba, B. L., Alger, S., Anderson, T. E., & Ravussin, E. (1991). Effect of endurance training on sedentary energy expenditure measured in a respiratory chamber. *American Journal of Physiology, 260,* E257–E261.

Webb, P. (1985). *Human calorimeters*. Westport, CT: Praeger.

Weigle, D. S. (1988). Contribution of decreased body mass to diminished thermic effect of exercise in reduced-obese men. *International Journal of Obesity, 12,* 567–578.

Weigle, D. S., Sande, K. J., Iverius, P. H., Monsen, E. R., & Brunzell, J. D. (1988). Weight loss leads to a marked decrease in nonresting energy expenditure in ambulatory human subjects. *Metabolism, 37,* 930–936.

Weinsier, R. L., Nelson, K. M., Hensrud, D. D., Darnell, B. E., Hunter, G. R., & Schutz, Y. (1995). Metabolic predictors of obesity: Contributions of resting energy expenditure, thermic effect of food, and fuel utilization to four-year weight gain in post-obese and never-obese women. *Journal of Clinical Investigation, 95,* 980–985.

Welle, S. L., & Campbell, R. G. (1983). Normal thermic effect of glucose in obese women. *American Journal of Clinical Nutrition, 37,* 87–92.

Weststrate, J. A. (1993). Resting metabolic rate and diet induced thermogenesis: A methodological reappraisal. *American Journal of Clinical Nutrition, 58,* 592–601.

Weyer, C., Pratley, R. E., Salbe, A., Bogardus, C., Ravussin, E., & Tataranni, P. A. (2000). Energy expenditure, fat oxidation, and body weight regulation: A study of metabolic adaptation to long term weight change. *Journal of Clinical Endocrinology and Metabolism, 85,* 1087–1094.

Weyer, C., Snitker, S., Rising, R., Bogardus, C., & Ravussin, E. (1999). Determinants of energy expenditure and fuel utilization in man: Effects of body composition, age, sex, ethnicity, and glucose tolerance in 916 subjects. *International Journal of Obesity, 23,* 715–722.

Wolf, A. M., & Colditz, G. A. (1996). Social and economic effects of body weight in the United States. *American Journal of Clinical Nutrition, 63*(Suppl. 3), 466S–469S.

World Health Organization. (1998). *Obesity, preventing and managing the global epidemic* (Publication No. WHO/NUT/NCD/98.1). Geneva: Author.

Yeo, G. S. H., Farooqi, I. S., Aminian, S., Halshall, D. J., Stanhope, R. G., & O'Rahilly, S. (1998). A frameshift mutation in MC4R associated with dominantly inherited human obesity. *Nature Genetics, 20,* 111–112.

Yost, T., Jensen, D. R., & Eckel, R. H. (1995). Weight regain following sustained weight reduction is predicted by relative insulin sensitivity. *Obesity Research, 3,* 583–587.

Zelewski, M., & Swierczynki, J. (1990). Comparative studies on lipogenic enzyme activities in the liver of human and some animal species. *Comparative Biochemistry and Physiology, 95,* 469–472.

Zhang, Y., Proenca, R., Maffei, M., Barone, M., Leopold, L., & Friedman, J. M. (1994). Positional cloning of the mouse obese gene and its human homologue. *Nature, 372,* 425–432.

Zurlo, F., Ferraro, R. T., Fontvieille, A. M., Rising, R., Bogardus, C., & Ravussin, E. (1992). Spontaneous physical activity and obesity: Cross-sectional and longitudinal studies in Pima Indians. *American Journal of Physiology, 263,* E296–E300.

Zurlo, F., Larson, K., Bogardus, C., & Ravussin, E. (1990). Skeletal muscle metabolism is a major determinant of resting energy expenditure. *Journal of Clinical Investigation, 86,* 1423–1427.

Zurlo, F., Lillioja, S., Esposito-Del Puente, A., Nyomba, B. L., Baz, I., Saad, M. F., Swinburn, B. A., Knowler, W. C., Bogardus, C., & Ravussin, E. (1990). Low ratio of fat to carbohydrate oxidation as a predictor of weight gain: Study of 24-h RQ. *American Journal of Physiology, 259,* E650–E657.

4

Genetics and Common Obesities: Background, Current Status, Strategies, and Future Prospects

R. ARLEN PRICE

We are in a period of rapid growth in our knowledge about genetic influences on obesity. That growth is likely to reach unprecedented levels over the next few years and there are several reasons for this. Genes for several Mendelian (single-gene) obesities have been identified and well characterized, resulting in the identification of key pathways that regulate energy intake, storage, and utilization. The Human Genome Project has finished a draft DNA sequence (Lander et al., 2001; Venter et al., 2001). Many technological innovations, such as high throughput, automated sequencing, genotyping, mutation, expression screening, and functional analysis, developed as a part of or concurrently with the Human Genome Project, are now generally available. In addition, the extremely large volume of data has stimulated the development of methods in bioinformatics needed for management and analysis. New methods of quantitative analyses for linkage disequilibrium and gene function have also been developed. Finally, several groups from around the world have developed large family cohorts, including extensive phenotypic and genotypic data. In spite of all this progress and promise, still very little is known about the specific genetic mechanisms that influence most human obesities. However, the tools at our disposal are powerful; the reagents and genetic data are extensive; and, not inconsequentially, we have much left to learn. It is difficult to imagine a more propitious time for studying the complex interplay of the multiple genes and environmental factors that influence common forms of human obesity.

Over 100 years' worth of scientific research has demonstrated that heredity plays a major role in the development of body size and obesity (Price & Lee, 2001; Price, Reed, & Guido, 2000). Surely plant and animal breeders have been aware of this relationship for much longer—at least since the domestication of multiple plant and animal species more than 10,000 years ago. However, it is only within the past few years, since the positional cloning of the mouse obese gene (Zhang et al., 1994), named the leptin gene, that we have begun to understand the role of specific genes in the development of obesity. In the brief intervening period, the identification and characterization of several genes, particularly leptin, the leptin receptor, and agouti-related protein, have made it possible to construct many of the key pathways in the regulation of energy balance (described by Chua & Leibel and by Tataranni & Ravussin in Chapters 2 and 3 of this volume, respectively). Perhaps because of the central importance of these regulatory mechanisms, mutations affecting the protein structures coded by these genes appear to occur only very rarely. After a worldwide search by many investigators, few obese individuals have been found who carry major gene mutations: about 50 individuals with 19 mutations in 6 genes (Perusse, Rice, et al., 2001). Obviously, these mutations are too infrequent to make any significant contribution to common forms of obesity.

The pattern of inheritance of obesity, combined with the absence of mutations in known major genes, suggests a complex mode of inheritance involving multiple genes. It is likely that many genes have relatively small effects on obesity phenotypes, and expression almost certainly depends on both genetic background and environmental conditions. The complexity of the phenotype not only presents difficulties for finding the relevant genes, but also is likely to challenge our previous notions about how genetic variability influences phenotype.

This chapter first reviews what we know about the inheritance of human obesity; it then discusses methodological obstacles, current status, strategies, and future prospects for identifying genes for common obesities.

THE FAMILIAL/GENETIC INHERITANCE OF HUMAN OBESITY

Human obesity has variously been attributed to inheritance and to individual character. Mild to moderate obesity clearly follows family lines and may more easily be accepted as beyond an individual's control. Extremely obese individuals, on the other hand, often stand out from other family members, and so their excess weight may more easily be attributable to character. Classical genetics has devised ways to explain such examples of heredity and variation. Genes passed from parents to children provide a basis for genetic inheritance, and gene segregation, the process by which only half of a parent's genes are passed on to each child, provides a mechanism for maintenance of genetic variation within families and populations. Differences in living conditions such as diet and exercise provide additional variation.

It is clear from a number of family studies that obesity and thinness follow family lines (Grilo & Pogue-Geile, 1991; Maes, Neale, & Eaves, 1997; Price, 1987). Correlations among first-degree relatives (parents, offspring, siblings, and dizygotic twins) generally range from .20 to .30, suggesting a moderate heritability. Correlations are slightly higher within than between generations, suggesting the possibility of nonadditive or even nongenetic inheritance.

Of course, the familial pattern alone is no guarantee of a genetic cause. Families share many things besides genes, and at least some nongenetic assets are transmitted across generations. Because of practical and ethical limitations on human experimentation, researchers have depended on the natural experiments of twinning and adoption to separate nature from nurture in humans. From the earliest reports, these studies have tended to support a genetic basis for obesity (Price, 1987). However, limitations in study size and design left many of the early reports open to different interpretations. During the 1960s and 1970s, it became fashionable to "debunk" biological explanations for behavioral traits, replacing them with environmental theories of sometimes questionable validity. We find, for example, published statements such as the following: "Family line resemblances in fatness, however striking, may be less the product of genes held in common than of the living-together effect" (Garn, 1985).

In fact, twin studies have found that identical twins are more highly correlated in body composition than are fraternal twins. Across multiple studies, correlations for adult monozygotic twins generally range from .60 to .70, with values being generally higher and more variable in younger twins. Correlations for dizygotic twins are similar to those of other first-degree relatives. Adoption studies have found that adoptees resemble their biological relatives in body composition, but not members of their adoptive families. These and later studies demonstrated that obesity is highly heritable, and that at least for adults, family environment appears to have a negligible influence. Studies of twins reared apart (Price & Gottesman, 1991; Stunkard, Harris, Pederson, & McClearn, 1990) have confirmed this pattern. Identical twins resemble each other to a similar degree, whether they are raised together or apart. On balance, genes appear to account for as much as two-thirds of individual differences in obesity in adults, with the remaining differences being due to idiosyncratic influences from outside the family.

Obesity measures have also been analyzed as qualitative traits (e.g., obesity vs. normal weight). The "heritability" in this case is best reflected by a comparison of familial and population affection rates, yielding an odds ratio or relative risk. Studies examining several obesity thresholds have found that the relative risk increases with more extreme obesity, from 1.5–3.0 for moderate obesity (90th percentile for body mass index [BMI] greater than 30) to 3.0–9.0 for extreme obesity (BMI greater than 40) (Lee, Reed, & Price, 1997; Price & Lee, 2001). It is not clear whether it is appropriate to extrapolate from the absence of shared environmental influences on the normal range of body fat to these extreme levels. If family environmental factors were minimal, the results would suggest that extreme obesity is strongly influenced by genes. It will be fortunate if this interpretation is true, for a higher heritability should facilitate the identification of causative genes.

Gender Differences

Women have a higher percentage of body fat than men; this increase in body fat for women is observed across many countries and seems stable across cultures and dietary habits (Bray, 1994). Female children are fatter than male children, so that behavioral differences between men and women (such as responsibility for food preparation) cannot account for gender difference in body fat (Forbes, 1972; Tanner, Hughes, & Whitehouse, 1981). The specific biological mechanisms that account for this difference remain to be determined. Family studies have revealed no general evidence for a pattern of transmission (e.g., X-linked dominant) that would explain the sex difference. As reviewed in a later section of this chapter, three groups have reported suggestive X linkage to quantitative trait loci influencing mild obesity and fat distribution. However, the influence of these genes, if they prove to be real, is likely to be small. One obvious explanation for the increased adiposity of women relative to men is that autosomal obesity genes interact with the sex hormones to favor the accumulation of body fat in women. Although these sorts of interactions are speculative, influences in the reverse direction are clear. Adipose tissue provides a signal for sexual maturity in both mice and humans through the secretion of leptin (Chehab, 2000).

Population Differences

Obesity is a disorder associated with the developed and developing world. Prosperity has produced many changes in the environment, including less physical work; more leisure time; more sedentary forms of entertainment, especially television; and an increased avail-ability of foods, especially those with high caloric content. Within the United States, obesity rates are highest in Native, African, and Hispanic Americans (Kuczmarski, Flegal, Campbell, & Johnson, 1994). Up to two-thirds of members of these groups are obese, as compared with about 30% of non-Hispanic European Americans.

Some of the highest rates of obesity occur in the Pima Indians of southern Arizona, where about two-thirds of adults in this group also have diabetes (Knowler et al., 1991). It is interesting that the increases in obesity and diabetes in the Pima closely parallel trends in acculturation during the past 50 years (Price, Charles, Pettitt, & Knowler, 1993). Obesity rates for Pima living in the Gila and Salt River areas of Arizona were apparently low early in the 20th century. A closely related Pima tribe that lives in Sonora, Mexico, and maintains a traditional lifestyle continues to have low obesity and diabetes rates today (Valencia et al., 1999), although the rates are still higher than in the neighboring Mexican population.

The differences in diabetes and obesity rates in Native Americans as compared with European Americans prompted anthropologist James Neel (1962) to hypothesize that Native Americans and some other groups possess a "thrifty" genotype, which has allowed them to survive periods of feast and famine by increased efficiency in energy storage and expenditure. Although energy efficiency must have been an evolutionary advantage in more difficult and unpredictable times, this advantage may have become a liability in modern times of relative plenty. Although all human populations evolved in a changeable environment, some may have experienced more extreme fluctuations than others. The high rates of obesity in Pima Indians, other Native American groups, several Pacific Islander groups, African Americans, and Hispanic groups with Native American admixtures are consistent with this hypothesis. However, to date no specific "thrifty" gene or genotype has been identified, but some have been suggested. Both leptin (Spiegelman & Flier, 2001) and melanocortin 3 receptor (MC3R; Chen et al., 2000) genes have been reported to influence energy efficiency, although the mechanisms are unknown and the case for MC3R remains controversial.

THE ROLE OF THE ENVIRONMENT IN HUMAN OBESITY

An intuitively compelling theory about the development of obesity is that it is due to patterns of diet and exercise that are learned in the home. This view has attractive features in that it provides a root cause, someone to blame, and a natural target for prevention. Some adoption studies do suggest that the family environment can influence level of obesity while children are living in the same home with their parents (Bouchard, Savard, Despres, Tremblay, & Leblanc, 1985). However, these effects do not appear to be long-lasting and do not persist into adulthood. Other studies of child adoptees suggest that the effects are negligible even at an early age.

Nonfamily environmental factors do influence obesity. Although genetically identical individuals tend to be similar in levels of obesity and thinness, they are rarely identical. Studies of monozygotic twins demonstrate that although there is high concordance in the presence of obesity, there can be large differences in the extent of obesity for individuals having the same genotype (Price & Stunkard, 1989), especially when the obesity in one or both twins is extreme. Presumably these discordances in level of obesity are due to differences in such factors as diet, exercise, and smoking that accumulate over a lifetime.

Nonfamily environmental influences can be powerful. Cultural changes appear to account for recent increases in the prevalence of obesity. The prevalence and extent of obesity in the United States have increased in more recent birth cohorts, especially among women (Kuczinarski et al., 1994). The rate of increase is striking, from a prevalence of about 25%

in 1980 to more than 30% in 1990. The increase has been particularly strong for African American women. Obesity also appears to be on the rise in European countries (James, 1995; Sørensen & Price, 1990). Most surveys have defined obesity as having a BMI greater than or equal to 27 kg/m². In a more recent survey (Mokdad et al., 1999), a lower BMI value of 25 kg/m² was used, resulting in an obesity prevalence of more than 50% in the United States. It has become abnormal to be thin.

We may be sure that the genetic compositions of these populations have not changed substantially over the past 10–20 years, so the obesity increases must be due to culturally mediated change in diet and exercise. Although no direct links are possible, population data largely support this view. The obesity increases have closely paralleled increases in dietary fat (Fujimoto et al., 1995) and in sedentary activities such as watching television (Jeffery & French, 1998). Furthermore, several groups have experienced increases in obesity following exposure to Western culture and diet, for example, the Pima Indians (Price et al., 1993) and Pacific Islanders (Hodge et al., 1994).

Genetic differences may mediate differential responses to cultural change through gene–environment interaction. Even following temporal increases, the heritability of obesity has remained substantial in all populations studied (Price, 1994). An obvious question that comes to mind is whether genes may play a role in determining the response to a changing diet and pattern of exercise. That is, do genes influence who gains the most weight in our obesity-promoting environment? There is at least some experimental evidence that such gene–environment interactions can occur. For example, in one study all identical twins who were overfed for up to 3 months gained weight (Bouchard et al., 1990). However, there were large differences in the extent of weight gain, with identical twin pairs gaining similar amounts of body fat. Animal studies confirm this pattern of gene–environment interaction observed in humans. Genetically different strains of mice also vary in weight gain in response to high-fat diets (Fenton & Dowling, 1953; Schemmel, Mickelsen, & Gill, 1970; West, Goudey-Lefevre, York, & Truett, 1994; West, Waguespack, York, Goudey-Lefevre, & Price, 1994). Studies such as these demonstrate that genetic predisposition can determine the magnitude of a response to a nongenetic influence such as diet composition. As sedentary lifestyles and high-caloric diets become more common, any preexisting differences among individuals in genetic predispositions to obesity should be magnified through gene–environment interactions.

Gene–Gene Interactions in Obesity

At least from animal studies, we know that gene–gene interactions may also occur and may be quite common. For example, the extent of obesity and diabetes resulting from a single gene mutant depends on genomic background (Coleman & Hummel, 1975). Gene–gene interactions have been reported for several human disorders as well. Of particular interest is the possible interaction of the gene Calpain-10 with an unknown gene on chromosome 15 in the predisposition to Type 2 diabetes and possibly obesity (Cox et al., 1999; Horikawa et al., 2000). Although we can only speculate at this point, the rich genetic diversity of human populations suggests that genetic interactions may be common for complex disorders such as obesity.

METHODOLOGICAL ISSUES AND OBSTACLES

Measuring Obesity

Obesity is an end result of long-term energy imbalance, which can be due to high caloric intake, low energy expenditure, or abnormal partitioning of energy into storage as body fat (see Chapters 2 and 3 in this volume). Factors influencing the energy equation (stored energy = intake − expenditure) are numerous and are often difficult to quantify because of unreliability (e.g., food intake, macronutrient choices, and physical activity), expense (indirect calorimetry and thermic effect of food), or accessibility (nutrient partitioning). Genetic studies generally must focus on the cumulative summation of this equation over a period of many years by measuring body composition through direct or indirect indices of the amount of body fat. The most accessible of these indices is BMI, a ratio of weight to height. Other common indices are derived from total body water by electrical impedance and from relative body density by underwater weighing. The amount of subcutaneous fat may be quantified through measures of skinfolds at various anatomical sites. There are formulas for combining skinfolds into an estimate of total body fat, and a simple sum works reasonably well. Direct imaging methods are also applicable, although limited by the expense of the procedures and the small size of most scanners relative to that of many extremely obese people. Fortunately, these obesity measures are moderately correlated (.65–.85), and so the more accessible and inexpensive ones can be used in large-scale studies (Warden et al., 1996).

Individual differences in body fat distribution or fat patterning, as opposed to overall amount of body fat, can also be measured through circumferences, skinfolds, and imaging. Several studies have demonstrated that fat distribution is largely uncorrelated with total body fat and is independently heritable (Borecki, Rice, Perusse, Bouchard, & Rao, 1994; Cardon, Carmelli, Fabsitz, & Reed, 1994; Hasstedt, Ramirez, Kuida, & Williams, 1989; Rice, Bouchard, Perusse, & Rao, 1995; Sellers et al., 1994). Because of the relation of abdominal fat to cardiovascular disease, it is of more than academic interest to study the genetics of fat patterning in humans.

Instability of the Obesity Phenotype

Obesity is an inherently changeable phenotype. Body weight fluctuates by 2%–3% during a normal day. Most people gain weight throughout much of their lifetimes, and it has been shown that this propensity to gain weight is heritable (Bouchard et al., 1990). However, not all obesity develops during adulthood. Between one-third and one-half of extremely obese people develop obesity in childhood or adolescence. Clearly, some overweight children eventually grow into lean adults; the more extreme the obesity, however, the better it tracks into adulthood. In addition, early-onset obesity has been reported to run in families, and to increase the risk that other relatives will be similarly obese (Price et al., 1990). The rates might simply appear higher because relatives with familial early-onset forms of obesity will tend to have more affected members in cross-sectional studies of individuals varying in age, even if censoring (an epidemiological control) is taken into account in a pooled sample. Lifetime rates estimated separately for early- and late-onset families could be similar. Whether genetic differences affect level of obesity or only timing of its development, age of onset of obesity has been shown to be a heritable trait (Price et al., 2000).

Identifying Genes for Common Obesities

Perusse, Chagnon, and colleagues (2001), in their annual summary of the status of the obesity gene map, report more than 250 genetic loci linked or associated with obesity. These include 10 major genes from animal models, 6 nonoverlapping major genes in humans, 24 genetic syndromes, 115 animal quantitative trait loci, 48 candidate genes with reported associations in humans, and 59 loci with at least one report of possible linkage. Even with

these comprehensive annual updates, the volume of new work makes ~~~~~
view to be completely current, and that is particularly true of a pu~~~~~
one. Therefore, in this chapter only consistent patterns are reported. ~~~~~
hensive Perusse and colleagues review are genes that have been we~~~~~
leptin and genetic loci that have only been inferred from genetic link~~~~~
of evidence for particular genes or genetic loci is quite variable, ran~~~~~
tion and functional characterization of specific single-gene mutatior~~~~~
of linkage and association.

One obvious question at the outset is whether 250 or more genes could influence obesity. Based purely on what we have learned about the biological complexity, we may confidently predict that at least this many genes may be involved and probably more. However, if we frame the question slightly differently and ask whether these particular 250-plus genes are the ones that account for individual human differences, we would say with equal confidence that they almost surely include a number of false-positives, while the effects of many other genes have yet to be detected. Finally, many of the genes implicated through animal models are so important that they appear to be largely invariable, and thus have little influence on common human obesity.

Multiple Testing for Multiple Genes

Since other chapters in this volume deal with plausible biological candidate genes and regulatory pathways, this chapter briefly considers the technical reasons for very high false-positive and false-negative rates and indicates how to distinguish the real or likely from the merely possible but unlikely. This technical discussion leads to a practical consideration of a few genomic regions for which there is emerging consensus.

Identifying the genetic loci influencing a multigenic trait such as obesity depends on many factors. If considered as a quantitative trait, power depends on the overall heritability and the proportion of trait variance due to a particular locus. For a qualitative dichotomization, power depends on the relative risk attributable to a locus. For a moderately heritable trait (approximately .40–.70), such as percentage of body fat or BMI, sample sizes that have been examined thus far could have expected to detect loci accounting for no less than about 15%–20% of the total trait variance. For qualitative traits, current sample sizes have the power to identify a gene with an attributable risk of no less than 1.5–2.0. In the context of an overall risk of 3.0–9.0 for obesity, identifying one or a few genes seems feasible; again, however, this will only be possible if some of the loci account for a sizable portion of the observable variance.

High rates of false-positive findings in genetic linkage and association studies are due to multiple testing in the extreme, basically to conducting a large number of tests of genes and markers over the entire human genome when the prior probability of any one gene's involvement is low. Given the size of the human genome, about 3 billion base pairs, there is no way to avoid the problem of multiple testing. For qualitative traits with clear phenotypes and single-gene inheritance, a nominal odds ratio favoring linkage of 3.0, roughly equivalent to a nominal p value of .001, was chosen in order to give a genome-wide posterior probability level of about 5%. For complex traits such as obesity, much higher odds ratios are needed because there are multiple genes to identify and variable phenotype definitions multiply the number of tests, making the false-positive rate still higher.

For association studies, the false-positives pose an even greater problem. The power to detect true associations is lower than for linkage, given equivalent sample sizes. It does not require any familiarity with genetics to know that low power and a high error rate make the

possible combination. One methodological study (Carey & Williamson, 1991) esti-
ed that as many as 80% of *replicated* association studies may be false! It is a sobering
oint that is well to keep in mind. Several multipoint tests of association have been devised
or are under development that appear to have greater power and may have lower error
rates; however, they have not yet been applied in any systematic way to obesity phenotypes.

Replication is the most obvious way around the false-positive problem, but repeating
linkage and association results has its own difficulties. For a single-gene trait without heterogeneity, the sample size needed for replication should be the same as or less than the
original. However, with a multigenic trait, the problem changes from finding at least one
gene out of many possibilities to finding exactly one gene previously identified. The difference is roughly analogous to the difference between finding any one of a number of needles
in a haystack compared to finding exactly the same needle that was identified previously
and then thrown back. A few years ago, Suarez, Hampe, and Van Eedewegh (1994) estimated that the time to replication (proportional to sample size) will at least double that of
the initial sample. One conclusion for a multigenic trait such as obesity is that replication
will be difficult and does not necessarily mean the original result is false. It is easy to see
that a temptation to invoke this principle to explain inconsistent results is a prescription for
scientific nihilism. For example, every geneticist could have his or her own gene with no expectation of replication. Obviously, this extreme view is scientifically unacceptable. On the
one hand, we should not dismiss unreplicated studies. On the other, we must insist on independent replication before accepting any result as true. However difficult, replication is the
only reasonably sure way to validate results from genetic studies.

Genome Scans for Obesity-Related Phenotypes

A genome scan tests for linkage between a phenotype (e.g., obesity) and evenly spaced markers spanning the genome such that no gene should be more distant than 5 million base pairs
from a marker. Typical scans for obesity used about 300 or more marker genotypes on 500
or more individuals for a minimum of 150,000 genotypes. A few scans used many more.

Results from the first nine scans are reviewed in this chapter with the understanding
that data collection, data analysis, and publication are ongoing for some of these and other
studies. In addition to full scans, there have been other linkage studies that focused on
smaller regions of the genome. This chapter reviews only selected studies that have supported results from the nine full scans.

Table 4.1 lists the samples examined in the scans. All nine scans found at least nominally significant results for one or more obesity-related phenotypes. In fact, there were 45
nominally positive linkage results for 37 genomic regions. The large number and genomic
dispersion of the results is a bit bewildering; however, 11 of the regions were independently
identified more than once and the largest number are concentrated in only three regions.
One of the regions, chromosome 18q21, was only weakly supported, for percent body fat in
the Quebec study and for a mild obesity phenotype in the Finnish study. The other two regions received strong support from at least one study and at least nominal support from
others. The two regions, along with obesity phenotypes and supporting samples, are summarized in Table 4.2.

The French group from Lille and Paris first reported linkage of obesity to chromosome
region 10p21 at about 55 cM (centamorgans, on average about 1 million base pairs per
cM) from the p (short arm) terminus (Hager, Dina, et al., 1998). Supporting studies followed from the Marburg (Hinney et al., 2000) and Philadelphia (Price, 2001) groups used
comparable phenotypes. The Heritage Family Study found support for linkage to this re-

TABLE 4.1. Samples Examined in the First Nine Obesity Genome Scans

Pima Indians (Phoenix Study)
(Hanson et al., 1998; Norman et al., 1997, 1998; Walder, Hanson, Kobes, Knowler, & Ravussin, 2000)

Mexican Americans (San Antonio Heart Study)
(A. G. Comuzzie et al., 1997; Hixson et al., 1999; Mitchell et al., 1999)

French families (Paris–Lille)
(Hager, Dina, et al., 1998)

European Americans and African Americans (Philadelphia)
(Lee et al., 1999)

European Americans (French Canadians, Quebec Family Study)
(Perusse, Rice, et al., 2001)

European Americans (Heritage Family Study)
(Bouchard et al., 2000; Chagnon et al., 2001)

Old Order Amish
(Hsueh et al., 2001)

European Americans (TOPS Study)
(Kissebah et al., 2000)

Finnish families
(Ohman et al., 2000; Perola et al., 2001)

gion using somewhat different phenotypes and analytic methods, variance component analyses of BMI and fat mass. Finally, the scan of the Old Order Amish sample supported linkage to leptin adjusted for BMI, perhaps a measure of leptin resistance that is commonly associated with obesity. Genomic sequence for this region is scant and there are few known genes, none of which are obvious candidates. While the absence of candidates may make it difficult to identify a specific gene in chromosome region 10p21, it also raises the possibility, and excitement, of finding something new and unexpected.

The San Antonio group reported linkage of plasma leptin to markers in 2p21 at about 57 cM from the p terminus (A. G. Comuzzie et al., 1997). The same group has presented additional support using augmented data from the original sample. Two other groups (one

TABLE 4.2. Genomic Regions with Most Consistent Support for Linkage to Obesity

Genomic region	Phenotype	Sample
10p15-p12	Obesity	French German European American (Philadelphia) African American (Philadelphia)
	BMI, fat mass	European American (Heritage Family Study)
	Leptin/BMI	Old Order Amish
2p21	BMI, FM, leptin	Mexican American (San Antonio Heart Study)
	Leptin	French African American (Chicago Study) European American (TOPS Study)

completely independent) have presented supportive results. The French group reported a replication that was strong in terms of support for linkage as well as for the congruence of the genomic location (Hager, Dina, et al., 1998). Results from separate African American samples analyzed by the San Antonio group also provide support for the 2p21 linkage, although the linkage was much weaker (Rotimi et al., 1999). This region centers on the genomic location of the gene for proopiomelanocortin (POMC), a precursor of melanocortins that interact with leptin. Although it is clear that POMC plays an important regulatory role in leptin-melanocortin pathways, the evidence that POMC gene variability accounts for linkage to the leptin phenotype is so far only circumstantial. No specific variability in coding or regulatory regions has been found, and many other genes lie within the linked interval. It is in any case an interesting coincidence.

The Pima group reported linkage of several obesity-related phenotypes to markers in 11q22–24. None of the eight other scans have reported linkage to this region. More will be said about this group later in the chapter.

Finally, our group in Philadelphia reported linkage of obesity to markers in 20q13 at about 71–85 cM from the p terminus (Lee et al., 1999). The location is close to previously reported linkages from the Quebec sample (Lembertas et al., 1997). There was some support from analyses of female sibling pairs in the French group; however, there was no linkage in the overall sample (Hager, Dina, et al., 1998). The Pima study reported linkage to 24-hour respiratory quotient, but the location is well centromeric of the 20q13 location (Norman et al., 1998). This region of the long arm of chromosome 20 is rich in known and orphan candidate genes, including the melacortin 3 receptor, CAAT enhancer binding protein beta, and a number of genes for DNA binding or signaling proteins. The region also includes genes for adenosine deaminase, agouti-signaling protein, and a gene for maturity-onset diabetes of the young. However, the linked region spans about 40 million base pairs, extending approximately from protein tyrosine phosphatase 1 beta in 20q11-12 to melanocortin 3 receptor in 20q13.

Overall, the agreement of results across multiple groups, samples, analytic methods, and related phenotypes is encouraging. Obviously, there are also many failures to replicate. The nonreplications may be explained in part by the relatively low sample sizes and correspondingly reduced power of all the studies. Particularly in the case of the Pima Indians, the differences in results may also be due in part to genetic heterogeneity among samples. Heterogeneity may also account, at least in part, for differences among seemingly similar samples of European Americans. If obesity is indeed caused by multiple genes with relatively small effects, random sampling theory would predict differences in the representation of particular genes across the various samples.

Only the the French and Finnish groups have published results on a full scan of the X chromosome (Hager, Dina, et al., 1998; Ohman et al., 2000), although the Philadelphia group has reported results at scientific meetings. In the original publication of the French scan, they reported a secondary linkage to Xp21. The Finnish group found no linkage in Xp, but a modest linkage result in Xq. The Philadelphia group found linkage to markers in Xp21 in two separate samples, one European American and one African American. However, the linkage results were for a measure of fat distribution and localized to a region several cM centromeric of those from the French sample. At the least, these ambiguous results support the need for other groups to examine the X chromosome.

Other Genomic Regions with Independent Support for Linkage

Although not identified in the context of a full genome screen, one other genomic location has received support from multiple independent groups. Several groups have reported linkage to markers flanking the leptin gene in 7q31 (Clement et al., 1996; Duggirala et al., 1996; Reed et al., 1996). Although there have also been negative reports, a meta-analysis found that the aggregate results were highly significant (Allison & Heo, 1998). Moreover, several groups have found evidence of associations or linkage disequilibrium between sequence variability 5′ of the leptin gene and obesity phenotypes, particularly for extreme obesity (Hager, Clement, et al., 1998; Li et al., 1999; Roth et al., 1998). The accumulated results suggest a gene of small effect, primarily on extreme obesity. It is still unclear whether the association is due to variation in the leptin promoter or some other nearby gene, since disequilibrium appears to extend over a large interval.

FUTURE STUDIES: HOW CAN WE IDENTIFY GENES FOR COMMON FORMS OF HUMAN OBESITY?

Additional Linkage Studies

Linkage studies represent the best way of regionally mapping new genes or genes with unanticipated effects on obesity phenotypes. It is important that additional linkage studies be completed, but future studies should have larger sample sizes in order to increase power and facilitate replication of existing linkages. Larger size can be achieved either by augmenting existing samples or by pooling data; the latter approach provides the largest samples, but the former permits independent replications. Given the large number of studies, it seems best to publish the primary results independently. Additional separate analyses may be coordinated among groups through the selection of comparable subsamples, phenotypes, and analyses. In some cases it may be appropriate to pool more disparate data. However, the analytic adjustment needed to achieve standardization among samples may ultimately be self-defeating, since any necessary assumptions will undermine confidence in the results.

Future linkage studies should also explore more complex models. For example, a genome scan of swine found that genomically imprinted genes are common. Several groups have developed linkage methods that incorporate parent-of-origin effects that would be expected with imprinting. However, there have been no published reports applied to obesity. In collaboration with Christopher Amos, we have conducted preliminary analyses of obesity phenotypes on one human chromosome. We found strong evidence for a maternal effect, but our results have not yet been published.

Another consideration that may be incorporated into linkage analyses is gene–gene interaction. Such interactions are common in animal models (Coleman & Hummel, 1975). My laboratory has completed preliminary work on five regions of three chromosomes that have been reported to be linked to obesity phenotypes. We found a strong interaction between two of the regions. The major difficulty with this approach that has not yet been solved is the familiar one of multiple testing. The scope of the problem is much greater in this case because the number of tests of interactions could be as high as the number of tests from a genome scan squared. For a modest example, consider a scan with 350 markers and 5 phenotypes; the potential number of interactions is over 3 million! Using split samples and requiring multiple replications is one approach; however, the reduced error rates will come at a great cost to power. The difficulties should not preclude this approach, since many or even most of the gene effects in human obesity may depend on the interactions of particular genes with genomic background. We cannot understand the genetics of common obesity without developing solutions to these inherent difficulties.

There are, however, limitations to linkage studies that will make it difficult to locate genes once linkage has been established. First, the resolution of linkage tends to be poor,

ue and potential pitfalls of genomic matching need to be established in practice, the high power of population studies appear to make them ideal for screening. Truth or falsehood of positive results can be established through replication or through more conservative family-based methods.

Family-Based Association Methods: Less Prone to Error

Family-based association methods were developed as an alternative to case–control studies. The basic idea was to avoid problems associated with population structure by substituting untransmitted parental alleles or haplotypes in place of unrelated controls. These methods differ from other tests of linkage, in that the focus of the analysis is on allele or haplotype sharing across families rather than on identity by descent within families.

Why Particularly High Levels of Statistical Significance Are Required for Association Studies

Linkage results between markers and a trait tend to be highly correlated when the markers are located very close together in the same chromosome region. This phenomenon occurs because large portions of chromosomes are passed on un-recombined, and any group of siblings will tend to share large chromosome segments identical by descent. However, linkage disequilibrium is due to the lack of recombination over large numbers of generations, and normally extends over very small regions of 200 kb or less in outbred populations (Lander & Schork, 1994). The median distance is only about 30 kb, but different genomic regions are extremely variable (Reich et al., 2001). For this reason, disequilibrium results usually will not be correlated for closely linked markers, and it will be necessary to apply a correction for multiple testing for each allele of each locus tested. Genome-wide significance levels of 10^{-9} (Risch & Merikangas, 1996) or less (Kruglyak, 1999) may be needed to reach empirical significance of even 5%. Without appropriate analyses and controls, 1 in a billion p value, which most researchers have seen only while asleep, may be no better than 1 in 20, a value they are well used to seeing while awake. Although it is possible to minimize the problem of multiple alleles by focusing on biallelic single-nucleotide polymorphisms, or by employing maximum-likelihood methods (Collins & Morton, 1998; Terwilliger, 1995), the problem of testing multiple loci in whole genome association scans remains a big one. One way of reducing the scope of the problem using currently available methods is to do "gene scans" rather than genome scans; although it may not always be possible to identify sufficient numbers of polymorphic genetic markers within or near all genes of interest.

In a study of 9.7 kb of the lipoprotein lipase (LPL) gene, 88 polymorphisms were detected (Clark et al., 1998; Nickerson et al., 1998). This rate is higher than previously supposed. Our own studies of the 5' region flanking the leptin gene found 16 polymorphisms (all biallelic) in 3 kb—less than the rate found for the LPL gene, but still much higher than expected (Li et al., 1999). Although many individual sites have limited frequency, variable sites may occur on average every 500 base pairs of DNA sequences (Nickerson et al., 1998).

In the published studies of the LPL gene and in our investigations of the leptin gene, many of the polymorphisms appear to be extremely old, most likely predating the spread of modern humans out of Africa and running much deeper into human evolutionary history. For example, in the report by Clark and colleagues (1998), one allele of each polymorphism was found in chimpanzees, making the polymorphisms somewhere between 100,000 and 4.5 million years old. Their rough estimate for the two "clades" (roughly meaning "root" or "branch") identified in their haplotype analysis was 1.2 million years, and most observed polymorphisms are probably more recent.

This work raises several issues for mapping complex traits through linkage disequilibrium. Over distances of even a few tens of thousands of bases, the number of haplotypes segregating in an outbred population will approach the number of chromosomes. Over large-enough distances, all chromosomes are likely to be unique. Although this latter statement seems self-evident, the scale of haplotype diversity was not apparent until recently. Another difficulty presented by these findings is that disequilibrium is highly variable across the genome (Reich et al., 2001) and may extend over distances of only a few thousand bases in some regions (Kruglyak, 1999), making linkage-disequilibrium-based genome scans difficult if not impractical, at least with current technology.

Yet another complication is that over small distances the extent of disequilibrium will be variable and can be discontinuous, making it difficult to identify sequence variability accounting for a phenotype association or linkage without some other insight into the nature of the particular sequences examined, for example, through information about population history. Clark and colleagues (1998) reported that the observed haplotypes showed considerable population structure. We also found differences between European and African Americans in our studies of the leptin gene. However, the Clark study found some population overlap in regions as small as 1–2 kb. On the other hand, they also noted the existence of two clades that extended over much of the 9.7-kb region. They drew the intriguing conclusion that there may be functional significance in patterns of non-protein-coding variation over large distances. Their conclusion is very speculative, but their results suggest the equivalent of DNA sequence interactions for patterns of variability in flanking and intronic regions of genes. It is well known that DNA, RNA, and amino acid sequence variability can affect transcription, processing, and protein folding, respectively. However, the nature of these long-distance interactions is as yet unknown. Although the extent of sequence variability is only beginning to emerge, it is apparent that it will be important to study the pattern of disequilibrium among multiple markers in any given region, in order to select haplotypes for studies of associations with complex phenotypes. These sequence polymorphisms may replace structural gene mutations in what we come to understand as "genes" for complex traits such as obesity.

CONCLUSION

Over the next few years, it should be possible to identify DNA sequence variability associated with common forms of obesity. However, larger-scale linkage studies and linkage disequilibrium studies will be needed. Much genetic variability is of ancient origin and probably existed before modern human groups left Africa 40,000–100,000 years ago. An intriguing hypothesis is that much of the sequence variability related to obesity evolved under selective pressure to promote metabolic efficiency and energy storage, leading to epidemic obesity in the presence of modern living conditions. We may need to reconsider the suggestion of James Neel (1962) regarding "thrifty genes" in some indigenous populations. It now appears that all existing populations are the closely related descendents of a few thousand modern humans. Thus, we must all carry a collection of ancient thrifty genes.

ACKNOWLEDGMENT

The preparation of this chapter was supported in part by National Institutes of Health Grants No. R01DK44073, No. R01DK48095, and No. R01DK56210 to R. Arlen Price. The review of linkage studies drew not only on the published literature cited in the references, but also on discussions with

Horikawa, Y., Oda, N., Cox, N. J., Li, X., Orho-Melander, M., Hara, M., Hinokio, Y., Lindner, T. H., Mashima, H., Schwarz, P. E., del Bosque-Plata, L., Oda, Y., Yoshiuchi, I., Colilla, S., Polonsky, K. S., Wei, S., Concannon, P., Iwasaki, N., Schulze, J., Baier, L. J., Bogardus, C., Groop, L., Boerwinkle, E., Hanis, C. L., & Bell, G. I. (2000). Genetic variation in the gene encoding calpain-10 is associated with type 2 diabetes mellitus. *Nature Genetics, 26*(2), 163–175.

Hsueh, W. C., Mitchell, B. D., Schnieder, J. L., St Jean, P. L., Pollin, T. I., Ehm, M. G., Wagner, M. J., Burns, D. K., Sakul, H., Bell, C. J., & Shuldiner, A. R. (2001). Genome-wide scan of obesity in the Old Order Amish. *Journal of Clinical Endocrinology Metabolism, 86*(3), 1199–1205.

James, W. P. T. (1995). A public health approach to the problem of obesity. *International Journal of Obesity and Related Metabolic Disorders, 19*(S3). S37–S45.

Jeffery, R. W., & French, S. A. (1998). Epidemic obesity in the United States: are fast foods and television viewing contributing? *American Journal of Public Health, 88*(2), 277–280.

Jorde, L. B. (1995). Linkage disequilibrium as a gene-mapping tool [Editorial]. *American Journal of Human Genetics, 56*(1), 11–14.

Jorde, L. B., Watkins, W. S., Carlson, M., Groden, J., Albertsen, H., Thliveris, A., & Leppert, M. (1994). Linkage disequilibrium predicts physical distance in the adenomatous polyposis coli region. *American Journal of Human Genetics, 54*(5), 884–898.

Khoury, M. J., & Yang, Q. (1998). The future of genetic studies of complex human diseases: an epidemiologic perspective. *Epidemiology, 9*(3), 350–354.

Kissebah, A. H., Sonnenberg, G. E., Myklebust, J., Goldstein, M., Broman, K., James, R. G., Marks, J. A., Krakower, G. R., Jacob, H. J., Wever, J., Martin, L., Blangero, J., & Comuzzie, A. G. (2000). Quantitative trait loci on chromosomes 3 and 17 influence phenotypes of the metabolic syndrome. *Proceedings of National Academy of Science USA, 97*(26), 14478–14483.

Knowler, W. C., Pettitt, D. J., Saad, M. F., Charles, M. A., Nelson, R. G., Howard, B. V., Bogardus, C., & Bennett, P. H. (1991). Obesity in the Pima Indians: its magnitude and relationship with diabetes. *American Journal of Clinical Nutrition, 53*(6 Suppl.) 1543S–1551S.

Kruglyak, L. (1999). Prospects for whole-genome linkage disequilibrium mapping of common disease genes. *Nature and Genetics, 22*(2), 139–144.

Kuczmarski, R. J., Flegal, K. M., Campbell, S. M., & Johnson, C. L. (1994). Increasing prevalence of overweight among US adults. *Journal of the American Medical Association, 272*(3), 205–211.

Lander, E. S., Linton, L. M., Birren, B., Nusbaum, C., Zody, M. C., Baldwin, J., Devon, K., Dewar, K., Doyle, M., FitzHugh, W., Funke, R., Gage, D., Harris, K., Heaford, A., Howland, J., Kann, L., Lehoczky, J., LeVine, R., McEwan, P., McKerman, K., Meldrim, J., Mesirov, J. P., Miranda, C., Morris, W., Naylor, J., Raymond, C., Rosetti, M., Santos, R., Sheridan, A., Sugnez, C., Stange-Thomann, N., Stojanovic, N., Subramanian, A., Wyman, D., Rogers, J., Sulston, J., Ainscough, R., Beck, S., Bentley, D., Burton, J., Clee, C., Carter, N., Coulson, A., Deadman, R., Deloukas, P., Dunham, A., Dunham, I., Durbin, R., French, L., Grafham, D., Gregory, S., Hubbard, T., Humphray, S., Hunt, A., Jones, M., Lloyd, C., McMurray, A., Matthews, L., Mercer, S., Milne, S., Mullikin, J. C., Mungall, A., Plumb, R., Ross, M., Shownkeen, R., Sims, S., Waterston, R. H., Wilson, R. K., Hillier, L. W., McPherson, J. D., Marra, M. A., Mardis, E. R., Fulton, L. A., Chinwalla, A. T., Pepin, K. H., Gish, W. R., Chissoe, S. L., Wendl, M. C., Dlehaunty, K. K., Miner, T. L., Delehaunty, A., Kramer, J. B., Cook, L. L., Fulton, R. S., Johnson, D. L., Minz, P. J., Clifton, S. W., Hawkins, T., Branscomb, E., Predki, P., Richardson, P., Wenning, S., Slezak, T., Doggett, N., Cheng, J. F., Olsen, A., Lucase, S., Elkin, C., Uberbacher, E., Frazier, M., Gibbs, R. A., Muzny, D. M., Scherer, S. E., Bouck, J. B., Sodergren, E. J., Worley, K. C., Rives, C. M., Gorrell, J. H., Metzker, M. L., Naylor, S. L., Kucherlapati, R. S., Nelson, D. L., Weinstock, G. M., Sakaki, Y., Fujiyama, A., Hattori, M., Yada, T., Toyoda, A., Itoh, T., Kawagoe, C., Watanabe, H., Totoki, Y., Taylor, T., Weissenbach, J., Heilig, R., Saurin, W., Artiguenave, F., Brottier, P., Bruls, T., Pelletier, E., Robert, C., Wincker, P., Smith, D. R., Doucette-Stamm, L., Rubenfield, M., Weinstock, K., Lee, H. M., Dubois, J., Rosenthal, A., Platzer, M., Nyakatura, G., Taudien, S., Rump, A., Yang, H., Yu, J., Wang, J., Huang, G., Gu, J., Hood, L., Rowen, L., Madan, A., Qin, S., Davis R. W., Federspiel, N. A., Abola, A. P., Proctor, M. J., Myers, R. M., Schmutz, J., Dickson, M., Gimwood, J., Cox, D. R., Olson, M. V., Kaul, R., Shimizu, N., Kawasaki, K., Minoshima, S., Evans, G. A., Athanasiou, M., Schultz, R., Roe, B. A., Chen, F., Pan, H., Ramser, J.,

Lehrach, H., Reinhardt, R., McCombie, W. R., de la Bastide, M., Dedhia, N., Blocker, H., Hornischer, K., Nordsiek, G., Agarwala, R., Aravind, L., Bailey, J. A., Bateman, A., Batzoglou, S., Birney, E., Bork, P., Brown, D. G., Gurge, C. B., Cerutti, L., Chen, H. C., Church, D., Clamp, M., Copley, R. R., Doerks, T., Eddy, S. R., Eichler, E. E., Furey, T. S., Galagan, J., Gilbert, J. G., Harmon, C, Hayashizaki, Y., Haussler, D., Hermjakob, H., Hokamp, K., Jang, W., Johnson, L. S., Jones, T. A., Kasif, S., Kaspryzk, A., Kennedy, S., Kent, W. J., Kitts, P., Koonin, E. V., Korf, I., Kulp, D., Lancet, D., Lowe, T. M., McLysaght, A., Mikkelsen, T., Moran, J. V., Mulder, N., Pollara, V. J., Ponting, C. P., Schuler, G., Schultz, J., Slater, G., Smit, A. F., Stupka, E., Szustakowski, J., Thierry-Mieg, D, Thierry-Mieg, J., Wagner, L., Wallis, J., Wheeler, R., Williams, A., Wolf, Y. I., Wolfe, K. H., Yang, S. P., Yeh, R. F., Collins, F., Guyer, M. S., Peterson J., Felsenfeld, A., Wetterstrand, K. A., Patrinos, A., Morgan, M. J., & Szustakowski, J. (2001). Initial sequencing and analysis of the human genome. *Nature, 409*(6822), 860–921.

Lander, E. S., & Schork, N. J. (1994). Genetic dissection of complex traits. *Science, 265*, 2037–2048.

Lee, J. H., Reed, D. R., Li, W-D., Xu, W., Joo, E-J., Kilker, R. L., Nanthakumar, E., North, M., Sakul, H., Bell, C., & Price, R. A. (1999). Genome scan for human obesity and linkage to markers in 20q13. *American Journal of Human Genetics, 64*(1), 196–209.

Lee, J. H., Reed, D. R., & Price, R. A. (1997). Familial risk ratios for extreme obesity: implications for mapping human obesity genes. *International Journal of Obesity Related Metabolic Disorders, 21*, 935–940.

Lembertas, A. V., Perusse, L., Chagnon, Y. C., Fisler, J. S., Warden, C. H., Purcell-Huynh, D. A., Dionne, F. T., Gagnon, J., Nadeau, A., Lusis, A. J., & Bouchard, C. (1997). Identification of an obesity quantitative trait locus on mouse chromosome 2 and evidence of linkage to body fat and insulin on the human homologous region 20q. *Journal of Clinical Investigation, 100*, 1240–1247.

Li, W., Reed, D., Lee, J., Xu, W., Kilker, R., Sodam, B., & Price, R. (1999). Sequence variants in the 5′ flanking region of the leptin gene are associated with obesity in women. *Annals of Human Genetics, 63*, 227–234.

Maes, H. H., Neale, M. C., & Eaves, L. J. (1997). Genetic and environmental factors in relative body weight and human adiposity. *Behavioral Genetics, 27*(4), 325–51.

Mitchell, B. D., Cole, S. A., Comuzzie, A. G., Almasy, L., Blangero, J., MacCluer, J. W., & Hixson, J. E. (1999). A quantitative trait locus influencing BMI maps to the region of the beta-3 adrenergic receptor. *Diabetes, 48*(9), 1863–1867.

Mokdad, A. H., Serdula, M. K., Dietz, W. H., Bowman, B. A., Marks, J. S., & Koplan, J. P. (1999). The spread of the obesity epidemic in the United States, 1991–1998. *Journal of the American Medical Association, 282*(16), 1519–1522.

Neel, J. V. (1962). Diabetes mellitus: a "thrifty" genotype rendered detrimental by "progress"? *American Journal of Human Genetics, 14*, 353–362.

Nickerson, D. A., Taylor, S. L., Weiss, K. M., Clark, A. G., Hutchinson, R. G., Stengard J., Salomaa, V., Vartiainen, E., Boerwinkle, E., & Sing, C. F. (1998). DNA sequence diversity in a 9.7-kb region of the human lipoprotein lipase gene. *Nature Genetics, 19*(3), 233–240.

Norman, R. A., Tataranni, P., Pratley, R., Thompson, D., Hanson, R., Prochazka, M., Baier, L., Ehm, M. G., Sakul, H., Foroud, T., Garvey, W. T., Burns, D., Knowler, W. C., Bennett, P. H., Bogardus, C., & Ravussin, E. (1998). Autosomal genomic scan for loci linked to obesity and energy metabolism in Pima Indians. *American Journal of Human Genetics, 62*(3), 659–668.

Norman, R. A., Thompson, D. B., Foroud, T., Garvey, W. T., Bennett, P. H., Bogardus, C., & Ravussin, E. (1997). Genomewide search for genes influencing percent body fat in Pima Indians: suggestive linkage at chromosome 11q21–q22. *American Journal of Human Genetics, 60*, 166–173.

Ohman, M., Oksanem, L., Kaprio, J., Koskenvuo, M., Mustajoki, P., Rissanen, A., Salmi, J., Kantula, K., & Peltonen, L. (2000). Genome-wide scan of obesity in Finnish sibpairs reveals linkage to chromosome Xq24. *Journal of Clinical Endocrinology Metabolism, 85*(9), 3183–3190.

Perola, M., Ohman, M., Hiekkalinna, T., Leppavuori, J., Pajukanta, P., Wessman, M., Koskenvuo, M., Palotie, A., Lange, K., Kaprio, J., & Peltonen, L. (2001). Quantitative-trait-locus analysis of body-mass index and of stature by combined analysis of genome scans of five Finnish study groups. *American Journal of Human Genetics, 69*(1), 117–123.

Wang, D. G., Fan, J. B., Siao, C. J., Berno, A., Young, P., Sapolsky, R., Ghandour, G., Perkins, N., Winchester, E., Spencer, J., Kruglyak, L., Stein, L., Hsie, L., Topaloglou, T., Hubbell, E., Robinson, E., Mittmann, M., Morris, M. S., Shen, N., Kilburn, D., Rioux, J., Nusbaum, C., Rozen, S., Hudson, T. J., Lander, E. S., et al. (1998). Large-scale identification, mapping, and genotyping of single-nucleotide polymorphisms in the human genome. *Science, 280*(5366), 1077–1082.

Warden, C. H., Bouchard, C., Friedman, J. M., Hebebrand, J., Hitman, G. A., Kozak, L. P., Leibel, R. L., Price, R. A., & Zechner, R. (1996). How can we best apply the tools of genetics to study body weight regulation? In C. Bouchard & G. A. Bray (Eds.), *Regulation of body weight: Biological and behavioral mechanisms* (pp. 289–309). Chichester, UK: Wiley.

West, D. B., Goudey-Lefevre, J., York, B., & Truett, G. E. (1994). Dietary obesity linked to genetic loci on chromosome 9 and 15 in a polygenic mouse model. *Journal of Clinical Investigation, 94,* 1410–1416.

West, D. B., Waguespack, J., York, B., Goudey-Lefevre, J., & Price, R. A. (1994). Genetics of dietary obesity in AKR/J X SWR/J mice: segregation of the trait and identification of a linked locus on chromosome 4. *Mammalian Genome, 5,* 546–552.

Williams, R. C., Long, J. C., Hanson, R. L., Sievers, M. L., & Knowler, W. C. (2000). Individual estimates of European genetic admixture associated with lower body-mass index, plasma glucose, and prevalence of type 2 diabetes in Pima Indians. *American Journal of Human Genetics, 66*(2), 527–538.

Zhang, Y., Proenca, R., Maffei, M., Barone, M., Leopold, L., & Friedman, J. M. (1994). Positional cloning of the mouse obese gene and its human homologue. *Nature, 372*(6505), 425–432.

5

Confronting the Toxic Environment: Environmental and Public Health Actions in a World Crisis

KATHERINE BATTLE HORGEN
KELLY D. BROWNELL

The rapid increase in the prevalence of obesity has led the World Health Organization (WHO) to declare a global obesity epidemic (WHO, 1998). Based on data from the National Health and Nutrition Examination Surveys, researchers at the National Center for Health Statistics report that almost 55% of U.S. adults are overweight (i.e., their body mass index [BMI] is greater than or equal to 25 kg/m²) and 22.5% are obese (i.e., their BMI is greater than or equal to 30 kg/m²) (Flegal, Carroll, Kuczmarski, & Johnson, 1998). The prevalence among middle-aged western Europeans is 15%–20%, while in eastern Europe some countries face rates as high as 40%–50% (Bjorntorp, 1997). As the availability of fast, inexpensive, energy-rich foods grows and physical activity declines, obesity rates continue to increase in countries across the world.

The prevalence of obesity increases even in the face of broad publicity about the problem, tremendous pressure to be thin, and multiple industries focused on dieting and weight control. In the United States alone, health clubs, diet centers, and low-fat snacks fuel a $33-billion-a-year weight control industry (Food and Nutrition Board, 1995), but obesity rates have grown in every segment of the population (Flegel et al., 1998).

In a U.S. population study comparing the period 1976–1980 to the period 1988–1991, investigators reported decreases in average daily fat intake from 41% to 36.6% of total calories and in daily caloric intake from 1,854 kilocalories (kcal) to 1,785 kcal (Heini & Weinsier, 1997). Yet there has been a dramatic rise in obesity (Food and Nutrition Board, 1995). Based on reports that the percentage of Americans consuming low-calorie products has risen from 19% in 1978 to 76% in 1991, and that the percentage of Americans leading a sedentary lifestyle (60%) did not change between 1986 and 1991, a *decrease* in the prevalence of obesity would be expected (Heini & Weinsier, 1997). Underreporting of fat and caloric intake may account for this anomaly, but it is clear that low-fat foods, health clubs, and weight loss programs are not solving the obesity crisis. Nothing is solving this crisis.

Researchers estimate the annual deaths in the United States attributable to obesity at approximately 325,000 (Allison, Fontaine, Manson, Stevens, & VanItallie, 1999). These mortality rates approach the approximately 400,000 tobacco-related deaths annually in the United States (Centers for Disease Control and Prevention, 2000). Obesity has been associated with coronary heart disease, diabetes, some cancers, stroke, hypertension, high blood cholesterol, gallbladder disease, respiratory disease, and arthritis (Must et al., 1999; Pi-Sunyer, 1995; see also Field, Barnoya, & Colditz, Chapter 1, this volume).

Wolf and Colditz (1998) estimated health care costs attributable to obesity at $99.2 billion in 1995. This figure represents approximately $51.6 billion in direct medical costs and $47.6 billion in indirect expenditures—a total that constitutes 5.7% of the annual U.S. health care cost. Over a 6-year period, the frequency of obesity-related doctor visits has increased 88% (Wolf, 1998).

LIMITATIONS OF TREATMENT

Nearly all approaches to weight loss focus on the individual. Even if these were effective, the number of people who receive treatment is small. Weight loss attempts that were initially considered successful frequently result in weight regain (Stunkard, 1996; Wing, 1998). Only surgery, recommended for the most extreme cases of morbid obesity, has shown long-term success on a broad level (Sjostrom, Lissner, Wedel, & Sjostrom, 1999; Stunkard, 1996). A study of weight loss through fasting found that 98% of the individuals had returned to pretreatment weight after 9 years (Drenick & Johnson, 1978), while an examination of behavioral self-management training showed that only about 5% of patients achieved long-term weight loss maintenance (Goodrick & Foreyt, 1991). Although some behavioral treatments show successful maintenance for up to 2 years, longer-term follow-up studies indicate a trend of gradual return to baseline weight over time (Wilson, 1995). Douketis, Feightner, Attia, and Feldman (1999) reviewed weight loss trials and also found a pattern of initial weight loss followed by gradual weight regain.

Several pharmacological treatments for obesity have been developed, and some have produced weight loss. However, the long-term effects of these drugs have not been studied, and given the chronic nature of obesity, it can only be assumed that weight regain will follow when the medication is discontinued. Obesity has many causes; hence it is unlikely that any medication can override all the relevant systems and provide a solution for the disease.

Treatment efficacy in studies is low, and treatment effectiveness for the general population is very low, as treatment for weight loss is costly and available to a select few (Horgen & Brownell, 1998). It is time to consider an alternative approach to the obesity epidemic.

THE INDIVIDUAL, BIOLOGY, AND THE ENVIRONMENT

There are three logical places to look when explaining the causes of obesity and identifying areas for its treatment or prevention: the individual, biology, and the environment. Obesity is multiply determined, so all these factors contribute to etiology. Every intervention derived for any of these areas should be enlisted in the fight. It is apparent, however, that if the tide of the obesity epidemic is to be halted (much less reversed), we must rely on advances in prevention, not treatment.

The question, then, is whether the individual, biology, or the environment offers the greatest hope for prevention. It would be hard to imagine more pressure on individuals to be thin. Nutrition and physical activity education programs in the schools, again aimed at individuals, have not been very effective. Were they effective, it is unlikely that schools, with the great demands placed on them, would place nutrition and physical activity as top priorities in any systematic way. Focusing on individuals may help selected people, but does not offer much hope for helping the obese society.

Biology is thought to explain 25%–40% of the variance in population body weight (Bouchard, 1995). At some point, biology may explain which individuals in an obesity-prone environment will in fact become obese, and may explain differences between people in the extent of obesity reached in response to a common environment. But biology does not explain the world problem any more than understanding biological vulnerabilities in individuals explains why there is so much lung cancer. There is so much lung cancer primarily because of tobacco, and there is so much obesity because of a dangerous food and physical activity environment.

THE ENVIRONMENT AS A CAUSAL FACTOR: WORLDWIDE EVIDENCE

The United States is not alone in its fight against obesity. During the past several years, obesity has hit epidemic proportions in both developed and developing countries, affecting residents of countries previously considered poor as well as those with higher income levels (VanItallie, 1994; WHO, 1998). Countries once plagued with issues of undernutrition must now face the problems associated with overweight (Popkin & Doak, 1998). The increasing prevalence of obesity in country after country suggests that the genesis of the problem supersedes biology. Although the problem exists in a wide range of environments, the underlying similarities are clear: shifts in physical activity and eating patterns (Popkin & Doak, 1998).

Popkin and Doak (1998) note that the increased level of obesity in countries as varied as Mexico, South Africa, Malaysia, and nations of the western Pacific underscores the need to focus on the underlying environmental causes of obesity rather than simply on genetic factors. In some Native American tribes and American Pacific Islanders, as well as in Australian Aborigines and Polynesians, obesity rates approaching 80% have been noted (Bjorntorp, 1997). Despite variations in socioeconomic and behavioral factors, countries across the world are moving toward environments that promote obesity (WHO, 1998). Bjorntorp (1997) notes that poverty is associated with greater prevalence of obesity in developed countries, but that affluence is linked to greater obesity prevalence in developing nations.

Research on a variety of cultures illustrates this diathesis–stress model of obesity. Many researchers cite migration studies as examples of the deleterious effects of Westernized eating habits on individuals. When Chinese, Japanese, or Filipina women move to the United States, their risk of breast cancer increases over several generations to equal that for women of European descent in the United States (who have rates traditionally four to seven times higher) (Ziegler et al., 1996). The investigators determined, after adjustment for breast cancer risk factors, that weight change is a critical factor in this increased risk for breast cancer (Ziegler et al., 1996). In a study of nutrition-related diseases and disorders among immigrants, Wandel (1993) focused on dietary change after migration and cited evidence that immigrants are especially susceptible to diseases related to overnutrition, such as coronary heart disease and non-insulin-dependent diabetes. In sum, immigrant groups tend to have more obesity than people remaining in their native countries.

The Pima Indians provide a basis for comparison between genetically similar people living in different environments. Ravussin, Valencia, Esparza, Bennett, and Schulz (1994) reported an average BMI of 35 kg/m² for Pima women living in Mexico, compared to 37 kg/m² for those living in Arizona. The average woman weighed 44 pounds more in Arizona. Bhatnagar, Anand, Durrington, Patel, and Wander (1995) found similar results when they compared individuals who had migrated to west London with biological relatives who remained in Punjab, India. When the environment changes, weight changes.

VanItallie (1994) proposes that migration, urbanization, new eating habits, and affluence may contribute to the growing prevalence of obesity in developing countries; he notes that the obesity epidemic will continue with inevitable modernization. In its recent report on the world obesity problem, the WHO (1998) concurs.

Even those who choose to remain in their countries of origin face growing exposure to Western culture. More processed, packaged, and high-calorie foods are becoming available. The eagerness of fast-food franchises to expand has led to their increased presence in countries across the globe. Although in Europe some groups have expressed concern about fast food impinging on the history and culture of the area, the job creation and promotional spending accompanying expansion—not to mention the cheap, tasty food—have enticed many to welcome fast-food chains (Tagliabue, 1999). As the French diet, once touted for its healthiness, has become "more Americanized" (Brody, 1999) to contain more snacks, more meat, and more fast foods, French cholesterol levels have risen. One expert predicts that the French will soon experience a rate of coronary death approaching that of Americans as the American diet and lifestyle continue to invade the country (Brody, 1999).

A study on the diet and activity of Chinese adults indicated that increased BMI paralleled increased energy and fat consumption (Paeratakul, Popkin, Keyou, Adair, & Stevens, 1998). The authors attributed the higher levels of obesity to increased fat consumption, which they noted can increase weight even in a survey population consisting primarily of rural residents with high levels of physical activity and physically demanding jobs. They noted that because obesity is often associated with affluence in China and many developing countries, those experiencing weight gain may not perceive the gain as a health hazard.

A prospective Japanese study concluded that childhood obesity is becoming a major public health concern in Japan, and that approximately 50% of children who were obese in primary school were obese at age 17 (Sugimori et al., 1999). In Kuwait, the high proportion of overweight children and adults has led the Ministry of Health to promote weight loss with the slogan "Food damages your health" (Kandela, 1999).

WHY THE ENVIRONMENT HAS BEEN IGNORED

As the environment worsens, so does obesity. Biology permits obesity to occur in individuals, but the environment causes obesity in the culture. The field has been preoccupied with why individuals are obese and how to help them, rather than with why society is obese and how to help it.

Cultural Attributions and Lack of Public Health Attention

We can only speculate why such obvious factors as a poor food and physical activity environment have been ignored. Part of the reason has been the cultural attribution of fault to obese individuals. This has led to widespread bias, stigma, and discrimination, but also— more pertinent to this chapter—to lack of attention to the environment. In addition, public health experts have focused primarily on infectious diseases and only more recently have begun to address chronic diseases. Only during the past few years have more than a handful of researchers and health officials called for obesity to be considered a chronic disease; attribution of the problem to the environment and calls for environmental action are even more recent (Brownell, 1994).

The Pervasiveness of the Toxic Environment

It is little wonder that approaches to weight loss focusing on the individual have yielded less than impressive results, given the environment. We (Brownell, 1994; Horgen & Brownell, 1998) have proposed that Americans are exposed to a "toxic environment," which pervasively surrounds them with inexpensive, convenient foods high in both fat and calories. Egger and Swinburn (1997) suggest that obesity is "a normal response to an abnormal environment" (p. 477).

There are many examples of the ever-worsening environment. Fast-food chains across the globe continue to increase serving sizes, inducing patrons to ingest extra fat and calories through packaged "value" meals. Many restaurants offer staggering portion sizes, sometimes large enough to feed two or three people, citing customers' appreciation for value.

Fast-food chains market directly to children with advertising campaigns using recognizable characters, such as cartoon and movie figures. Hager (1998) noted Burger King executive Richard Tyler's statement that "Providing kids with twice the number of toys . . . doubles the reasons for kids to visit our restaurant," and the manager of Burger King's Youth and Family Division's claim that "Kids of all ages will be able to share in the excitement generated by the MIB [Men in Black] phenomenon . . . what kid would want to be without the official Men in Black gear or other official MIB toys that will be offered with every kid's meal?" Ronald McDonald is known to 96% of children in the United States and across the globe, and he speaks over 20 different languages (Hager, 1998, p. 758).

Young children may not be capable of distinguishing between television programming and advertising (Martin, 1997). Research has indicated a link between obesity and television viewing, showing a dose–response relationship between hours of television viewed and obesity (Dietz & Gortmaker, 1985). The majority of television advertisements are for food products, and most of the foods advertised are sugared cereals, fast food, candy, and soft drinks (Dibb, 1996). Studies have shown that television viewing hours are related to caloric intake of children as well as to food requests by children and food purchases by parents (Taras, Sallis, Patterson, Nader, & Nelson, 1989). Television contributes to obesity both by encouraging children to buy food of low nutritional value, and by enticing them to spend time in a sedentary activity rather than doing something that burns calories (Horgen, Choate, & Brownell, 2001). Not only are children sitting inactive while watching television, but they are also likely to be snacking while doing so.

Several advocacy groups have formed to encourage regulation of advertising to children. In 1996, the Federal Communications Commission strengthened the Children's Television Act of 1990 by requiring broadcasters to show a specific amount (at least 3 hours per week) of programming designed to "educate and inform" (Center for Media Education [CME], 1999, p. 1) children aged 2–16. The CME (1999) issued a report that reviewed the various methods broadcast stations have chosen for complying with the regulations, and that encouraged parents to be actively involved in monitoring broadcasters' compliance.

Some children are barraged by food advertisements in school as well as at home. Schools broadcast Channel One—a 10-minute news program with 2 minutes of commercials—to over 8 million middle and high school children, in return for televisions, VCRs, and satellite dishes for the schools (Consumers Union, 1996; Mifflin, 1998). Brand and Greenberg (1994) found that 69% of the 45 commercials shown on Channel One during a 4-week period were for food products such as fast food, gum, candy, soft drinks, and snack chips. The study also found that advertising contributed to students' positive attitudes to-

(1997) found that when the prices of low-fat foods in a vending machine were reduced by 50%, sales of the low-fat items increased from 25.7% of machine sales to 45.8%, then decreased to 22.8% when the prices returned to normal. A cafeteria study reduced fruit and salad prices by 50% and found that sales of these items increased threefold while sales of other items remained constant (Jeffery, French, Raether, & Baxter, 1994). Lower price decreases have also been effective in encouraging healthier choices. A restaurant study lowering prices 20%–30% found that sales increased significantly over those at baseline and decreased when prices returned to normal (Horgen, 2000).

6. *Tax unhealthy foods.* Taxes can encourage healthy eating, both by providing money for subsidies of healthy foods and by discouraging the consumption of foods low in nutritional value. Previous food taxes have not been earmarked for subsidies for healthy foods, and they have been criticized as regressive. One could argue that the current pricing structure, which makes healthy foods more expensive than less healthy foods, forces those with lower incomes to eat poorly and is itself regressive. A tax on unhealthy foods with revenues designated for subsidies could reverse this harmful pricing structure. Such taxes have been enacted in several states, but they have not been well received. In 1991, California levied an 8.25% tax on "nonessential" foods (Zuck, 1992). Although the tax generated approximately $200 million during the first year, it was largely unpopular and was repealed in December 1992. Maryland's 5% snack food tax was enacted in 1992 (Abramowitz, 1995; Harrison, 1993) and repealed effective July 1997 (Maryland Comptroller of the Treasury, 2000). The tax received widespread opposition from the Snack Food Association, which represents snack manufacturers and suppliers to the snack food industry. Maine imposed a 7% tax on "nonnutritious" foods, instituted in 1991 (Zuck, 1992). Maine lawmakers repealed the tax in 2000 (Higgins, 2001).

Critics have attacked the taxes as regressive (Lozano, 1991), arbitrary in their classification of foods (Garry, 1992), and difficult for retailers to impose (Gasparello, 1991). The taxes were never evaluated, but judging by the fierceness of the opposition from snack food companies, they might be expected to have an effect. Although there is much room for improvement in the design of such taxes, it is also clear that they generate substantial revenue. They might be improved through a classification system based on clearer nutritional guidelines and a designation of revenues for healthy food and exercise projects.

There is also the possibility, if taxes large enough to change food consumption are not acceptable, of using smaller taxes to generate funds for programs aimed at altering diet and activity patterns. Jacobson and Brownell (2001) have noted that a number of cities and states have imposed taxes on soda pop or snack foods. The taxes are small enough (usually several cents per can or bottle) to minimize resistance, but the consequence has been many millions of dollars in revenue. Currently the monies are earmarked for work irrelevant to diet and physical activity (e.g., building roads), or are not earmarked at all. Jacobson and Brownell (2001) propose specific earmarking of such money for nutrition education or other similar programs.

7. *Increase awareness of the obesity epidemic.* Twenty years ago, few would have heeded warnings about tobacco or believed that smoking would be illegal in many public places. Only through widespread education about the health and financial costs of the problem did the campaign against tobacco gain public support. With mortality from obesity approaching that related to tobacco, and health care costs increasing, an analogy between smoking and obesity is not only useful but unavoidable.

8. *Involve parents in the protection of their children.* Many parents do not know that their children are targets of advertising in school. They are also unaware of the extent of the focus on their children by the fast-food industry. Children who are obese are

at increased risk of becoming obese adults (Whitaker, Wright, Pepe, Seidel, & Dietz, 1997), and parents can play a role in helping their children avoid a painful struggle with obesity.

FUTURE DIRECTIONS

By drawing attention to the toll that obesity takes on America's physical and mental health, as well as on the American health care budget, public advocates can gain support for action at the environmental level. A survey of community attitudes toward public policy approaches to alcohol, tobacco, and food control indicated that the public favored regulatory controls in all three areas, although support was greater for alcohol and tobacco regulation than for food control intervention (Jeffery et al., 1990). The regulation most strongly supported was that designed to protect children, followed by advertising restriction and control over sales conditions.

A survey of over 700 mothers of elementary school children revealed significant concerns with the nutritional content shown in food advertising toward children (Grossbart & Crosby, 1984). The authors delineate suggestions to food advertisers, including direct appeals to children to be conscious about nutrition and to be responsible consumers. They also advocate advertising messages showing respect for parental authority.

An overview of health psychology and public policy noted that from 1985 to 1995, health care costs grew more than any other segment of the economy (DeLeon, Frank, & Wedding, 1995). The researchers cite efforts to contain health care costs through public and preventive measures as paramount. We agree, and feel that the obesity field is in desperate need of such a mentality.

It is clear that obesity has become a national epidemic, and that worldwide rates of obesity continue to expand at alarming rates. The limited success of interventions focused on the individual indicates that it is time to approach the problem from a different perspective. The environment provides numerous opportunities for intervention and stands as a largely untapped resource for relief from the obesity epidemic.

REFERENCES

Abramowitz, M. (1995, May 8). Snack tax crunched. *The Washington Post,* p. BO3.

Allison, D. B., Fontaine, K. R., Manson, J. E., Stevens, J., & VanItallie, T. B. (1999). Annual deaths attributable to obesity in the United States. *Journal of the American Medical Association, 282,* 1530–1538.

Bhatnagar, D., Anand, I. S., Durrington, P. N., Patel, D. J., & Wander, G. S. (1995). Coronary risk factors in people from the Indian subcontinent living in west London and their siblings in India. *Lancet, 345,* 405–409.

Bjorntorp, P. (1997). Obesity. *Lancet, 350,* 423–426.

Bouchard, C. (1995). Genetic influences on body weight and shape. In K. D. Brownell & C. G. Fairburn (Eds.), *Eating disorders and obesity: A comprehensive handbook* (pp. 21–26). New York: Guilford Press.

Brand, J., & Greenberg, B. (1994, January). Commercials in the classroom: The impact of Channel One advertising. *Journal of Advertising Research, 34,* 18–23.

Brody, J. E. (1999, June 22). Paradox or not, cholesterol in France is on the rise. *The New York Times,* p. F1.

Brownell, K. D. (1994, December 15). Get slim with higher taxes [Editorial]. *The New York Times,* p. A29.

motion and disease prevention objectives (DHHS Publication No. 91-50213). Washington, DC: U.S. Government Printing Office.

VanItallie, T. B. (1994). Worldwide epidemiology of obesity. *Pharmacoeconomics, 5*(Suppl. 1), 1–7.

Wandel, M. (1993). Nutrition-related diseases and dietary change among Third World immigrants in northern Europe. *Nutrition and Health, 9*(2), 117–133.

Whitaker, R. C., Wright, J. A., Pepe, M. S., Seidel, K. D., & Dietz, W. H. (1997). Predicting obesity in young adulthood from childhood and parental obesity. *New England Journal of Medicine, 337*(13), 869–873.

Wilson, G. T. (1995). Behavioral approaches to the treatment of obesity. In K. D. Brownell & C. G. Fairburn (Eds.), *Eating disorders and obesity: A comprehensive handbook* (pp. 479–483). New York: Guilford Press.

Wing, R. R. (1998). Behavioral approaches to the treatment of obesity. In G. A. Bray, C. Bouchard, & W. P. James (Eds.), *Handbook of obesity* (pp. 855–873). New York: Marcel Dekker.

Wolf, A. M. (1998). What is the economic case for treating obesity? *Obesity Research, 6*(Suppl., 1), 2S–7S.

Wolf, A. M., & Colditz, G. A. (1998). Current estimates of the economic cost of obesity in the United States. *Obesity Research, 6*(2), 173–175.

World Health Organization (WHO). (1998). *Obesity: Preventing and managing the global epidemic. Report of a WHO Consultation on Obesity, Geneva, June 3–5, 1997* (Publication No. WHO/NUT/NCD/98.1). Geneva: Author.

Ziegler, R. G., Hoover, R. N., Nomura, A. M., West, D. W., Wu, A. H., Pike, M. C., Lake, A. J., Horn-Ross, P. L., Kolonel, L. N., Siteri, P. K., & Fraumeni, J. F. (1996). Relative weight, weight change, height, and breast cancer risk in Asian-American women. *Journal of the National Cancer Institute, 88*(10), 650–660.

Zuck, R. A. (1992). What balancing acts follow tax on snacks? *Paper, Film, and Foil Converter, 66,* 4.

6

Binge-Eating Disorder and the Night-Eating Syndrome

ALBERT J. STUNKARD

This chapter describes the relationship of obesity to the eating disorders. For many years this relationship has been unclear. At times even obesity itself was considered an eating disorder—a result of disordered overeating that affected all obese persons indiscriminately. This view became particularly popular during the 1970s, when the advent of behavior therapy had effects on food intake and body weight, almost regardless of differences among obese persons. As we learned more about eating disorders, however, it became clear that there were major differences in eating behavior among obese individuals. For the majority, overeating fitted no specific pattern. For a minority, however, two eating disorders that contribute to obesity have been identified: binge-eating disorder and the night-eating syndrome.

BINGE-EATING DISORDER

Diagnostic Criteria

Among disorders of eating, binge eating (or its cognate, bulimia) has by far the longest history. Bulimia (literally, "ox hunger") was recognized by Hippocrates as a sick hunger, distinct from normal hunger (Stunkard, 1993). Reports during the past century have mentioned bulimia, usually as eating binges, but at times also as the associated vomiting and purging. In 1959 a diagnosis, binge-eating syndrome, was proposed (Stunkard, 1959). The cardinal feature of this syndrome was bingeing, which has been defined as "eating, in a discrete period of time . . . , an amount of food that is definitely larger than most individuals would eat under similar circumstances" (American Psychiatric Association [APA], 1994, p. 731).

The concept of binge eating, without the purging, vomiting, exercise, and fasting associated with bulimia nervosa, was advanced by the proposal by Spitzer and colleagues (1992) of the diagnosis of binge-eating disorder. The proposal was based on data from a

A great deal of attention has been directed toward the possibility that dieting is a risk factor for binge-eating disorder. Thus it has been proposed that binge eating is a result of dieting (Herman & Polivy, 1980, 1990), that dieting is a "precondition" for the development of binge eating (Marcus et al., 1988), and that attempts at weight loss may exacerbate binge eating (Garner & Wooley, 1991; Polivy & Herman, 1985).

Interest in the possibility that dieting is a risk factor for binge-eating disorder arose from its similarity to bulimia nervosa. Dieting has been implicated in the genesis of bulimia nervosa (Polivy & Herman, 1985; Polivy, Herman, Olmsted, & Jazwinski, 1984), and since bingeing occurs in both, it seemed reasonable to implicate dieting in the genesis of binge-eating disorder. This implication has been the subject of considerable study, focused particularly on the question of which comes first—bingeing or dieting? In binge-eating disorder, very frequently dieting follows bingeing and thus can hardly have caused it.

Spitzer and colleagues' first papers on binge-eating disorder (Spitzer et al., 1992; Spitzer, Yanovski, et al., 1993), described binge eating as occurring before the first diet. Wilson and colleagues (1993) reported that bingeing preceded dieting in 64% of their subjects, and no more than 9% reported that they had been on a strict diet at the time they began bingeing. Five subsequent reports have confirmed this sequence (Abbott et al., 1998; Berkowitz, Stunkard, & Stallings, 1993; Grilo & Masheb, 2000; Mussell et al., 1997; Spurrell, Wilfley, Tanofsky, & Brownell, 1997).

In the face of this evidence, what was the basis for the idea that dieting led to bingeing? The idea seems to have arisen from the finding that dieting led to an increase in the Restraint factor of the Herman and Polivy (1980) Restraint Scale, and that this "restraint" was elevated in bulimia nervosa as well as in unsuccessful dieting (Herman & Polivy, 1990; Polivy & Herman, 1993). But this "restraint" is a misnomer. The Scale's two subscales appear to measure not restraint, but *disinhibition* of eating behavior. The Weight Fluctuation subscale is associated with greater weight and the weight fluctuations that accompany this greater weight, as well as with dietary lapses. The Concern with Dieting subscale measures the kind of rigid dieting that has been found (Westenhoefer, Stunkard, & Pudel, 1999) to be associated with a poor outcome of dieting, and in fact this subscale is associated with unsuccessful dieting (Charnock, 1989; Gorman & Allison, 1995). A key experiment in the development of the Herman and Polivy (1980) Restraint Scale showed (significantly) that in response to a preload of food by persons who scored high on the scale, restraint was disinhibited, and subjects overate.

The development of a later scale, the Eating Inventory (Stunkard & Messick, 1985), built upon the Herman and Polivy (1980) scale to address problems with it. Instead of focusing on a single factor of restrained eating, construction of the Eating Inventory began with literature-based items that tapped several aspects of eating behavior. These items were administered to large groups of persons selected as being high or low in dietary restraint. Factor analysis of their responses yielded three factors, prominent among which was a factor designated Disinhibition. It corresponded to the Concern with Dieting subscale in the Herman and Polivy scale, and performed clinically in much the same way. A second factor on the Eating Inventory reflected Restraint, but a restraint far different from the Restraint factor of the Herman and Polivy scale and one that predicted successful dieting (Charnock, 1989; Gorman & Allison, 1995).

The differing implications of "restraint" as conceptualized by the two scales was demonstrated in the study by Yanovski and Sebring (1994). When persons with binge-eating disorder were placed on reducing diets, their Restraint factor scores on the Eating Inventory increased significantly during precisely the time when their rate of bingeing decreased dramatically. These authors concluded that disinhibition, rather than restraint, is a major contributor to binge eating.

Prevalence

A benefit of the delineation of binge eating has been to encourage study of its prevalence. The study is still in its infancy, as illustrated by widely varying estimates. The first estimates, in the original Spitzer and colleagues papers, were that 29%–30% of obese people seeking treatment for their obesity had binge-eating disorder, with the disorder being about 1.5 times more common in overweight women than in overweight men (Spitzer et al., 1992). These estimates were based upon self-report questionnaires. Later interview-based studies of treatment-seeking obese persons have found a far lower prevalence. For example, my colleagues and I found ·it necessary to screen 1,450 obese women, who had identified themselves as bingeing, in order to recruit 50 subjects who met interview-based criteria for binge-eating disorder (Stunkard, Berkowitz, Tanrikut, Reiss, & Young, 1996). Among patients seeking treatment for obesity in other studies, the prevalences were 7.6% (Stunkard, Berkowitz, Wadden, et al., 1996), 8.9% (Basdevant, Pouillon, & Lahlon, 1995), and 18.8% (Brody, Walsh, & Devlin, 1994). In community studies, the prevalences were 2% (of whom only half were obese; Spitzer et al., 1992) and 1.8% (Bruce & Agras, 1992).

Treatment

A flood of reports of treatment for binge-eating disorder followed publication of the Spitzer and colleagues papers. These treatments have often followed the precedent of treatments for bulimia nervosa. The most distinctive have involved the use of cognitive-behavior therapy.

Psychological Treatments: Cognitive-Behavior Therapy and Interpersonal Therapy

In 1993 Fairburn revised his manual for the treatment of bulimia nervosa to include treatment of binge-eating disorder (Fairburn, Marcus, & Wilson, 1993). Wilfley and colleagues (1993), Wilfley and Cohen (1997), and Marcus (1997) have further adapted this approach, which focuses first on the eating disturbance and the associated problematic cognitions and attitudes about eating, body shape, and weight. It emphasizes moderation in food intake so that it is neither over- nor underrestrictive, and recommends increased physical activity. Fairburn and others maintain that control of binge eating is necessary before obese persons can lose weight, and that attempts at weight loss should be deferred until binge eating has been controlled. Cognitive-behavior therapy consistently produces clinically significant reductions (from 48% to 98%) in binge eating (Marcus et al., 1996; Smith, Marcus, & Kaye, 1992; Telch, Agras, Rossiter, Wilfley, & Kenardy, 1990; Wilfley & Cohen, 1997; Wilfley et al., 1993).

An important extension of cognitive-behavior therapy was pioneered by Carter and Fairburn (1998), who assessed its effectiveness in a 12-week program when delivered with little or no professional attention. In this study, patients with binge-eating disorder were given Fairburn's (1995) book *Overcoming Binge Eating*. Then they either were given instructions to read and apply the contents (pure self-help), or received six to eight 25-minute sessions with a nonprofessional "facilitator." The results were comparable to those of face-to-face treatments, with reductions in the frequency of binge eating of 53% in the pure self-help condition and 76% in the guided self-help condition.

A second psychological treatment (also following the precedent with bulimia nervosa) is interpersonal therapy, modified by Wilfley and colleagues (1993) for application to binge-eating disorder. It too produced a clinically significant reduction (71%) in binge eating, with maintenance of these effects at a 1-year follow-up (Wilfley et al., 1993, 2000).

It is worthy to note that, despite the reduction in binge eating, neither cognitive-behavior therapy nor interpersonal therapy for binge-eating disorder has produced significant weight loss. There are two possible explanations of this surprising finding. First, the excess caloric intake of the binges may be so small as to make negligible or no contribution to body weight. Second, nutrient intake that would have been consumed in binges may be redistributed to the non-binge-eating caloric intake.

Pharmacotherapy

Pharmacotherapy has also reduced the frequency of binge eating. The first controlled trial (Alger, Schwalberg, Bigaoutte, Michalek, & Howard, 1991) found that, compared to a placebo control, neither naltrexone nor imipramine reduced the frequency of binges. However, a significant reduction in bingeing was found in small, short-term trials of three antidepressants—desipramine (McCann & Agras, 1990), fluvoxamine (Hudson et al., 1998) and sertraline (McElroy et al., 2000)—and in one trial of the appetite suppressant dexfenfluramine (Stunkard, Berkowitz, Tanrikut, et al., 1996). Two of the studies reported weight loss (Hudson et al., 1998; McElroy et al., 2000), but two did not (McCann & Agras, 1990; Stunkard, Berkowitz, Tanrikut, et al., 1996). In the latter two studies, the efficacy of the drugs was shown by the prompt recurrence of bingeing when medication was discontinued (McCann & Agras, 1990; Stunkard, Berkowitz, Tanrikut, et al., 1996). Presumably medication could be used over the long term, but such use has never been attempted.

Standard Weight Reduction Programs

A surprising finding has been the effectiveness of traditional behavioral weight loss programs that ignore the issue of binge eating. Agras and colleagues (1994) found that such programs reduced binge eating as adequately as pharmacotherapy did, and Marcus, Wing, and Fairburn (1995) found that a behavioral weight loss program reduced the number of binge days from 21.6 per 28 days to 2.7 per 28 days. Four previous reports on the use of very-low-calorie diets together with behavioral treatment found that the presence of binge eating did not affect weight loss, adherence to diet, or attrition, and that the frequency of binge eating decreased (Laporte, 1992; Telch & Agras, 1993; Wadden, Foster, & Letizia, 1992; Wadden et al., 1994). Ho, Nichaman, Taylor, Lec, and Foreyt (1995) have shown that those with binge eating were actually only half as likely as those without it to drop out of a large treatment program for obesity. Assessing the outcome of a behavioral treatment that also included no special provision for binge eating, Gladis and colleagues (1998) found that patients with binge-eating disorder lost significantly more weight than those without the disorder, and had comparable attrition rates and decreases in depression. The table in Porzelius, Houston, Smith, Arfkin, and Fisher (1995) shows that a standard behavioral treatment was as effective as a "binge-eating weight loss treatment" in reducing bingeing and body weight in persons with moderate and severe binge-eating disorder.

These studies have clearly laid to rest one of the concerns that had motivated the development of cognitive-behavior therapy—namely, that dietary restriction might exacerbate problems with binge eating. It should be noted that few studies have addressed the long-term effects of behavioral treatment on binge eating; the limited effects on weight loss are all too well known.

Binge-Eating Disorder: A Reassessment

The surprising effectiveness of programs that have ignored the issue of binge eating calls for a reassessment of the nature of binge-eating disorder. In this reassessment, two types of studies are useful: those of placebo responsiveness and those of untreated subjects.

The first type of research concerns the remarkable placebo responsiveness of binge-eating disorder. In the study by Alger and colleagues (1991) described above, placebo responsiveness was 68%, not significantly less than the 79% and 88% reductions produced by active medication. In the Hudson and colleagues (1998) study, among patients receiving placebo, binges per week fell 41% (from 5.3 ± 2.5 to 3.1 ± 3.0; J. I. Hudson, personal communication), and 44% of these patients showed a greater than 50% reduction in binges per week. This placebo response was also sufficient to affect the results: A difference between fluvoxamine and placebo was statistically significant only in a completer analysis, not in a last-observation-carried-forward analysis. Similarly, in the McElroy and colleagues (2000) study, among patients receiving placebo, binges per week fell 46% (from 7.2 ± 5.8 to 3.9 ± 3.8) (S. L. McElroy, personal communication). Once again, the placebo response was large enough to affect the results: The difference between sertraline and placebo was statistically significant only in a last-observation-carried-forward analysis, not in a completer analysis. A fourth study assessed placebo responsiveness by means of a 4-week placebo run-in period. During this period, binges fell from 6.0 to 1.8 per week—a reduction of 70% (Stunkard, Berkowitz, Tanrikut, et al., 1996). Figure 6.1 illustrates the findings. But the placebo responsiveness was as great as any in the medical literature.

The second kind of study assessed the fate of binge-eating disorder among persons who received no treatment at all, either as waiting-list control subjects or as members of a community survey. The shortest such duration was the 12 weeks of the minimal-treatment program of Carter and Fairburn (1998). Among subjects in the waiting-list control group, binge eating fell by 38%. In the second longest period with no treatment, the 6-month community survey of Cachelin and colleagues (1997), partial remission was reported in 48% of persons who had been diagnosed with binge-eating disorder. In a second community study, Fairburn, Cooper, Doll, Norman, and O'Connor (in press) reported that only 10% of sub-

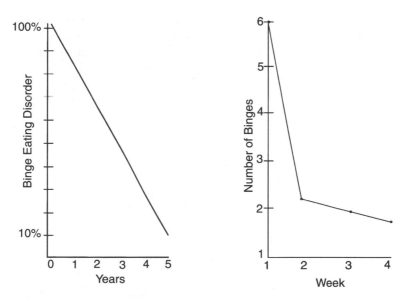

FIGURE 6.1. Two illustrations of the unstable nature of binge-eating disorder. The panel on the left shows the 90% decline in persons diagnosed as having binge-eating disorder during a 5-year period when they received no treatment. The panel on the right shows the 70% decline in the frequency of binge eating during a 4-week period when subjects received only placebo. Data from Stunkard, Berkowitz, Tanrikut, Reiss, and Young (1996).

jects diagnosed with binge-eating disorder at the beginning of the survey received this diagnosis 5 years later. Fairburn and colleagues (in press) concluded that, unlike bulimia nervosa, binge-eating disorder "is an unstable state with a strong tendency toward spontaneous remission."

These two types of studies help to explain the results with binge-eating disorder of traditional weight loss programs that have ignored binge eating. These studies and their results raise serious doubt that control of binge eating is necessary before obese persons can lose weight, and that attempts at weight loss should be deferred until binge eating is controlled. In fact, it has been argued that "standard behavioral treatments are better able to address all of the treatment needs of this [binge-eating] group" (Gladis et al., 1998, p. 383).

If binge-eating disorder is an unstable state with a strong tendency toward spontaneous remission, should it be the object of special treatment? Probably not for the binge eating. Traditional weight loss programs appear fully able to cope with both the overweight and the binge eating of persons with this disorder.

The diagnosis of binge-eating disorder, however, may serve another function: identification of persons whose comorbidity deserves treatment. Such treatment, however, should be directed toward the specific comorbid conditions, not toward the binge eating. In the last analysis, this may be the major value of the diagnosis of binge-eating disorder—as a marker for other psychological problems that deserve consideration in their own right.

NIGHT-EATING SYNDROME

Whereas binge-eating disorder is the oldest of the eating disorders, the night-eating syndrome is the youngest. It was described for the first time in 1955 as a syndrome comprising the triad of morning anorexia, evening hyperphagia, and insomnia (Stunkard, Grace, & Wolff, 1955). Although this was not a defining characteristic, the disorder included depression with an unusual circadian pattern: The depression was minimal in the morning and increased during the evening and night. Clinical investigation revealed that it occurred disproportionately among obese persons during periods of life stress and was alleviated with the alleviation of the stress. In the 1955 publication, the night-eating syndrome was suggested to be a special diurnal response to stress characteristic of some obese persons.

Although it has not been included in any edition of the DSM, studies of the prevalence of the night-eating syndrome have revealed that it is uncommon in the general population (1.5%; Rand, Macgregor, & Stunkard, 1997). Like that of binge-eating disorder, prevalence of the night-eating syndrome increases with increasing weight—to 8.9% in an obesity clinic (Stunkard, 1959), and to a peak of 27% among obese persons in a clinic for the surgical treatment of obesity (Rand et al., 1997).

Much of what we know about the night-eating syndrome was reported by Birketvedt and colleagues (1999). This study confirmed the elements of the night-eating syndrome previously reported, including night eating, evening hyperphagia, and insomnia. The list of provisional criteria for the syndrome developed by these authors is provided in Table 6.2. Birketvedt and colleagues (1999) also quantified the evening hyperphagia, showing that daily food intake, which continued later than that of obese control subjects, was 2,930 kilocalories (kcal) compared to 2,334 for the control subjects ($p < .055$). Figure 6.2 shows that the cumulative caloric intake of the night-eating subjects lagged behind that of the obese control subjects so that at 6:00 P.M. they had consumed only 37% of their daily intake, compared to 74% for the controls ($p < .001$). The food intake of the control subjects then slowed, while that of the night-eating subjects continued at a rapid pace until after midnight. During the period from 10:00 P.M. to 6:00 A.M., the night-eating subjects consumed

TABLE 6.2. Provisional Criteria for the Night-Eating Syndrome

A. Morning anorexia, even if the subject eats breakfast
B. Evening hyperphagia. At least 50% of the daily caloric intake is consumed in snacks after the last evening meal
C. Awakenings at least once a night at least three nights a week
D. Consumption of high calorie snacks during the awakenings on frequent occasions
E. The pattern occurs for a period of at least 3 months
F. Subjects do not meet criteria for any other eating disorders

Note. From Birketvedt et al. (1999). Copyright 1999 by the American Medical Association. Reprinted by permission.

56% of their caloric intake, compared to 15% for the control subjects (*p* < .001). As reported also in the Stunkard and colleagues (1955) paper, Figure 6.2 shows that the mood of the night-eating subjects was lower than that of the control subjects during the morning, and that it fell significantly during the evening and night.

The night-eating subjects studied by Birketvedt and colleagues (1999) suffered from both sleep onset and sleep maintenance insomnia, awakening 3.6 times per night, compared to 0.3 for the control subjects (*p* < .001). Half of the 178 awakenings of the night-eating subjects were associated with food intake, while none of the controls ate while they were

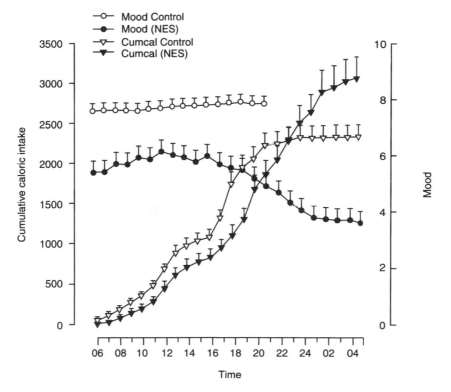

FIGURE 6.2. Twenty-four-hour pattern of mean cumulative energy intake and mood for a 5-day period. The intake of the night-eating subjects lags behind that of control subjects until 10:00 P.M. and then greatly exceeds it (*p* < .001). Daytime mood of the night-eating subjects is lower than that of the control subjects (*p* < .001) and falls even lower during the evening and night (*p* < .001). Error bars represent *SEM* in all figures. NES indicates night-eating syndrome. From Birketvedt et al. (1999). Copyright 1999 by the American Medical Association. Reprinted by permission.

awake. The nighttime snacks of the night-eating subjects were not binges but of only moderate size, averaging 271 kcal. The carbohydrate content of these nighttime snacks was very high (70% of caloric intake), compared to 47% for their food intake during the rest of the day ($p < .001$). Furthermore, the carbohydrate-to-protein ratio of the nighttime snacks was also very high—7:1. This nutrient pattern of a high carbohydrate-to-protein ratio increases the availability of tryptophan for transport into the brain and conversion into serotonin with its sleep-promoting properties (Berry, Growdon, Wurtman, Caballero, & Wurtman, 1991; Yokogoshi & Wurtman, 1986). This sequence makes it appear that the nighttime snacks are a form of self-medication for insomnia.

The behavioral study was complemented by a neuroendocrine study conducted in the Clinical Research Center of the University Hospital in Tromsø, Norway, where subjects were admitted for 24-hour periods (Birketvedt et al., 1999). All subjects were women, and both the night-eating and control groups included both overweight and normal-weight subjects, matched for body mass index and age. Unlike the usual nighttime eating of the night-eating subjects, all subjects received four meals of 400 kcal at 8:00 A.M., 12:00 noon, 4:00 P.M., and 8:00 P.M.

Among the night-eating subjects, both overweight and normal-weight, there was a marked blunting of plasma melatonin levels at night ($p < .001$). As expected, plasma leptin levels were considerably higher among overweight subjects than among normal-weight ones in both groups. In contrast to the expected rise in leptin at night among the control subjects, there was no increase in leptin among the night-eating subjects, either overweight or normal-weight. Confirming the earlier clinical impression that the night-eating syndrome was associated with stress, plasma cortisol levels of the night-eating subjects were higher than those of control subjects for most of the 24 hours (see Figure 6.3).

The night-eating syndrome appears to be a unique combination of an eating disorder, a sleep disorder, and a mood disorder. The distinctive neuroendocrine findings are closely associated in a pattern that helps to link these findings with the behavior characteristic of this syndrome. Thus the blunting of the nighttime rise in melatonin may contribute to the sleep maintenance insomnia, as suggested by Hajak and colleagues (1995), and to depression, as suggested by Kennedy, Garfinkel, Parienti, Costa, and Braun (1989). The failure of leptin to rise at night must limit its usual nighttime suppression of appetite and may permit the breakthrough of hunger impulses, further disrupting sleep. The elevated levels of cortisol reflect the clinical impression that night eating occurs during periods of life stress.

The first step in defining a disease or disorder has been taken in the case of the night-eating syndrome: It is readily recognized by persons manifesting the disorder, and physicians are becoming familiar with it. There have been no studies of treatment to date, but research on this topic is currently underway. The nature of the symptoms suggests the use of melatonin and selective serotonin reuptake inhibitors.

The night-eating syndrome appears to differ from binge-eating disorder both in the far greater frequency of nighttime awakenings and in the modest amount of the food ingested—270 kcal, compared to the 1,300 kcal ingested during eating binges reported by Grilo and Schiffman (1994). It appears to differ also from the "nocturnal sleep-related eating disorders" reported in sleep research clinics and characterized by eating upon awakening from sleep, often in association with sleepwalking and related sleep disturbances. The relation between these disorders and the night-eating syndrome is unclear, in part because of the uncertainty regarding the nature of the former disorders. Thus Schenk and Mahowald (1994) reported only 38 (0.5%) cases out of approximately 8,000 polysomnographic examinations, and in 84% the night eating occurred during total or partial unconsciousness. Manni, Ratti, and Tartara (1997), on the other hand, reported

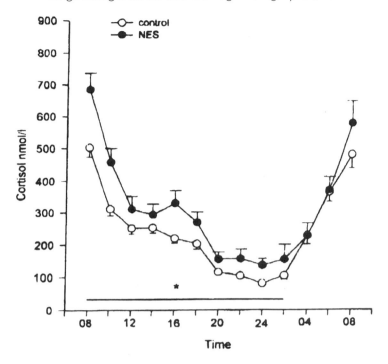

Figure 6.3. Twenty-four-hour mean plasma cortisol levels in subjects with (*n* = 12) and without (*n* = 21) night-eating syndrome (NES). The asterisk and line indicate a significant difference between the levels of the two groups (*p* < .001). From Birketvedt et al. (1999). Copyright 1999 by the American Medical Association. Reprinted by permission.

that 5.8% of 120 persons referred for insomnia manifested night eating during full consciousness.

SUMMARY AND CONCLUSIONS

The identification of two different eating disorders helps to define two subsets of obese persons who may benefit from special attention. Studies of binge-eating disorder show that traditional behavioral weight reduction programs reduce binge eating and body weight and are the treatment of choice. The diagnosis of binge-eating disorder may be most useful as a marker for the other psychological problems that frequently affect those who binge-eat, and that deserve treatment in their own right.

Identification of the night-eating syndrome provides information that may be useful in the care of persons afflicted with this disorder. Treatment of the night-eating syndrome has not been assessed since the initial report (Stunkard et al., 1955). In that report, it was noted that long-term psychodynamic psychotherapy was associated with improvement in the night eating behaviors of some patients.

Anecdotal reports from persons with night-eating syndrome who have explored treatment options suggest that selective serotonin reuptake inhibitors have been helpful, as might be expected from their effects on disturbances in mood and sleep. In view of the lack of rise in nighttime melatonin, provision of such agents at bedtime would seem a rational option.

Mitchell, J. E., & Mussell, M. P. (1995). Comorbidity and binge eating disorder. *Addictive Behaviors, 20,* 725–732.

Mussell, M. P., Mitchell, J. E., Fenna, C. J., Crosby, R. D., Miller, J. P., & Hoberman, H. M. (1997). A comparison of onset of binge eating versus dieting in the development of bulimia nervosa. *International Journal of Eating Disorders, 12,* 353–360.

Polivy, J., & Herman, C. P. (1985). Dieting and bingeing: A causal analysis. *American Psychologist, 40,* 193–201.

Polivy, J., & Herman, C. P. (1993). Etiology of binge eating: Psychological mechanisms. In C. G. Fairburn & G. T. Wilson (Eds.), *Binge eating: Nature, assessment, and treatment* (pp. 173–205). New York: Guilford Press.

Polivy, J., Herman, C., Olmsted, M., & Jazwinski, C. (1984). Restraint and binge eating. In R. C. Hawkins, W. J. Frenow, & P. P. Clement (Eds.), *The binge–purge syndrome: Diagnosis, treatment and research* (pp. 104–122). New York: Springer.

Porzelius, L. K., Houston, C., Smith, M., Arfkin, C., & Fisher, E. (1995). Comparison of a standard behavioral weight loss treatment and a binge eating weight loss treatment. *Behavior Therapy, 26,* 119–134.

Rand, C. S. W., Macgregor, M. D., & Stunkard, A. (1997). The night eating syndrome in the general population and among post-operative obesity surgery patients. *International Journal of Eating Disorders, 22,* 65–69.

Schenk, C. H., & Mahowald, M. W. (1994). Review of nocturnal sleep-related eating disorders. *International Journal of Eating Disorders, 16,* 343–356.

Smith, D. E., Marcus, M. D., & Kaye, W. (1992). Cognitive-behavioral treatment of obese binge eaters. *International Journal of Eating Disorders, 12,* 257–262.

Spitzer, R. L., Devlin, M., Walsh, B. T., Hasin, D., Wing, R., Marcus, M., Stunkard, A. J., Wadden, T., Yanovski, S., Agras, S., Mitchell, J., & Nonas, C. (1992). Binge eating disorder: A multisite field trial of the diagnostic criteria. *International Journal of Eating Disorders, 11,* 191–203.

Spitzer, R. L., Stunkard, A. J., Yanovski, S., Marcus, M. D., Wadden, T. A., & Wing, R. R. (1993). Binge-eating disorder should be included in DSM-IV: A reply to Fairburn et al.'s "The classification of recurrent overeating: The 'binge-eating disorder' proposal." *International Journal of Eating Disorders, 13,* 161–169.

Spitzer, R. L., Yanovski, S., Wadden, T. A., Wing, R., Marcus, M. D., Stunkard, A. J., Devlin, M., Mitchell, J., Hasin, D., & Horne, R. L. (1993). Binge-eating disorder: Its further validation in a multisite study. *International Journal of Eating Disorders, 13,* 137–150.

Spurrell, E. B., Wilfley, D. E., Tanofsky, M. B., & Brownell, K. D. (1997). Age of onset for binge eating disorder: Are there different pathways to binge eating? *International Journal of Eating Disorders, 21,* 55–65.

Stunkard, A. J. (1959). Eating patterns and obesity. *Psychiatric Quarterly, 33,* 284–294.

Stunkard, A. J. (1993). A history of binge eating. In C. G. Fairburn & G. T. Wilson (Eds.), *Binge eating: Nature, assessment, and treatment* (pp. 15–34). New York: Guilford Press.

Stunkard, A. J., Berkowitz, R., Tanrikut, C., Reiss, E., & Young, L. (1996). D-Fenfluramine treatment of binge eating disorder. *American Journal of Psvchiatrv, 153,* 1455–1459.

Stunkard, A. J., Berkowitz, R., Wadden, T., Tanrikut, C., Reiss, E., & Young, L. (1996). Binge eating disorder and the night eating syndrome. *International Journal of Obesity, 20,* 1–6.

Stunkard, A. J., Grace, W. J., & Wolff, H. G. (1955). The night-eating syndrome: A pattern of food intake among certain obese patients. *American Journal of Medicine, 19,* 78–86.

Stunkard, A. J., & Messick, S. (1985). The Three-Factor Eating Questionnaire to measure dietary restraint, disinhibition and hunger. *Journal of Psvchosomatic Research, 29,* 71–83.

Tanofsky, M. B., Wilfley, D. E., Spurrell, E. B., Welch, R., & Brownell, K. D. (1997). Comparison of men and women with binge eating disorder. *International Journal of Eating Disorders, 21,* 49–54.

Telch, C. F., & Agras, W. S. (1993). The effects of a very low calorie diet on binge eating. *Behavior Therapy, 24,* 177–193.

Telch, C. F., Agras, W. S., & Rossiter, F. M. (1988). Binge eating increases with increasing adiposity. *International Journal of Eating Disorders, 7,* 115–119.

Telch, C. F., Agras, W. S., Rossiter, F. M., Wilfley, D. E., & Kenardy, J. (1990). Group cognitive behavioral treatment for non-purging bulimics: An initial evaluation. *Journal of Consulting and
Clinical Psychology, 58*, 629–635.

Wadden, T. A., Foster, G. D., & Letizia, K. A. (1992). Response of obese binge eaters to treatment by
behavior therapy combined with very low calorie diet. *Journal of Consulting and Clinical Psychology, 60*, 808–811.

Wadden, T. A., Foster, G. D., & Letizia, K. A. (1994). One-year behavioral treatment of obesity:
Comparison of moderate and severe caloric restriction and the effects of weight maintenance
therapy. *Journal of Consulting and Clinical Psychology, 62*, 165–171.

Westenhoefer, J., Stunkard, A. J., & Pudel, V. (1999). Validation of flexible and rigid control dimensions of dietary restraint. *International Journal of Eating Disorders, 26*, 53–64.

Wilfley, D. E., Agras, W. S., Telch, C. F., Rossiter, E. M., Schneider, J. A., Cole, A. G., Sifford, L., &
Raeburn, S. D. (1993). Group cognitive-behavioral therapy and group interpersonal psychother-
apy for the nonpurging bulimic individual: A controlled comparison. *Journal of Consulting and
Clinical Psychology, 61*, 296–305.

Wilfley, D. E., & Cohen, L. R. (1997). Psychological treatment of bulimia nervosa and binge eating
disorder. *Psychopharmacology Bulletin, 33*, 437–454.

Wilfley, D. E., Schwartz, M. H., Spurrell, E. B., & Fairburn, C. G. (2000). Using the Eating Disorders
Examination to identify specific psychopathology of binge eating disorder. *International Journal
of Eating Disorders, 27*, 259–269.

Wilson, G. T., Nonas, C. A., & Rosenblum, G. D. (1993). Assessment of binge eating in obese patients. *International Journal of Eating Disorders, 150*, 1472–1479.

Yanovski, S. Z. (1993). Binge eating disorder: Current knowledge. *Obesity Research, 1*, 306–324.

Yanovski, S. Z., Nelson, J. E., Dubbert, B. K., & Spitzer, R. L. (1993). Association of binge eating disorder and psychiatric comorbidity in obese subjects. *American Journal of Psychiatry, 150*,
1472–1479.

Yanovski, S. Z., & Sebring, N. G. (1994). Recorded food intake of obese women with binge eating
disorder before and after weight loss. *International Journal of Eating Disorders, 15*, 135–150.

Yokogoshi, H., & Wurtman, R. J. (1986). Meal composition and plasma amino acid ratios: Effects of
various proteins or carbohydrates, and of various protein concentrations. *Metabolism, 35*,
637–642.

7

The Relationship of Intentional Weight Loss to Disease Incidence and Mortality

EDWARD W. GREGG
DAVID F. WILLIAMSON

Obesity is related to many adverse health outcomes, including cardiovascular disease (CVD), diabetes, cancer, osteoarthritis, sleep apnea, and mortality (National Institutes of Health Consensus Development Panel on the Health Implications of Obesity, 1985; Pi-Sunyer, 1993a). Weight loss, on the other hand, is known to improve physiological risk factors such as impaired glucose tolerance (IGT), hyperlipidemia, and high blood pressure over the short term (Maggio & Pi-Sunyer, 1997; Pi-Sunyer, 1993b). Despite these benefits, epidemiological studies have generally failed to show that weight loss reduces disease incidence or mortality, but have instead suggested that the greatest longevity results from stable weight or slight weight gain (Andres, Muller, & Sorkin, 1993; Lee & Paffenbarger, 1996). Others have suggested that repeated weight loss and regain may actually be detrimental (Blair, Shaten, Brownell, Collins, & Lissner, 1993; Hamm, Shekelle, & Stamler, 1989; Lissner et al., 1991). Thus a quandary exists: It is clear that obesity is bad, but do we know whether intentional weight loss is good?

The contradictory reports of the effects of weight loss may stem from the fact that there are many different circumstances of weight loss. For instance, weight loss may be deliberate or intentional, as achieved through lifestyle or medical interventions. Weight loss may also be unintentional, but resulting from a deliberate process to improve health, such as through physical activity or dietary change. Finally, weight loss may occur unintentionally due to known disease processes, mental illness, stressful life events, aging, or unknown circumstances. Estimates from epidemiological studies suggest that unintentional weight loss is almost as common as intentional weight loss (Williamson, 1997). National estimates have shown that among those reporting weight loss, about 60% lost the weight intentionally and 40% unintentionally (Meltzer & Everhart, 1995).

Obesity has become increasingly prevalent and costly, affecting approximately one-fourth of U.S. adults and leading to over $50 billion in direct medical costs (Flegal, Carroll,

found weight loss to be associated with reduced mortality (Hammond & Garfinkel, 1969), but as indicated by several extensive review articles, many more studies have found weight loss to be associated with *increased* mortality (Andres et al., 1993; Lee & Paffenbarger, 1996; Williamson & Pamuk, 1993). For example, Lee and Paffenbarger (1996) reported that only 3 out of 17 epidemiological studies found weight loss to be associated with increased longevity; mortality tended to be highest among people who had lost or gained substantial weight during their lives, and lowest among those whose weight had remained stable. The authors pointed out, however, that these studies are limited by lack of data on weight loss intention, and in some cases by failure to rule out coexisting disease or to control adequately for smoking and other behavioral confounders.

Two recent epidemiological studies, however, suggest that the association of weight loss and longevity depends on the composition of the weight that is lost. Allison and colleagues (1999) used skinfold thickness measures to estimate change in body fat in two population-based cohort studies (Framingham, Massachusetts, and Tecumseh, Michigan). Although each additional standard deviation of weight loss (4.6 kg–7.6 kg in the two studies) was associated with a 28%–39% increase in mortality rates, each additional standard deviation of *fat* loss was associated with about a 16% *reduction* in mortality rates in the two studies. In support of the view that loss of body fat increases longevity, Heitmann, Erikson, Ellsinger, Mikelsen, and Larsson (2000) followed up a cohort of 60-year-old Swedish men 22 years after their body composition had been measured by potassium counting. They found that men with lower lean body mass had increased mortality, but men with lower fat mass had decreased mortality.

There may be reason to believe that weight loss could have either beneficial or detrimental effects on musculoskeletal outcomes, disability, and quality of life. In the Framingham Knee Osteoarthritis Study, weight loss during the previous 10 years was associated with a 59% reduction in risk for symptomatic knee osteoarthritis among overweight women (Felson, Zhang, Anthony, Naimark, & Anderson, 1992). Although obesity has also been related to an increased risk of disability (Launer, Harris, Rumpel & Madans, 1994), weight loss can result in loss of lean mass and bone mineral density, which could lead to adverse consequences, particularly among the elderly. This is evident in at least three cohort studies of older adults—the Study of Osteoporotic Fractures, the Established Populations for Epidemiologic Study of the Elderly, and the National Health and Examination Survey Follow-Up Study I—in which weight loss between middle age and later years was associated with at least a twofold increased relative risk of hip fracture and loss of mobility (Ensrud, Cauley, Lipshutz, & Cummings, 1997; Langlois et al., 1998; Launer et al., 1994).

One population-based study has assessed the relationship between weight change and change in health-related quality of life. Among women participating in the Nurses' Health Study, weight loss over 4 years was associated with improved physical function and vitality, particularly among the most obese women (Fine et al., 1999). The only exception was among lean women (BMI < 25 kg/m²), for whom weight loss was associated with worsening scores on physical functioning, freedom from bodily pain, vitality, and mental health. The authors conjectured that among the lean group in particular, weight loss was probably largely unintentional and a marker of physical or mental illness.

METHODOLOGICAL LIMITATIONS OF THE EPIDEMIOLOGICAL STUDIES OF GENERAL WEIGHT LOSS

A key limitation of the epidemiological literature on general weight loss summarized above is the lack of information on weight loss intention (Williamson, 1996). Several studies have shown that in addition to being common, unintentional weight loss is associated with older age, negative health behaviors, and poor health status (French, Jeffery, Folsom, Williamson, & Byers, 1995; McGuire, Wing, & Hill, 2000; McGuire, Wing, Klem, & Hill, 1999; Meltzer & Everhart, 1995, 1996; Williamson et al., 1995). Weight loss may be related to depression or may be part of the natural history (particularly the end stages) of conditions such as cancer, diabetes, coronary heart disease, cerebrovascular disease, obstructive pulmonary disease, and dementia (Marton, Sox, & Krupp, 1981; Thompson & Morris, 1991). Thus inclusion of people who had unintentional weight loss in the studies discussed above could have spuriously increased disease incidence and mortality among those losing weight.

Observational studies of weight loss and disease are plagued by other seemingly obvious, but confusing, methodological dilemmas. First, obese people, those who smoke, and those with preexisting disease are more likely to lose weight during their lives than healthy people who are of normal weight (French et al., 1995; Meltzer & Everhart, 1995). Thus the interpretation of studies relating weight loss to an increased risk of diseases such as diabetes and heart disease should acknowledge that people who lost weight were likely at higher risk for disease and death in the first place. This points to the need for careful stratification and/or control for initial body weight and health status. For example, in a report from the Nurses' Health Study, a weight loss (intent unknown) of ≥11 kg was related to an almost twofold *increased* risk of diabetes (Colditz, Willett, Rotnitzky, & Manson, 1995). After initial BMI was controlled for, however, weight loss was associated with about an 80% *reduced* risk of diabetes. Second, people who lose weight are also more likely to experience weight cycling (French et al., 1995). Since some have argued that weight cycling may have its own adverse effects on metabolism and health outcomes independent of weight loss (National Task Force on the Prevention and Treatment of Obesity, 1994), weight cycling could also confound relationships between weight loss and disease. The reader is referred to several extensive reviews of the epidemiology of general weight loss and disease (Andres et al., 1993; Lee & Paffenbarger, 1996; Williamson, 1996; Williamson & Pamuk, 1993).

STUDIES OF INTENTIONAL WEIGHT LOSS

Because of the limitations of observational studies of general weight loss, we have focused the remainder of this review on studies in which weight loss intention was assessed directly or was part of controlled weight loss or lifestyle interventions. The limitations of observational studies point toward RCTs as an appropriate alternative to assessing the causal impact of intentional weight loss on health outcomes (Yanovski, Bain, & Williamson, 1999). However, with the exception of hypertension and diabetes studies, few RCTs have specifically examined the impact of weight loss approaches on morbidity or mortality. Thus evidence for evaluating whether a causal relationship between intentional weight loss and health outcomes comes from three types of studies: (1) observational cohort studies that include direct self-report of weight loss intention; (2) nonrandomized controlled trials (NCTs) of weight loss interventions; and (3) RCTs of lifestyle interventions in which weight loss was a secondary objective.

Observational Cohort Studies

Six prospective cohort studies and one retrospective cohort study have examined the relationship between intentional weight loss and mortality in middle-aged and older populations (Table 7.1).

Mortality

In prospective studies of approximately 100,000 enrolled in the Cancer Prevention Study I, intentional weight loss was related to a 20% reduction in all-cause mortality and 30%–40% reductions in diabetes and cancer mortality among women, as well as one-third reduction in diabetes-related mortality among men (Williamson et al., 1995, 2000). These reductions were greater for those who lost 1–9 kg than for those who lost more than 9 kg and were only observed among those with preexisting conditions such as heart disease, diabetes, and hypertension. However, there were no associations between intentional weight loss and CVD mortality in these studies.

In a study specifically conducted among overweight diabetic persons in the Cancer Prevention Study, intentional weight loss was associated with about 25% reduced risk of all-cause, cardiovascular, and diabetes-related mortality (Williamson et al., 2000). Weight loss of up to 50 lbs was associated with reduced mortality, with greatest reductions observed among those losing 10%–15% of initial weight. In contrast, intentional weight loss of >70 lbs and unintentional weight loss and weight gain are associated with small increases in mortality.

A report of approximately 26,000 women aged 55–69 years in the Iowa Women's Health Study found that intentional weight loss of more than 9 kg during any of three periods of adulthood (ages 18–39, 40–54, or 55+ years) was unrelated to total CVD or all-cause mortality (French, Folsom, Jeffery, & Williamson, 1999). Those who had unintentionally lost more than 9 kg, however, were at 40%–60% increased risk of CVD or all-cause mortality.

One study has assessed intentional weight loss and mortality among older adults. In a 5-year follow-up of 5,204 adults aged 65 years or older enrolled in the Cardiovascular Health Study, the 5-year cumulative mortality among men with an intentional 4.4-kg (10-pound) weight loss (16.4%) was equivalent to that for those with stable weight (16.1%), but mortality was over twice as high (33%) among those with an unintentional 4.4-kg weight loss (Diehr et al., 1998). Among women, those with an intentional 4.4-kg weight loss had a slightly lower 5-year mortality incidence (5%) than those with stable weight (7.4%), and they had only one-third the mortality of those with unintentional weight loss (16.2%).

Yaari and Goldbourt (1998) conducted an 18-year follow-up of more than 9,000 Israeli men aged 40–65 years and found that, overall, weight loss of at least 5 kg was associated with a 20%–40% greater risk of mortality than that associated with stable weight. The study also reported that, compared to men with stable weights, those who had lost at least 5 kg and reported being on a "slimming diet" to lose weight had a twofold higher mortality risk. However, these analyses based on dieting status did not control for body weight and important comorbidities such as hypertension and coronary heart disease, so it is unclear whether the increased mortality risk was due to underlying disease among those trying to lose weight.

Thus, of the six prospective epidemiological studies that have assessed the relationship of intentional weight loss to mortality, one found benefits on all-cause, cancer, and diabetes mortality among women with preexisting disease (Williamson et al., 1995); one also found benefits on diabetes mortality among men (Williamson et al., 1999); and one found reduced CVD and all-cause mortality among men and women with diabetes (Williamson et al., 2000). Three studies found that intentional weight loss neither increased nor decreased all-cause or CVD mortality among older adult men (Diehr et al., 1998; French et al., 1999; Williamson et al., 1999); and one (Yaari & Goldbourt, 1998) found an increased risk of all-cause mortality. Although these studies did not consistently find that intentional weight loss was associated with decreased mortality, they suggest that the earlier epidemiological studies relating weight loss of unknown intention to increased mortality were confounded by unintentional weight loss.

One retrospective cohort study assessed mortality among 233 patients with Type 2 diabetes who had received intensive dietary counseling after their disease was diagnosed (Lean, Powrie, Anderson, & Garthwaite, 1990). Mean weight change was −3.5 kg in men and −2.3 kg in women. For the entire sample, life expectancy was 2.5 months longer for each kilogram of weight loss, and it was 3.6 months longer per kilogram of weight loss among those with a BMI greater than 25 kg/m^2.

Osteoporotic Fractures

Only one study has assessed the relationship of intentional weight loss to risk of musculoskeletal outcomes. A report by Ensrud and colleagues (1997) found that older women who had a 10% unintentional weight loss had a significant 80% increased risk of osteoporotic fracture, but those who lost weight intentionally did not have an increased fracture risk. Both intentional and unintentional weight loss were associated with slight but statistically significant (relative risk = 1.16–1.18) increased risks of falling, however.

NCTs of Weight Loss Interventions

Several NCTs have examined the effects of weight loss on diabetes incidence and mortality (Table 7.2). Such trials are hampered by the fact that systematic differences in health status and behavior may exist between people who agree to undergo difficult weight loss interventions and those who do not.

Diabetes

The Malmö Prevention Trial (Eriksson & Lindgärde, 1991) recruited 785 men aged 47–49 years and enrolled them in a nonrandomized manner into four groups: (1) a 6-year diet and exercise intervention for people with IGT; (2) a usual-care condition for those with IGT; (3) the same diet-plus-exercise intervention conducted among people with diabetes; and (4) a control condition for persons with normal glucose tolerance. Percentages of BMI change among the IGT intervention, IGT control, diabetes, and normal glucose tolerance groups after 6 years were −2.3%, 0.5%, −3.7%, and 1.7%, respectively. Thus the IGT intervention group had a net 2.8% BMI decrease (−2.3% vs. 0.5%), compared to the IGT control group. After 6 years, those with IGT in the intervention group had a 63% reduction in diabetes incidence (11%), compared to the nonrandomized control group of people with IGT (29%).

Two studies found reduced incidence of diabetes among individuals who underwent surgical treatment for obesity. A study of 109 patients undergoing gastric bypass surgery (Long et al., 1994) and 27 nonrandomized controls found a strong protective effect of surgery on diabetes risk. The surgery group lost more than 50% of excess weight after a year, and had only one incident case of diabetes among treated individuals (incidence = 0.15 per 100 person-years) after 6 years. By comparison, 6 out of the 27 control subjects (4.7 per 100 person-years) developed diabetes. A follow-up examination of the surgical patients reported 30% loss of body weight after 7.6 years (Pories et al., 1995), and among those with diabetes, a reduction in diabetic medication use and overall mortality compared to those not receiving surgery (MacDonald et al., 1997). These studies, however, were limited by their design, which included an unmatched and nonrandomized control group.

In the Swedish Obese Subjects study, 845 individuals had bariatric surgery that was ac-

TABLE 7.3. Summary of Randomized Controlled Trials (RCTs) of Lifestyle Interventions: Effects on Disease Incidence and Mortality

Author(s)	Design, mean follow-up	Outcome	Population	Definition of weight loss	Weight change comparison	Effect[a]	Effect of weight loss relative to control
TOHP Collaborative Research Group (1992)	RCT, 1.5 yr	Hypertension incidence	2,182 men and women aged 30–54 yr with high-normal diastolic blood pressure	Diet and exercise intervention vs. control	Net 4% loss vs. control	+	34% ↓ hypertension incidence.
TOHP Collaborative Research Group (1997)	RCT, 4 yr	Hypertension incidence	2,382 overweight men and women aged 30–54 yr with high-normal diastolic blood pressure	Diet and exercise intervention vs. control	Net 2% loss vs. control at 3 yr	+	21% ↓ hypertension incidence.
Whelton et al. (1998)	RCT, 2.5 yr	Hypertension and CVD events	585 obese hypertensive men and women aged 60–80 yr	Diet and exercise intervention vs. control	Net 4% loss vs. control	+	30% ↓ combined hypertension and CVD outcomes.
Pan et al. (1997)	RCT, 6 yr	Diabetes incidence	577 men and women (mean age 45 yr) with IGT	Diet, exercise, and diet + exercise interventions vs. control	Net 2% weight loss among diet plus exercise; no weight change in other groups	+	29%, 32%, and 33% ↓ diabetes incidence in diet, exercise, and diet + exercise groups, respectively.
Wing et al. (1998)	RCT, 2 yr	Diabetes incidence	154 men and women aged 40–55 yr	Diet, exercise, and diet + exercise interventions vs. control	Net 2% weight loss vs. control	Ø +	No significant association with diabetes incidence. 4.5-kg weight loss related to 30% ↓ diabetes incidence in post hoc analyses.
Singh et al. (1992)	RCT, 1 yr	Cardiac events, mortality	406 men and women aged 50+ yr with coronary heart disease	Cardioprotective diet intervention vs. control	Net 6% weight loss vs. control	+	40% ↓ cardiac events; 45% ↓ total mortality; nonsignificant 51% ↓ stroke deaths.
Tuomilehto et al. (2001)	RCT, 3.2 yr	Diabetes incidence	522 overweight, glucose intolerant men and women (mean age 55 ± 7 yr)	Diet and exercise vs. control	Net 3.8% weight loss at 1 yr vs. control	+	58% ↓ diabetes incidence.

[a]See footnote to Table 7.1.

(14.3%) and usual-care (16.7%) conditions. At the end of the 2.5-year study, 39% of those in the weight loss intervention were medication- and event-free, compared to 26% of those getting usual care.

Diabetes

A study of 577 people with IGT randomly assigned to diet, exercise, or diet-plus-exercise groups in the Da Qing IGT and Diabetes Study in China resulted in 2%–5% reductions in BMI and 29%–33% reductions in diabetes incidence relative to controls over 6 years (Pan et al., 1997). Six-year cumulative incidence of diabetes ranged from 44% to 47% among lifestyle conditions, compared to 66% among controls. However, these effects appeared to be independent of weight loss. Only overweight individuals in the diet plus exercise condition had lost weight (5.5% decrease in BMI) compared to controls (3.2% decrease in BMI). Paradoxically, individuals who developed diabetes in the four groups had higher mean weight loss (0.9 kg) than those who did not develop diabetes (0.3 kg). It is possible, however, that in many individuals weight loss occurred after being diagnosed with diabetes.

Wing and colleagues (1998) conducted a four-arm, 2-year intervention trial in which 154 individuals aged 40–55 years were randomly assigned to control, diet, exercise, or diet-plus- exercise groups. Relative to controls, the diet and diet-plus-exercise interventions achieved approximately 9% weight loss after 6 months and 5%–7% weight loss after 1 year. The initial 6-month weight loss was accompanied by significant improvements in several cardiovascular risk factors. However, after 2 years, the net weight loss among intervention groups was only 2%; most risk factor advantages had disappeared; and the incidence of diabetes was paradoxically higher ($p = .08$) in the intervention groups (diet, 30%; exercise, 14%; diet plus exercise, 16%) than in the control group (7%). However, in post hoc analyses, those who lost at least 4.5 kg in each of the treatment conditions had a 25%–30% reduction in diabetes risk, compared to those who lost no weight. This study suggests that substantial benefits may be achieved among those successful at losing weight, but that the overall benefit in clinical trials may be diluted by those who do not maintain weight loss.

More recently, results from the Finnish Diabetes Prevention Study provide yet more evidence that modest weight loss reduces the risk of Type 2 diabetes (Tuomilehto et al., 2001). The study randomized 522 middle-aged, overweight men and women with glucose tolerance to an intensive diet and exercise-based lifestyle intervention or a control group. Participants in the intervention group lost 4.7% (4.2 kg) of their body weight after 1 year, compared to 0.9% (0.8 kg) in the control condition. After an average follow-up of 3.2 years, the intervention group had a 58% reduced risk of diabetes compared to the control group. The 4-year cumulative incidence of diabetes was 11% for intervention participants, compared to 23% for participants in the control group.

CVD and Mortality

An RCT of a lifestyle intervention (Singh et al., 1992) among 406 patients with coronary heart disease resulted in a 9% weight loss (vs. 3% in the control group), as well as significant improvements in lipid and blood pressure levels. The study also observed 40%–45% reductions in cardiac events and all-cause mortality, and a 50% reduction in deaths from stroke relative to controls. Post hoc analyses conducted among intervention participants indicated that the reduction in events was primarily driven by those who had lost weight during the year. These findings are consistent with the Lifestyle Heart Trial (Ornish et al., 1990, 1998), which showed that intensive lifestyle changes were associated with 8% net weight loss and significant reductions in coronary stenosis over 5 years. It is important to note, however, that these lifestyle interventions were multifaceted and included a low-fat, high-fiber, and antioxidant-rich diet, along with counseling for smoking cessation, alcohol, stress, and exercise. Thus the extent to which health benefits were primarily due to weight loss or to dietary and behavioral changes is unclear.

Interpretation of the RCTs is complicated by the fact that some of these trials were not weight loss studies per se, but instead were lifestyle interventions wherein weight loss was one of several effects. Because physical activity and dietary factors such as fat and sodium intake can influence health outcomes independently of body weight, it is difficult to separate the effects of these behaviors from the effects of weight loss. Knowing the independent effects of weight loss, physical activity, and dietary change on health outcomes is important for understanding biological mechanisms. From a public health perspective, however, identifying the feasible and appropriate interventions that improve long-term health status may be more important than isolating the mechanisms for their effects.

SUMMARY

Several conclusions may be drawn from our review of the effects of weight loss on disease incidence and mortality:

1. *Weight loss is related to many short-term benefits, primarily in terms of reduced risk factors for CVD and diabetes.* These benefits have been consistently observed in studies of 3 to 12 months' duration, but rarely have been tested for more than 2 years.

2. *Intentional weight loss does not increase mortality but may decrease mortality, especially among people with obesity-related health conditions.* Although three observational studies and one NCT of lifestyle intervention suggest that weight loss enhances longevity among high-risk populations, more studies are needed to confirm this. Previous observations relating weight loss of unknown intent to increased mortality are probably explained by unintentional weight loss associated with preexisting disease.

3. *Modest weight loss and lifestyle interventions can prevent hypertension and diabetes among those at high risk for these diseases.* Benefits of modest weight loss (e.g., 2%–6%) on hypertension and diabetes have been demonstrated in RCTs. A combination of NCTs of surgical and lifestyle interventions have also suggested that diabetes may be prevented.

4. *It is unclear whether intentional weight loss reduces CVD incidence.* One RCT and one NCT have suggested that weight loss reduces CVD incidence and mortality, but observational studies have not found that intentional weight loss reduces CVD incidence.

5. *There is a lack of studies on the effects of intentional weight loss on important health outcomes.* RCTs would be an ideal approach to assess the effects of intentional weight loss on physical disability, osteoporotic fractures, and health-related quality of life. There is also a need for well-designed observational studies of this issue.

Many fundamental questions about unintentional weight loss remain unanswered. Do the physiological benefits of short-term weight loss translate into long-term benefits on CVD incidence and mortality? Are there particular populations, such as elderly persons or those with preexisting diseases, among whom the health effects of intentional weight loss are enhanced or diminished? What is the impact of different weight loss modalities, such as dietary restriction and exercise, on quality-of-life? Could the quality-of-life benefits of intentional weight loss justify possible null effects on disease incidence and mortality? Finally, can weight loss interventions be implemented with reasonable effectiveness, safety, and cost through clinical and public health efforts?

Clearly, RCTs of the long-term impact of intentional weight loss on disease incidence and mortality are needed, and several ongoing trials may provide some answers to these questions. The Look AHEAD (Action for Health in Diabetes) trial, a multicenter clinical trial funded by the National Institutes of Health, was recently initiated to study the effects of weight loss on cardiovascular and other outcomes among overweight persons with Type 2 diabetes over a planned follow-up period of 11.5 years (Yanovski et al., 1999). The Diabetes Prevention Program, currently underway in the United States, is designed to estimate the impact of lifestyle interventions on the incidence of diabetes in overweight persons with IGT (Diabetes Prevention Program Research Group, 1999).

Regardless of the results of ongoing RCTs, debates about the long-term health impact of intentional weight loss are likely to continue. Perhaps the scientific focus of obesity research will begin to move toward the question of whether obesity prevention is ultimately more effective than obesity treatment in reducing disease incidence and mortality.

ACKNOWLEDGMENTS

We thank Dr. Henry Kahn for his insightful comments on an earlier draft of this chapter.

REFERENCES

Agurs-Collins, T. D., Kumanyika, S. K., Ten Have, T. R., & Adams-Campbell, L. L. (1997). A randomized controlled trial of weight reduction and exercise for diabetes management in older African-American subjects. *Diabetes Care, 20,* 1503–1511.

Allison, D. B., Zannolli, R., Faith, M. S., Heo, M., Pietrobelli, A., VanItallie, T. B., Pi-Sunyer, F. X., & Heymsfield, S. B. (1999). Weight loss increases and fat loss decreases all-cause mortality rate: Results from two independent cohort studies. *International Journal of Obesity, 23,* 603–611.

Andersen, R. E., Wadden, T. A., Bartlett, S. J., Vogt, R. A., & Weinstock, R. S. (1995). Relation of weight loss to changes in serum lipids and lipoproteins in obese women. *American Journal of Clinical Nutrition, 62,* 350–357.

Andres, R., Muller, D. C., & Sorkin, J. D. (1993). Long-term effects of change in body weight on all-cause mortality: A review. *Annals of Internal Medicine, 119,* 737–743.

Blair, S. N., Shaten, J., Brownell, K., Collins, G., & Lissner, L. (1993). Body weight change, all-cause mortality, and cause-specific mortality in the Multiple Risk Factor Intervention Trial. *Annals of Internal Medicine, 119,* 749–757.

Centers for Disease Control and Prevention. (1997). Cardiac valvulopathy associated with exposure to fenfluramine or dexfenfluramine: U. S. Department of Health and Human Services interim public health recommendation, November 1997. *Morbidity and Mortality Weekly Report, 46,* 1061–1065.

Centers for Disease Control and Prevention. (1998). Hyperthermia and dehydration-related deaths associated with intentional rapid weight loss in three collegiate wrestlers—North Carolina, Wisconsin, and Michigan, November–December 1997. *Morbidity and Mortality Weekly Report, 47,* 105–108.

Colditz, G. A., Willett, W. C., Rotnitzky, A., & Manson, J. E. (1995). Weight gain as a risk factor for clinical diabetes mellitus in women. *Annals of Internal Medicine, 122,* 481–486.

Dengel, J. L., Katzel, L. I., & Goldberg, A. P. (1995). Effect of an American Heart Association diet, with or without weight loss, on lipids in obese middle-aged and older men. *American Journal of Clinical Nutrition, 62,* 715–721.

Diabetes Prevention Program Research Group. (1999). The Diabetes Prevention Program: Design and methods for a clinical trial in the prevention of Type 2 diabetes. *Diabetes Care, 22,* 623–634.

Diehr, P., Bild, D. E., Harris, T. B., Duxbury, A., Siscovick, D., & Rossi, M. (1998). Body mass index and mortality in nonsmoking older adults: The Cardiovascular Health Study. *American Journal of Public Health, 88,* 623–629.

Dublin, L. I. (1953). Relation of obesity to longevity. *New England Journal of Medicine, 248,* 971–974.

Dublin, L. I., & Marks, H. H. (1951). Mortality among insured overweights in recent years. *Transactions of the Association of Life Insurance Medical Directors of America, 35,* 235–263.

Ensrud, K. E., Cauley, J. A., Lipschutz, R., & Cummings, S. R. (1997). Weight change and fractures in older women. *Archives of Internal Medicine, 157,* 857–863.

Eriksson, K.-F., & Lindgärde, F. (1991). Prevention of Type 2 (non-insulin-dependent) diabetes mellitus by diet and physical exercise. *Diabetologia, 34,* 891–898.

Eriksson, K.-F., & Lindgärde, F. (1998). No excess 12-year mortality in men with impaired glucose tolerance who participated in the Malmö Preventive Trial with diet and exercise. *Diabetologia, 41,* 1010–1016.

Eriksson, J., Lindström, J., Valle, T., Aunola, S., Hämäläinen, H., Ilanne-Parikka, P., Keinänen-Kiukaanniemi, S., Laakso, M., Lauhkonen, M., Lehto, P., Lehtonen, A., Louheranta, A., Mannelin, M., Martikkala, V., Rastas, M., Sundvall, J., Turpeinen, A., Viljanen, T., Uusitupa, M., & Tuomilehto, J. (1999). Prevention of Type II diabetes in subjects with impaired glucose tolerance: The Diabetes Prevention Study (DPS) in Finland. *Diabetologia, 42,* 793–801.

Felson, D. T., Zhang, Y., Anthony, J. M., Naimark, A., & Anderson, J. J. (1992). Weight loss reduces the risk for symptomatic knee osteoarthritis in women. *Annals of Internal Medicine, 116,* 535–539.

Fine, J. T., Colditz, G. A., Coakley, E. H., Moseley, G., Manson, J. E., Willett, W. C., & Kawachi, I. (1999). A prospective study of weight change and health-related quality of life in women. *Journal of the American Medical Association, 282,* 2136–2142.

Flegal, K. M., Carroll, M. D., Kuczmarski, R. J., & Johnson, C. L. (1998). Overweight and obesity in the United States: Prevalence and trends, 1960–1994. *International Journal of Obesity, 22,* 39–47.

French, S. A., Folsom, A. R., Jeffery, R. W., & Williamson, D. F. (1999). Prospective study of intentionality of weight loss and mortality in older women: The Iowa Women's Health Study. *American Journal of Epidemiology, 149,* 504–514.

French, S. A., Jeffrey, R. W., Folsom, A. R., Williamson, D. F., & Byers, T. (1995). Relation of weight variability and intentionality of weight loss to disease history and health-related variables in a population-based sample of women aged 55–69 years. *American Journal of Epidemiology, 142,* 1306–1314.

Hamm, P. B., Shekelle, R. B., & Stamler, J. (1989). Large fluctuations in body weight during young adulthood and 25-year risk of coronary death in men. *American Journal of Epidemiology, 129,* 312–318.

Hammond, E. C., & Garfinkel, L. (1969). Coronary heart disease, stroke, and aortic aneurysm. *Archives of Environmental Health, 19,* 167–182.

Heitmann, B. L., Erikson, H., Ellsinger, B., Mikelsen, K. L., & Larsson, B. (2000). Mortality associated with body fat, fat-free mass and body mass index among 60-year-old Swedish men—a 22-year follow-up: The study of men born in 1913. *International Journal of Obesity, 24,* 33–37.

Karason, K., Wallentin, I., Larsson, B., & Sjöström, L. (1997). Effects of obesity and weight loss on left ventricular mass and relative wall thickness: Survey and intervention study. *British Medical Journal, 315,* 912–916.

Katzel, L. I., Bleecker, E. R., Colman, E. G., Rogus, E. M., Sorkin, J. D., & Goldberg, A. P. (1995). Effects of weight loss vs. aerobic exercise training on risk factors for coronary disease in healthy, obese, middle-aged and older men. *Journal of the American Medical Association, 274,* 1915–1921.

Kuczmarski, R. J., Flegal, K. M., Campbell, S. M., & Johnson, C. L. (1994). Increasing prevalence of overweight among US adults: The National Health and Nutrition Examination Surveys, 1960 to 1991. *Journal of the American Medical Association, 272,* 205–211.

Langlois, J. A., Visser, M., Davidovic, L. S., Maggi, S., Li, G., & Harris, T. B. (1998). Hip fracture risk in older white men is associated with change in body weight from age 50 years to old age. *Archives of Internal Medicine, 158,* 990–996.

Launer, L. J., Harris, T., Rumpel, C., & Madans, J. (1994). Body mass index, weight change, and risk of mobility disability in middle-aged and older women. *Journal of the American Medical Association, 271,* 1093–1098.

Lean, M. E. J., Powrie, J. K., Anderson, A. S., & Garthwaite, P. H. (1990). Obesity, weight loss and prognosis in Type 2 diabetes. *Diabetic Medicine, 7,* 228–233.

Lee, I., & Paffenbarger, R. S. (1996). Is weight loss hazardous? *Nutrition Reviews, 54,* S116–S124.

Liddle, R. A., Goldstein, R. B, & Saxton, J. (1989). Gallstone formation during weight reduction dieting. *Archives of Internal Medicine, 149,* 1750–1753.

Lissner, L., Odell, P. M., D'Agostino, R. B., Stokes, J., III, Kreger, B. E., Belanger, J. A., & Brownell, K. D. (1991). Variability of body weight and health outcomes in the Framingham population. *New England Journal of Medicine, 324,* 1839–1844.

Long, S. D., O'Brien, K., MacDonald, K. G., Leggett-Frazier, N., Swanson, M. S., Pories, W. J., & Caro, J. F. (1994). Weight loss in severely obese subjects prevents the progression of impaired glucose tolerance to Type II diabetes. *Diabetes Care, 17,* 372–375.

MacDonald, K. G., Long, S. D., Swanson, M. S., Brown, B. M., Morris, P., Dohm, G. L., & Pories, W. J. (1997). The gastric bypass operation reduced the progression and mortality of non-insulin-dependent diabetes mellitus. *Journal of Gastrointestinal Surgery, 1,* 213–220.

Maggio, C. A., & Pi-Sunyer, F. X. (1997). The prevention and treatment of obesity: Application to Type 2 diabetes. *Diabetes Care, 20,* 1744–1766.

Marton, K. I., Sox, H. C., & Krupp, J. R. (1981). Involuntary weight loss: Diagnostic and prognostic significance. *Annals of Internal Medicine, 95,* 568–574.

McGuire, M. T., Wing, R. R., & Hill, J. O. (2000). The prevalence of weight loss maintenance among American adults. *International Journal of Obesity, 23,* 1314–1319.

McGuire, M. T., Wing, R. R., Klem, M. L., & Hill, J. O. (1999). The behavioral characteristics of individuals who lose weight unintentionally. *Obesity Research, 7,* 485–490.

McMahon, S., Cutler, J., Brittain, E., & Higgins, M. (1987). Obesity and hypertension: epidemiological and clinical issues. *European Heart Journal, 150,* 153–162.

Meltzer, A. A., & Everhart, J. E. (1995). Unintentional weight loss in the United States. *American Journal of Epidemiology, 142,* 1039–1046.

Meltzer, A. A., & Everhart, J. E. (1996). Correlations with self-reported weight loss in overweight U. S. adults. *Obesity Research, 4,* 479–486.

National Institutes of Health Consensus Development Panel on the Health Implications of Obesity. (1985). Health implications of obesity: National Institutes of Health Consensus Development Conference statement. *Annals of Internal Medicine, 103,* 1073–1077.

National Task Force on the Prevention and Treatment of Obesity. (1994). Weight cycling. *Journal of the American Medical Association, 272,* 1196–1202.

Pan, X., Li, G.-W., Hu, Y.-H., Wang, J.-X., Yang, W.-Y., An Z.-X., Hu, Z.-X., Lin, J., Xiao, J.-Z., Cao, H.-B., Liu, P.-A., Jiang, X.-G., Jiang, Y.-Y., Wang, J.-P., Zheng, H., Zhang, H., Bennett, P. H., & Howard, B. V. (1997). Effects of diet and exercise in preventing NIDDM in people with impaired glucose tolerance. *Diabetes Care, 20,* 537–544.

Pi-Sunyer, F. X. (1993a). Medical hazards of obesity. *Annals of Internal Medicine, 119*(7, Pt. 2), 655–660.

Pi-Sunyer, F. X. (1993b). Short-term medical benefits and adverse effects of weight loss. *Annals of Internal Medicine, 119*(7, Pt. 2), 722–726.

Pories, W. J., Swanson, M. S., MacDonald, K. G., Long, S. B., Morris, P. G., Brown, B. M., Barakat, H. A., deRamon, R. A., Israel, G., Dolezal, J. M., & Dohm, L. (1995). Who would have thought it? An operation proves to be the most effective therapy for adult-onset diabetes mellitus. *Annals of Surgery, 3,* 339–352.

Ornish, D., Brown, S. E., Scherwitz, L. W., Billings, J. H., Armstrong, W. T., Ports, T. A., McLanahan, S. M., Kirkeeide, R. L., Brand, R. J., & Gould, K. L. (1990). Can lifestyle changes reverse coronary heart disease? *Lancet, 336,* 129–133.

Ornish, D., Scherwitz, L. W., Billings, J. H., Gould, K. L., Merritt, T. A., Sparler, S., Armstrong, W.

8

Psychosocial Consequences of Obesity and Weight Loss

THOMAS A. WADDEN
LESLIE G. WOMBLE
ALBERT J. STUNKARD
DREW A. ANDERSON

Stereotypes about obesity abound. This is particularly true concerning psychological characteristics attributed to obese persons and to the effects of weight loss. In many cases, popular views are contradictory. Overweight individuals are frequently portrayed as jolly, but equally often as depressed or anxious. Advertisements picture dieters as brimming with self-confidence, energy, and sex appeal, while some researchers contend instead that they are vulnerable to binge eating, irritability, and emotional distress.

This chapter reviews empirical studies of the psychosocial consequences of obesity and weight loss. Studies are described under four general categories: (1) the prejudice and discrimination to which obese individuals are subjected; (2) the effects of this hostile environment on their psychological functioning; (3) the behavioral and psychosocial effects of dieting and weight loss; and (4) the consequences of the all-too-frequent occurrence of weight loss and regain (i.e., weight cycling).

PREJUDICE AND DISCRIMINATION AGAINST OBESE INDIVIDUALS

Prejudice

History shows that prejudice against obese individuals is not simply a product of society's current worship of a thin ideal. As early as the 12th century, Buddhists stigmatized obesity as the karmic consequence of moral failing (Stunkard, LaFleur, & Wadden, 1998). In the Christian culture, gluttony was considered one of the seven deadly sins, and Adam was labeled a glutton for eating the apple (Stunkard et al., 1998). Today obesity is known to have a significant genetic component; yet disparagement of overweight and obese individuals persists as what Sobal and Stunkard (1989) have called "the last socially acceptable form of prejudice" (p. 417).

Such prejudice has been observed in children as young as 6 years of age, who labeled silhouettes of an overweight child as "lazy, dirty, stupid, ugly, cheats, and lies" (Staffieri, 1967). When shown black-and-white line drawings of an obese child and children with various handicaps, including missing hands and facial disfigurement, both children and adults rated the obese child as the one with whom they least wished to play (Goodman, Dornbusch, Richardson, & Hastorf, 1963; Richardson, Goodman, Hastorf, & Dornbusch, 1961). In a similar study, college students rated embezzlers, cocaine users, shoplifters, and blind people as more suitable marriage partners than obese individuals (Venes, Krupka, & Gerard, 1982). Almost all obese and overweight adolescent girls in one sample reported having been verbally abused (Neumark-Sztainer, Story, & Faibisch, 1998). Prejudice against the obese extends to health care professionals. Numerous studies have reported that physicians have negative attitudes toward obesity (Harris, Hamaday, & Mochan, 1999; Maddox, Back, & Liederman, 1968; Maddox & Liederman, 1969; Olson, Schumaker, & Yawn, 1994; Rand & Macgregor, 1990).

Discrimination

Prejudice against obese individuals is associated with discrimination that affects virtually every domain of life. An exemplary study by Gortmaker, Must, Perrin, Sobol, and Dietz (1993) followed 10,039 overweight and normal-weight adolescents for 7 years. At the end of this time, overweight females had completed significantly fewer months of school, were less likely to be married, and had lower household incomes than nonoverweight females, despite comparable intellectual aptitudes. Overweight males were less likely to be married than were their nonoverweight peers. By contrast, people with other chronic conditions such as asthma, rheumatoid arthritis, and cerebral palsy did not differ from the nonoverweight participants on any of these outcomes. Other studies similarly found that obese individuals had lower acceptance rates into prestigious colleges than nonobese students did, despite comparable scholastic performance in the two groups (Canning & Mayer, 1966; Pargaman, 1969).

Studies from the 1960s and 1970s found evidence of weight-related discrimination in the workplace. Sixteen percent of employers interviewed by Roe and Eichwort (1976) reported that they would not hire obese individuals under any conditions, and an additional 44% would hire them only under special circumstances. A study in 1974, when salaries were lower, revealed that only 9% of executives who earned $25,000–$50,000 were more than 10 pounds overweight, whereas 39% of those earning $10,000–$20,000 were similarly overweight ("Fat Execs Get Slimmer Paychecks," 1974). The authors of this study calculated that each pound of fat cost an executive $1,000 per year.

More recent laboratory studies, which have experimentally manipulated job applicants' perceived weights, have found a strong bias against obese individuals in almost every stage of employment—selection, placement, compensation, promotion, discipline, and discharge (Frieze, Olson, & Good, 1990; Roehling, 1999). This bias seems to be more pronounced for women than for men. A study, for example, by Pingitore, Dugoni, Tindale, and Spring (1994) asked participants to rate videotaped job interviews of actors who appeared to be of normal weight or were made up to look overweight. The applicant's apparent weight was the strongest determinant of the hiring decision, accounting for 35% of the variance. The same applicant, when made to look overweight, was selected significantly less often than when he or she appeared to be of average weight. This bias was stronger against overweight-appearing women than against such men.

Field studies, which usually involve national samples of self-reported survey data, have yielded similar but less consistent results (Roehling, 1999). A longitudinal survey by Averett and Korenman (1996) found that the wages of obese European American women were lower than those of their average-weight peers. This effect was not found in African American females. By contrast, among overweight and underweight men, there was weaker and less consistent evidence of a wage penalty.

Despite evidence of discrimination against obese persons in the workplace, regrettably, such practice does not appear to violate current federal law (Roehling, 1999). Title VII, which safeguards employees from discrimination, does not designate obesity as a protected characteristic. Under Title VII, disparate treatment occurs when an employer treats people differently because of race, color, religion, sex, or national origin. In a few cases, obese individuals have prevailed when their weight was associated with a protected characteristic. In 1982, a court determined that Continental Airlines applied its weight restriction policy only to female employees, and therefore the policy resulted in discrimination based on gender (*Gerdom v. Continental Airlines*, 1982).

Obesity has, in a few instances, been protected as a disability under federal law. To attain this status, a person must be either extremely obese (100% above ideal weight) or obese because of a physiological condition (Roehling, 1999). Because less than 3% of the obese population is extremely obese, this leaves the great majority of obese individuals vulnerable to discrimination. Similarly, although obesity is known to be under significant genetic control, only rare circumstances (such as absolute leptin deficiency or Cushing's disease) would allow a practitioner to attribute a patient's obesity 100% to a physiological condition.

Studies clearly demonstrate that obese people bear overt discrimination and prejudice in today's society. However, despite the preponderance of evidence, this discrimination is rarely considered illegal according to federal law. Some states and municipalities have passed laws barring discrimination based on weight (Roehling, 1999). We believe that it is time for the federal government to do the same.

PSYCHOSOCIAL STATUS OF OBESE INDIVIDUALS

Given the ubiquitous prejudice and discrimination that obese persons endure, it would not be surprising to discover that they experience greater psychological distress than their nonobese peers. This appears to be the case with individuals who seek weight reduction; distress is probably one of the factors that leads them to seek weight loss. This section reviews the psychosocial status of obese individuals encountered in clinical settings, as well as that of unselected obese individuals from the general population.

Psychosocial Status of Obese Individuals in the General Population

Psychological Functioning

Several early studies found few differences in psychological functioning between obese and nonobese individuals in the general population (Friedman & Brownell, 1995; Stunkard & Wadden, 1992; Wadden & Stunkard, 1985). For example, Moore, Stunkard, and Srole (1962) examined 1,660 people in midtown Manhattan and found that obese individuals scored significantly higher than nonobese persons on only three of nine measures of psychological functioning—immaturity, suspiciousness, and rigidity. Differences between groups on these measures were so small, however, as to be judged clinically insignificant. Stewart and Brook (1983) similarly observed only small differences between obese and nonobese subjects. In a study of 5,817 persons, obese individuals were significantly less depressed and anxious than were their nonobese counterparts. Results of two British studies (Crisp & McGuiness, 1976; Silverstone, 1968) and three European investigations (Hallstrom & Noppa, 1981; Kittel, Rustin, Dramaix, DeBacker, & Kornitzer, 1978; Larsson, 1978) also found few differences in psychological status between obese and nonobese persons in the general population.

The finding of essentially normal psychological functioning in obese individuals is heartening. As reviewed by Friedman and Brownell (1995), however, some of these early investigations had shortcomings that included (1) the study of small convenience samples rather than nationally representative surveys; (2) the use of variable criteria to define overweight and obesity; (3) the often limited assessment of psychological status by paper-and-pencil inventories that did not yield clinical diagnoses; and (4) the failure to include appropriate control groups. Similarly, Wadden and Stunkard (1985) noted that women appeared to be at higher risk than men of emotional complications because of the greater social pressures on females to be thin. Many early studies, however, did not adequately examine gender differences, particularly at the highest weight levels.

At least two studies have addressed these limitations. In a nationally representative sample of 32,000 persons 25–74 years of age, Istvan, Zavela, and Weidner (1992) found a positive (though weak) relation in women between body mass index (BMI) and symptoms of depression, as measured by the Center for Epidemiologic Studies Depression (CES-D) scale (Radloff, 1977). As shown in Figure 8.1, women in the highest BMI quintile who had ever smoked (in the past or present) had significantly higher CES-D total scores than did women of similar smoking status who fell in the lower BMI quintiles. No relationship, however, was found between BMI and CES-D scores in women who had never smoked. Istvan and colleagues (1992) hypothesized that depression in obese women who had ever smoked might have resulted from the failure of smoking to reduce weight, as these women might have expected it to. In contrast to women, no relationship was observed in men between body weight and CES-D scores, regardless of smoking status.

Carpenter, Hasin, Allison, and Faith (2000) used a structured interview to establish a diagnosis of major depression in a nationally representative sample of 40,289 persons. They used criteria comparable to those proposed in the *Diagnostic and Statistical Manual of Mental Disorders,* fourth edition (DSM-IV). They found that obese women, as defined by having a BMI $\geq$ 30 kg/m^2, were 37% more likely to have experienced major depression in the past year than were average-weight women (defined as having a BMI between 20.8 and 29.9 kg/m^2). Obese women also were significantly more likely to report suicidal ideation and suicide attempts (see Table 8.1 for odds ratios). By contrast, in men, obesity was associated with significantly *reduced* risks of major depression and suicide attempts. Being underweight (defined as having a BMI < 20.8 kg/m^2), not obese, was associated with an increased risk of all three adverse events in men.

These last two studies clearly suggest that excess weight has different psychosocial consequences in males and females (in the general population), as reviewed by other investigators (Polivy & Herman, 1985; Striegel-Moore, 1993). Women and teenage girls appear to be particularly vulnerable to symptoms of low self-esteem and depression when they fail, in their own eyes, to measure up to the thin ideal that haunts them on video screens and magazine covers. Their perception that they are overweight, rather than their actual body weight, may well be the more important factor in precipitating emotional complications (Wadden, Foster, Stunkard, & Linowitz, 1989). Women of upper-middle to upper socioeconomic status (SES) would appear to be particularly vulnerable to weight-related distress,

require professional attention, but nonetheless are likely to detract from the individuals' enjoyment of work and leisure activities. Further studies are needed to identify those individuals who are at greatest risk of progressing from decreased quality of life to clinically significant anxiety or depression. As discussed later, our clinical impression is that these individuals are likely to be heavier (i.e., BMI > 40 kg/m^2) and to have more serious health complications.

Psychological Status of Obese Individuals in Clinical Populations

In contrast to population studies, investigations of obese individuals in clinical settings have consistently reported significant psychopathology (Friedman & Brownell, 1995; Stunkard & Wadden, 1992; Wadden & Stunkard, 1985). Reports in the 1950s by psychodynamically oriented psychiatrists described patients' unconscious conflicts and difficulties in establishing intimate relationships, which purportedly resulted in pathological eating and obesity. The 1960s and 1970s witnessed the publication of at least 10 studies that described elevations in obese individuals on the Depression, Hypochondriasis, and Impulsivity scales of the Minnesota Multiphasic Personality Inventory (MMPI; Hathaway & McKinley, 1967) (for a review, see Wadden & Stunkard, 1985). In their review of the literature, Friedman and Brownell (1995) found a moderate effect size (mean d = 0.52) for differences in rates of depression between population controls and obese individuals presenting for treatment.

Wadden and Stunkard (1985) and Friedman and Brownell (1995) noted that these early clinical studies had numerous shortcomings, among which was the failure, reported before, to include appropriate control groups. Increased anxiety and depression, for example, are routinely observed in patients who seek medical care, regardless of their body weight. Swenson, Pearson, and Osborne (1973) administered the MMPI to 18,328 women who underwent general medical or surgical procedures. Mean scores on the Hypochondriasis and Depression scales were 61 and 60, respectively, equal to one standard deviation above the mean. This was the criterion used to define psychopathology in the studies of obese individuals described above. This finding does not diminish the distress experienced by obese individuals who seek weight reduction. It does, however, place it in context; untoward emotional responses to medical conditions are not unique to obese individuals.

One of the most thorough studies of psychopathology was conducted by Fitzgibbon, Stolley, and Kirschenbaum (1993), who examined the psychological status of obese persons who did (n = 57) or did not (n = 57) seek weight reduction, as well as that of nonobese individuals (n = 57) who were not seeking medical care. The obese treatment-seeking patients reported significantly greater symptoms of distress, as measured by the Borderline Symptom Inventory (Conte, Plutchik, Karaus, & Jerrett, 1980), than did either the obese or nonobese individuals who did not seek treatment. These latter two groups did not differ significantly from each other. Obese persons seeking treatment also reported significantly greater psychopathology than nonobese individuals, as assessed by the Symptom Checklist 90 (Derogatis, Lipman, & Covi, 1973), with no other differences between groups.

This study clearly indicates that obese individuals who seek treatment are likely to have higher rates of psychopathology than are obese individuals in the general population. Significant emotional distress (i.e., symptoms of depression or anxiety) is likely to be one of the factors that prompts people to seek professional assistance. In addition to mood disorders, these individuals appear more likely than obese individuals in the general population to suffer from binge-eating disorder (BED) and body image dissatisfaction.

Binge-Eating Disorder

As reviewed by Stunkard in Chapter 6 of this volume, binge eating is characterized by the consumption of an objectively large amount of food in a brief period (i.e., less than 2 hours), during which the individual experiences a subjective loss of control. With BED, overeating is not followed by purging or other compensatory behavior, which distinguishes this condition from bulimia nervosa. BED was originally estimated, by self-report, to occur in approximately 30% of obese individuals who sought treatment (Spitzer et al., 1992, 1993). When diagnosed by expert examiners, however, the prevalence appears to be as low as 10%–15% (Stunkard, Chapter 6, this volume). This reduced rate is still several times greater than that observed in the general population, again suggesting that the presence of BED motivates patients to seek treatment (Spitzer et al., 1992).

Binge eating appears to account for increased rates of depression within the population of obese individuals who seek weight reduction. Several early studies found that patients with severe binge eating, as diagnosed by the Binge Eating Scale (BES; Gormally, Black, Daston, & Rardin, 1982), reported significantly greater symptoms of depression, as measured by the Beck Depression Inventory (BDI; Beck & Steer, 1987), than did obese individuals with moderate or no binge eating. As shown in Table 8.2, the mean BDI scores of patients with severe binge eating, as determined in three studies, ranged from 14.1 to 17.5. These scores are indicative of mild depression and reflect the need for further clinical evaluation. By contrast, the scores of obese individuals without severe binge eating fell in the normal range.

Two of three later studies also found greater depression in patients who were diagnosed with BED, as defined by Spitzer and colleagues (1992). Obese patients with BED studied by Kuehnel and Wadden (1994) and by Mussell, Peterson, and colleagues (1996) scored in the mildly depressed range and at least 5 points higher than obese individuals without BED, who in both studies scored in the normal range. By contrast, patients diagnosed with BED by Brody, Walsh, and Devlin (1994) did not score in the depressed range or even significantly higher than obese patients without BED.

The overwhelming majority of research in this area indicates that, compared to obese persons without BED, obese individuals with BED are more likely to report not only increased symptoms of depression but also lower self-esteem, greater symptoms of borderline personality disorder, and a significantly greater lifetime prevalence of any Axis I disorder,

TABLE 8.2. Mean BDI Scores of Binge-Eating and Non-Binge-Eating Patients as Assessed by Self-Report or Interview

			BDI score	
Study	Method of assessment	n	Binge-eating	Non-binge-eating
Marcus, Wing, & Hopkins (1988)	BES	56	17.5 ± 5.4	7.7 ± 5.2
Telch & Agras (1994)	BES	107	14.1 ± 7.3	10.2 ± 6.0
Wadden, Foster, Letizia, & Wilk (1993)	BES	86	17.0 ± 8.4	7.0 ± 4.7
Brody, Walsh, & Devlin (1994)	QEWP with interview	69	8.7 ± 6.5	7.8 ± 5.1
Kuehnel & Wadden (1994)	QEWP with interview	70	15.5 ± 6.9	8.1 ± 5.3
Mussell, Peterson, et al. (1996)	SCID—Patient Version	128	11.4 ± 7.3	6.1 ± 4.5

Note. QEWP, Questionnaire on Eating and Weight Patterns (Spitzer et al., 1992); SCID, Structured Clinical Interview for DSM-III-R (Spitzer, Williams, Gibbon, & First, 1990); BES, Binge Eating Scale (Gormally, Black, Daston, & Rardin, 1982); BDI, Beck Depression Inventory (BDI; Beck & Steer, 1987).

to pay particular attention to the psychological status of extremely obese individuals. As BMI increases beyond 40 kg/m², these individuals are increasingly likely to experience health complications that limit their functioning at work and at home, and thus precipitate depression or other untoward psychological reactions. Binge eating also appears to be common in these individuals (Hsu, Betancourt, & Sullivan, 1996), and two studies have reported higher-than-expected rates of sexual abuse in persons with extreme obesity (Brewerton, O'Neil, Dansky, & Kilpatrick, 1999; Felitti, 1991). Wadden, Sarwer, Arnold, Gruen, and O'Neil (2000) have described elsewhere the psychological status and assessment of obese individuals who seek bariatric surgery.

PSYCHOSOCIAL EFFECTS OF DIETING AND WEIGHT LOSS

Dieting, the principal treatment for obesity, has been the subject of significant controversy during the past decade, as discussed by Foster and McGuckin in Chapter 24 of this volume. Several critics have charged that "diets don't work," because most people regain their lost weight within 5 years (Garner & Wooley, 1991; Goodrick & Foreyt, 1991). It has also been charged that dieting is associated with adverse emotional responses (e.g., depression) and may precipitate binge eating (Polivy & Herman, 1985). These charges appear to be without merit. In a recent review, the National Task Force on the Prevention and Treatment of Obesity (2000) concluded that dieting in overweight and obese individuals is not associated with adverse psychosocial or behavioral effects. The second half of this chapter briefly examines the data on which these conclusions were based, and also assesses the effects of weight loss on quality of life and body image. The review is limited to weight loss efforts by overweight individuals, not by average-weight teenage girls, who often diet aggressively and unwisely in pursuit of an ever-thinner ideal. Dieting clearly may contribute to eating disorders in these individuals, although it is not a sufficient cause of such complications, as reviewed by Wilson (1993).

The term "dieting," as used here, refers to "the intentional and sustained restriction of caloric intake for the purpose of reducing body weight or changing body shape. The restriction of caloric intake results in significant negative energy balance" (National Task Force, 2000, p. 2582). The effects of dieting on psychological status may differ from those of restrained eating, a separate topic that is not discussed here (Lowe, 1993). Separating the effects of dieting from those of weight loss is also not discussed, since the two usually go hand in hand.

Effects of Dieting on Mood

Concerns that dieting precipitates depression and other adverse emotional reactions resulted from two now classic reports. The first, from Minnesota, was an experiment in which normal-weight male volunteers reduced their initial body weight by 25% during 6 months of marked caloric restriction (Keys, Brozek, Henschel, Mickelsen, & Taylor, 1950). This loss resulted in a body weight lower than that required for a diagnosis of anorexia nervosa (i.e., a weight ≥15% below normal), and the men displayed many of the psychological symptoms of this disorder, including depressed mood, apathy, and preoccupation with food. Findings of this study are frequently used to warn of potential dangers of dieting in obese individuals. These findings, however, are more relevant to the experiences of average-weight teenage girls (who diet aggressively) than they are to obese adults who seek weight reduction.

The second investigation found that 54% of obese patients who were treated in a hospital nutrition clinic reported retrospectively that they had experienced symptoms of weakness, nervousness, irritability, or fatigue at some time when previously dieting (Stunkard, 1957). These individuals did not report symptoms of depression, although the journal article that described these findings was titled "The Dieting Depression." The title was derived from observations of a second group of 25 individuals who were treated on an inpatient unit for both their psychiatric illness and obesity. Other early investigations, reviewed by Stunkard and Rush (1974), also reported negative emotional responses to dieting.

In contrast to these early findings, numerous studies published in the past 25 years have reported reductions in symptoms of depression and anxiety—or, at a minimum, no worsening in affect—in obese patients who lost weight with behavior modification combined with a low-calorie diet (Taylor, Ferguson, & Reading, 1978; Wadden & Stunkard, 1986; Wing, Blair, Marcus, Epstein, & Harvey, 1994; Wing, Marcus, Epstein, & Kupfer, 1983), a very-low-calorie diet (VLCD) (Wadden, Foster, & Letizia, 1994; Wadden & Stunkard, 1986; Wing et al., 1994; Wing, Marcus, Blair, & Burton, 1991), or weight loss medications (Brownell & Stunkard, 1981; Craighead, Stunkard, & O'Brien, 1981; Wadden, Vogt, et al., 1997). Several factors appear to explain the discrepancy between the early and later findings. Reports in the 1950s and 1960s were based principally on patients who had been referred to psychiatrists and were thus more likely to have had significant emotional disturbance prior to weight loss (Smoller, Wadden, & Stunkard, 1987; Wing, Epstein, Marcus, & Kupfer, 1984). By contrast, more recent investigations, since 1975, have included obese individuals who volunteered specifically for weight reduction; a majority of these individuals are known to be free of clinically significant depression (Telch & Agras, 1994). In addition, most patients in the more recent studies received both group support and cognitive-behavioral therapy, each of which may favorably influence mood (Smoller et al., 1987; Wing et al., 1984). A review by Smoller and colleagues (1987), showed that studies that included patients who were treated in behaviorally or medically oriented programs reported uniformly favorable changes in mood, whereas investigations of obese patients who received psychiatric care found uniformly negative outcomes.

The difference in findings may also reflect differences in the frequency with which mood was assessed. Behavioral studies typically evaluated mood only before and after treatment—an assessment that may capture primarily the positive effects of losing weight, which often include looking and feeling better, receiving compliments from family and friends, or being able to wear fashionable clothing (Smoller et al., 1987; Wadden, Stunkard, & Smoller, 1986). More frequent assessment, as included in early studies, may detect daily stresses and strains of dieting, which may include feeling hungry, having to monitor food intake, or missing out on food-related celebrations. A pilot study revealed partial support for this hypothesis (Wadden et al., 1986): A handful of patients reported clinically significant increases in dysphoria at some point while dieting, but mean depression scores were significantly below baseline at the end of the 26-week weight loss program. Smoller and colleagues (1987) identified other methodological factors that appeared to account for the differences reported in early and later studies.

Clinical Issues

The vast majority of findings indicate that obese individuals who lose weight are likely to experience improvements in mood. Improvements, however, are generally modest. As discussed previously, obese individuals who do not binge-eat usually score in the nondepressed range on the BDI and similar inventories. With weight loss they report even fewer symptoms of dysphoria, but such changes are probably not of clinical significance, given the normal baseline levels. Larger reductions in depression are likely to be observed in obese indi-

In contrast to these findings, Telch and Agras (1993) reported an increase in binge eating after 12 weeks' consumption of a liquid VLCD. Nearly 60% of patients who at baseline had been classified as not binge-eating, reported occasional binge episodes in the 9 months following consumption of the VLCD. At a final assessment, 12 months after severe caloric restriction, 15% of these individuals met criteria for BED. (Surprisingly, 39% of patients who met criteria for BED before treatment no longer did so at the final assessment.) These findings are cause for concern, but must be interpreted cautiously. Except for the baseline and final assessments, all measurements of binge eating were based on patients' self-reports, which are likely to overestimate the occurrence of binge episodes (see Stunkard, Chapter 6, this volume). This finding underscores the need to use uniform criteria in assessing binge eating.

Data on the relationship between severe caloric restriction and binge eating are contradictory, and thus cannot provide definitive clinical guidance. Smith and Wing (1991), for example, found no greater rate of reported dietary lapses in patients treated by moderate versus severe caloric restriction. In addition, patients with BED generally lose as much weight on a VLCD as those who are free of this disorder (LaPorte, 1992; Telch & Agras, 1993; Wadden, Foster, & Letizia, 1992; Yanovski et al., 1994). Prudence, however, suggests not prescribing VLCDs to patients with a history of BED or bulimia nervosa. Moreover, our research team has obtained excellent weight losses with the use of a 925–1,000 kcal/day diet that combines four servings a day of a nutritional supplement with an evening meal of a frozen food entree (Wadden, Vogt, et al., 1997). Patients treated by this diet reported few worries about resuming consumption of conventional foods after the period of marked caloric restriction. This is often a period of high anxiety when a traditional liquid VLCD is used (Wadden & Bartlett, 1992).

Bariatric Surgery

Concerns have also been expressed that surgical procedures for obesity, including vertical banded gastroplasty and gastric bypass, may precipitate eating disorders. Postoperative vomiting is a direct, involuntary consequence of gastric restriction and serves as a stimulus to reduce the amount consumed, as well as the consumption of certain items (e.g., steak) (Kral, 1998; Sugerman et al., 1992). Although it is aversive to patients, such vomiting is not comparable to that observed with bulimia nervosa or anorexia nervosa, in which patients report losing control of their food intake and then intentionally purging to prevent feared weight gain.

Three studies found that approximately 25%–47% of patients reported binge eating twice weekly or more before surgery (Adami, Gandolfo, Bauer, & Scopinaro, 1995; Hsu, et al., 1996; Kalarchian, Wilson, Brolin, & Bradley, 1998). Hsu and colleagues (1996), for example, estimated that 37% of their patients met criteria for BED preoperatively. After surgery, none of their patients reported eating an unusually large amount of food in a discrete period of time, because their reduced stomach capacity prevented such overeating. Thus surgery appeared to ameliorate excessive eating, although 20% of patients still reported subjective loss of control of their food intake, as they did prior to surgery. The few data available do not indicate that bariatric surgery is associated with the precipitation or exacerbation of eating disorders, although further study is required.

Effects of Weight Loss on Body Image

Several studies have reported improvements in body image in obese individuals who lost weight with behavioral treatment (Cash, 1994; Foster, Wadden, & Vogt, 1997; Rosen,

Orosan, & Reiter, 1995), as well as with bariatric surgery (Adami et al., 1998). Foster, Wadden, and Vogt (1997), for example, found that patients' scores on the Appearance Evaluation and Body Areas Satisfaction scales of the Multidimensional Body–Self Relations Questionnaire (Brown, Cash, & Mikulka, 1990) increased by a full standard deviation, bringing values to "normal." Surprisingly, larger losses were not associated with greater improvements in body image.

This finding suggests the possibility of a weight loss threshold: Small losses may yield substantial improvements in body image, but no further improvements may occur with additional weight reduction. Alternatively, the finding suggests that factors other than weight (or weight loss), such as self-esteem or attributional style, may affect changes in body image. Rosen and colleagues (1995), for example, found that a cognitive-behavioral intervention that was designed to modify negative weight-related thoughts, but did not induce weight loss, produced significant improvements in body image—comparable to those produced by weight reduction.

Studies have also shown that body image dissatisfaction may persist despite weight loss. Cash and colleagues (1990) compared body dissatisfaction in normal-weight women without a history of obesity, currently normal-weight women with a history of obesity, and women who were currently overweight. Obese women reported a stronger drive for thinness, more negative body image affect (associated with weight and overall appearance), more discrepant weight ideals, and higher anxiety while being weighed than did nonobese women without a history of obesity. However, normal-weight women with a history of obesity, compared with those without such a history, also reported significantly higher levels of body dissatisfaction, greater anxiety while being weighed, and a larger discrepancy between their current and ideal weights.

Adami and colleagues (1995) found that age of onset of obesity was a critical determinant of changes in body image satisfaction following bariatric surgery. After weight loss, the body image of individuals with adult-onset obesity did not differ from that of normal-weight controls. In contrast, those with early-onset obesity were significantly less satisfied with their weight and shape than were those with adult-onset obesity and normal-weight controls. The authors argued, similar to Stunkard and Mendelson (1961), that body image crystallizes during childhood and adolescence, and that persons with early-onset obesity may retain a negative internalized body image despite the reduction in their BMI to normal levels.

Effects of Weight Loss in Extremely Obese Individuals

Improvements in Mood

The most dramatic improvements in psychosocial functioning are likely to be observed in extremely obese individuals who undergo bariatric surgery. This is because, prior to surgery, they generally experience the most adverse psychosocial and physical consequences of obesity; thus they have the greatest potential for improvement. Solow, Siberfarg, and Swift (1974) described very favorable changes in their patients following bariatric surgery:

> Previously housebound patients began to go out shopping; several took up athletic activities, and one even developed an enthusiasm for motorcycling. . . . A virtuous circle seemed operating here: as social withdrawal declined and social contacts developed, patients experienced novel positive feedback. Rather than feeling themselves objects of ridicule and contempt, they came to appreciate the respect and positive regard shown them. (p. 301)

Positive changes in mood have been reported by others (Powers, Rosemurgy, Boyd, & Perez, 1997; Stunkard, Stinnett, & Smoller, 1986; Waters et al., 1991). As shown in Figure 8.3, sur-

Wing, Jakicic, Butler, & Marcus, 1996; Wadden, Bartlett, et al., 1992). The studies consistently found no significant differences in depression between subjects with and without a history of weight cycling. These investigations have been criticized because they did not assess differences in mood prior to weight loss and because they used varying definitions of weight cycling (Foster, Sarwer, & Wadden, 1997; Friedman, Schwartz, & Brownell, 1998). However, several prospective studies that followed patients through a cycle of weight loss and regain also failed to find adverse effects of weight cycling on mood (Brownell & Stunkard, 1981; Foster et al., 1996; Wadden, Sternberg, et al., 1989). The most thorough study, which examined patients who lost and regained 21.9 kg over a period of approximately 4 years, observed a mean BDI score of 9.3 at follow-up, compared with a score of 12.7 at baseline (Foster et al., 1996).

Taken together, the results of cross-sectional and longitudinal studies indicate that weight cycling is not associated with clinically significant depression. It would be a mistake, however, to conclude that weight cycling does not have adverse emotional consequences. Patients evaluated by Wadden, Stunkard, and Liebschutz (1988) reported that weight regain had a moderately to very negative effect on their satisfaction with appearance, self-esteem, and self-confidence. Weight cycling may affect dimensions of personal experience that simply are not assessed by standard depression scales. The generally positive findings reported here should not lead practitioners to minimize the shame and distress that so many patients report concerning their failed efforts to control their weight.

Relation of Weight Cycling to Binge Eating

Cross-sectional studies have consistently found a positive relationship between weight cycling and binge eating (Bartlett et al., 1996; Spitzer et al., 1992; Venditti et al., 1996; Yanovski & Sebring, 1994). Thus the greater the number of weight loss efforts, the greater the likelihood (or severity) of binge eating. These studies, however, cannot address the casual relation between these two variables. Rather than weight cycling causing binge eating, it is possible that binge eating leads to obesity, which is followed by efforts to lose weight and later to weight regain. In a thorough longitudinal investigation of this issue, Foster and colleagues (1996) observed reductions, rather than increases, in symptoms of binge eating in women who lost and regained 21.6 kg. Moreover, patients reported reductions in dietary disinhibition.

Clinical Implications of Findings

Taken as a whole, the literature indicates that neither dieting nor weight cycling has serious adverse effects on the psychosocial functioning or eating habits of the great majority of overweight and obese individuals. Given the clear adverse health effects of excess weight, we do not believe that obese individuals should be dissauded from trying to lose weight because of fears of negative behavioral consequences. There is, however, a clear and pressing need to identify new treatments that will confer long-term weight control, and thus spare obese individuals from the frustration and dismay that accompany weight cycling.

SUMMARY AND CONCLUSIONS

Obesity is an exceptionally heterogeneous disorder in terms of its etiology, physical and behavioral presentation, and association with adverse health events. This heterogeneity is particularly evident when one considers the psychosocial status of overweight and obese individuals. The great majority of these persons appear to have essentially normal psychological functioning, despite their daily exposure to weight-related prejudice and discrimination in a society that glorifies thinness. Among persons encountered in clinical settings, approximately 10%–20% are likely to suffer from clinically significant symptoms of depression, negative body image, or impaired health-related quality of life. Such problems are most likely to occur in women (particularly from higher SES levels), in those with BED, and in those with extreme obesity (i.e., BMI $\geq$ 40 kg/m^2) and its attendant health complications. Thus practitioners should be particularly sensitive to the emotional well-being of obese women who present with any of these additional risk factors.

Practitioners, however, must balance the need for attentiveness with the equally important need not to stereotype their obese patients—not to attribute psychopathology or other shortcomings to them. The most satisfactory approach is to encourage patients to tell their own stories concerning how weight has affected their lives. Most welcome this opportunity. More often than not, we are impressed not by patients' emotional problems but by their resilient spirit and tenacious efforts to control their weight. These are the very qualities that should guide practitioners' care of their patients.

REFERENCES

Adami, G. F., Gandolfo, P., Bauer, B., & Scopinaro, N. (1995). Binge eating in massively obese patients undergoing bariatric surgery. *International Journal of Eating Disorders, 17,* 45–50.

Adami, G. F., Gandolfo, P., Campostano, A., Meneghelli, A., Ravera, G., & Scopinaro, N. (1998). Body image and body weight in obese patients. *International Journal of Eating Disorders, 24,* 299–306.

Agras, W. S., Telch, C. F., Arnow, B., Eldredge, K. L., Wilfley, D., Raeburn, S. D., Henderson, J., & Marnell, M. (1994). Weight loss, cognitive-behavioral, and desipramine treatments in binge eating disorder: An additive design. *Behavior Therapy, 25,* 225–238.

American Psychiatric Association. (1994). *Diagnostic and statistical manual of mental disorders* (4th ed.). Washington, DC: Author.

Averett, S., & Korenman, S. (1996). The economic reality of the beauty myth. *Journal of Human Resources, 31,* 304–329.

Barofsky, I., Fontaine, K. R., & Cheskin, L. J. (1998). Pain in the obese: Impact on health-related quality of life. *Annals of Behavioral Medicine, 19,* 408–410.

Bartlett, S. J., Wadden, T. A., & Vogt, R. A. (1996). Psychosocial consequences of weight cycling. *Journal of Consulting and Clinical Psychology, 64,* 587–892.

Beck, A. T., & Steer, R. A. (1987). *Manual for the Beck Depression Inventory.* New York: Psychological Corporation.

Berkowitz, R. I., Stunkard, A. J., & Stallings, V. A. (1993). Binge eating disorder in obese adolescent girls. *Annals of the New York Academy of Sciences, 699,* 200–296.

Brewerton, T. D., O'Neil, P. M., Dansky, B. S., & Kilpatrick, D. G. (1999). Links between morbid obesity, victimization, PTSD, major depression, and bulimia in a national sample of women. *Obesity Research, 7*(Suppl.), 56S.

Brody, M. L., Walsh, T., & Devlin, M. J. (1994). Binge eating disorder: Reliability and validity of a new diagnostic category. *Journal of Consulting and Clinical Psychology, 62,* 381–386.

Brown, T. A., Cash, T. F., & Mikulka, P. J. (1990). Attitudinal body image assessment: Factor analysis of the Body–Self Relations Questionnaire. *Journal of Personality Assessment, 55,* 135–144.

Brownell, K. D., & Stunkard, A. J. (1981). Couples training, pharmacotherapy, and behavior therapy in the treatment of obesity. *Archives of General Psychiatry, 38,* 1224–1232.

Brownell, K. D., & Wadden, T. A. (1991). The heterogeneity of obesity: Fitting treatments to individuals. *Behavior Therapy, 22,* 153–177.

Canning, H., & Mayer, J. (1966). Obesity: Its possible effects on college admissions. *New England Journal of Medicine, 275,* 1172–1174.

Lean, M. E., Han, T. S., & Seidell, J. C. (1999). Impairment of health and quality of life using new US federal guidelines for the identification of obesity. *Archives of Internal Medicine, 159,* 837–843.

LePen, C., Levy, E., Loos, F., Banzet, M. N., & Basdevant, A. (1998). "Specific" scale compared with "generic" scale: A double measurement of the quality of life in a French community sample of obese subjects. *Journal of Epidemiology and Community Health, 52,* 445–450.

Lowe, M. R. (1993). The effects of dieting on eating behavior: A three-factor model. *Psychological Bulletin, 114,* 100–121.

Maddox, G. L., Back, K., & Liederman, V. (1968). Overweight as social deviance and disability. *Journal of Health and Social Behavior, 9,* 287–298.

Maddox, G. L., & Liederman, V. (1969). Overweight as a social disability with medical implications. *Journal of Medical Education, 44,* 214–220.

Manson, J. E., Willett, W. C., Stampfer, M. J., Colditz, G. A., Hankinson, C. H., & Speizer, F. E. (1995). Body weight and mortality among women. *New England Journal of Medicine, 333,* 677–685.

Marcus, M. D., Wing, R. R., & Fairburn, C. G. (1995). Cognitive treatment of binge eating v. behavioral weight control in the treatment of binge eating disorder [Abstract]. *Annals of Behavioral Medicine, 17,* S090.

Marcus, M. D., Wing, R. R., & Hopkins, J. (1988). Obese binge eaters: Affect, cognitions, and response to behavioral weight control. *Journal of Consulting and Clinical Psychology, 56,* 433–439.

Moore, M. E., Stunkard, A. J., & Srole, L. (1962). Obesity, social class and mental illness. *Journal of the American Medical Association, 181,* 962–966.

Mussell, M. P., Mitchell, J. E., de Zwaan, M., Crosby, R. D., Seim, H. C., & Crow, S. J. (1996). Clinical characteristics associated with binge eating in obese females: A descriptive study. *International Journal of Obesity, 20,* 324–331.

Mussell, M. P., Peterson, C. B., Weller, C. L., Crosby, R. D., de Zwann, M., & Mitchell, J. E. (1996). Differences in body image and depression among obese women with and without binge eating disorder. *Obesity Research, 4,* 431–439.

National Task Force on the Prevention and Treatment of Obesity. (2000). Dieting and the development of eating disorders in overweight and obese adults. *Archives of Internal Medicine, 160,* 2581–2589.

Neumark-Sztainer, D., Story, M., & Fabisch, L. (1998). Perceived stigmatization among overweight African American and Caucasian adolescent girls. *Journal of Adolescent Health, 23,* 264–270.

Olson, C. L., Schumaker, H. D., & Yawn, B. P. (1994). Overweight women delay medical care. *Archives of Family Medicine, 10,* 888–892.

O'Neill, M. (1990, April 1). Dieters, craving balance, are battling fears of food. *The New York Times,* p. 1.

Pargaman, D. (1969). The incidence of obesity among college students. *Journal of School Health, 29,* 621–625.

Pingitore, R., Dugoni, B. L., Tindale, R. S., & Spring, B. (1994). Bias against overweight job applicants in a simulated employment interview. *Journal of Applied Psychology, 79,* 909–917.

Polivy, J., & Herman, C. P. (1985). Dieting and binging: A causal analysis. *American Psychologist, 40,* 193–201.

Porzelius, L. K., Houston, C., Smith, M., Arfkin, C., & Fisher, E. (1995). Comparison of standard behavioral weight loss treatment and a binge eating weight loss treatment. *Behavior Therapy, 26,* 199–134.

Powers, P. S., Rosemurgy, A., Boyd, F., & Perez, A. (1997). Outcome of gastric restriction procedures: Weight, psychiatric diagnoses, and satisfaction. *Obesity Surgery, 7,* 471–477.

Radloff, S. (1977). The CES-D scale: A self-report depression scale for research in the general population. *Application for Psychological Measurement, 1,* 385–401.

Rand, C. S. W., Kowalske, K., & Kuldau, J. M. (1984). Characteristics of marital improvement following obesity surgery. *Psychosomatics, 25,* 221–226.

Rand, C. S. W., & Macgregor, A. M. C. (1990). Morbidly obese patients' perceptions of social discrimination before and after surgery for obesity. *Southern Medical Journal, 83,* 1390–1395.

Richardson, S. A., Goodman, N., Hastorf, A. H., & Dornbusch, S. M. (1961). Cultural uniformity in reaction to physical disabilities. *American Sociological Review, 26,* 241–247.

Rippe, J. M., Price, J. M., Hess, S. A., Kline, G., DeMers, K. A., Damitz, S., Kreidieh, I., & Freedson, P. (1998). Improved psychological well-being, quality of life, and health practices in moderately overweight women. *Obesity Research, 6*(3), 208–218.

Rodin, J. (1993). Cultural and psychosocial determinants of weight concerns. *Annals of Internal Medicine, 119,* 643–645.

Roe, D. A., & Eickwort, K. R. (1976). Relationships between obesity and associated health factors with unemployment among low-income women. *Journal of the American Medical Women's Association, 31,* 193–204.

Roehling, M. V. (1999). Weight-based discrimination in employment: Psychological and legal aspects. *Personnel Psychology, 52,* 969–1016.

Rosen, J. C., Orosan, P., & Reiter, J. (1995). Cognitive behavior therapy for negative body image in obese women. *Behavior Therapy, 26,* 25–42.

Rosen, J. C., & Reiter, J. (1996). Development of the Body Dysmorphic Disorder Examination. *Behaviour Research and Therapy, 34,* 755–766.

Rosenberg, M. (1965). *Society and the adolescent self-image.* Princeton, NJ: Princeton University Press.

Sarwer, D. B., Wadden, T. A., & Foster, G. D. (1998). Assessment of body image dissatisfaction in obese women: Specificity, severity, and clinical significance. *Journal of Consulting and Clinical Psychology, 66,* 651–654.

Seligman, M. E. P., & Csikszentmihalyi, M. (2000). Positive psychology. *American Psychologist, 55,* 5–14.

Sherwood, N. E., Jeffery, R. W., & Wing, R. R. (1999). Binge status as a predictor of weight loss treatment outcome. *International Journal of Obesity, 23,* 485–493.

Silverstone, J. T. (1968). Psychosocial aspects of obesity. *Proceedings of the Royal Society of Medicine, 61,* 371–375.

Smith, D. E., & Wing, R. R. (1991). Diminished weight loss and behavioral compliance during repeated diets in obese patients with type II diabetes. *Health Psychology, 10,* 378–383.

Smoller, J. W., Wadden, T. A., & Stunkard, A. J. (1987). Dieting and depression: A critical review. *Journal of Psychosomatic Research, 31,* 429–440.

Sobal, J., & Stunkard, A. J. (1989). Socioeconomic status and obesity: A review of the literature. *Psychological Bulletin, 105,* 260–275.

Solow, C., Silberfarg, P. M., & Swift, K. (1974). Psychological effects of intestinal bypass surgery for severe obesity. *New England Journal of Medicine, 290,* 300–303.

Specker, S., de Zwann, M., Raymond, N., & Mitchell, J. (1994). Psychopathology in subgroups of obese women with and without binge eating disorder. *Comprehensive Psychiatry, 35,* 185–190.

Spitzer, R. L., Devlin, M., Walsh, B. T., Hasin, D., Wing, R. R., Marcus, M. D., Stunkard, A., Wadden, T., Yanovski, S., Agras, W. S., Mitchell, J., & Nonas, C. (1992). Binge eating disorder: A multisite field trial of the diagnostic criteria. *International Journal of Eating Disorders, 12,* 191–203.

Spitzer, R. L., Williams, S. B. W., Gibbon, M., & First, M. (1990). *Structured Clinical Interview for DSM-III-R: Patient edition* (SCID-P, Version 1. 0). Washington, DC: American Psychiatric Press.

Spitzer, R. L., Yanovski, S., Wadden, T., Wing, R., Marcus, M. D., Stunkard, A., Devlin, M., Mitchell, J., Hasin, D., & Horne, R. L. (1993). Binge eating disorder: Its further validation in a multisite study. *International Journal of Eating Disorders, 13,* 137–153.

Spurrell, E. B., Wilfley, D. E., Tanofsky, M. B., & Brownell, K. D. (1997). Age of onset for binge eating disorder: Are there different pathways to binge eating? *International Journal of Eating Disorders, 21,* 55–65.

Staffieri, J. R. (1967). A study of social stereotype of body image in children. *Journal of Personality and Social Psychology, 7,* 101–104.

Stewart, A. L., & Brook, R. H. (1983). Effects of being overweight. *American Journal of Public Health, 73,* 171–178.

Striegel-Moore, R. J. (1993). Etiology of binge eating: A developmental perspective. In C. G. Fairburn

PART III

ASSESSMENT OF
THE OBESE ADULT

chapter describes the medical evaluation of obese patients who seek weight reduction. It is aimed at the practicing physician and attempts to provide a logical, stepwise progression in the medical evaluation, with special reference to complications associated with obesity. These complications may be overlooked in an examination that is not focused on obesity.

HISTORY OF THE PATIENT'S OBESITY

A thorough history is the most important part of the initial evaluation. This includes both the usual medical history and an evaluation of obesity-specific factors. Since obesity is the chief complaint, it is necessary to take a history of the patient's development of this disorder.

Onset and Progression of Obesity

The clinician should ask when the patient first become overweight or obese, and whether there were any events that might be implicated in the etiology, as discussed below. Changes in body weight over time, with weights at such milestones as puberty, high school or college graduation, pregnancy, or menopause, may give clues about the etiology. It is important to record the lifetime maximum weight, because if the patient is significantly below that weight, it may indicate that he or she is engaging in restrained eating and is maintaining a weight below the level that the body defends (i.e., the body weight set point). This may have implications for treatment, as described below. A history of events surrounding rapid weight gain or loss should be elicited. For females, prepregnancy weight and weight 6 months after delivery are useful.

Family History of Obesity

A family history of obesity provides an indication of the genetic contribution to the patient's obesity (Bray, 1998b). Also, a family history of complications such as diabetes, hypertension, heart disease, or stroke should prompt a careful evaluation for the presence of these in the patient. A family history of complications mandates educating patients about the signs and symptoms to which they should pay attention. It may also prompt more aggressive initial or long-term therapy.

ASSESSMENT OF THE ETIOLOGIES OF OBESITY

Obesity may have many different etiologies. Decisions on treatment may be influenced by an understanding of the underlying mechanisms in the individual patient.

Endocrine Dysfunction

Endocrine dysfunction is among the most rare causes of obesity, but critically important, because treating the underlying disease may improve or resolve the obesity. The endocrine diseases associated with obesity are as follows:

1. Thyroid disease: Hyperthyroidism and hypothyroidism
2. Syndromes of excess insulin: Insulinoma, nesidioblastosis
3. Cushing's syndrome: Adrenocorticoid excess

4. Polycystic ovary syndrome
5. Hypogonadism
6. Hypothalamic damage or disease
7. Growth hormone deficiency
8. Leptin deficiency or receptor defect
9. Pseudohypoparathyroidism

Failure to diagnose an underlying endocrine disorder may have major implications for health and even survival. Research suggests that obese patients often suffer discrimination from health care professionals (Maddox & Leiderman, 1969; Price, Desmond, Krol, Snyder, & O'Connell, 1987). Physical complaints that in a lean individual might be taken seriously are often ignored in obese patients. Complaints uncommon in obese people, such as documented hypoglycemia, bone fractures in younger individuals, or cold intolerance, may point to insulinoma, Cushing's syndrome, or hypothyroidism.

Genetic Background

Single-gene defects as etiologies of obesity are exceedingly rare, but do occur (Bouchard et al., 1998; Chagnon et al., 2000). Most cases of obesity due to genetic factors are associated with multiple-gene defects or differences (Bouchard et al., 1998; Chagnon et al., 2000). When a clinician is faced with a massively obese patient or an individual who is gaining weight very rapidly, particularly a child, genetic defects should be considered. Several syndromes of obesity are associated with specific findings, such as mental retardation, short stature, small hands and feet, hypogonadism, ophthalmic disorders, and voracious appetite (Bouchard et al., 1998). These include genetic or dysmorphic syndromes (e.g., Prader–Willi, Bardet–Biedl, Ahlstrom, Cohen, and Carpenter syndromes; see Bray, 1998a), as well as endocrine dysfunction sydromes. If there is a suspicion of a genetic disorder or a specific syndrome, referral to a specialist in obesity or pediatric obesity may be indicated. These patients are remarkably difficult to treat, and aggressive therapy, such as drugs or surgery, may be indicated.

Environmental Contributors to Obesity

All obese individuals have had an imbalance in energy intake and expenditure during accumulation of their excess adiposity. Thus either intake has been excessive, or expenditure has been inadequate. Often obese patients will clearly identify their problem as an excessive intake or a very sedentary lifestyle. A careful evaluation of customary diet and physical activity patterns, as described below, may reveal these common causes of excess energy balance. Ethnic or social identity may be associated with particular patterns of food intake or types of foods that enhance the likelihood of developing obesity (Kumanyika, 1987).

A careful evaluation may reveal other factors or events that have contributed to obesity. Some severely obese people, particularly women, give a history of sexual abuse in childhood or adolescence that may have contributed to their weight gain; in such cases, the obesity serves either a protective or a comforting function (Felitti et al., 1998). Patients rarely volunteer this information, so it is important to inquire. Unresolved issues may require referral for psychological or psychiatric counseling.

Few individuals have any knowledge of their mothers' pregnancy histories, but malnutrition during pregnancy is known to produce obesity and other complications in the offspring (Silverman et al., 1998; Stanner et al., 1997; Strauss, 1997). Thus inquiries about this topic may be revealing. Low-birthweight and small-for-gestational-age babies have been shown to have a higher prevalence of obesity in later life (Forsen et al., 2000), so inquiries about birthweight may be helpful. An increased prevalence of obesity after tonsillectomy (Lang, Sebok, & Katona, 1986) validates the anecdotal stories that many patients tell of obesity's starting after a surgical procedure. Similar anecdotes about obesity's beginning after the "flu" or other infection gain credibility with the reports of obesity in animals due to infectious agents (Carter et al., 1983; Dhurandhar et al., 1992; Dhurandhar, 1992, 2000, 2001; Gosztonyi & Ludwig, 1995; Lyons et al., 1982).

ASSESSMENT OF WEIGHT LOSS EFFORTS, DIET, AND PHYSICAL ACTIVITY

The clinician should inquire, for several reasons, about previous weight loss efforts. A history of repeated failure with diet and exercise therapy may be a justification for more aggressive treatment, or may require a more careful history to determine whether the programs were sufficiently comprehensive. My own belief is that past failure in a comprehensive program predicts future failure. It may be necessary to proceed to pharmacological therapy, or even to obesity surgery if the patient qualifies for it. If a particular pharmacological agent has been used unsuccessfully in the past or with only modest effects, this may be an indication to start combination therapy. Other important aspects of past weight loss efforts are the occurrence of any complications, such as gout, gallbladder attack, bulimia, psychological or emotional problems, or other less frequent adverse events.

Current Efforts to Control Body Weight

Often patients are already using weight control methods when they are evaluated by the clinician. It is important to know not only about physician-directed treatments, but particularly about self-treatment with special diets, diet supplements, or over-the-counter (OTC) weight loss aids. A list of the medications the patient takes is obviously needed, but often patients will not volunteer that they are taking OTC preparations unless specifically asked. OTC preparations with substances such as ephedra and caffeine, St. John's wort, or phenyl-propanolamine should not be used with certain weight loss drugs. Some OTC preparations contain diuretics that may promote loss of potassium or magnesium, and may influence the selection of obesity medications or prompt careful attention to cardiac function and electrolyte concentrations. Fad diets that restrict or increase intake of individual nutrients, such as low-carbohydrate diets, high-protein diets, or very-low-calorie diets, need to be evaluated to determine the most appropriate treatment regimen.

Dietary Assessment

Although a physician should be able to obtain at least a cursory diet history, a careful assessment of dietary intake probably is best done by a dietitian. It is useful to have patients keep a 3-day food diary to ascertain their customary intake, but since most individuals underestimate their calorie intake, and particularly their fat intake, these diet records should be interpreted cautiously (Livingstone, 1995). Dietitians have experience in assessing the accuracy of diet records and are valuable colleagues in the treatment of obese patients. The impact of the advent of the Internet on diet analysis programs has not been adequately evaluated. For intelligent and perceptive patients who are computer-literate, such programs may offer another option for obtaining a diet history. Physicians should note the daily intake of fat, protein, and fiber, as these are most often altered in dieting patients. It may be useful to pay particular attention to the consumption of fruits and vegetables, since high intake of these foods is associated with a reduced risk of obesity, heart disease, strokes, and cancer.

Physical Activity Assessment

Several studies have now shown that the level of daily physical activity correlates with body mass index (BMI) in the population and is critical for long-term weight maintenance (Coakley, Rimm, Colditz, Kawachi, & Willett, 1998; McGuire, Wing, Klem, Seagle, & Hill, 1998; Sarlio-Lahteenkorva & Rissanen, 1998; Schoeller, Shay, & Kushner, 1997). Many obese people do not exercise and are not active in their daily lives. The reasons for this are unclear, but Sims and colleagues (1973) noted that overfed volunteers reduced their physical activity as they gained weight, so it is likely that this is a physiological response to increasing adiposity. There are suggestions that obese people are more sensitive to pain than are lean individuals (Pradalier, Dry, Willer, & Boureau, 1980), so perhaps exercise is more uncomfortable.

Questions should be directed not only toward the amount and types of exercise that patients engage in each week, but toward their activities of daily living. Zurlo and colleagues (1992) and Levine, Eberhardt, and Jensen (1999) have shown that spontaneous physical activity or "fidgeting" is a source of significant energy expenditure and varies dramatically among individuals. A history of a very sedentary lifestyle may alter the treatment regimen prescribed.

Since aerobic and resistance exercise produce different effects on body composition (Garrow & Summerbell, 1995; Walberg, 1989), it is useful to obtain a history of the types of exercise in which patients engage. Swimming produces good cardiovascular conditioning, but some studies suggest that it does not produce as much weight loss as does weight-bearing exercise (Garrow & Summerbell, 1995; Gwinup, 1987; Walberg, 1989).

ASSESSMENT OF COMPLICATIONS OF OBESITY

Obesity is associated with numerous health complications, as listed in Table 9.1. Patients may not be aware of these conditions or of their association with obesity. Complications that frequently go unrecognized by a patient are sleep apnea, diabetes mellitus, hypertension, gallbladder disease, gout, and hyperlipidemia. If these conditions are identified, coordination of their treatment with the patient's primary care physician is mandatory. If the condition is already known, the patient may be on medications. Since weight loss reduces or sometimes resolves some of these conditions, medication dose may need to be adjusted. With weight loss, patients may develop hypoglycemia on diabetes medications or hypotension on antihypertensives. Thus frequent assessment of blood glucose by home glucose monitoring and of blood pressure is necessary.

Sleep apnea deserves special mention, since it is common in obese individuals and frequently is not recognized. The major symptoms include morning headache, daytime hypersomnolence, restless sleep, nightmares, nocturnal awakening with dyspnea, and dramatically loud snoring. Family members may give a history of apneic episodes if asked (Guilleminault, 1989; Phillipson, 1993; Schwab, Goldberg, & Pack, 1998). A suspicious history for sleep apnea should prompt consideration of referral to a sleep laboratory for formal evaluation.

Other complications seen commonly in obese people that should be sought are a history of gastroesophageal reflux disease (GERD), urinary incontinence, sexual or reproductive dysfunction, symptoms of gout, and symptoms of the increased intra-abdominal pressure

TABLE 9.1. Complications of Obesity

1. Diabetes mellitus, insulin resistance, hyperinsulinemia	12. Urinary incontinence
2. Hypertension	13. Reproductive dysfunction
3. Dyslipoproteinemia	14. Gout
4. Heart disease: Atherosclerotic disease, congestive heart failure	15. Increased intra-abdominal pressure (IAP) syndrome
5. Cerebrovascular disease	16. Pseudotumor cerebri
6. Lung disease: Sleep apnea, restrictive lung disease	17. Adiposis dolorosa (Dercum's disease)
7. Cancer: Breast, uterus, colon, prostate, renal, others	18. Pregnancy risks: Toxemia, diabetes
8. Gallbladder disease: Stones, infection	19. Surgery risks: Pneumonia, wound infection, thrombophlebitis
9. Degenerative arthritis	20. Psychological and emotional problems
10. Venous stasis and edema	21. Social and economic problems
11. Gastroesophageal reflux disease (GERD)	22. Premature mortality

(IAP) syndrome (Sugerman, Bloomfield, & Saggi, 1999). Sugerman and colleagues have published several studies of morbidly obese people that have documented the presence of increased IAP, which may include symptoms of hypertension, urinary incontinence, GERD, headaches, increased intracranial pressure, and pseudotumor cerebri (Bloomfield, Ridings, Blocher, Marmarou, & Sugerman, 1997; Sugerman, Bloomfield, & Saggi, 1999; Sugarman, Felton, Salvant, Sismanis, & Kellum, 1995; Sugerman, Felton, et al., 1999). IAP responds very well to massive weight loss after gastric bypass surgery, so documentation of its presence is a strong indication for such treatment.

General Medical History

Once the history of obesity and its complications has been obtained, a general medical history, appropriate for all patients, should be taken. The presence of other diseases (such as arthritis, fibromyalgia, neuropathy, and gastrointestinal disorders) may influence the diet, physical activity, or medication regimens prescribed. It is imperative to determine the medications the patient is taking, since there may be drug interactions with obesity drugs. Of particular note are drugs that affect the central nervous system (CNS), since this is the mechanism of action of most obesity drugs. The patient's use of antidepressant medications should be assessed. Fluoxetine and sertraline are associated with weight loss, at least over the short term (Goldstein & Potvin, 1994; Goldstein et al., 1993, 1995; Wadden et al., 1995). It may be useful to switch to these drugs (from the older noradrenergic agents) if the depression can be controlled with their use. Conversely, antidepressants that are selective serotonin reuptake inhibitors or adrenergic stimulating agents may preclude use of some of the obesity drugs, such as sibutramine, phentermine, or other CNS agents.

PHYSICAL EXAMINATION

As with the history, there are features specific to obesity that should be assessed in the course of a complete physical examination.

Anthropometric Measurements

Obesity is an excess of adipose tissue, and virtually all obese people also are overweight. On every patient, but particularly every obese patient, height and weight should be measured.

Patients give inaccurate values for both height and weight, so self-reports are not sufficient. Assessment of body fat is better than simple height and weight, and there are simple to very complicated methods of assessing fat (Pietrobelli, Wang, & Heymsfield, 1998), as discussed later.

Perhaps the most global method of estimating body fat is with the BMI, which is calculated as weight in kilograms divided by height in meters squared. The BMI is highly correlated with measures of body fat and predicts both morbidity and mortality. Figure 9.1 allows determination of BMI, based on the patient's height in inches and weight in pounds.

According to the National Heart, Lung, and Blood Institute (1998; see also Table 18.2 in Aronne, Chapter 18, this volume), a BMI of 18.5–24.9 kg/m² falls in the "normal" range, while persons with a BMI of 25.0–29.9 kg/m² are considered "overweight." "Obesity" begins at a BMI of 30 kg/m², with "extreme obesity" defined as a BMI ≥ 40 kg/m². The

BODY MASS INDEX (BMI) CHART

HEIGHT (inches, meters)

Inches	58	59	60	61	62	63	64	65	66	67	68	69	70	71	72	73	74	75	76
Meters	1.47	1.50	1.52	1.55	1.57	1.60	1.63	1.65	1.68	1.70	1.73	1.75	1.78	1.80	1.83	1.85	1.88	1.91	1.93

Pounds	Kg																		
100	45.5	21	20	20	19	18	18	17	17	16	16	15	15	14	14	14	13	13	13	12
105	47.7	22	21	21	20	19	19	18	18	17	16	16	16	15	15	14	14	14	13	13
110	50.0	23	22	22	21	20	20	19	18	18	17	17	16	16	15	15	15	14	14	13
115	52.3	24	23	23	22	21	20	20	19	19	18	18	17	17	16	16	15	15	14	14
120	54.5	25	24	23	23	22	21	21	20	19	19	18	18	17	17	16	16	15	15	15
125	56.8	26	25	24	24	23	22	22	21	20	20	19	18	18	17	17	17	16	16	15
130	59.1	27	26	25	25	24	23	22	22	21	20	20	19	19	18	18	17	17	10	10
135	61.4	28	27	26	26	25	24	23	23	22	21	21	20	19	19	18	18	17	17	16
140	63.6	29	28	27	27	26	25	24	23	23	22	21	21	20	20	19	19	18	18	17
145	65.9	30	29	28	27	27	26	25	24	23	23	22	21	21	20	19	19	18	18	18
150	68.2	31	30	29	28	27	27	26	25	24	24	23	22	22	21	20	20	19	19	18
155	70.5	32	31	30	29	28	28	27	26	25	24	24	23	22	22	21	20	20	19	19
160	72.7	34	32	31	30	29	28	28	27	26	25	26	24	23	22	22	21	21	20	20
165	75.0	35	33	32	31	30	29	28	28	27	26	25	24	24	23	22	22	21	21	20
170	77.3	36	34	33	32	31	30	29	28	27	27	26	25	24	24	23	22	22	21	21
175	79.5	37	35	34	33	32	31	30	29	28	27	27	26	25	24	24	23	23	22	21
180	81.8	38	36	35	34	33	32	31	30	29	28	27	27	26	25	24	24	23	23	22
185	84.1	39	37	36	35	34	33	32	31	30	29	28	27	27	26	25	24	24	23	23
190	86.4	40	38	37	36	35	34	33	32	31	30	29	28	27	27	26	25	24	24	23
195	88.6	41	39	38	37	36	35	34	33	32	31	30	29	28	27	27	26	25	24	24
200	90.9	42	40	39	38	37	36	34	33	32	31	30	30	29	28	27	26	26	25	24
205	93.2	43	41	40	39	38	36	35	34	33	32	31	30	29	29	28	27	26	26	25
210	95.5	44	43	41	40	38	37	36	35	34	33	32	31	30	29	29	28	27	26	26
215	97.7	45	44	42	41	39	38	37	36	35	34	33	32	31	30	29	28	28	27	26
220	100.0	46	45	44	42	40	39	38	37	36	35	34	33	32	31	30	29	28	28	27
225	102.3	47	46	44	43	41	40	39	38	36	35	34	33	32	31	31	30	29	28	27
230	104.5	48	47	45	44	42	41	40	38	37	36	35	34	33	32	31	30	30	29	28
235	106.6	49	48	46	44	43	42	40	39	38	37	36	35	34	33	32	31	30	29	29
240	109.1	50	49	47	45	44	43	41	40	39	38	37	36	35	34	33	32	31	30	29
245	111.4	51	50	48	46	45	43	42	41	40	38	37	36	35	34	33	32	32	31	30
250	113.6	52	51	49	47	46	44	43	42	40	39	38	37	36	35	34	33	32	31	30
255	115.9	53	52	50	48	47	45	44	43	41	40	39	38	37	36	35	34	33	32	31
260	118.2	54	53	51	49	48	46	45	43	42	41	40	38	37	36	35	34	33	33	32
265	120.5	56	54	52	50	49	47	46	44	43	42	40	39	38	37	36	35	34	33	32
270	122.7	57	55	53	51	49	48	46	45	44	42	41	40	39	38	37	36	35	34	33
275	125.0	58	56	54	52	50	49	47	46	44	43	42	41	40	38	37	36	35	34	34
280	127.3	59	57	55	53	51	50	48	47	45	44	43	41	40	39	38	37	36	35	34
285	129.5	60	58	56	54	52	51	49	48	46	45	43	42	41	40	39	38	37	36	35
290	131.8	61	59	57	55	53	51	50	48	47	46	44	43	42	41	39	38	37	36	35
295	134.1	62	60	58	56	54	52	51	49	48	46	45	44	42	41	40	39	38	37	36
300	136.4	63	61	59	57	55	53	52	50	49	47	46	44	43	42	41	40	39	38	37
305	138.6	64	62	60	58	56	54	52	51	49	48	46	45	44	43	41	40	39	38	37
310	140.9	65	63	61	59	57	55	53	52	50	49	47	46	45	43	42	41	40	39	38
315	143.2	66	64	62	60	58	56	54	53	51	49	48	47	45	44	43	42	41	39	38
320	145.5	67	65	63	61	59	57	55	53	52	50	49	47	46	45	43	42	41	40	39
325	147.7	68	66	64	62	60	58	56	54	53	51	50	48	47	45	44	43	42	41	40

WEIGHT (lb, Kg)

FIGURE 9.1. Guide for calculating body mass index (BMI), with a BMI ≥ 30 kg/m² considered as obesity.

risks of health complications, including Type 2 diabetes, hypertension, and cardiovascular disease, increase with increasing obesity.

In patients with a BMI of 25.0–34.9 kg/m², risk is increased further by the presence of upper-body fat distribution. Upper-body fat is usually indicative of increased abdominal obesity, which is associated with increased morbidity and mortality (Pi-Sunyer, 1993). Body fat distribution may be estimated by the waist circumference, which should be measured at the iliac crest. Upper-body obesity is indicated in men by a waist circumference over 40 inches, and in women by a value over 35 inches.

The waist-to-hip circumferences ratio has fallen out of favor and no longer is recommended as a tool for evaluating morbidity risk. Skinfold thickness may be measured with special calipers, but the accuracy and reproducibility in obese patients, particularly in massively obese individuals, is not adequate.

Specific Evaluation for Obesity-Related Complications

A clinician performing a physical exam on an obese person should pay special attention to certain features. These include the impact of obesity on the patient's ability to walk, sit in a chair, or move about. The exam should proceed from head to toe. First, the fundi should be examined for any evidence of increased intracranial pressure such as blurred disc margins or papilledema, which may be present in the increased intra-abdominal pressure syndrome. The mouth exam may reveal carious teeth due to increased sugar or soft drink consumption, or eroded teeth due to gastric acid exposure with bulimia. Also, the uvula and tonsils should be evaluated to see whether the airway is narrowed, as this may exacerbate sleep apnea. A careful thyroid exam is necessary, since 5% or more of obese people will have an enlarged or nodular thyroid. Wheezing on examination of the lungs may signal obesity-induced asthma.

Obese people are more susceptible to cardiac disease, including arrhythmias, so careful examination of the heart is mandatory (Bray, 1998b). For patients who have been on fenfluramine or dexfenfluramine, assessment of aortic or mitral regurgitation may be revealing. Breast cancer is more common in obese women, so a breast exam should be methodical in covering the four quadrants of each breast (Pi-Sunyer, 1993). Gallbladder disease is much more common in obesity, so evaluation of abdominal pain or discomfort in the right upper quadrant should be performed. Thrombophlebitis is common in obesity, so a calf exam should evaluate for Homan's sign. The presence of stasis changes of the lower legs and any edema should be noted. Edema is present in a large majority of patients with a BMI over 40 kg/m². Since diabetes is common in obesity, evaluation of the legs and feet for infection or skin lesions should be performed (Bray, 1998b; Pi-Sunyer, 1993).

Adiposis dolorosa is an unusual syndrome that occurs in obesity and is almost always missed unless specifically sought (Atkinson, 1982). This syndrome is characterized by pain on palpation of subcutaneous fat. The pain may be very severe, and patients typically have sought increasingly potent analgesics without effect. It often occurs on the trunk, as abdominal pain, flank pain, or occasionally across-the-back pain. Pain in the fat pads around the knees is reportedly common (Atkinson, 1982). I have seen three patients who had surgery or were scheduled for surgery (i.e., laparotomy, gallbladder surgery) and whose symptoms were due to adiposis dolorosa. This syndrome has a dramatic effect on quality of life, and most patients with it are miserable, particularly since their physicians have usually dismissed them as having psychological problems. Adiposis dolorosa responds in a high percentage of cases to intravenous infusions of lidocaine (Petersen & Kastrup, 1987). Relief may be temporary, but with repeated infusions, many patients have permanent resolution. The etiology of this syndrome is unknown.

General Physical Exam

The remaining elements of a general physical exam should be performed in obese individuals to identify other conditions that may have an impact on the treatment regimen selected.

LABORATORY TEST AND ASSESSMENTS OF BODY COMPOSITION

Laboratory Tests

An extensive set of laboratory tests is recommended for the initial evaluation of obese patients, because so many different systems may be affected by obesity. A complete blood count (CBC) documents any anemia, but obese patients with sleep apnea may have polycythemia with an elevated hemoglobin level because of the chronic hypoxemia. A white blood cell differential analysis may uncover smoldering cholecystitis or cellulitis secondary to venous stasis. Electrolytes, calcium, and magnesium should also be checked, because obese people are more prone to cardiac arrhythmias. The presence of hypertension often mandates treatment with diuretics, which may alter results of these tests. Diet restriction, if severe, may also alter results of testing.

Some obese patients have a high alcohol intake, which may alter electrolytes, magnesium, calcium, and phosphorus levels. Liver and renal function may be abnormal in obesity and should be checked. A blood glucose level and a lipid panel are mandatory because of the high frequency of abnormalities in obese individuals. An elevated uric acid level should alert the physician to evaluate the patient for a history of gout and to follow the patient more closely during weight loss for any evidence of an acute attack of gout. Proteinuria, urinary tract infections, and renal cancer may occur in obesity, so a urinalysis is indicated. Because the prevalence of heart disease is more common in obesity, an electrocardiogram is indicated, and if there are any symptoms, consideration should be given to performing a cardiac stress test before instituting an exercise program.

The follow-up laboratory assessment depends on the treatment regimen. Very-low-calorie diets are not often used today, but additional lab tests are indicated in those cases (National Task Force on the Prevention and Treatment of Obesity, 1993). Since obese people, as noted, are at increased risk for diabetes, hypertension, cardiac disease, and gallbladder disease, tests that assess these problems should be performed during weight reduction. Rapid weight loss regimens require more tests, including electrolytes, liver function tests (to assess gallbladder disease), and electrocardiogram rhythm strips. A CBC every 3–6 months to check for anemia in food-restricted obese patients is advisable.

Methods of Assessing Body Composition

Determination of body composition is becoming easier with the introduction of relatively inexpensive bioelectric impedance analysis (BIA) machines (Pietrobelli et al., 1998). BIA may be affected by a variety of factors, such as time from last meal, posture, and perhaps body habitus. Nevertheless, it may be a useful tool with which to follow changes in body composition with weight loss. The cost of dual-energy X-ray absorptiometry and of air displacement is falling with the introduction of these machines into more hospitals. Both give a better estimate of body composition than anthropometric measurements or BIA (Pietrobelli et al., 1998). Underwater weighing is available in some hospitals or research facilities, but is not generally available to the public.

For selected patients at high risk for cardiac or vascular disease and diabetes, measurement of visceral fat may be helpful. Computerized tomography (CT) or magnetic resonance imaging (MRI) scans allow calculation of visceral fat (Pietrobelli et al., 1998). Single-cut CT across the fourth and fifth lumbar vertebrae is becoming a standard method of assessing visceral fat, and is relatively less expensive.

Assessment of Factors that Might Affect Obesity Treatment

It is useful, upon completing the history and physical examination, for the clinician to reflect on the information learned that may affect the weight loss treatment prescribed. This is particularly true if other medical conditions, complications of obesity, or medications that may provoke drug interactions have been identified. Lack of any prior weight loss efforts may favor using less aggressive weight reduction regimens, such as conventional diet and exercise prescriptions. Conversely, repeated failure may prompt use of obesity drugs or surgery with appropriate individuals.

SUMMARY

In summary, obesity is a disease of multiple etiologies. Careful attention to potential pathogenic factors, as well as to the possibility of obesity-related complications, is necessary during the medical evaluation of an obese person. Evaluation for common complications, such as diabetes, hypertension, and cardiac disease, is part of every history and physical examination. Less common conditions, such as sleep apnea, adiposis dolorosa, and increased intra-abdominal pressure syndrome, must be specifically evaluated when one is seeing an obese patient. A wide assortment of laboratory tests may be justified because of the protean nature of the complications of obesity. Finally, specific laboratory tests to assess body fat or components of body fat, such as visceral fat, may be indicated for individual patients.

ACKNOWLEDGMENTS

Preparation of this chapter was supported in part by funds from the Beers–Murphy Clinical Nutrition Center, University of Wisconsin–Madison, and by National Institutes of Health Grants No. R01-DK5227 and No. R01-DK44937.

REFERENCES

Allison, D. B., Fontaine, K. R., Manson, J. E., Stevens, J., & VanItallie, T. B. (1999). Annual deaths attributable to obesity in the United States. *Journal of the American Medical Association, 282*(16), 1530–1538.

Atkinson, R. L. (1982). Intravenous lidocaine for the treatment of intractable pain of adiposis dolorosa. *International Journal of Obesity, 6,* 351–357.

Bloomfield, G. L., Ridings, P. C., Blocher, C. R., Marmarou, A., & Sugerman, H. J. (1997). A proposed relationship between increased intra-abdominal, intrathoracic, and intracranial pressure. *Critical Care Medicine, 25,* 496–503.

Bouchard, C., Perusse, L., Rice, T., & Rao, D. C. (1998). The genetics of human obesity. In G. A. Bray, C. Bouchard, & W. P. T. James (Eds.), *Handbook of obesity* (pp. 157–190). New York: Marcel Dekker.

Bray, G. A. (1998a). Classification and evaluation of the overweight patient. In G. A. Bray, C. Bouchard, & W. P. T. James (Eds.), *Handbook of obesity* (pp. 831–854). New York: Marcel Dekker.

Bray, G. A. (1998b). *Contemporary diagnosis and management of obesity.* Newton, PA: Handbooks in Health Care.

Carter, J. K., Ow, C. L., & Smith, R. E. (1983). Rous-associated virus Type 7 induces a syndrome in chickens characterized by stunting and obesity. *Infection and Immunity, 39,* 410–422.

Chagnon, Y. C., Perusse, L., Weisnagel, S. J., Rankinen, T., & Bouchard, C. (2000). The human obesity gene map: The 1999 update. *Obesity Research, 8,* 89–117.

Coakley, E. H., Rimm, E. B., Colditz, G., Kawachi, I., & Willett, W. (1998). Predictors of weight change in men: Results from the Halth Professionals Follow-Up Study. *International Journal of Obesity, 22,* 89–96.

Dhurandhar, N. V., Israel, B. A., Kolesar, J. M., Cook, M. E., & Atkinson, R. L. (2000). Increased adiposity in animals due to a human virus. *International Journal of Obesity, 24,* 989–996.

Dhurandhar, N. V., Israel, B. A., Kolesar, J. M., Mayhew, G., Cook, M. E., & Atkinson, R. L. (2001). Transmissibility of adenovirus-induced adiposity in a chicken model. *International Journal of Obesity, 25,* 990–1006.

Dhurandhar, N. V., Kulkarni, P. R., Ajinkya, S. M., & Sherikar, A. A. (1992). Effect of adenovirus infection on adiposity in chickens. *Veterinary Microbiology, 31,* 101–107.

Dhurandhar, N. V., Kulkarni, P. R., Ajinkya, S. M., Sherikar, A. A., & Atkinson, R. L. (1997). Association of adenovirus infection with human obesity. *Obesity Research, 5,* 464–469.

Drent, M. L. (1998). Effects of obesity on endocrine function. In G. A. Bray, C. Bouchard, & W. P. T. James (Eds.), *Handbook of obesity* (pp. 753–773). New York: Marcel Dekker.

Felitti, V. J., Anda, R. F., Nordenberg, D., Williamson, D. F., Spitz, A. M., Edwards, V., Koss, M. P., & Marks, J. S. (1998). Relationship of childhood abuse and household dysfunction to many of the leading causes of death in adults: The Adverse Childhood Experiences (ACE) Study. *American Journal of Preventive Medicine, 14,* 245–58.

Forsen, T., Eriksson, J., Tuomilehto, J., Reunanen, A., Osmond, C., & Barker, D. (2000). The fetal and childhood growth of persons who develop Type 2 diabetes. *Annals of Internal Medicine, 133,* 176–182.

Garrow, G., & Summerbell, C. D. (1995). Meta-analysis: Effect of exercise, with or without dieting, on the body composition of overweight subjects. *European Journal of Clinical Nutrition, 49,* 1–10.

Goldstein, D. J., & Potvin, J. H. (1994). Long-term weight loss: The effect of pharmacologic agents. *American Journal of Clinical Nutrition, 60,* 647–657.

Goldstein, D. J., Rampey, A. H., Dornseif, B. E., Levine, L. R., Potvin, J. H., & Fludzinski, L. A. (1993). Fluoxetine: A randomized clinical trial in the maintenance of weight loss. *Obesity Research, 1,* 92–98.

Goldstein, D. J., Rampey, A. H., Roback, P. J., Wilson, M. G., Hamilton, S. H., Sayler, M. E., & Tollefson, G. D. (1995). Efficacy and safety of long-term fluoxetine treatment of obesity: Maximizing success. *Obesity Research, 3*(Suppl. 4), 481S–490S.

Gosztonyi, G., & Ludwig, H. (1995). Borna disease: Neuropathology and pathogenesis. *Current Topics in Microbiology and Immunology, 190,* 39–73.

Guilleminault, C. (1989). Clinical features and evaluation of obstructive sleep apnea. In M. H. Kryger, T. Roth, & W. C. Dement (Eds.), *Principles and practice of sleep medicine* (pp. 667–677). Philadelphia: W. B. Saunders.

Gwinup, G. (1987). Weight loss without dietary restriction: Efficacy of different forms of aerobic exercise. *American Journal of Sports Medicine, 15,* 275–279.

Kumanyika, S. (1987). Obesity in black women. *Epidemiologic Reviews, 9,* 31–50.

Lang, K., Sebok, A., & Katona, G. (1986). The role of tonsillectomy in the development of childhood obesity. *Orvosi Hetilap, 127*(38), 2303–2305.

Levine, J. A., Eberhardt, N. L., & Jensen, M. D. (1999). Role of nonexercise activity thermogenesis in resistance to fat gain in humans. *Science, 283*(5399), 212–214.

Livingstone, M. B. (1995). Assessment of food intakes: Are we measuring what people eat? *British Journal of Biomedical Science, 52,* 58–67.

Lyons, M. J., Faust, I. M., Hemmes, R. B., Buskirk, D. R., Hirsch, J., & Zabriskie, J. B. (1982). A virally induced obesity syndrome in mice. *Science, 216,* 82–85.

Maddox, G. L., & Leiderman, V. (1969). Overweight as a social disability with medical implications. *Journal of Medical Education, 44,* 214–220.

McGuire, M. T., Wing, R. R., Klem, M. L., & Hill, J. O. (1999). Behavioral strategies of individuals who have maintained long-term weight losses. *Obesity Research, 7,* 334–341.

McGuire, M. T., Wing, R. R., Klem, M. L., Seagle, H. M., & Hill, J. O. (1998). Long-term maintenance of weight loss: Do people who lose weight through various weight loss methods use different behaviors to maintain their weight? *International Journal of Obesity, 22,* 572–577.

National Heart, Lung, and Blood, Institute. (1998). Clinical guidelines on the identification, evaluation, and treatment of overweight and obesity in adults: The evidence report. *Obesity Research,* 6(Suppl.), 51S–210S.

National Task Force on the Prevention and Treatment of Obesity. (1993). Very low calorie diets. *Journal of the American Medical Association, 270,* 967–974.

Petersen, P., & Kastrup, J. (1987). Dercum's disease (adiposis dolorosa): Treatment of the severe pain with intravenous lidocaine. *Pain, 28,* 77–80.

Phillipson, E. A. (1993). Sleep apnea: A major public health problem. *New England Journal of Medicine, 328,* 1271–1273.

Pi-Sunyer, F. X. (1993). Medical hazards of obesity. *Annals of Internal Medicine, 119,* 655–660.

Pietrobelli, A., Wang, Z., & Heymsfield, S. B. (1998). Techniques used in measuring human body composition. *Current Opinion in Clinical Nutrition and Metabolic Care, 1,* 439–448.

Pradalier, A., Dry, J., Willer, J. C., & Boureau, F. (1980). Obesity and the nociceptive reflex. *Pathologie Biologie, 28,* 462–464.

Price, J. H., Desmond, S. M., Krol, R. A., Snyder, F. F., & O'Connell, J. K. (1987). Family practice physicians' beliefs, attitudes, and practices regarding obesity. *American Journal of Preventive Medicine, 3,* 339–345.

Sarlio-Lahteenkorva, S., & Rissanen, A. (1998). Weight loss maintenance: Determinants of long-term success. *Eating and Weight Disorders, 3,* 131–135.

Schoeller, D. A., Shay, K., & Kushner, R. F. (1997). How much physical activity is needed to minimize weight gain in previously obese women? *American Journal of Clinical Nutrition, 66,* 551–556.

Schwab, R. J., Goldberg, A. N., & Pack, A. I. (1998). Sleep apnea syndromes. In A. P. Fishman (Ed.), *Fishman's pulmonary diseases and disorders* (pp. 1617–1637). New York: McGraw-Hill.

Silverman, B. L., Rizzo, T. A., Cho, N. H., & Metzger, B. E. (1998). Long-term effects of the intrauterine environment. *Diabetes Care, 21*(Suppl. 2), 142–149.

Sims, E. A. H., Danforth, E. Horton, E. S., Bray, G. A., Glennon, J. A., & Salans, L. B. (1973). Endocrine and metabolic effects of experimental obesity in main. *Recent Progress in Hormone Research, 29,* 457–496.

Stanner, S. A., Bulmer, K., Andres, C., Lantseva, O. E., Borodina, V., Poteen, V. V., & Yudkin, J. S. (1997). Does malnutrition *in utero* determine diabetes and coronary heart disease in adulthood?: Results from the Leningrad siege study, a cross sectional study. *British Medical Journal, 315*(7119), 1342–1348.

Strauss, R. S. (1997). Effects of the intrauterine environment on childhood growth. *British Medical Bulletin, 53*(1), 81–95.

Sugerman, H. J., Bloomfield, G. L., & Saggi, B. W. (1999). Multisystem organ failure secondary to increased intraabdominal pressure. *Infection, 27*(1), 61–66.

Sugerman, H. J., Felton, W. L., Salvant, J. B., Sismanis, A., & Kellum, J. M. (1995). Effects of surgically induced weight loss on idiopathic intracranial hypertension in morbid obesity. *Neurology, 45,* 1655–1659.

Sugerman, H. J., Felton, W. L., Sismanis, A., Kellum, J. M., DeMaria, E. J., & Sugerman, E. L.

(1999). Gastric surgery for pseudotumor cerebri associated with severe obesity. *Annals of Surgery, 229,* 634–640.

Wadden, T. A., Bartlett, S. J., Foster, G. D., Greenstein, R. A., Wingate, B. J., Stunkard, A. J., & Letizia, K. A. (1995). Sertraline and relapse prevention training following treatment by very-low-calorie diet: A controlled clinical trial. *Obesity Research, 3*(6), 549–557.

Walberg, J. (1989). Aerobic exercise and resistance weight-training during weight reduction: Implications for obese persons and athletes. *Sports Medicine, 47,* 343–356.

Zurlo, F., Ferraro, R. T., Fontvieille, A. M., Rising, R., Bogardus, C., & Ravussin, E. (1992). Spontaneous physical activity and obesity: Cross-sectional and longitudinal studies in Pima Indians. *American Journal of Physiology, 263,* E296–E300.

range by losing just 10 to 15 pounds. Would you like to consider this?" These approaches show respect for the patient and underscore the importance of inviting the individual's participation in treatment.

Reviewing BEST Treatment

In this chapter, we review biological, environmental, social, and timing factors in that order (the same in which they are assessed by the WALI), and then discuss the selection of the best treatment option. Practitioners, however, may cover the "BEST" items however they wish, particularly if a patient is eager to discuss a particular topic at the outset of the interview.

BIOLOGICAL FACTORS

Classification

The National Heart, Lung, and Blood Institute (NHLBI, 1998) guidelines, reviewed by Atkinson in Chapter 9 of this volume, classify patients into different categories of overweight and obesity based on body mass index (BMI). In addition, the waist circumference may be used to assess whether the individual has upper-body fat distribution. These two simple measures provide an estimate of the patient's risk of weight-related health complications.

Fat Cell Size and Number

Body weight also provides a rough estimate of whether a patient's obesity is characterized by an increase in fat cell size (hypertrophic obesity), by an increase in fat cell number (hyperplastic obesity), or by both. Fat cell weight in nonobese individuals is approximately 0.4–0.5 μg, but with weight gain it may reach 1.0–1.2 μg (Bjorntorp, 1975). Once cells reach this latter size, additional weight gain appears to result in an increase in fat cell number. Thus, when an individual achieves a fat mass approximately twice the normal size, the likelihood of hyperplastic obesity increases significantly. As shown in Figure 10.1, the greater the excess weight (and fat), the greater the hyperplasia. An average-weight person has about 25–35 billion fat cells (Leibel, Berry, & Hirsch, 1983), whereas a person with a body mass index ≥ 40 kg/m^2 may have as many as 100–150 billion cells (Leibel et al., 1983; Sjöström, 1980).

Persons with hypertrophic obesity alone have a reasonable prognosis for reaching "average" weight because cell hypertrophy is reversible (Krotkiewski et al., 1977). By contrast, fat cell number does not appear to be reversible (Naslun, Hallgreen, & Sjöström, 1988). Thus, even with weight reduction (achieved by reducing cell hypertrophy), patients with severe, hyperplastic obesity are likely to have two to three times the normal number of fat cells and a fat mass that is increased by the same proportion. These patients appear to stop losing weight when they achieve normal fat cell size, even though they may remain 50% or more overweight (because of their increased cell number) (Bjorntorp et al., 1975; Krotkiewski et al., 1977). This finding appears to explain why extremely obese patients do not achieve statistically average weight, even when treated with bariatric surgery.

Fat cell size and number can only be measured in research settings. Cell number, however, can be estimated from the data in Figure 10.1. Patients suspected of having hyperplastic obesity can be informed that there may be limits to their weight loss.

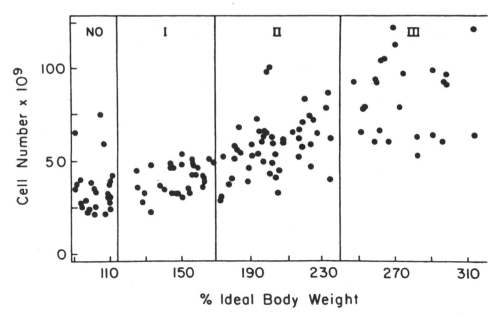

FIGURE 10.1. The relationship between fat cell number (in billions) and percent of ideal body weight (as determined by the 1959 Metropolitan Life Insurance Co. height and weight tables). I, II, and III refer to three groups of subjects with increasing severity of obesity. NO refers to nonobese subjects. From Leibel, Berry, and Hirsch (1983). Copyright 1983 by Raven Press. Reprinted by permission.

Genetic Factors

As reviewed by Price in Chapter 4 of this volume, family and adoption studies suggest that genetic factors account for an estimated 20%–40% of the variance in body weight. Estimates from some twin studies are even higher, reaching 70% (Allison et al., 1996; Stunkard, Harris, Pederson, & McClearn, 1990). Body fat distribution also appears to be heritable (Bouchard, 1995; Bouchard, Despres, & Mauriege, 1993).

The specific genes that contribute to common forms of human obesity have yet to be identified, and there are likely to be dozens, if not hundreds, that interact (Price, Chapter 4). A defect in a single gene, leptin, is sufficient to produce obesity in humans, but only a handful of such cases have been identified worldwide (Montague et al., 1997; Strobe, Issad, Camoin, Ozata, & Strosberg, 1997). Other genes may influence resting energy expenditure (Argyropoulos, Brown, & Willi, 1998; Bogardus, Lillioja, Ravussin, & Abbott, 1986; Bouchard et al., 1989), dietary-induced thermogenesis (Bouchard et al., 1990), and metabolic responses to overfeeding (Bouchard et al., 1990).

Currently, there are not adequate methods to assess an individual's genetic predisposition to obesity. However, several factors are likely to suggest an increased role of biological as compared to environmental influences in the etiology of obesity. These variables can be assessed by obtaining a detailed weight and dieting history:

1. *Age of onset of obesity.* Childhood onset and adolescent onset of obesity are generally associated with greater body weight as an adult and with increased fat cell number (Bjorntorp, 1975; Sjöström, 1980). In addition, onset of obesity by age 10 was found in one study to be associated with an increased relative risk of this condition in adult first-degree relatives (Price et al., 1990). Childhood onset doubles the risk of obesity in adulthood (Ser-

dula et al., 1993), and the risk increases further if an individual is obese as an adolescent (Guo, Roche, Chumlea, Gardner, & Siervogel, 1994; Whitaker, Wright, Pepe, Seidel, & Dietz, 1997). Age of onset can be assessed by taking a careful weight history, as captured by items B1 and B6 of the WALI (i.e., section B of the WALI, items 1 and 6). Persons with childhood or adolescent onset of their obesity can lose large amounts of weight but are unlikely to reach statistically average weight, as noted previously.

2. *Family history.* A family history of obesity also appears to be a marker for a biological predisposition. As noted, obesity runs in families, and it is now clear that this is due in part to shared genetic characteristics (Stunkard et al., 1986). Obesity in one parent more than doubles the risk that a child will be obese as an adult (Whitaker et al., 1997); the risk is even greater if both parents are obese (Lake, Power, & Cole, 1997; Whitaker et al., 1997). The strongest predictor of adult obesity is the combination of childhood or adolescent onset with a family history of obesity; 70%–75% of children with these two risk factors become obese as adults.

Maternal obesity appears to be a stronger risk factor than paternal obesity (Hashimoto, Kawasaki, Kikuchi, Takahashi, & Uchiyama, 1995; Mafeis, Talamini, & Tato, 1998; Noble, 1997). Family history may be assessed by obtaining a patient's reports of the weights and heights of his or her mother, father, and siblings (items C1 and C2 of the WALI). Weights of maternal and paternal grandparents should also be assessed. The use of silhouettes, included in the WALI, helps to confirm the presence of overweight and obesity in relatives.

3. *Weight loss history.* Obese individuals who regain weight rapidly after treatment are likely to have increased fat cell number (Krotkieweski et al., 1977; Sjöström, 1980). Some investigators have also suggested that weight cycling is a marker of an elevated body weight set point; weight loss is quickly reversed by compensatory biological mechanisms (including reductions in leptin and in resting and nonresting energy expenditure) that serve to restore weight to pretreatment levels (Keesey, 1986; Stunkard, 1982). Regardless of whether a history of weight cycling is a marker for a biological predisposition to obesity, before prescribing yet another course of treatment, the practitioner will want to know what weight loss methods the patient has tried. Weight loss history may be assessed by item E1 of the WALI, which inquires about the number of diets that resulted in a weight loss of 10 pounds (4.2 kg) or more. This method has adequate reliability (Wadden, Bartlett, et al., 1992). Patients in one of our studies reported an average of 4.9 ± 0.5 weight loss efforts, with a cumulative loss of 55.9 ± 6.0 kg (Wadden, Bartlett, et al., 1992). This careful analysis revealed that most persons had not lost and regained hundreds of pounds, despite frequent anecdotal reports to this effect.

Summarizing the Role of Biological Factors

Some patients will present histories that clearly suggest a biological (i.e., genetic) predisposition to obesity, but other cases will be less clear. For example, a patient with a BMI of 40 kg/m^2, childhood onset of obesity, and a positive family history is likely to have hyperplastic obesity and a genetic predisposition to this disorder. The presence of a biological predisposition is harder to judge in a male with a BMI of 40 kg/m^2 who became obese as an adult; has lost and regained weight only once; and, as a result of adoption, knows nothing about the weights of his biological parents.

At least three issues should be discussed with patients in whom a marked biological predisposition to obesity is suspected. The first is that even though obesity is a heritable disorder, it is not inherited in the same manner as eye color (in which a person is born with blue, green, or brown eyes, with little influence of the environment). By contrast, genes probably confer the potential for obesity, but it is the environment that determines whether and the extent to which this potential is realized. As G. A. Bray (personal communication, 1997) has stated, "Genes load the gun; the environment pulls the trigger." A second point is that by changing their personal environment—their eating and activity habits—patients can lose weight, even if they cannot achieve a statistically average weight. Third, information about biological contributions to obesity can be used to assuage the feelings of guilt and shame that so burden some patients. Studies such as that by Bouchard and colleagues (1990) have shown clearly that some persons gain more weight than others when overfed by the same number of calories. This finding resonates with the experiences of many obese people, who are perplexed by their body weight when they compare their eating and activity habits with those of lean friends. The message here is that patients are not to blame for their excess weight, even though they are still responsible for adopting healthier eating and activity habits.

ENVIRONMENTAL FACTORS

Environmental factors are clearly more responsible than genetic influences for the increased prevalence of obesity observed in industrialized nations in the past 10–20 years (Horgen & Brownell, Chapter 5, this volume). This makes it imperative to assess eating and activity habits to determine their possible contribution to a patient's obesity. Such an assessment will also reveal areas for intervention. This portion of the assessment should provide a sketch of the patient's daily eating pattern, approximate calorie intake, problem eating, and physical activity. Assessment of these variables typically continues throughout treatment.

Food Intake

Number of Meals and Snacks a Day

A key task is to determine the number of meals and snacks the patient consumes each day (as covered by item H2 of the WALI). This includes assessing when meals and snacks are consumed and evaluating the consistency of the meal pattern. Individuals who skip meals (Schlundt, Hill, Sbrocco, Pope-Cordle, & Kasser, 1990) or have highly variable eating patterns (Roger, 1999) report greater hunger and disinhibition. A principal goal of treatment is to establish a structured meal plan.

Calorie Intake

A rough estimate of the patient's calorie intake can be obtained by reviewing food intake for a typical weekday and a typical weekend day (see section I of the WALI). The goal is to determine whether the patient's calorie intake is consistent with elevated body weight or is reportedly lower than would be expected. (Formulas for estimating energy requirements are provided by Melanson and Dwyer in Chapter 12 of this volume.) We also frequently ask, "Do you think you eat the same amount as people of average weight, more than such people, or less than people of average weight?" Patients who report, usually with embarrassment, that they eat large amounts of food (or have a high calorie intake) can be told that this is actually good news, because treatment can help them reduce their intake. By contrast, persons who report an unexpectedly low energy intake should be told that it is difficult to count portion sizes and to keep track of calories. This statement is based on the results of studies with doubly labeled water, which have shown that obese individuals typically underestimate their calorie intake by 30%–50%; nonobese individuals underestimate by approximately 20% (Lichtman et al., 1992; Schoeller, 1988, 1995; Schoeller & Field, 1991). Doubly labeled water is the preferred method of assessing energy requirements, but is too expensive for use in clinical care practice.

Diet Composition

The composition of the diet can also be estimated by examining a typical weekday and weekend day, as well as the patient's favorite foods. The goal again is to determine (in broad terms) whether the patient eats a high-fat diet, or instead one that is consistent with the Food Guide Pyramid (Agricultural Research Service, 1995). A useful starting point for intervention is to determine how many fruits and vegetables the individual consumes a day, and to increase this number gradually to at least five a day. Alcohol intake should also be assessed, (i.e., item G3), given the effects of alcohol consumption on dietary disinhibition and overall energy intake (Melanson & Dwyer, Chapter 12, this volume).

Diet composition can be assessed more fully by a registered dietitian or by the use of a food frequency questionnaire, such as that developed by Block, Woods, Potosky, and Clifford (1990). The questionnaire by Block and colleagues is easily administered and can be machine-scored for a fee. Readers should know that no measure of dietary intake has fully adequate reliability or validity (Melanson & Dwyer, Chapter 12). The behavioral assessment can provide only an impression of the patient's food intake that can be further refined during treatment.

Environmental Cues

For some individuals, eating is strongly influenced by environmental cues, including times, people, places, emotions, and activities (Brownell, 2000; Schlundt et al., 1990). Practitioners should attempt to identify cues that are reliably associated with overeating. Environmental cues are covered by item H1 (L–X) of the WALI, but should also be assessed on an ongoing basis during treatment.

Appetite

Many individuals who binge-eat report that they overeat because of emotional distress. Some individuals who do not binge-eat, however, also report eating large amounts of food, principally because they have trouble feeling full at mealtimes. Such individuals appear to have impaired satiation, a problem that may be treated by behavioral intervention, but also by pharmacological agents such as sibutramine (Hansen, Toubro, Stock, Macdonald, & Astrup, 1999). Similarly, it is useful to determine whether the individual reports significant hunger or cravings and, if so, what times and places are associated with these events. These variables are assessed by item H1 (G–J) of the WALI, as well as by the Eating Inventory (Stunkard & Messick, 1988).

Problem Eating

As reviewed by Stunkard in Chapter 6 of this volume, as many as 30% of participants who seek weight reduction report significant symptoms of binge eating, and 10%–15% meet criteria for binge-eating disorder (BED) as confirmed by a diagnostic interview. BED is characterized by the consumption of an objectively large amount of food in a short period of time

(2 hours) with an accompanying subjective loss of control (Spitzer et al., 1992). Individuals with BED are more likely to report symptoms of depression and other psychopathology (Marcus, Wing, & Hopkins, 1988; Sherwood, Jeffery, & Wing, 1999; Spitzer et al., 1992, 1993; Telch & Agras, 1994; Wadden, Foster, Letizia, & Wilk, 1993).

Binge eating can be assessed by the Questionnaire on Eating and Weight Patterns—Revised (QEWP-R; Spitzer et al., 1992; Yanovski, 1993), which is easily administered and provides decision rules for diagnosing BED, bulimia nervosa, and related eating disorders. (The QEWP-R is included in the WALI in items J1–J17.) The practitioner should confirm reports of binge eating by having patients describe two or more recent binge episodes, to determine that they ate an objectively large amount of food and experienced loss of control. As Stunkard (Chapter 6, this volume) has noted, however, if BED is present, the patient's mood disturbance may be more significant in planning treatment than is the binge eating. Most studies have found no differences in weight loss between obese individuals with and without BED (Gladis et al., 1998; Sherwood et al., 1999; Wadden, Foster, & Letizia, 1992). In addition, binge-eating episodes decline quickly with the introduction of a structured diet (Stunkard, Chapter 6).

Symptoms of night-eating syndrome are assessed by section K of the WALI. This eating pattern was first described by Stunkard, Grace, and Wolff (1955) almost 50 years ago. Studies are being conducted to define better its principal characteristics, prevalence, and etiology.

Physical Activity

The increased prevalence of obesity has been paralleled by the proliferation of energy-saving devices, including automobiles, televisions, computers, and remote control devices (Hill & Melanson, 1999; Hill, Wyatt, & Melanson, 2000; Prentice & Jebb, 1995; Weinsier, Hunter, Heini, Goran, & Sell, 1998). Sedentary behavior is now a recognized risk factor for cardiovascular disease (Ravussin et al., 1997) and is significantly related to increased weight (Brownell, 1995). Increased physical activity is not only the single best predictor of the maintenance of weight loss (Pronk & Wing, 1994); as reviewed by Blair and Leermakers in Chapter 13 of this volume, it appears to decrease the risk of morbidity and mortality, independently of weight loss.

The goal in assessing physical activity is to locate patients on a continuum that ranges from "couch potato" to "marathon athlete." This can be done by inquiring about general level of daily activity, including number of blocks walked, flights of stairs climbed, and hours of television watched. This provides an estimate of the individual's lifestyle activity (Andersen et al., 1999). Programmed or purposeful activity can be assessed by inquiring about the patient's frequency of walking (or jogging) and participation in other aerobic or anaerobic activities. Physical activity is covered by items L1–L9 of the WALI.

More formal assessment of physical activity is provided by the Physical Activity Recall, which is available in both questionnaire and interview versions (Blair, 1984). This instrument assesses occupational and leisure activities over the previous 7 days and categorizes activities by their intensity. The instrument has acceptable test–retest reliability (Blair, 1984). Alternatively, the Paffenbarger Physical Activity Questionnaire is a one-page inventory that assesses habitual daily and weekly activity (Paffenbarger, Wing, & Hyde, 1978).

Informal assessment reveals that most of our patients are very sedentary. Their physical activity often consists of little more than getting into the car to drive to work, the mall, or the supermarket. When patients report with shame or chagrin that they are "couch pota-

Mood Disorder

* *"Does the individual have a mood disorder or other psychiatric condition?"* Approximately 20% of obese women who seek weight reduction report significant symptoms of depression, although fewer than 10% are likely to meet the *Diagnostic and Statistical Manual of Mental Disorders,* fourth edition (DSM-IV; American Psychiatric Association, 1994) criteria for a major depressive episode (Wadden, Anderson, et al., 2000) (see Table 10.1). We routinely assess mood with the BDI-II. Scores of 13 or under on the BDI-II are generally not of clinical concern, unless the patient reports suicidal ideation (Beck et al., 1996). With scores over 13, we review some of the individual items to assess more fully the patient's affect, behavior, and cognition. Scores of 29 or over indicate severe depression that definitely requires professional attention. Mood may also be assessed informally by asking patients to describe, for the past month, their mood, sleep, energy level, and satisfaction with work, leisure activities, and personal relationships. (Items O3–O5 of the WALI assess depressed affect.)

TABLE 10.1. Diagnostic Criteria for Major Depressive Episode

A. Five (or more) of the following symptoms have been present during the same 2-week period and represent a change from previous functioning; at least one of the symptoms is either (1) depressed mood or (2) loss of interest or pleasure.

Note: Do not include symptoms that are clearly due to a general medical condition, or mood-incongruent delusions or hallucinations.

(1) depressed mood most of the day, nearly every day, as indicated by either subjective report (e.g., feels sad or empty) or observation made by others (e.g., appears tearful). **Note:** In children and adolescents, can be irritable mood.

(2) markedly diminished interest or pleasure in all, or almost all, activities most of the day, nearly every day (as indicated by either subjective account or observation made by others)

(3) significant weight loss when not dieting or weight gain (e.g., a change of more than 5% of body weight in a month), or decrease or increase in appetite nearly every day. **Note:** In children, consider failure to make expected weight gains.

(4) insomnia or hypersomnia nearly every day

(5) psychomotor agitation or retardation nearly every day (observable by others, not merely subjective feelings of restlessness or being slowed down)

(6) fatigue or loss of energy nearly every day

(7) feelings of worthlessness or excessive or inappropriate guilt (which may be delusional) nearly every day (not merely self-reproach or guilt about being sick)

(8) diminished ability to think or concentrate, or indecisiveness, nearly every day (either by subjective account or as observed by others)

(9) recurrent thoughts of death (not just fear of dying), recurrent suicidal ideation without a specific plan, or a suicide attempt or a specific plan for committing suicide

B. The symptoms do not meet criteria for a Mixed Episode. . . .

C. The symptoms cause clinically significant distress or impairment in social, occupational, or other important areas of functioning.

D. The symptoms are not due to the direct physiological effects of a substance (e.g., a drug of abuse, a medication) or a general medical condition (e.g., hypothyroidism).

E. The symptoms are not better accounted for by Bereavement, i.e., after the loss of a loved one, the symptoms persist for longer than 2 months or are characterized by marked functional impairment, morbid preoccupation with worthlessness, suicidal ideation, psychotic symptoms, or psychomotor retardation.

Note. From American Psychiatric Association (1994). Copyright 1994 by the American Psychiatric Association. Reprinted by permission.

Persons suffering from major depression should be treated for their mood disorder prior to undertaking weight loss. In this regard, they should be treated in the same manner as persons of average weight who present with major depression. Weight reduction will not ameliorate major depression, despite some patients' protests to the contrary, and it could exacerbate it (Wadden & Bartlett, 1992).

Rather than major depression, practitioners may be more likely to encounter dysthymic disorder in obese individuals. Dysthymic disorder is a chronic low-grade depression, as defined in DSM-IV and described in Table 10.2. It is frequently accompanied by binge eating and reports of distress with work or personal relationships (Stunkard, Chapter 6, this volume). These complications are not a contraindication to weight reduction; these individuals can lose weight and will experience improvements in mood (Gladis et al., 1998). It is unlikely, however, that weight reduction will result in lasting improvements in mood. These

TABLE 10.2. Diagnostic Criteria for Dysthymic Disorder

A. Depressed mood for most of the day, for more days than not, as indicated either by subjective account or observation by others, for at least 2 years. **Note:** In children and adolescents, can be irritable and duration must be at least 1 year.

B. Presence, while depressed of two (or more) of the following:

   (1) poor appetite or overeating
   (2) insomnia or hypersomnia
   (3) low energy or fatigue
   (4) low self-esteem
   (5) poor concentration or difficulty making decisions
   (6) feelings of hopelessness

C. During the 2-year period (1 year for children or adolescents) of the disturbance, the person has never been without the symptoms in Criteria A and B for more then 2 months at a time.

D. No Major Depressive Episode . . . has been present during the first 2 years of the disturbance (1 year for children and adolescents); i.e., the disturbance is not better accounted for by chronic Major Depressive Disorder, or Major Depressive Disorder, In Partial Remission.

   Note: There may have been a previous Major Depressive Episode provided there was a full remission (no significant signs or symptoms for 2 months) before development of the Dysthymic Disorder. In addition, after the initial 2 years (1 year in children or adolescents) of Dysthymic Disorder, there may be superimposed episodes of Major Depressive Disorder, in which case both diagnoses may be given when the criteria are met for a Major Depressive Episode.

E. There has never been a Manic Episode . . . , a Mixed Episode . . . , or a Hypomanic Episode . . . , and criteria have never been met for Cyclothymic Disorder.

F. The disturbance does not occur exclusively during the course of a chronic Psychotic Disorder, such as Schizophrenia or Delusional Disorder.

G. The symptoms are not due to the direct physiological effects of a substance (e.g., a drug of abuse, a medication) or a general medical condition (e.g., hypothroidism).

H. The symptoms cause clinically significant distress or impairment in social, occupational, or other important areas of functioning.

Specify if:
   Early Onset: if onset is before age 21 years
   Late Onset: if onset is age 21 years or older

Specify (for most recent 2 years of Dysthymic Disorder):
   With Atypical Features . . .

Note. From American Psychiatric Association (1994). Copyright 1994 by the American Psychiatric Association. Reprinted by permission.

free of major life stressors. We have found that protracted stress in intimate or professional relationships, as well as life crises (i.e., death of a parent, financial or legal problems, etc.), disrupt patients' weight reduction efforts (Wadden & Letizia, 1992). In one study, patients who discontinued treatment during the first 2 months of a multicenter trial endorsed more stressors at baseline (as measured by items P1–P4 of the WALI) than persons who remained in treatment. The distinguishing stressors were "relationship with significant other," "events related to parents," and "financial or legal difficulties" (Wadden & Letizia, 1992).

Persons who report that they are experiencing high stress, as compared to their usual levels, should consider delaying weight reduction until the stressor has passed. For example, an accountant might wait until after tax season to lose weight, or a mother of three young children might wait until after her kitchen remodeling has been completed. The goal during the interlude is to maintain a stable body weight. If, however, patients with stressful lives insist that they can meet the demands of treatment, we usually defer to their judgment. Some report that weight is the one thing they can control in a life that otherwise feels out of control.

The patient's travel or vacation schedule should also be considered. Preferably, the individual should have a 2- to 3-month block in which to attend treatment regularly. If a behavioral intervention is to be used, the individual should be able to attend the clinic at least every other week and preferably on a weekly basis. Thus, for instance, a business woman who is going to be in town for the next 2 weeks but away for the following 3 weeks should probably wait until her return to begin weight loss. It is critical that patients get off to a successful start, which is facilitated by continuity of care during the first few months. Initial success (with weight loss) is associated with long-term success (Jeffery, Wing, & Mayer, 1998; Wadden & Letizia, 1992). False starts are demoralizing to both patients and providers and are often the result of missed visits early in treatment.

Summarizng Temporal Factors

Patients who seek weight reduction are usually "ready" for treatment, as reflected by their having taken the initiative to contact a health care provider. Thus it is not surprising, in this self-selected sample, that tests of weight loss readiness generally do not predict attrition or weight loss (Fontaine, Cheskin, & Allison, 1997). Nevertheless, a practitioner should determine that a patient has selected a propitious time to lose weight. In the minority of cases in which timing does not appear favorable, the practitioner might remark, "You clearly are motivated to lose weight and have given this issue a lot of thought. As we look at the next month, however, it seems that you're going to be very busy. What do you think about waiting until after your business trip to begin your program? Your goal until that time would be to remain weight-stable."

Tests of weight loss readiness are likely to be of greater benefit to primary care physicians, most of whom have hundreds of overweight and obese patients in their practices. Some of these individuals are likely to be motivated to lose weight, but have stopped talking with their primary care providers about weight control (Wadden, Anderson, et al., 2000). These individuals may be able to reduce successfully with some support and structure.

The greater challenge is to motivate patients who appear to be uninterested in weight control, either because they have made previous unsuccessful attempts or because they do not believe that obesity is a serious problem. Women appear to fall more often into the first category, and men into the second. With those who feel frustrated with weight loss, the practitioner should acknowledge, "I know how frustrated you are with your weight. You have worked so hard on it. There are some new approaches that could be of help. I would be pleased to discuss them if you would like." With males who appear unconcerned about their weight, a different approach may be useful: "You seem like a guy who's determined to be successful in life. Tell me why you're not more interested in your weight. It's a key to health success." This approach, which borrows from motivational interviewing, is designed to elicit patients' curiosity about their inconsistent or contradictory behavior (Smith, Heckemeyer, Kratt, & Mason, 1997).

SUMMARY AND IDENTIFICATION OF TREATMENT GOALS

We conclude the behavioral assessment by briefly summarizing what we have learned about contributors to the patient's obesity, and about the individual's psychosocial status and the timing of the current weight loss effort. In reviewing biological factors, a practitioner might remark: "You have been overweight since you were 12 years old, and you noted that your mother had a weight problem all of her life, as did her mother. In addition, you have lost and regained weight on several occasions. These factors suggest that you have a biological (or genetic) tendency toward obesity—a tendency that probably makes weight control more difficult for you than for the next person. This does not mean that you cannot lose weight; you certainly can. You may not, however, be able to reach as low a weight as you would like. We can discuss how much weight you can expect to lose and keep off."

The practitioner should then summarize findings from the other "BEST" components, as described previously. Patients should be encouraged to ask questions or to comment.

Identifying Goals of Treatment

Patient and practitioner are likely to have discussed the patient's goals of treatment throughout the interview. However, these should be clarified; patients often have implicit assumptions or goals that need to be articulated.

The immediate goal of treatment would appear to be to help patients lose weight. As noted previously, however, obese individuals often seek weight loss as a means to another goal. In our clinic, their principal motivations are to improve their health and/or appearance (Foster, Wadden, Vogt, & Brewer, 1997). Many hope that weight loss will improve self-esteem, body image, or a failing marriage. In such cases, we ask patients to rate (on a 1–10 scale) the likelihood that they will obtain the desired psychosocial outcomes if they lose weight. We also ask how much weight they think they need to lose to achieve these outcomes, and whether weight loss on previous occasions yielded the benefits desired.

We tell patients that weight loss typically does not change personality or intimate relationships. It may improve body image, self-esteem, or mood, but these events are also influenced by factors other than weight (Foster, Wadden, & Vogt, 1997; Wadden, Steen, Wingate, & Foster, 1996). Thus, if changes in these areas are the principal ones desired, the patient should consider the benefits of cognitive-behavioral therapy, interpersonal psychotherapy, or other interventions. Body image, for example, improves with cognitive-behavioral therapy in the absence of weight loss (Rosen, Orosan, & Reiter, 1995; Sarwer & Thompson, Chapter 21, this volume).

By contrast, weight loss more reliably improves health complications of obesity, including hypertension, hypercholesterolemia, and Type 2 diabetes (NHLBI, 1998; World Health Organization, 1998). Losses of 5%–10% of initial weight are sufficient to improve these disorders, although larger losses usually have a greater impact (Sjöström, Lissner, & Sjöström, 1998; Wing et al., 1987). Atkinson (1993) has provided criteria for assessing medical success. In addition to health changes, we ask patients to think of lifestyle changes that they would like to achieve as a result of weight loss. These might include walking stairs more easily, having the energy to play with children or grandchildren, or being able to enjoy

Finally, we hope that patients leave feeling that they have been treated with respect and understanding. It is hard to grasp, in only 60 minutes, the many years of effort that most obese individuals have already devoted to weight control. So many have experienced sadness and frustration each time they lost and regained weight, in full view of family, friends, and coworkers. Few health problems are as public as obesity. Practitioners must look to the future, to renew their patients' hope with the promise of new treatments. But they must also look to the past with respect and admiration for the individuals' previous efforts.

REFERENCES

Agricultural Research Service. (1995). Report of the Dietary Guidelines Advisory Committee: Dietary guidelines for Americans. *Nutrition Reviews, 53,* 376–379.

Allison, D. B., Kaprio, J., Korkeila, M., Koskenvuo, M., Neale, M. C., & Hayakawa, K. (1996). The heritability of body mass index among an international sample of monozygotic twins reared apart. *International Journal of Obesity, 20,* 501–506.

American Psychiatric Association. (1994). *Diagnostic and statistical manual of mental disorders* (4th ed.). Washington, DC: Author.

Andersen, R. E., Wadden, T. A., Bartlett, S. J., Zemel, B. S., Verde, T. J., & Franckowiak, S. C. (1999). Effects of lifestyle activity vs. structured aerobic exercise in obese women: A randomized trial. *Journal of the American Medical Association, 287,* 335–340.

Argyropoulos, G., Brown, A. M., & Willi, S. M. (1998). Effects of mutations in the human uncoupling protein 3 gene on the respiratory quotient and fax oxidation in severe obesity and type 2 diabetes. *Journal of Clinical Investigation, 102,* 1345–1351.

Atkinson, R. L. (1993). Proposed standards for judging the success of the treatment of obesity. *Annals of Internal Medicine, 119,* 677–680.

Barofsky, I., Fontaine, K. R., & Cheskin, L. J. (1998). Pain in the obese: Impact on health related quality of life. *Annals of Behavior Medicine, 19,* 408–410.

Beck, A. T., Steer, R. A., & Brown, G. K. (1996). *Beck Depression Inventory—II (BDI-II) manual.* San Antonio, TX: Harcourt Brace.

Bjorntorp, P. (1975). When should obesity be treated? *Nordisk Medicin, 90,* 129–30.

Bjorntorp, P., Carlgren, G., Isaksson, B., Krotiewski, M., Larsson, B., & Sjöström, L. (1975). The effect of an energy reducing dietary regime in relation to adipose tissue cellularity in obese women. *American Journal of Clinical Nutrition, 28,* 445–452.

Blair, S. N. (1984). How to assess exercise habits and physical fitness. In J. D. Matarazzo, S. M. Weiss, J. A. Herd, & N. E. Miller (Eds.), *Behavioral health: A handbook of health enhancement and disease prevention* (pp. 424–427). New York: Wiley.

Blair, S. N., Kohl, H. W., Paffenbarger, R. S., Clark, D. G., Cooper, K. H., & Gibbons, L. W. (1989). Physical fitness and all-cause mortality: A prospective study of healthy men and women. *Journal of the American Medical Association, 262,* 2395–2401.

Block, G., Woods, M., Potosky, A., & Clifford, C. (1990). Validation of a self-administered diet history questionnaire using multiple diet records. *Journal of Clinical Epidemiology, 43,* 1327–1335.

Bogardus, C., Lillioja, S., Ravussin, E., & Abbott, W. G. H. (1986). Familial dependence of the resting metabolic rate. *New England Journal of Medicine, 315,* 96–100.

Bouchard, C. (1995). Genetic influence on body weight and shape. In K. D. Brownell & C. G. Fairburn (Eds.), *Eating disorders and obesity: A comprehensive handbook* (pp. 21–26). New York: Guilford Press.

Bouchard, C., Despres, J. P., & Mauriege, P. (1993). Genetic and nongenetic determinants of regional fat distribution. *Endocrine Reviews, 14,* 72–93.

Bouchard, C., Tremblay, A., Despres, J., Nadeau, A., Lupien, P. J., Theriault, G., Dussault, J., Moorjani, S., Pineault, S., & Fournier, A. (1990). The response to long-term overfeeding in identical twins. *New England Journal of Medicine, 322,* 1477–1482.

Bouchard, C., Tremblay, A., Naudeau, A., Despres, J., Theriault, G., Boulay, M., Lortie, G., Leblanc,

C., & Fournier, G. (1989). Genetic effects in resting and exercise metabolic rates. *Metabolism, 38*, 364–370.

Brewerton, T. D., O'Neil, P. M., Dansky, B. S., & Kilpatrick, D. G. (1999). Links between morbid obesity, victimization, PTSD, major depression and bulimia in a national sample of women. *Obesity Research, 7*(Suppl.), 56S.

Brownell, K. D. (1995). Exercise in the treatment of obesity. In K. D. Brownell & C. G. Fairburn (Eds.), *Eating disorders and obesity: A comprehensive handbook* (pp. 437–438). New York: Guilford Press.

Brownell, K. D. (2000). *The LEARN program for weight management 2000.* Dallas, TX: American Health.

Cash, T. F. (1994). *What do you see when you look in the mirror?* New York: Bantam Books.

Clark, M. M., Abrams, D. B., Niaura, R. S., Eaton, C. A., & Rossi, J. S. (1991). Self-efficacy in weight management. *Journal of Consulting and Clinical Psychology, 59*, 739–744.

Epstein, L. H., Wing, R. R., Koeske, R., & Valoski, A. (1985). A comparison of lifestyle exercise, aerobic exercise and calisthenics on weight loss in obese children. *Behavior Therapy, 16*, 345–356.

Felitti, V. J. (1993). Childhood sexual abuse, depression, and family dysfunction in obese persons. *Southern Medical Journal, 86*, 732–736.

Fontaine, K. R., Cheskin, L. J., & Allison, D. B. (1997). Predicting treatment attendance and weight loss: Assessing the psychometric properties and predictive validity of the Dieting Readiness Test. *Journal of Personality Assessment, 68*, 173–183.

Foster, G. D., Wadden, T. A., & Vogt, R. A. (1997). Body image before, during, and after weightloss treatment. *Health Psychology, 16*, 226–229.

Foster, G. D., Wadden, T. A., Vogt, R. A., & Brewer, G. (1997). What is a reasonable weight loss?: Patients' expectations and evaluations of obesity treatment outcomes. *Journal of Consulting and Clinical Psychology, 65*, 79–85.

Friedman, M. A., & Brownell, K. D. (1995). Psychological correlates of obesity: Moving to the next research generation. *Psychological Bulletin, 117*, 3–20.

Gladis, M. M., Wadden, T. A., Vogt, R. A., Foster, G. D., Kuehnel, R. H., & Bartlett, S. J. (1998). Behavioral treatment of obese binge eaters: Do they need different care? *Journal of Psychosomatic Research, 44*, 375–384.

Glynn, S. M., & Ruderman, A. J. (1986). The development and validation of an eating self-efficacy scale. *Cognitive Therapy and Research, 10*, 403–420.

Grilo, C. M., Wilfley, D. E., Brownell, K. D., & Rodin, J. (1994) Teasing, body image, and self-esteem in a clinical sample of obese women. *Addictive Behaviors, 19*, 443–450.

Guo, S. S., Roche, A. F., Chumlea, W. C., Gardner, J. C., & Siervogel, R. M. (1994). The predictive value of childhood body mass index values for overweight at age 35. *American Journal of Clinical Nutrition, 59*, 810–819.

Hansen, D. L., Toubro, S., Stock, M. J., Macdonald, I. A., & Astrup, A. (1999). The effect of sibutramine on energy expenditure and appetite during chronic treatment without dietary restriction. *International Journal of Obesity, 23*, 1016–1024.

Hashimoto, N., Kawasaki, T., Kikuchi, T., Takahashi, H., & Uchiyama, M. (1995). Influence of parental obesity on the physical constitution of preschool children in Japan. *Acta Paediatrica Japonica, 37*, 150–153.

Hill, J. O., & Melanson, E. L. (1999). Overview of the determinants of overweight and obesity: Current evidence and research issues. *Medicine and Science in Sports and Exercise, 31*, S515–S521.

Hill, J. O., Wyatt, H. R., & Melanson, E. L. (2000). Genetic and environmental contributions to obesity. *Medical Clinics of North America, 84*, 333–346.

Jeffery, R. W., Wing, R. R., & Mayer, R. R. (1998). Are smaller weight losses or more achievable weight loss goals better in the long term for obese patients? *Journal of Consulting and Clinical Psychology, 66*, 641–645.

Keesey, R. (1986). A set-point theory of obesity. In K. D. Brownell, & J. P. Foreyt (Eds.), *Handbook of eating disorders: Physiology, psychology, and treatment of obesity, anorexia, and bulimia* (pp. 63–87). New York: Basic Books

Klem, M. L., Wing, R. R., McGuire, M. T., Seagle, H. M., & Hill, J. O. (1997). A descriptive study of

Valley, V., & Grace, M. (1987). Psychosocial risk factors in gastric surgery for obesity: Identifying guidelines for screening. *International Journal of Obesity, 11,* 105–113.

Wadden, T. A., Anderson, D. A., Foster, G. D., Bennett, A., Steinberg, C., & Sarwer, D. (2000). Obese women's perceptions of their physician's weight management attitudes and practices. *Archives of Family Medicine, 9,* 854–860.

Wadden, T. A., & Bartlett, S. J. (1992). Very low calorie diets: An overview and appraisal. In T. A. Wadden & T. B. Vanltallie (Eds.), *Treatment of the seriously obese patient* (pp. 44–79). New York: Guilford Press.

Wadden, T. A., Bartlett, S., Letizia, K. A., Foster, G. D., Stunkard, A. J., & Conill, A. (1992). Relationship of dieting history to resting metabolic rate, body compostition, eating behavior, and subsequent weight loss. *American Journal of Clinical Nutrition, 56,* 203S–208S.

Wadden, T. A., Berkowitz, R. I., Sarwer, D. B., Prus-Wisniewski, R. P., & Steinberg, C. (2001). Benefits of lifestyle modification in the pharmacological treatment of obesity: A randomized trial. *Archives of Internal Medicine, 161,* 218–227.

Wadden, T. A., Berkowitz, R. I., Womble, L. G., Sarwer, D. B., Arnold, M. E., & Steinberg, C. M. (2000). Effects of sibutramine plus orlistat in obese women following 1 year of treatment by sibutramine alone: A placebo-controlled trial. *Obesity Research, 8,* 431–437.

Wadden, T. A., & Foster, G. D. (2001). *Weight and Lifestyle Inventory.* Philadelphia: University of Pennsylvania.

Wadden, T. A., Foster, G. D., & Letizia, K. A. (1992). Response of obese binge eaters to treatment by behavior therapy combined with very low calorie diet. *Journal of Consulting and Clinical Psychology, 60,* 808–811.

Wadden, T. A., Foster, G. D., Letizia, K. A., & Wilk, J. E. (1993). Metabolic, anthropometric, and psychological characteristics of obese binge eaters. *International Journal of Eating Disorders, 14,* 17–25.

Wadden, T. A., & Letizia, K. A. (1992). Predictors of attrition and weight loss in persons treated by moderate and severe caloric restriction. In T. A. Wadden & T. B. VanItallie (Eds.), *Treatment of the seriously obese patient* (pp. 383–410). New York: Guilford Press.

Wadden, T. A., Steen, S. N., Wingate, B. J., & Foster, G. D. (1996). Psychosocial consequences of weight reduction: How much weight loss is enough? *American Journal of Clinical Nutrition, 63*(3, Suppl.), 461S–465S.

Wadden, T. A., Vogt, R. A., Andersen, R. E., Bartlett, S. J., Foster, G. D., Kuehnel, R. H., Wilk, J., Weinstock, R., Buckenmeyer, P., Berkowitz, R. I., & Steen, S. N. (1997). Exercise in the treatment of obesity: Effects of four interventions on body composition, resting energy expenditure, appetite, and mood. *Journal of Consulting and Clinical Psychology, 65,* 269–277.

Ware, J. E., & Sherbourne, C. D. (1992). The MOS 36-Item Short-Form Health Survey (SF–36): I. Conceptual framework and item selection. *Medical Care, 30,* 473–483.

Weinsier, R. L., Hunter, G. R., Heini, A. F., Goran, M., & Sell, S. (1998). The etiology of obesity: Relative contribution of metabolic factors, diet, and physical activity. *American Journal of Medicine, 105,* 145–150.

Whitaker, R. C., Wright, J. A., Pepe, M. S., Seidel, K. D., & Dietz, W. H. (1997). Predicting obesity in young adulthood from childhood and parental obesity. *New England Journal of Medicine, 25,* 869–873.

Wiederman, M. W., Sansone, R. A., & Sansone, L. A. (1999). Obesity among sexually abused women: An adaptive function for some? *Women and Health, 29,* 29–100.

Wing, R. R., Koeske, R., Epstein, L. H., Nowalk, M. P., Gooding, W., & Becker, D. (1987). Long-term effects of modes weight loss in type 2 diabetic patients. *Archives of Internal Medicine, 147,* 1749–1753.

World Health Organization. (1998). *Obesity: Preventing and managing the global epidemic* (Publication No. WHO/NUT/NCD/98.1). Geneva: Author.

Yanovski, S. Z. (1993). Binge eating disorder: Current knowledge. *Obesity Research, 1,* 306–324.

Young, J. B., & Macdonald, I. A. (1992). Sympathoadrenal activity in human obesity: Heterogeneity of findings since 1980. *International Journal of Obesity, 16,* 959–967.

APPENDIX 10.1. WEIGHT AND LIFESTYLE INVENTORY (WALI)

The WALI is designed to obtain information about your weight and dieting histories, your eating and exercise habits, and your relationships with family and friends. Please complete the questionnaire carefully and make your best guess when unsure of the answer. Feel free to use the margins and bottom of pages when you need more space for your answers. You will have an opportunity to review your answers with a member of our professional staff.

Please allow 1.5 hours to complete this questionnaire. Your answers will help us better identify problem areas and plan your treatment accordingly. Please be assured the information you provide will be regarded as strictly confidential and will only be available to our treatment staff. Thank you for taking the time to complete this questionnaire.

Section A: Identifying Information

¹Name   ²Social Security #   ³Date

⁴Date of Birth   ⁵Age   ⁶Weight ____lbs   ⁷Height ____ft ____inches

⁸Address

⁹Phone: Day   ¹⁰Phone: Evening   ¹¹Occupation/# of yrs at job ____/____

¹²Highest year of school completed (circle one):
1 2 3 4 5 6 7 8 9 10 11 12 13 14 15 16   Master's   Doctorate
                        High school   College

¹³Ethnicity (*circle*):   American Indian   Asian   African American   Hispanic   White
Other:_____

¹⁴How did you hear about our program?
___Newspaper   ___Physician   ___Other professional   ___Web site
___Friend   ___Employer   ___Other (please specify): _____

Section B: Weight History

1. At what age were you first overweight by 10 lbs or more? _____ yrs old
   How do you remember that you were overweight at this time? (e.g., pictures, clothes size, others telling you)_____

2. What has been your highest weight after age 21? _____lbs at _____yrs old

3. What has been your lowest weight (not due to illness) after age 21, which you have maintained for at least 1 year? _____lbs at _____yrs old, maintained for _____yrs

   Was this weight reached after a weight loss effort? _____Yes _____No

4. Check the statement that best describes you: "During the past 6 months my weight has . . ."
   __ decreased more than 10 lbs or more.
   __ decreased 5 to 10 lbs.

Note. The WALI as a whole is adapted from Wadden and Foster (2001). Copyright 2001 by the authors. Adapted by permission. Section J of the WALI comprises the Questionnaire on Eating and Weight Patterns—Revised (QEWP-R; Yanovski, 1993).

__ been relatively stable.

__ increased by 5 to 10 lbs.

__ increased by more than 10 lbs. or more.

5. What was your weight: 6 months ago? _____lbs

                           1 year ago? _____lbs

                           2 years ago? _____lbs

6. For each time period shown below, please list your maximum weight. *If you cannot remember what your maximum was, make your best guess and mark "G" (for guess) next to your answer.* In addition, please note any events related to your gaining weight during this period. For ages 16 and beyond, please identify the figure that most resembles yours at that time. Record the number of the figure.

Age	Maximum Weight	Figure #	Events Related to Weight Gain
A. 5–10			
B. 11–15			
C. 16–20			
D. 21–25			
E. 26–30			
F. 31–35			
G. 36–40			
H. 41–50			
I. 51–60			
J. 61–70			

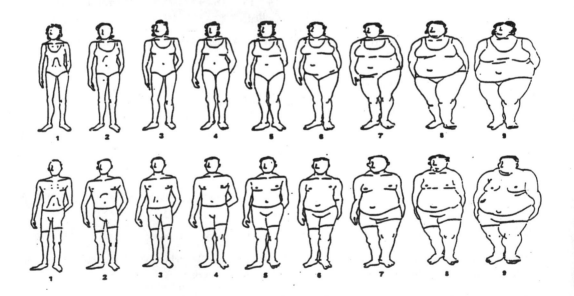

Section C: Family Weight History

1. Please indicate the average height and weight of your biological mother and father *during their middle-age years*. Also, please select, from the figures provided in Section B, the ones that are most similar to your parents' body shapes. If you do not know your biological parents' height and weights, please mark NA (not applicable) in the spaces.

Parent	Height (ft + in)	Weight (lbs)	Current Age (or year of death)	Figure #
A. Mother	_____	_____	_____	_____
B. Father	_____	_____	_____	_____

2. Please indicate the height and weight of the following members of your immediate family.

Family Member	Height (ft + in)	Weight (lbs)	Current Age (or year of death)	Figure #
A. Spouse/ Significant Other	_____	_____	_____	_____
B. Oldest Brother	_____	_____	_____	_____
C. 2nd Oldest Brother	_____	_____	_____	_____
D. 3rd Oldest Brother	_____	_____	_____	_____
E. Oldest Sister	_____	_____	_____	_____
F. 2nd Oldest Sister	_____	_____	_____	_____
G. 3rd Oldest Sister	_____	_____	_____	_____

Section D: Weight, Pregnancy, and Menstrual Cycle

(*For Women Only*)

1. Do you have children? ____Yes ____No   *If yes,*
   A. What was your weight at the start of your pregnancy? _____lbs
      What was your weight at delivery? _____lbs
      What was your lowest weight after delivery? _____lbs

   B. What was your weight at the start of your second pregnancy? _____lbs
      What was your weight at delivery? _____lbs
      What was your lowest weight after delivery? _____lbs

   C. What was your weight at the start of your third pregnancy? _____lbs
      What was your weight at delivery? _____lbs
      What was your lowest weight after delivery? _____lbs

   D. What was your weight at the start of your fourth pregnancy? _____lbs
      What was your weight at delivery? _____lbs
      What was your lowest weight after delivery? _____lbs

Please turn to the last page if you need more space.

2. Do you experience a regular menstrual cycle? _____ Yes _____ No   *If yes,*
   A. Describe your eating around the time of your menstruation (*circle one*):
      Eat much less   Eat less   No change   Eat more   Eat much more

   B. Do you crave particular foods around the time of your menstruation?
      ____Yes ____No

   C. If yes, which foods do you crave?
      _____
      _____

Section E: Weight Loss History

1. Please record each major weight loss (i.e., diet, exercise, moderation, etc.) *that resulted in a weight loss of 10 pounds or more.* Take time to think over your previous efforts, starting with the first

_____ H. Eating because I crave certain foods
_____ I. Continuing to eat because I don't feel full after a meal
_____ J. Eating because I can't stop once I've begun
_____ K. Eating because of the good taste of foods
_____ L. Eating in response to the sight or smell of food
_____ M. Eating while cooking or preparing food
_____ N. Eating when anxious
_____ O. Eating when tired
_____ P. Eating when bored
_____ Q. Eating when stressed
_____ R. Eating when angry
_____ S. Eating when depressed/upset
_____ T. Eating when socializing/celebrating
_____ U. Eating when happy
_____ V. Eating when alone
_____ W. Eating with family/friends
_____ X. Eating at business functions

Please indicate any other factors that contribute a moderate amount or more to your weight gain.

_____

_____

_____

2. How many days a week do you eat the following meals? Write the number of days in the space and the usual time of each meal.

A. Breakfast: _____days a week   Time: _____   Morning snack: _____days a week
B. Lunch: _____days a week   Time: _____   Afternoon snack: _____ days a week
C. Dinner: _____days a week   Time: _____   Evening snack: _____ days a week

3. Who prepares meals at your home? _____

4. Who does the food shopping? _____

5. Please list your five favorite foods: _____

_____

6. Do you have any food allergies? _____Yes _____No   *If yes,* please specify the food and the allergic reactions.

_____

7. Please specify the amount (in 8-oz cups) of the following fluids you typically consume a day.
_____Skim milk   _____Lowfat milk   _____Whole milk   _____Seltzer water
_____Fruit juice   _____Water   _____Tea   _____Coffee   _____Diet soda
_____Sugared soda   _____Beer   _____Wine   _____Hard liquor   _____Other

8. During a typical week, how many meals do you eat at a fast-food restaurant (including drive-through and convenience stores)?
Breakfast: _____ meals a week
Lunch: _____ meals a week
Dinner: _____ meals a week

9. During a typical week, how many meals do you eat at a traditional restaurant, coffee shop, cafeteria, or similar establishment?
Breakfast: _____ meals a week

Lunch: _____ meals a week
Dinner: _____ meals a week

10. How many times a week do you typically eat out with others (including family)? _____

Section I: Food Intake Recall

Please indicate the foods you consume on a typical weekday.

Meal	Time	Location	Food and Beverages Consumed	Amount
Breakfast				
Morning snack				
Lunch				
Afternoon snack				
Dinner				
Evening snack				

Please indicate the foods you consume on a typical weekend day.

Meal	Time	Location	Food and Beverages Consumed	Amount
Breakfast				
Morning snack				
Lunch				
Afternoon snack				
Dinner				
Evening snack				

13. During the past 3 months, did you ever take more than twice the recommended dose of laxatives in order to avoid gaining weight after binge eating? *Circle one:*

Yes   No

If yes: How often, on average, was that?

A. Less than once a week
B. Once a week
C. Two or three times a week
D. Four or five times a week
E. More than five times a week

14. During the past 3 months, did you ever take more than twice the recommended dose of diuretics (water pills) in order to avoid gaining weight after binge eating? *Circle one:*

Yes   No

If yes: How often, on average, was that?

A. Less than once a week
B. Once a week
C. Two or three times a week
D. Four or five times a week
E. More than five times a week

15. During the past 3 months, did you ever fast (not eat anything at all for at least 24 hours) in order to avoid gaining weight after binge eating? *Circle one:*

Yes   No

If yes: How often, on average, was that?

A. Less than once a week
B. Once a week
C. Two or more times a week
D. Four or five times a week
E. More than five times a week

16. During the past 3 months, did you ever exercise for more than 1 hour specifically in order to avoid gaining weight after eating? *Circle one:*

Yes   No

If yes: How often, on average, was that?

A. Less than once a week
B. Once a week
C. Two or three times a week
D. Four or five times a week
E. More than five times a week

17. During the past 3 months, did you ever take more than twice the recommended dosage of a diet pill in order to avoid gaining weight after binge eating? *Circle one:*

Yes   No

If yes: How often, on average, was that?

A. Less than once a week
B. Once a week
C. Two or three times a week
D. Four or more times a week
E. More than five times a week

Section K: Eating Patterns III

In reference to the past 6 months, please circle ONE answer for each question, except where directed otherwise on questions 2, 3, and 11.

1. What level of appetite do you usually have in the morning?

0	1	2	3	4
None	Very low	Low	Moderate	High

2. When do you usually eat for the first time? (Mark an X on the line where appropriate.)

6 A.M.	9 A.M.	Noon	3 P.M.	6 P.M. or later

3. How much of your daily food intake do you consume *after* supper? (Mark an X on the line where appropriate.)

0%	25%	50%	75%	100%

4. How often do you have trouble getting to sleep?

0	1	2	3	4
Never	Sometimes	Half the time	Usually	Always

5. How often do you get up in the middle of the night?

0	1	2	3	4
Never	Once/month	Once/week	Once/night	More than once/night

6. When you get up in the middle of the night, how often to you snack?

0	1	2	3	4
Never	Sometimes	Half the time	Usually	Always

7A. To what extent do you have cravings or urges to eat snacks after supper, but before bedtime?

0	1	2	3	4
None at all	A little	Somewhat	Very much so	Extremely so

B. To what extent do you have cravings or urges to eat snacks when you wake up at night?

0	1	2	3	4
None at all	A little	Somewhat	Very much so	Extremely so

8. To what extent do you believe you need to eat in order to get back to sleep when you awake at night?

0	1	2	3	4	___ Check here if
None at all	A little	Somewhat	Very much so	Extremely so	you did not get up

9. If you snack in the middle of the night, how aware are you of your eating?

0	1	2	3	4	___ Check here if
Unaware	Mostly unaware	Partially aware	Mostly aware	Completely aware	you don't snack in the middle of the night

10. Are you feeling blue or down in the dumps?

0	1	2	3	4
None at all	A little	Somewhat	Very much so	Extremely

Section N: Self-Perceptions

1. How satisfied are you with your current weight? (*Check one*)

   _____Very satisfied
   _____Moderately satisfied
   _____Slightly satisfied
   _____Neutral
   _____Slightly dissatisfied
   _____Moderately dissatisfied
   _____Very dissatisfied

2. How satisfied are you with your current shape (i.e., figure or physique)? (*Check one*)

   _____Very satisfied
   _____Moderately satisfied
   _____Slightly satisfied
   _____Neutral
   _____Slightly dissatisfied
   _____Moderately dissatisfied
   _____Very dissatisfied

3. How satisfied are you with your current overall appearance? (*Check one*)

   _____Very satisfied
   _____Moderately satisfied
   _____Slightly satisfied
   _____Neutral
   _____Slightly dissatisfied
   _____Moderately dissatisfied
   _____Very dissatisfied

4. Pick the one sentence that best describes your *overall* feelings about yourself: "In general, I am . . ."

   _____very happy with who I am.
   _____happy with who I am.
   _____OK with who I am, but have some mixed feelings.
   _____unhappy with who I am.
   _____very unhappy with who I am.

5. Pick the one sentence that best describes you: "As compared with most people, I think I have . . ."

   _____very good self-esteem.
   _____good self-esteem.
   _____average self-esteem.
   _____poor self-esteem.
   _____very poor self-esteem.

6. Pick the one sentence that best describes your feelings about the way you looked the last time you lost a lot of weight: "I was . . ."

   _____very happy with the way I looked.
   _____happy with the way I looked.
   _____OK with the way I looked, but with some mixed feelings.
   _____unhappy with the way I looked.
   _____very unhappy with the way I looked.

7. How much weight did you lose? _____lbs And at what weight did you start to diet during this time? _____lbs

Section O: Psychological Factors

1. Have you ever had any problems at any time with depression, anxiety, or other emotions that disrupted your normal functioning?

    _____Yes   _____No

2. Have you ever sought professional help for emotional problems? *If yes,* please specify below.

Problem	Year	Duration (wks)	Type of Professional Help
_____	____	_____	_____
_____	____	_____	_____
_____	____	_____	_____

3. During the past month, have you felt depressed, sad, or blue much of the time? (*Circle one*)

    Yes   No

4. During the past month, have you often felt hopeless about the future? (*Circle one*)

    Yes   No

5. During the past month, have you had little interest or pleasure in doing things? (*Circle one*)

    Yes   No

6. Have you ever been subjected to physical abuse? _____Yes _____No

7. Have you ever been subjected to sexual abuse? _____Yes _____No

8. Are any of your immediate family members alcoholic? _____Yes _____No

Section P: Timing

1. Please indicate if you are currently experiencing any stress in your life related to the following events. Complete each item by checking the appropriate box.

    A.   Work: _____ Yes ____ No

    B.   Health: _____ Yes ____ No

    C.   Relationship with spouse/significant other: _____ Yes ____ No

    D.   Activities related to your children: _____ Yes ____ No

    E.   Activities related to your parents: _____ Yes ____ No

    F.   Legal/financial trouble: _____ Yes ____ No

    G.   School: _____ Yes ____ No

    H.   Moving: _____ Yes ____ No

    I.   Other:_____

    Please explain in a sentence any items to which you responded yes:

    _____

    _____

    _____

2. List all medications being taken (including vitamins and supplements). Please indicate the dosage and frequency of each medication.

Medication	Dosage	Frequency	Reason for Taking
_____	_____	_____	_____
_____	_____	_____	_____
_____	_____	_____	_____
_____	_____	_____	_____

Please indicate your primary care physician's name, telephone number, and address here.

Name: _____ Phone: _____

Address: _____

_____

PART IV

TREATMENT OF ADULT OBESITY

Treatment Algorithms

Aronne (Chapter 18, this volume) has reviewed the NHLBI and NAASO (2000) algorithm for selecting therapy (see Table 18.4 on page 396). Persons with a BMI of 25.0–29.9 kg/m^2 who have two or more risk factors are encouraged to consume a balanced low-calorie diet, to increase their physical activity (so that they eventually exercise 30 minutes a day most days of the week), and to modify inappropriate eating habits. Alternatively, prevention of weight gain is recommended for persons in the same BMI range who are not motivated to reduce or who have fewer than two risk factors. As BMI increases, so generally do the health complications of obesity and the need for more intensive intervention. Pharmacotherapy is an option for persons with a BMI $\geq$ 30 kg/m^2 (or a BMI $\geq$ 27 kg/m^2 in the presence of comorbid conditions) and who have failed to reduce using more conservative measures. Bariatric surgery is reserved for individuals with a BMI $\geq$ 40 kg/m^2 or those with a BMI $\geq$ 35 kg/m^2 who have significant comorbid conditions.

Wadden, Brownell, and Foster (in press) have proposed a stepped-care algorithm that, similar to that developed by the NHLBI and NAASO (2000) panel, recommends treatment based on the patient's BMI and risk of health complications (see Figure 11.1). The principal difference between the two schemes is the greater number of treatment options listed by the former algorithm and the stronger encouragement for persons with a BMI of 27–29 kg/m^2 to lose weight. The presence of a single risk factor, such as hypertension or Type 2 diabetes, would appear to provide ample reason to undertake weight loss. Moreover, prevention of weight gain for individuals who fall into the BMI range of 27–29 kg/m^2 is likely to require periodic bouts of caloric restriction, as well as increased physical activity, to reverse weight gain that occurs over the winter months or at other times. In overweight and obese adults, intentional weight loss, even when followed by weight regain, does not appear to be associated with (1) increased risks of morbidity or mortality, (2) adverse effects on metabolism or energy expenditure, or (3) the precipitation of eating disorders or depression (Foster, Sarwer, & Wadden, 1997; Gregg & Williamson, Chapter 7, this volume; National Task Force on the Prevention and Treatment of Obesity, 1994, 2000; Wadden, Foster, Stunkard, & Conill, 1996). Thus there do not appear to be strong reasons to dissuade persons with a BMI of 27–29 kg/m^2 from attempting to lose weight.

Treatment Selection

Treatment selection should be guided not only by the individual's BMI and health risks, but also by the patient's history of weight loss efforts. For example, we have encountered many obese males (BMI $\geq$ 30 kg/m^2) who were eligible for pharmacotherapy but who had never participated in a traditional behavioral program of diet and physical activity. The latter intervention is less expensive than pharmacotherapy and is associated with fewer risks of health complications. Pharmacotherapy may be useful with these individuals for maintaining weight loss, but is not necessary to induce it. By contrast, it is hard to argue that a woman with a BMI of 35 kg/m^2, Type 2 diabetes, and a marked history of weight cycling should enroll in yet another diet and exercise program. She is more likely to achieve long-term success with long-term pharmacotherapy or with bariatric surgery. Diet and activity modification will remain an important focus of treatment, but they would need to be supported by these other interventions. Patients should have tried a less intensive treatment option once or twice before selecting a more aggressive therapy, but it is not necessary to try the less intensive option again with each new practitioner.

Treatment options must also be selected with consideration of their safety, efficacy, and cost. Self-help programs, for example, are very attractive because of their safety and low cost, but they usually produce minimal weight loss (Womble, Wang, & Wadden, Chap-

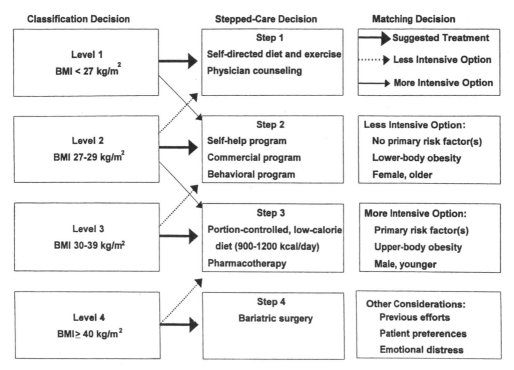

FIGURE 11.1. A conceptual scheme showing a three-stage process for selecting treatment. The first step, the Classification Decision, divides people into four levels based on body mass index (BMI). This level indicates which of four classes of interventions are likely to be most appropriate in the second stage, the Stepped-Care Decision. The interventions range from low-intensity, low-cost approaches, such as self-directed diet-and-exercise programs, to extremely aggressive and expensive interventions such as bariatric surgery. All individuals are encouraged to control their weight by increasing their physical activity and consuming an appropriate diet. When this approach is not successful, more intensive intervention may be warranted, with the most conservative treatment (i.e., lowest cost and risks of side effects) tried next. The thick, solid arrows between the boxes shows the class of treatments that is usually most appropriate for an individual when less intensive interventions have not been successful. The third stage, the Matching Decision, is used to make a final treatment selection, based on the individual's prior weight loss efforts, treatment preferences, and need for weight reduction (as judged by the presence of comorbid conditions or other risk factors). The dashed arrows point to treatment options for persons with a reduced need for weight reduction because of a reduced risk of health complications. The thin arrows show the more intensive treatment options for persons who, despite relatively low BMI levels, have increased risks of health complications. Adjunct nutritional or psychological counseling is recommended for patients who report marked problems with meal planning, depression, body image, or like difficulties. From Wadden, Brownell, and Foster (in press). Copyright by the American Psychological Association. Reprinted by permission.

ter 19, this volume). Thus such programs may not be a good choice for an individual who needs to lose approximately 10% of initial weight to improve a weight-related health complication.

Individual preferences also must be considered. Given that patients must actively participate in their weight management (i.e., by modifying eating and activity habits and/or by taking medications), they must find the therapy acceptable. Concerns about the safety of some approaches, including pharmacotherapy or surgery, must be respected in view of the history of complications associated with these interventions. Similarly, patients may raise objections to specific diet or exercise regimens. A health care provider can suggest that a pa-

greater weight loss than are most commercial programs, although this hypothesis has not been tested in randomized trials.

There are numerous accounts of the components of behavioral treatment, which include self-monitoring, stimulus control, problem solving, cognitive restructuring, social support, nutrition education, physical activity, and the use of reinforcement contingencies (Brownell, 2000; Wadden & Foster, 2000; Wing, 1998). Brownell (2000) has provided a 16-week, step-by-step manual that covers these topics in a detailed but user-friendly manner. Rather than repeat this description, this section briefly discusses some of the mechanics of behavioral treatment that we believe contribute to its successful induction of weight loss. This begins with the fact that behavioral treatment is very goal-oriented. Participants are given homework assignments (for changing eating, activity, and thinking habits), which are specified in terms that can be easily operationalized and measured. This is true whether the goal is walking after dinner five times a week for 20 minutes, keeping a daily record of food intake, decreasing the number of self-critical statements, or limiting breakfast to 275 kilocalories (kcal). Treatment sessions eschew lecturing by the group leader and instead are devoted principally to reviewing patients' completion of homework assignments and helping them find solutions to barriers.

Frequent Visits

Behavior change is facilitated by meeting with patients on a weekly basis. Frequent visits provide not only more opportunities for instruction, but also more opportunities for staff to review and reinforce patients' completion of food and activity records. Anticipation of weekly weigh-ins motivates most patients to adhere to the prescribed behaviors, and weight change provides a crude but critical measure of adherence. The failure to weigh participants each week is likely to result in suboptimal weight loss, as suggested by the results of a study by Goodrick, Poston, Kimball, Reeves, and Foreyt (1998).

Time-Limited Therapy

Most behavioral programs last 16–26 weeks. Treatment (at least during the weight loss induction phase) has a clear beginning and end, which appears to help patients pace themselves. They can set their sights on a specific date to complete treatment and achieve a sense of accomplishment, compared with the practice in open-ended therapy of having participants attend sessions indefinitely. Identifying a "treatment end date," however, is clearly a misnomer, given that patients require long-term behavioral or pharmacological treatment to maintain their weight loss. Even knowing this, patients usually prefer to divide maintenance therapy into time-limited blocks; this is similar to enrolling in a course for a semester, with the knowledge that additional courses will be needed.

Group Treatment

Behavioral treatment is typically delivered to groups of 10–20 persons. The use of closed treatment groups, in which the same patients begin and end treatment together, appears preferable to the use of open groups, in which new members may be added to the group at any point in treatment. The addition of new members after the first few weeks impairs the development of group cohesiveness and may contribute to the high attrition rates that characterize commercial programs that use open groups (Volkmar, Stunkard, Woolston, & Bailey, 1981). Moreover, it is difficult to establish a curriculum of behavior change, in which one week's session builds upon another, if patients in the same group are at different stages of treatment.

Group treatment is not only more cost-effective than individual therapy but also may produce larger weight losses. A recent study found that persons who requested individual therapy but were randomly assigned to group treatment nevertheless achieved significantly greater weight losses than participants who requested individual therapy and received it (Renjilian et al., 2001). The benefits of group treatment may derive not only from the support that patients provide each other, but also from a healthy dose of competition. Patients may push themselves to keep up with the group norm.

Treatment Flexibility

Although behavioral treatment as described here is highly structured, the treatment principles can be used to help patients adopt a variety of different eating and activity plans. Traditional behavioral interventions, for example, encourage patients to consume a balanced-deficit diet of approximately 1,200–1,800 kcal/day, as described by Melanson and Dwyer in Chapter 12 of this volume. Behavioral principles, however, can be used to facilitate adherence to diets that vary dramatically in their macronutrient or calorie content, including very-low-calorie diets (VLCDs) or plans that allow *ad libitum* intake of carbohydrate with only small amounts of fat. The same behavioral principles can be used to increase programmed exercise, lifestyle activity, or both, as described by Wing (Chapter 14, this volume). Thus "behavioral treatment" refers to the principles and techniques that are used to change eating and activity habits, rather than to the specific diet or exercise plan that is to be adopted.

Limitation of Behavioral Treatment

Traditional group behavioral treatment is appropriate for overweight or obese individuals who have failed to reduce on their own or who have not been successful with self-help or commercial programs. The greater intensity and structure provided by this approach should be of benefit. The greatest drawback of group behavioral treatment is its limited availability. Health care providers (in the United States) are encouraged to contact their local hospital, university psychology clinic, sports medicine clinic, or YMCA to determine whether they offer a closed-group behavioral program as described above. A local registered dietitian may also offer such treatment. In the absence of referral sources, practitioners may wish to use *The LEARN Program for Weight Management 2000* (Brownell, 2000). (The manual may be ordered at 800-736-7323.)

TREATMENT OPTIONS: BMI OF 30–39 kg/m^2

One-quarter of U.S. adults have a BMI $\geq$ 30 kg/m^2, which places them in the "obese" category. The algorithm in Figure 11.1 lists two options for persons with a BMI of 30–39 kg/m^2 who have failed to reduce using the less intensive (and less expensive) options described previously. The options are (1) a low-calorie, portion-controlled diet; and (2) pharmacotherapy.

Low-Calorie, Portion-Controlled Diet

The NHLBI (1998) recommended that persons with a BMI of 27–35 kg/m^2 who wish to lose weight reduce their intake by 300–500 kcal/day, with the goal of losing 10% of initial weight in 6 months. Persons with a BMI over 35 kg/m^2 are encouraged to reduce their intake by 500–1,000 kcal/day in order to achieve a comparable reduction in the same time. Caloric intake is restricted more severely with heavier individuals because they have to lose more weight (in absolute terms) to achieve a 10% reduction.

TABLE 11.1 Comparison of Very-Low-Calorie Diets (VLCDs) versus Balanced-Deficit Diets (BDDs) providing 1,000–1,6000 kcal/day

Reference	Subjects	Mean pretreatment weight (kg)	Mean age (yr)	Treatment regimen	Mean treatment duration (wk)	Maximum mean weight loss (kg)	Mean weight loss at follow-up (kg)
Ryttig, Flaten, & Rossner (1997)	44 F, 37 M (42)	114.2	42.5	1. BDD (1,600 kcal/day) for 112 wk.	112	Wk 8: 7.2[a]	112 wk: 5.5
				2. VLCD (420 kcal/day) for 8 wk, followed by BDD (1,600 kcal/day) for 104 wk.	112	Wk 8: 9.2[b]	112 wk: 5.9
				3. VLCD for 8 wk, followed by BDD using nutrient packets for 104 wk.	112	Wk 8: 9.2[b]	112 wk: 5.7
Togerson et al. (1997)	74 F, 39 M (87)	110.9 126.15	47.1	1. VLCD (456 kcal/day for women, 608 for men) + BT for 12 wk, followed by BDD (1,200–1,800 kcal/day) + BT for 92 wk.	104	Wk 26: 15.9[a]	104 wk: 9.2
				2. BT + BDD for 104 wk.	104	Wk 26: 8.6[b]	104 wk: 6.2
Wadden, Foster, & Letizie (1994)	49 F (37)	106.3	39.3	1. BDD (1,200 kcal/day) + BT.	52	Wk 26: 11.9[a]	78 wk: 12.2
				2. BDD for 1 wk; VLCD (420 kcal/day) for wk. 2–17; BDD (1,000–1,200 kcal/day) for wk 18–52.	52	Wk 26: 21.5[b]	78 wk: 10.9
Wing et al. (1994)	93 F (74)	106.75	51.8	1 BDD (1,000–1,200 kcal/day) + BT for 1 yr.	50	Wk 26: 14.5	104 wk: 5.7
				2. VLCD (400–500 kcal/day) for wk 1–12 and 24–36 + BT.	50	Wk 26: 16.8	104 wk: 7.2

Note. F, female; M, male; number in parentheses = subjects remaining at longest follow-up; BT, behavior therapy. Values of maximum mean weight loss with different superscripts (a vs. b) are significantly different from each other.

238

In this volume, Bray (Chapter 15) has reviewed current and potential agents for the treatment of obesity, and Aronne (Chapter 18) has discussed the prescription of weight loss agents by primary care physicians. Several other thoughtful reviews of this topic are available (Atkinson & Hubbard, 1994; Bray, 1993; Bray & Greenway, 1999; National Task Force, 1996). Thus the present discussion is limited to four related issues: (1) the size of the weight losses to be expected with medication, (2) the relation between behavioral and pharmacological interventions, (3) methods to facilitate medication adherence, and (4) the long-term use of pharmacotherapy.

Size of Weight Losses

Sibutramine and orlistat induce mean reductions of approximately 7%–10% of initial weight during the first 6 months of treatment—a loss nearly identical to that produced by traditional behavioral treatment. Weight loss usually stops (i.e., plateaus) at this time, despite patients' remaining on medication (for up to 2 years). As many as 40% of participants treated by either medications may lose 10% or more of initial weight, but even the most successful individuals fall far short of the 25% reduction in initial weight that patients expect to achieve (Wadden, Berkowitz, Sarwer, Prus-Wisniewski, & Steinberg, 2001). Efforts to increase weight losses by combining sibutramine and orlistat (which have different and potentially complementary mechanisms of action) were not successful in a pilot study of this approach, but further studies are needed (Wadden, Berkowitz, et al., 2000). Combining weight loss medications with a strong behavioral program may yield larger weight loss.

Relation of Behavioral and Pharmacological Treatment

Currently approved pharmacological agents induce weight loss by modifying *internal* signals that regulate hunger and/or satiety (as with sibutramine) or by causing nutrient malabsorption (as with orlistat) (Wadden et al., 2001). Medications in the first group may reduce the desire to initiate (or to continue) eating. Behavior modification, by contrast, induces weight loss by helping patients modify the *external* environment (Craighead & Agras, 1991). For example, patients are instructed to select smaller portion sizes, to avoid convenience stores and fast-food restaurants, to store foods out of sight, and to avoid engaging in other activities while eating. The desire to eat is controlled by limiting exposure to events that precipitate eating. Thus pharmacotherapy and behavior therapy would appear to induce weight loss by different but potentially complementary mechanisms. Combining these two approaches could be expected to induce larger weight losses than either intervention used alone.

This belief is supported by the results of a study by Craighead, Stunkard, and O'Brien (1981). Patients who were treated weekly for 26 weeks by group behavior modification alone (i.e., without medication) lost an average of 10.9 kg (about 11% of initial weight). Those treated by pharmacotherapy alone (120 mg/day of fenfluramine), in brief monthly office visits, lost a significantly smaller 6.0 kg (about 7%). The combination of medication plus weekly group behavior modification resulted in a mean weight loss of 15.3 kg (about 16%). Thus medication and behavior therapy appeared to have additive effects.

The withdrawal from the market of fenfluramine and dexfenfluramine, because of their association with valvular heart disease, obviously limits the clinical significance of these findings (Connolly et al., 1997). A recent study, however, of sibutramine and behavior modification (the latter therapy is now often referred to as "lifestyle modification") yielded similar findings (Wadden et al., 2001). A total of 53 obese women were randomly assigned to one of three conditions, all of which received 1 year of treatment. Those in the first group (i.e., drug-alone condition) were prescribed 15 mg/day of sibutramine and were instructed to consume 1,200 kcal/day and to exercise four to five times a week for 30 minutes per bout. Patients had 10 brief physician visits during the year to check their blood pressure and any side effects; however, they received no formal instruction in modifying their eating or activity habits. Patients in a second group (i.e., drug plus lifestyle) also received 15 mg/day of sibutramine and the same diet and exercise prescription. These participants, however, also attended weekly group sessions during the first 5 months at which they were instructed in behavioral methods of weight control, including keeping daily records of their food intake and physical activity. Sessions were led by psychologists, who followed *The LEARN Program for Weight Control* (Brownell & Wadden, 1998). Participants attended monthly meetings from months 5 to 12. Participants in the third group (i.e., combined treatment) received the same program, except during the first 4 months, they consumed 1,000 kcal/day of a portion-controlled diet. This consisted of four servings/day of a liquid diet (OPTIFAST 800), combined with an evening meal of a frozen food entree and a vegetable and a fruit serving. This diet was included to induce a larger initial weight loss, given previous findings that obese women were disappointed by modest weight losses (Foster, Wadden, Vogt, & Brewer, 1997).

Figure 11.2 shows that the addition of group lifestyle modification to sibutramine increased weight loss almost threefold. Patients who received the drug alone lost 4.1% of initial weight at the end of the year, compared with a loss of 10.8% for those who received the drug plus lifestyle modification. Women who received the drug plus the portion-controlled diet (i.e., combined treatment) lost 16.5% of initial weight—an outcome similar to that re-

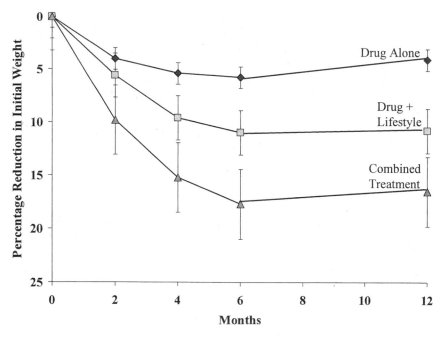

FIGURE 11.2. Percentage reduction in initial weight for women treated by sibutramine alone (i.e., drug alone) (*n* = 19), sibutramine plus group lifestyle modification (i.e., drug plus lifestyle) (*n* = 17), or sibutramine plus group lifestyle modification combined with a portion-controlled diet providing 1,000 kcal/day (i.e., combined treatment) (*n* = 17). From Wadden, Berkowitz, Sarwer, Prus-Wisniewski, and Steinberg (2001). Copyright 2001 by the American Medical Association. Reprinted by permission.

ported in a sibutramine trial that included a 1-month VLCD (Apfelbaum et al., 1999). These results show that although sibutramine alone (as typically prescribed in primary care practice) will induce weight loss, substantially better results are likely to be achieved by combining the medication with a patient's own efforts to modify eating and activity habits. Weight loss medications may facilitate the consumption of a healthier diet, but should not be considered a substitute for the patient's own efforts in this regard. A key challenge is to find effective ways of providing lifestyle modification during primary care visits (Wadden et al., 1997). Physicians who do not believe that they have the time or expertise to provide such counseling may wish to prescribe medication but refer patients to a dietitian or self-help program to obtain the lifestyle modification.

Combining pharmacotherapy with a group program of lifestyle modification required more time and effort of patients. However, the greater weight loss significantly improved patients' satisfaction with their treatment outcomes, including satisfaction with changes in their health and fitness, self-esteem, and body image. Satisfaction with all outcomes, including that with the medication, was positively related to patients' meeting their weight loss expectations. Prior to treatment, the women reported the number of pounds they expected to lose after 1, 3, 6, and 12 months of treatment. Patients, on average, expected at 1 year to lose the equivalent of 25% of their initial weight—a loss that eluded even patients who received combined treatment. However, the greater the percentage of their expected weight loss patients achieved, the greater their satisfaction with changes in their weight, health and fitness, body image, and related outcomes. (Correlations ranged from $r = .62$ to .72.)

Facilitating Medication Adherence

In addition to improving patients' eating and exercise habits, behavioral principles may be used to facilitate adherence to weight loss medications. This is an important issue, given findings, for example, that as many as half of persons prescribed antihypertensive agents do not achieve optimal control of blood pressure because of inadequate medication adherence (Dunbar & Stunkard, 1979). When prescribing weight loss agents, practitioners may wish to review several issues with patients. These include:

1. Explaining the mechanisms by which the weight loss medication works. This includes describing what the medication will do (i.e., increase satiety or block fat absorption), as well as what the patient should do (i.e., decrease exposure to food triggers, record food intake, etc.).

2. Describing the medication's possible side effects and how the patient should respond to them. This includes having the patient call the practitioner before he or she stops taking the medication.

3. Inquiring whether the patient or the patient's family members have any health concerns about the use of medications (particularly in view of the adverse effects of the fenfluramines) or about costs of medications (which are not covered by most insurance plans).

4. Describing the course of treatment (at least for the first year), outlining medication use and the frequency of office visits, and discussing behavioral goals of treatment.

5. Developing a medication schedule that identifies when and where patients will take their medication and what they should do in the event of missed doses. The more concrete the schedule, the better patients' adherence.

6. Having patients keep a daily medication log, at least during the first few months. This log should be reviewed at subsequent office visits.

7. Reviewing how much weight patients can realistically expect to lose during the first

6 months of treatment, and helping them define success in terms of non-weight-related outcomes. These might include improvements in health complications, increased fitness and mobility, or the ability to enjoy recreational or social activities that the individual has forgone because of excess weight (Wadden et al., 2001).

Long-Term Medication Use

Practitioners will also need to prepare patients for the slowdown in weight loss that typically occurs between the fourth and sixth months, after which most individuals stop losing weight altogether, despite remaining on medication. As shown in Figure 11.3, obese women treated by Wadden and colleagues (2001) expected to continue to lose weight from months 6 to 12. They were totally unprepared for the weight loss plateau that occurred at month 6, which is illustrated in Figure 11.2. Practitioners should inform patients that the weight loss plateau is to be expected (although it is not easily explained), and that medications work after the first 6 months to maintain the weight loss that has been achieved. This last point is critical, because most patients interpret the lack of continued weight loss as a sign that the medication is no longer working, and this leads them to discontinue therapy.

Discontinuing medication usually results in rapid regaining of lost weight, which paradoxically illustrates how well the medication was working to maintain weight loss. This finding was observed in a recent study, in which 24 patients who had completed 68 weeks of treatment with sibutramine were encouraged by their physician to remain on the medication indefinitely to facilitate weight maintenance (Womble, Wadden, Berkowitz, Sarwer, & Rothman, in press). As shown in Figure 11.4, the five women who remained on medication

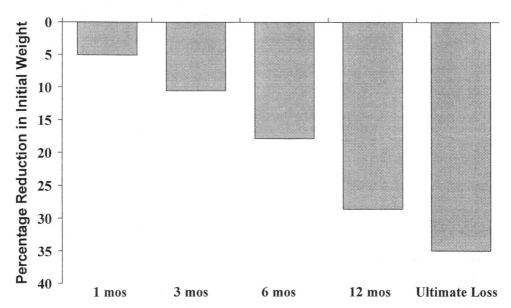

FIGURE 11.3. Patients' expected reduction in initial weight after 1, 3, 6, and 12 months of treatment. Prior to treatment, participants reported the cumulative number of pounds they expected to lose by each period. These values were converted to percentage reduction in initial weight. "Ultimate loss" reflects the weight loss patients hoped ultimately to achieve, even if not during the 12-month study. From Wadden, Berkowitz, Sarwer, Prus-Wisniewski, and Steinberg (2001). Copyright 2001 by the American Medical Association. Reprinted by permission.

at the 104-week assessment maintained their full end-of-treatment weight loss, whereas those who discontinued medication at week 68 or shortly thereafter regained about 6 kg from week 68 to week 104.

In order to be used on a long-term basis, weight loss medications must be both safe and effective. Orlistat and sibutramine both appear to be effective, as judged by 2-year placebo-controlled trials (Davidson et al., 1999; James et al., 2000; Sjöström et al., 1998). Both also appear to be generally safe, although sibutramine is associated in some patients with significant increases in blood pressure and pulse, and thus must be monitored closely (Hansen, Tourbo, Stock, Macdonald, & Astrup, 1999; Wadden et al., 2001). Studies are now needed to determine the best schedule for maintaining patients on medication over the long term in order to maintain their weight losses over the long term. For example, it may be possible to limit medication use to every other month, as shown with phentermine (Munro, MacCuish, Wilson, & Duncan, 1968) or to prescribe medication primarily during high-risk periods for weight gain, such as during the winter holidays. Regardless of whether we consider current medications or those yet to be discovered, they will have to be used on a long-term basis in the same fashion as agents for other chronic disorders, including hypertension, hyperlipidemia, and diabetes.

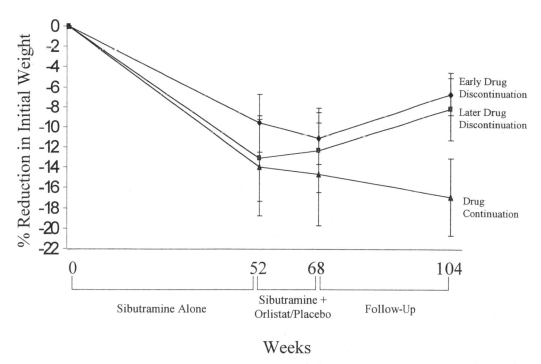

FIGURE 11.4. Change in body weight over 2 years in patients who discontinued sibutramine at week 68 (i.e., early drug discontinuation) (*n* = 13), who discontinued medication between weeks 68 and 104 (i.e., later drug discontinuation) (*n* = 6), and who continued medication until week 104 (i.e., drug continuation) (*n* = 6). During weeks 0–52, all participants received sibutramine. During weeks 52–68, all patients received sibutramine, while half were randomly assigned to orlistat and half to placebo. At the study's conclusion (week 68), all patients were encouraged to continue taking sibutramine to facilitate the maintenance of weight loss. Data from Womble, Wadden, Berkowitz, Sarwer, and Rothman (in press).

TREATMENT OPTIONS: BMI $\geq$ 40 kg/m^2

Persons with a BMI $\geq$ 40 kg/m^2 deserve special attention from health care providers. This is because extremely obese individuals typically experience more serious health complications, as well as more adverse psychosocial consequences, than do persons with lesser degrees of excess weight. The physical and psychosocial complications of extreme obesity are discussed in this volume by Field, Barnoya, and Colditz (Chapter 1), Latifi, Kellum, De Maria, and Sugerman (Chapter 16), and Wadden, Womble, Stunkard, and Anderson (Chapter 8). Practitioners must ensure that these individuals receive the medical care that they need, independent of their need for weight reduction.

Latifi and colleagues (Chapter 16) have described surgical interventions for the management of obesity, including vertical banded gastroplasty, gastric bypass, and gastric banding procedures. The gastric bypass would appear to be the treatment of choice for extremely obese individuals, given that the procedure induces an average loss of 25%–30% of initial weight and is associated with excellent long-term weight loss and improvements in comorbid conditions (Albrecht & Pories, 1999; Latifi et al., Chapter 16). Patients, however, must be fully informed of the risks of the procedures, which include an operative mortality rate of approximately 0.5%–1.0%. In addition, surgical candidates must understand that the gastric bypass will radically change their eating, in terms of reducing the amounts and types of foods that they can consume (particularly sweets and meats). At our program at the University of Pennsylvania, all candidates are screened not only by a surgeon and specialist in internal medicine, but also by a behavioral psychologist and dietitian. The latter two staff members describe the eating and activity habits that must be adopted after surgery; they assess the patients' readiness to make these changes (Wadden, Sarwer, et al., 2001).

Our opinion of bariatric surgery has changed dramatically over the past 20 years, from thinking that it bordered on the barbaric to now believing that the approach is underutilized. Bariatric surgery should be considered with all individuals who have serious obesity-related health complications and a BMI > 35 kg/m^2 (or a BMI > 40 kg/m^2 in the absence of major health complications). Candidates should have tried to lose weight using the safer, more traditional options of diet, exercise, and weight loss medication. Those, however, with a marked history of weight cycling (i.e., lost and regained a total of 50 kg or more) should consider bariatric surgery before embarking on another weight loss effort with traditional therapy.

IMPROVING THE MAINTENANCE OF WEIGHT LOSS

Bariatric surgery receives high marks because it is associated with excellent maintenance of weight loss for up to 15 years after surgery (Albrecht & Pories, 1999; Latifi et al., Chapter 16, this volume). By contrast, weight regain remains the Achilles's heel of both behavioral and pharmacological interventions. Remarkably little is known about the specific physiological and behavioral factors that contribute to weight regain, despite the reliability with which this occurrence is observed. By contrast, factors associated with the maintenance of weight loss are well known and include high levels of physical activity; consumption of a low-calorie, low-fat diet; regular monitoring of weight and food intake; and the use of positive coping strategies in response to lapses in diet and exercise adherence (Jeffery, Wing, Thorson, & Burton, 1998; Klem, Wing, McGuire, Seagle, & Hill, 1997; Wadden, 1995).

In this volume, Perri and Corsica (Chapter 17), as well as Wing (Chapter 14), discuss methods of facilitating patients' long-term adherence to these critical behaviors. Cooper and Fairburn (Chapter 22) propose a cognitive model that attributes weight regain in part to patients' negative body image. Obese individuals who are dissatisfied with their weight and shape are unable to accept the modest 10% weight loss that behavioral and pharmacological therapies typically produce. Their frustration and disappointment ultimately lead them to abandon efforts needed to maintain the modest weight losses they have achieved. Several of the therapeutic interventions proposed by Cooper and Fairburn (Chapter 22) are used in nondieting approaches to weight management, as discussed by Foster and McGuckin (Chapter 24).

LOOKING AHEAD

This chapter has been written with the knowledge that the interventions described are likely to benefit the individuals who receive them but are inadequate to solve our nation's growing epidemic of obesity. This is because weight reduction therapy is currently available only to a minority of obese individuals, typically those who can pay out of pocket. Even with these persons, earnest efforts to modify eating and activity habits usually are no match in the long term for a toxic environment that explicitly encourages the consumption of large portions of high-fat, high-sugar foods and implicitly discourages physical activity, as a result of fundamental changes in the nation's work and leisure habits. Clearly, efforts are needed to improve the treatment of obesity, as well as to obtain recognition and reimbursement of this disorder. But far greater attention now must be devoted to the prevention of obesity, as described in this volume by Horgen and Brownell (Chapter 5) and Schmitz and Jeffery (Chapter 27), and to the treatment of childhood obesity, as discussed by Goldfield, Raynor, and Epstein (Chapter 26). Such efforts must attack the environment that lies at the heart of this disorder. This will require investigators and practitioners to work not only in the laboratory and consulting room but also in schools, workplaces, and other community settings. Those interested in the treatment of obesity must realize that the objects of their care are not only the individuals who present to them for treatment, but also the larger social and economic forces that shape our nation's eating and activity habits.

REFERENCES

Albrecht, R. J., & Pories, W. J. (1999). Surgical intervention for the severely obese. *Ballière's Clinical Endocrinology and Metabolism, 13,* 149–172.

Anderson, J. W., Vichitbandra, S., Qian, W., & Kryscio, R. J. (1999). Long-term weight maintenance after an intensive weight-loss program. *Journal of the American College of Nutrition, 18,* 620–627.

Apfelbaum, M., Vague, P., Ziegler, O., Hanotin, C., Thomas, F., & Leutenegger, E. (1999). Long-term maintenance of weight loss after a very-low-calorie diet: A randomized blinded trial of the efficacy and tolerability of sibutramine. *American Journal of Medicine, 106,* 179–184.

Atkinson, R. L., & Hubbard, V. S. (1994). Report on the NIH workshop on pharmacologic treatment of obesity. *American Journal of Clinical Nutrition, 60,* 153–156.

Bandini, L. G., Schoeller, D. A., Cyr, H. N., & Dietz, W. H. (1990). Validity of reported energy intake in obese and non-obese adolescents. *American Journal of Clinical Nutrition, 52,* 421–425.

Bray, G. A. (1993). Use and abuse of appetite-suppressant drugs in the treatment of obesity. *Annals of Internal Medicine, 119,* 707–713.

Bray, G. A., & Greenway, F. L. (1999). Current and potential drugs for treatment of obesity. *Endocrine Reviews, 20,* 805–875.

Broomfield, P. H., Chopra, R., Sheinbaum, R. C., Bonorris, G. G., Silverman, A., Schoenfield, L. J., & Marks, J. W. (1988). Effects of ursodeoxycholic acid and aspirin on the formation of lithogenic bile and gallstones during loss of weight. *New England Journal of Medicine, 319,* 1567–1572.

Brownell, K. D. (2000). *The LEARN program for weight management 2000.* Dallas, TX: American Health.

Volkmar, F. R., Stunkard, A. J., Woolston, J., & Bailey, B. A. (1981). High attrition rates in commercial weight reduction programs. *Archives of Internal Medicine, 141,* 426–428.

Wadden, T. A. (1995). Characteristics of successful weight loss maintainers. In F. X. Pi-Sunyer & D. B. Allison (Eds.), *Obesity treatment: Establishing goals, improving outcomes, and reviewing the research agenda* (pp. 111–118). New York: Plenum Press.

Wadden, T. A., Anderson, D. A., Foster, G. D., Bennett, A., Steinberg, C., & Sarwer, D. B. (2000). Obese women's perceptions of their doctors' weight management attitudes and behaviors. *Archives of Family Medicine, 9,* 854–860.

Wadden, T. A., & Bartlett, S. J. (1992). Very low calorie diets: An overview and appraisal. In T. A. Wadden & T. B. VanItallie (Eds.), *Treatment of the seriously obese patient* (pp. 44–79). New York: Guilford Press.

Wadden, T. A., & Berkowitz, R. I. (2001). Very low calorie diets. In C. G. Fairburn & K. D. Brownell (Eds.), *Eating disorders and obesity* (2nd ed., pp. 529–533). New York: Guilford Press.

Wadden, T. A., Berkowitz, R. I., Sarwer, D. B., Prus-Wisniewski, R., & Steinberg, C. (2001). Benefits of lifestyle modification in the pharmacologic treatment of obesity. *Archives of Internal Medicine, 161,* 218–227.

Wadden, T. A., Berkowitz, R. I., Vogt, R. A., Steen, S. N., Stunkard, A. J., & Foster, G. D. (1997). Lifestyle modification in the pharmacologic treatment of obesity: A pilot investigation of a potential primary care approach. *Obesity Research, 5,* 218–226.

Wadden, T. A., Berkowitz, R. I., Womble, L. G., Sarwer, D. B., Arnold, M., & Steinberg, C. (2000). Effects of sibutramine plus orlistat in obese women following one year of treatment by sibutramine alone: A placebo-controlled trial. *Obesity Research, 8,* 431–437.

Wadden, T. A., Brownell, K. D., & Foster, G. D. (in press). Obesity: Responding to the global epidemic. *Journal of Consulting and Clinical Psychology.*

Wadden, T. A., & Foster, G. D. (2000). Behavior therapy for obesity. *Medical Clinics of North America, 84,* 441–461.

Wadden, T. A., Foster, G. D., & Letizia, K. A. (1994). One-year behavioral treatment of obesity: Comparison of moderate and severe caloric restriction and the effects of weight maintenance therapy. *Journal of Consulting and Clinical Psychology, 62,* 165–171.

Wadden, T. A., Foster, G. D., Stunkard, A. J., & Conill, A. (1996). Effects of weight cycling on resting metabolic rate and body composition of obese women. *International Journal of Eating Disorders, 19,* 5–12.

Wadden, T. A., Sarwer, D. B., & Berkowitz, R. I. (1999). Behavioral treatment of the overweight patient. *Ballière's Clinical Endocrinology and Metabolism, 13,* 93–107.

Wadden, T. A., Sarwer, D. B., Womble, L. G., Foster, G. D., McGuckin, B. G., & Schimmel, A. (2001). Psychological aspects of obesity and obesity surgery. *Surgical Clinics of North America, 81,* 1001–1024.

Wadden, T. A., Sternberg, J. A., Letizia, K. A., Stunkard, A. J., & Foster, G. D. (1989). Treatment of obesity by very low calorie diet, behavior therapy, and their combination: A five-year perspective. *International Journal of Obesity, 13,* 39–46.

Wing, R. R. (1998). Behavioral approaches to the treatment of obesity. In G. A. Bray, C. Bouchard, & W. P. T. James (Eds.), *Handbook of obesity* (pp. 855–873). New York: Marcel Dekker.

Wing, R. R., Blair, E., Marcus, M., Epstein, L. H., & Harvey, J. (1994). Year-long weight loss treatment for obese patients with Type II diabetes: Does including an intermittent very-low-calorie diet improve outcome? *American Journal of Medicine, 97,* 354–362.

Wing, R. R., Marcus, M. D., Salata, R., Epstein, L. H., Miaskiewicz, S., & Blair, E. H. (1991). Effects of a very-low-calorie diet on long-term glycemic control in obese Type 2 diabetic subjects. *Archives of Internal Medicine, 151,* 1334–1340.

Womble, L. G., Wadden, T. A., Berkowitz, S., Sarwer, D. B., & Rothman, R. A. (in press). Continued use of medication facilitates weight maintenance [Letter to the editor]. *Obesity Research.*

World Health Organization. (1998). *Obesity: Preventing and managing the global epidemic* (Publication No. WHO/NUT/NCD/98.1) Geneva: Author.

12

Popular Diets for Treatment of Overweight and Obesity

KATHLEEN MELANSON
JOHANNA DWYER

Millions of individuals in industrialized societies are constantly attempting to lose excess weight, either on their own, under their physicians' care, or through other programs (Galuska, Will, Serdula, & Ford, 1999). However, most fail in the process, often growing more discouraged and even more obese as a result (National Heart, Lung, and Blood Institute [NHLBI], 1998; Pasman, Saris, & Westerterp-Plantenga, 1999). The myriad claims of advocates of different weight loss approaches lead many dieters to choose inappropriate options (Galuska et al., 1999). In an effort to clarify this confusion, this chapter focuses on popular diets used to treat overweight and obesity. It begins by examining criteria for evaluating weight loss and maintenance strategies, and applying these to some popular diets. Diet foods and products, as well as special ingredients and techniques for achieving weight control, are discussed. Readers desiring a review of the physiological basis of weight loss, as well as the regulation of macronutrient intake, are directed to Appendix 12.1.

CRITERIA FOR EVALUATING WEIGHT LOSS STRATEGIES

During the hypocaloric phase of weight control efforts, there are seven criteria that the eating plan must meet. These are called the "seven C's," and are summarized in Table 12.1. The last three C's also apply to maintenance of a healthier weight, once it has been achieved.

Calories

The size of the caloric deficit, and thus the amount of weight that will be lost, depend on the difference between the individual's usual food intake and the calorie level of the reducing diet. The energy needs of a person in energy balance can be estimated by using a formula

phosphorus, potassium, and vitamins follow the loss of lean tissue. Loss of more than 40% of the initial lean body mass in a normal healthy individual is life-threatening (Roubenoff & Kehayias, 1991). Lesser losses of lean body mass can also be hazardous, affecting cardiovascular function, exercise tolerance, and possibly immune responses, and thus should be avoided.

As a rule of thumb, a minimum of 65–70 g of protein is needed daily. On a VLCD, 1.5 g of high-quality protein per kilogram of ideal body weight per day is desirable, with intakes no less than about 65–70 g. Intakes may need to be even higher if the dieter suffers from certain diseases or is physically stressed, since nitrogen losses may rise further in these states. On 800–1,200 kcal/day, daily protein intake should be at least 1 g/kg ideal body weight. Reducing diets over 1,200 kcal/day should provide protein at a rate of at least 0.8 g/kg ideal body weight. Levels should remain this high after weight loss has stopped and maintenance has begun.

Electrolytes and Water

Electrolyte levels are important, especially in fasting and on VLCDs; cardiac arrhythmias have resulted from hypokalemia on such regimens (Amatruda, Biddle, Patton, & Lockwood, 1982). Since hypocalemia can be fatal, electrolyte levels must always be monitored.

Hydration is also important, both to slake thirst and to avoid dehydration, particularly in hot climates or with physical exertion. Much of the very rapid weight loss that occurs in the first few days of dieting is due to diuresis and dehydration, particularly when ketogenic, very-low-carbohydrate, low-calorie diets (LCDs) are employed. As mentioned earlier, losses of body glycogen and protein are accompanied by losses of body water. Thus intake of low- or no-calorie fluids such as water should be emphasized. Beverages containing caffeine and alcohol should not be encouraged, since they increase diuresis. When the individual engages in very vigorous physical activity, electrolytes and water should be monitored. Often the fatigue that some dieters associate with hypocaloric diets is actually due, at least in part, to dehydration. Body water losses of as little as 2% have been associated with decreased physical and mental performance, as well as with impaired thermoregulation (Kleiner, 1999). The daily recommendation of at least 8 glasses of water is especially important for dieters; they often require even more. Thus a fluid intake plan should be incorporated in every weight loss regimen.

Vitamins and Minerals

Vitamins and minerals are also critical on reducing diets. The recommended dietary allowance for an individual's age and sex must be met in both usual and reducing diets. The lower the diet is in calories, the more likely it is that other essential nutrients and electrolytes (such as potassium, magnesium, vitamin B_6, iron, and calcium) will be low. As a rule of thumb, diets below 1,200 kcal/day are likely to require vitamin and mineral supplements. Above 1,200 kcal/day, iron and calcium supplements may still be needed by women in the reproductive age groups, but most other nutrient needs can be met by a well-balanced diet that follows the Dietary Guidelines for Americans (U.S. Department of Agriculture [USDA] & U.S. Department of Health and Human Services [USDHHS], 2000). For this reason, foods with high micronutrient density but low energy density are especially important on a reducing diet.

The guidelines for the composition of weight-reducing diets, as discussed above, are outlined in Table 12.2.

TABLE 12.2. Guidelines for Composition of Healthy Weight Control Plans

Carbohydrate
  VLCD: ≥50 g/day
  LCD: ≥100 g/day

Protein
  VLCD: 1.5 g/kg body wt. (≥65–70 g/day)
  LCD: 1.0 g/kg body wt.
  BDD: 0.8 g/kg body wt.

Fat
  ≤30% of dietary energy from total fat
  ≤10% of dietary energy from saturated fat

Fiber
  20–30 g/day

Water
  8 glasses (~2 quarts or 2 liters)
  More needed with exercise and/or heat

Vitamins/minerals
  Supplemented on VLCD and LCD (to recommended daily allowance)
  Iron and calcium for women of reproductive age

Alcohol
  Minimal to none

Note. VLCD, very-low-calorie diet (<800 kcal/day); LCD, low-calorie diet (800–1,200 kcal/day); BDD, balanced-deficit diet (>1,200 kcal/day).

Cost

The cost of weight loss programs is probably one of the reasons why so many Americans use popular diet books. Obesity, uncomplicated by other comorbidities, is not considered a reimbursable expense by most insurance companies and health maintenance organizations. Therefore, a dieter must usually pay out of pocket for all or most of the cost of treatment. Billions of dollars are spent each year on obesity treatment, with charges ranging from modest to exorbitant.

Unfortunately, there is no *Consumer Reports* list that summarizes the effectiveness and costs of different programs. Standardized information, including disclosure of the effectiveness and cost of different approaches, is not available. Therefore, the buyer must beware. Some professional societies, such as local chapters of the American Dietetic Association, the American Medical Association, and the North American Society for the Study of Obesity, are good sources to consult if questions arise about a particular program.

Consumer Friendliness

Health is a social good. The fact that health care, including obesity treatment, also represents a commercial transaction does not exempt it from the need for ethical and humanistic marketing and treatment practices. Therefore, consumers of obesity treatment programs have the right to be treated respectfully and with safe treatments. In the early 1990s, congressional hearings examined the misleading advertising claims used by some commercial weight loss programs. As a result of these hearings, the Federal Trade Commission recently encouraged commercial weight loss programs to voluntarily disclose their costs and results of treatment, so that consumers can make informed decisions when selecting treatment.

often gain large amounts of weight in a few days, due to restoration of water balance to more normal levels. Because VLCDs are so different from usual dietary intakes, instruction is necessary to avoid overindulgence when a dieter returns to regular eating patterns. The characteristics and problems of VLCDs, as well as examples of popular diets based on them, are discussed elsewhere in greater detail (Dwyer & Lu, 1993; Kanders & Blackburn, 1994; National Task Force, 1993).

Low-Calorie Diets

LCDs, providing 800–1,200 kcal/day, are still below the RMR for most adults, but they have less pronounced effects on metabolism than do VLCDs. Many meal replacement products, designed for use in LCDs, are now available in supermarkets and drugstores. Examples include SlimFast and Ultra SlimFast, as well as the Cambridge Food for Life Program. These products are specially formulated foods or powders that are designed as meal replacements; if label directions are followed, intakes should average approximately 1,100–1,200 kcal/day. Deviation from these recommened levels could be associated with adverse consequences, as discussed later.

Frozen low-calorie main dishes are also popular among dieters. These include Healthy Choice, Ultra SlimFast Frozen Entrees, Weight Watchers entrees (e.g., Smart Ones), Stouffer's Lean Cuisine, Budget Gourmet Light, and many others. Most of them provide about 200–300 kcal/serving, are low in fat and cholesterol, are relatively high in carbohydrate, and vary in their vitamin and mineral contributions. All of these products provide convenient, portion-controlled, quick-to-prepare entrees that are useful adjuncts to a total weight management program. However, there is no guarantee that individuals will devise and follow an appropriate plan on their own. Therefore, some medical assistance is advisable. Similar meals are sold as part of commercial weight loss programs, such as nutrisystem.com, Jenny Craig Weight Loss Centres, and Intelligent Cuisine. These products have the advantage of being part of broader and more comprehensive programs, but the total costs of the programs are also greater.

Several commercial programs, including Weight Watchers, Diet Workshop, and Diet Center, also provide (or have provided) LCDs that use conventional (table) foods. Many of these regimens begin with a low-carbohydrate, hypocaloric diet of 900–1,000 kcal/day to stimulate diuresis and rapid weight loss in the first few weeks. Calorie intake is then increased to 1,200 kcal/day or more. Usually multivitamin and mineral supplements, and for women calcium and iron supplements, are recommended. Most of the programs also include group support, some nutrition education, and a program of physical activity.

Books that advocate LCDs are also plentiful. "Unbalanced-deficit diets" are currently popular. Deficits in calories are accompanied by a radical redistribution of the energy-providing nutrients to emphasize low carbohydrate, high protein, and relatively low fat, in comparison to usual dietary intakes. The advantages of such regimens are that they are novel; the energy level is usually low enough to cause weight loss, but not so low as to induce troublesome metabolic side effects; and they stimulate a rapid diuresis with welcome loss of weight, albeit water weight. This may encourage dieters to continue their efforts. Several such diets are discussed below, and others are analyzed elsewhere (Dwyer, 1992; Dwyer & Lu, 1993).

Balanced-Deficit Diets

Diets that provide 1,200 kcal/day or more and are suitably formulated are probably the most benign if not the most popular of the self-prescribed diets that Americans undertake.

They are sometimes referred to as "balanced-deficit diets." They tend to be lower in calories but have a "balanced" profile of calories that provides nutrients and foods closer to the profile recommended for good health among nondieters. That is, they are relatively low in fat (<30% calories), high in complex carbohydrate (>55% calories), moderate in protein (10–15% calories), devoid of or very low in alcohol, and high in fiber (25–30 g/day).

Various nutritionally adequate well-planned regimens are available. They include the regimens recommended by nonprofit weight loss groups, by professionals such as registered dietitians, and by most programs based in hospitals or health centers (other than the VLCD programs). Balanced-deficit diets may also be offered by commercial programs such as the Diet Center, Physicians' Weight Loss Centers, and Weight Watchers. For those who cannot afford such programs, two self-help programs, Take Off Pounds Sensibly (TOPS) and Overeaters Anonymous (OA), may be helpful. Several popular diet books also promote reasonable, moderately-low-calorie diets. These books include *The Callaway Diet* (Callaway with Whitney, 1990), *The T-Factor Diet* (Katahn, 1989), and *The Fat Attack Plan* (Natow & Heslin, 1990).

The higher calorie levels of balanced-deficit diets (relative to VLCDs and LCDs) make compliance easier, minimize undesirable metabolic side effects, eliminate the need for special foods, and permit dietary and eating reeducation to occur during the weight loss process. In addition, exercise tolerance is good on a balanced-deficit diet. An aerobic exercise program can be a helpful adjunct to counteract the decrease in RMR induced by a hypocaloric diet and to further increase weight loss without excessive dietary deprivation. Furthermore, loss of metabolically active tissue is minimized when the weight loss strategy includes exercise (Marks, Ward, Morris, Castellani, & Rippe, 1995).

The major disadvantage of balanced-deficit diets is that weight loss is somewhat slower than on the more drastic regimens, and thus motivation, patience, and adherence may be low. The key to success, as it is on any weight loss program, is adherence. To facilitate adherence, some regimens restrict choice to a preplanned menu or an exchange plan that allows a dieter to select only certain alternatives. Other regimens restrict choice to a set menu. For these approaches, one should always be sure that no major food group is completely excluded. In addition, dieters should choose the dieting approach that best suits their needs and preferences.

DIET BOOKS AND REGIMENS

Diets Based on the Glycemic Index

The "glycemic index" (GI) is a dietary concept that has become very popular recently. The GI describes the blood glucose response resulting from consumption of a defined amount of carbohydrate (usually 50 g) from a given food, relative to the same amount of carbohydrate from a control food (Wolever, Jenkins, Jenkins, & Josse, 1991). The control food may be pure glucose or white bread, although the latter is preferred due to problems with osmolarity of glucose solutions. The GI concept was first developed as a strategy to help guide patients with diabetes in maintaining stable blood glucose. The pros (Brand-Miller & Foster-Powell, 1999; Wolever, 1999) and cons (Beebe, 1999; Franz, 1999) of its applicability are still being discussed in the literature.

Recently the GI has been suggested as a tool for the treatment and prevention of overweight and obesity (Ludwig et al., 1999). It is purportedly the basis for the diets outlined in the books *Dr. Bob Arnot's Revolutionary Weight Control Program* (Arnot, 1998) and *The Glucose Revolution* (Brand-Miller, Wolever, Colagiuri, & Foster-Powell, 1999). Other, less

diets is that carbohydrate consumption in excess of this stimulates the release of insulin, an anabolic hormone that functions to promote the storage of metabolic fuels, thus leading to weight gain. This is an oversimplification of very complex metabolic processes. The crucial fact that is missing from the theory is that metabolic fuels will only be stored under conditions of energy surplus, not during an energy deficit. Insulin itself will not promote body fatness if there is no energy available to be stored. The reasons these diets work are their energy deficits (most provide about 1,200 kcal/day or less) and the fact that they are ketogenic and lead to a state of relative dehydration. Weight loss is not the result of alterations in insulin metabolism that the diets engender.

In the absence of medical supervision, any diet that promotes a state of ketosis should be avoided as potentially dangerous. Even if these diets lead to initial loss of relatively large amounts of water, they should not be encouraged because prolonged adherence to high-protein diets may lead to calcuria, to kidney stones in those who are prone to them, and to high blood urea nitrogen in those with undiagnosed kidney problems. The increased nitrogenous load caused by the combination of high protein intake and a high rate of gluconeogenesis results in an elevated obligatory urine volume, and thus may lead to dehydration. This can have deleterious effects on physical and mental health. However, dieters may perceive the weight loss associated with dehydration as beneficial, and thus may think the diet is particularly effective. This may be a factor in the popularity of high-protein diets.

High-protein diets are often high in fat and in saturated fat, and because high-saturated-fat diets are well established as atherogenic, they are inappropriate over the long run. In addition, many high-protein, very-low-carbohydrate plans have lists of "forbidden foods" that include potatoes, pasta, rice, white bread, bagels, carrots, corn, and watermelon. This is one reason why the diets may be lacking in such nutrients as calcium, magnesium, manganese, and potassium; the B vitamins; dietary fiber; and water. Vitamin D levels, as well as calcium, may be low if milk products are prohibited because of the lactose (a sugar) they contain. Many professional organizations, including the American College of Sports Medicine, the American Dietetic Association, the Women's Sports Foundation, and the Cooper Institute for Aerobics Research, have all issued statements that high-protein plans are the answer neither for weight loss nor for improving athletic performance. Indeed, they can cause harm.

An important aspect of any weight loss regimen is that it must provide strategies for maintenance of weight loss after a healthier weight is achieved. This is critical, considering the extremely high relapse rates as individuals move from weight loss into weight management (Pasman et al., 1999). In order to prevent weight regain, permanent changes in diet and lifestyle must be learned and adopted. Long-term adherence (i.e., over several months) to a low-carbohydrate, high-protein diet that is also high in fat and saturated fat could pose significant health risks, as previously described. Furthermore, the protective effects of a diet high in whole grains, fruits and vegetables, soluble and insoluble fiber, and antioxidant nutrients would be missed. This could increase the risk of a number of chronic degenerative diseases, including certain cancers and diverticulosis. Long-term data on the effectiveness and safety of 40/30/30 plans are lacking, but because the risks associated with high-protein and high-fat diets in general are well established, these diets are not recommended. The fact that a high-protein, low-carbohydrate diet does not teach healthful lifelong eating habits is a strong argument against such a regimen.

Low-Protein Diets

Fortunately, low-protein diets are not presently in vogue. Low-protein regimens are a serious concern, because protein needs are higher in hypocaloric states than they are in energy balance. As noted earlier, significant health risks and undesirable metabolic effects are associated with insufficient protein intake during weight loss. Protein deficiency can result in hair loss, lethargy, exercise intolerance, edema, fluid and electrolyte imbalances, cardiac and kidney problems, depressed immunity, and skin abnormalities. These diets may also be lacking in vitamin B_{12}, zinc, calcium, and some fat-soluble vitamins. Recommendations for appropriate amounts of protein are provided in preceding sections.

High-Fat Diets

The Montignac Method

A weight loss strategy particularly popular among upper-class Europeans is the Montignac Method, created by the French chef Michel Montignac (Montignac, 1999a, 1999b). The diet includes foie gras, creme brûlée, souffle, chocolate truffles, and wine daily. However, fat and carbohydrate are not permitted at the same meal because (according to the plan's "metabolic synopsis") increases in blood glucose cause fat to be stored in the body. The author states that hyperinsulinemia is the cause of obesity rather than a consequence. This is an erroneous, oversimplified interpretation of the relationship and the direction of causality. If the diet does cause weight loss, it is because the diet is hypocaloric, not because it plays "metabolic tricks." Perhaps the appeal of the intriguing French cuisine enhances adherence.

According to Montignac's theories, individuals can lose weight and become healthier without restricting quantities of food intake, exercising, or being concerned about dietary fat and cholesterol. One part of the rationale is that French people are thin despite a rich diet. Montignac claims that habits such as eating the biggest meal at lunchtime rather than at dinner and avoiding snacks between meals must be responsible. This correlational evidence cannot prove causality. Clearly, other lifestyle factors (including habitual physical activity) play roles in determining levels of adiposity. Another part of the Montignac plan is based on the GI, listing "bad" and "good" carbohydrates. Any food with a GI above 50 is forbidden. This is arbitrary, because many GI lists have very different values for the same foods. Thus a food may be "good" according to some lists and "bad" according to others. Furthermore, many of the foods on the "bad" lists are nourishing foods that are rich in vitamins, minerals, and fiber. Examples include carrots, beets, potatoes, corn, rice, popcorn, rice cakes, watermelon, bananas, raisins, and cantaloupe. These foods do not deserve a bad name. As indicated earlier, lists of "bad" and "good" foods are warning signs that a diet is unreasonable, especially if fruits and vegetables are considered "bad" foods.

The Atkins Diets

The popular Atkins diets (Atkins, 1981, 1992, 1999), which are also high in fat (and low in carbohydrate), encourage a state of ketosis. In fact, dieters are told that they are doing something wrong if they are not ketotic; they are told to stimulate ketosis. According to Atkins, the best diet is high in fat and moderate in protein, with zero carbohydrate. Parts of this diet include 20 g of carbohydrate daily. This low level causes extreme ketosis, which can be hazardous, especially in the absence of medical supervision. Furthermore, these types of diets are lacking in several vitamins, antioxidants, and calcium. In addition to being potentially threatening to cardiovascular health, these regimens do not teach a proper lifelong diet.

Low-Carbohydrate Diets

Low-carbohydrate diets come in many forms, but should not be recommended under most circumstances. Carbohydrate levels are important in LCDs, because adequate carbohydrate

benefit is that whole grains, fruits, and vegetables have also been implicated in the prevention of heart disease and some cancers.

Other Diet Books

In recent decades, numerous weight loss plans have been published, some more reasonable and sound than others. Some books that offer less sound or otherwise inappropriate diets include *Eat Right 4 Your Type* (D'Adamo, 1997), *The New Beverly Hills Diet* (Mazel with Wyatt & Sokol, 1996), *The 5-Day Miracle Diet* (Puhn, 1996), *Fit for Life* (Diamond & Diamond, 1985), *The Hilton Head Over-35 Diet* (Miller, 1989), and *The Rotation Diet* (Katahn, 1987). These have been reviewed in detail elsewhere (Burland, 1986; Dwyer & Lu, 1993). *Eat Right 4 Your Type* (D'Adamo, 1997) is a weight loss plan based on blood type, which is scientifically unfounded, lacking in research to substantiate the author's claims, and unduly limited in the foods it permits. The regimen described in *The New Beverly Hills Diet* (Mazel et al., 1996) restricts different food groups at different times of day, based on erroneous assumptions about the metabolism of certain combinations of foods. Moreover, this diet does not account for individual differences in energetic needs. Puhn (1996), in *The 5-Day Miracle Diet,* describes a potentially dangerous VLCD (800 kcal/day) when self-administered without medical supervision. Although the diet's recommended duration is only 5 days, the likelihood that people will follow it longer, or repeatedly, is almost certain. This probability is high because such a diet sets one up for failure, so a dieter tends to attempt it repeatedly. Most of the early weight loss probably consists of water, and it is unlikely to be maintained. The diet described in *Fit for Life* (Diamond & Diamond, 1985) should likewise be avoided, since it excludes some food groups and lacks variety, which is necessary for adherence. In addition to this diet's being high in fat (>40%), its metabolic basis is unfounded; the authors claim that fat deposits result from improper food combinations. Diets that advocate variations in energy intakes in order to prevent declines in RMR are also based on unfounded assumptions for which there is no ample scientific evidence. In fact, if they lead to weight cycling, decreases in percentage of lean tissue can result, leading to depressions in metabolic rate that make further weight loss attempts more difficult. These include the regimens outlined in *The Hilton Head Over-35 Diet* (Miller, 1989) and *The Rotation Diet* (Katahn, 1986). Both of these diets are also lacking in some of the food groups.

Weight Loss Books with Less Diet Emphasis

Weight loss books recommending sound nutrition and lifestyle changes to promote healthful habits and strategies for weight maintenance include *The Solution* (Meillin, 1997), *Intuitive Eating* (Tribole & Resch, 1995), *Habits, Not Diets: The Secret to Lifetime Weight Control* (Ferguson & Ferguson, 1997), *The Complete Idiot's Guide to Losing Weight* (McQuillan, 1998), and *Dieting for Dummies* (Kirby, 1998). *The Solution* (Meillin, 1997) describes a nondiet approach that focuses on addressing the underlying causes for obesity or overweight, not the symptoms. It encourages the reader to understand why he or she overeats and to address those issues. This may be a good book for chronic dieters. *Intuitive Eating* (Tribole & Resch, 1995) instructs readers to listen to internal hunger and satiety signals as cues for food ingestion rather than being controlled by external cues. This is potentially a good book for individuals who binge-eat, or who eat in response to circumstances such as stress, loneliness, boredom, or depression. *Habits, Not Diets* (Ferguson & Ferguson, 1997) promotes the use of such tools as food intake and activity journals and self-evaluations. Teaching commitment to change and self-discipline, this book's structured approach may not be for everyone, but its underlying principles are sound. *The Complete Idiot's Guide to Losing Weight* (McQuillan, 1998) and *Dieting for Dummies* (Kirby, 1998) are well-rounded books that include sensible weight loss strategies, tips for spotting fraudulent fad diets, and healthy approaches to long-term lifestyle changes promoting weight maintenance. It should be noted, however, that the approaches described above are supported by minimal or no data. A thorough review of nondieting approaches to weight control is provided by Foster and McGuckin in Chapter 24 of this volume.

DIET FOODS AND PRODUCTS

Powdered-Diet Formulas and Meal Replacement Products

Over-the-counter diet products have a place in weight reduction strategies, but they often lend themselves to misuse, especially if consumers do not follow label directions. The oldest such product was Metrecal, a milk-based, low-kilocalorie meal replacement that was popular in the 1960s. Later, SlimFast, Ultra SlimFast, and similar powdered-diet formulas were placed on the market. Recently these products have become available ready-prepared in single-serving cans. The manufacturers of these products recommend the replacement of breakfast and dinner with one of their shakes (the powders are mixed with low-fat milk or water). These shakes are supplemented to include most of the daily required micronutrients (as well as fiber, in the case of Ultra SlimFast), and provide 190–220 kcal. In addition to the meal replacements, manufacturers recommend that dieters consume one piece of fruit and a low-calorie dinner (about 410 kcal), for a total daily energy intake of 1,100–1,200 kcal.

Instructions are included with the meal replacement products. If these are followed incorrectly, however, the results could be hazardous, especially in the absence of medical supervision. Some dieters believe that they can be more ambitious than the instructions suggest and try to restrict themselves more than is recommended. This can lead to micronutrient deficiencies, undesirable metabolic effects (as described earlier in regard to severe hypocaloric intakes), dietary imbalances, and an accumulation of hunger that can lead to subsequent overconsumption.

The rationale behind these meal replacement weight loss products is that because they are monotonous and measured, they relieve the dieter from having to make daily food choices. If the number of kilocalories and sufficiency of micronutrients are already accounted for by the manufacturer, then a step is saved for the dieter. However, this does not teach proper dietary habits, since once the diet is over, the dieter must learn to choose appropriate breakfast and dinner items that contain the appropriate amounts of kilocalories and micronutrients.

Newer diet formulas have come onto the market in recent years, which promise a quick start to the dieting process. These include such products as SlimFast's Jump Start, which suggests the consumption of three meal replacement shakes (210 kcal each) plus two pieces of fruit and a salad as the daily consumption. Thus this regimen qualifies as an LCD, but since the product is purchased over the counter, it could be dangerous in the absence of medical supervision. The SlimFast Jump Start meals are sold as 5-day kits, and are much more costly than their longer-term counterparts. Statements such as "Lose 5 pounds in 5 days" are listed on the label. If this loss was all body fat, it would require a deficit of 3,500 kcal/day. Thus, if a person were to consume the suggested maximum of 1,000 kcal/day, an expenditure of 4,500 kcal in some other manner such as physical activity would be required for the claim to be true. A person would have to be abnormally active and/or large in order to expend so much energy daily. Obviously, the major weight loss on such a diet is mostly water and glycogen, not body fat. Water weight returns upon refeeding and restoration of glycogen stores.

Meal Replacement Bars

Meal replacement bars have appeared on the market as alternatives to meal replacement shakes. These include SlimFast and Pounds-Off bars. Like meal replacement shakes, these bars contain about 200 kcal apiece, and are supplemented with certain micronutrients. However, some of these bars are sold individually with little or no dietary advice or instructions. Their labels may state that the bars should replace breakfast and lunch, and that a normal dinner should be consumed. Providing the dieter with little guidance, this approach can be either hazardous or useless. If the dieter were to consume one of these bars in place of breakfast and lunch for a total of about 420 kcal, then he or she would be ravenous by dinnertime. If the dieter were to succumb to the natural feelings of hunger, it is possible that a dinner of excess calories would be consumed, defeating the purpose of the diet. The opposite scenario is also possible; that is, an overly ambitious dieter may consume a dinner of 400 kcal or less, in the caloric range of a VLCD or LCD, which can be potentially hazardous when unsupervised. Like meal replacement shakes, these bars also do not teach lifelong healthy eating habits.

Another type of meal replacement bar accommodates individuals who are following high-protein, low-carbohydrate diets. These include several brands of bars that all contain proportions of the macronutrients in the range of the high-protein plans described earlier. The labels on these bars also contain little nutrition advice, and so they are particularly prone to misuse, especially if they are used as the sole source of nourishment. The bars are too low in carbohydrate, too high in protein, and potentially too hypocaloric for a sound reducing regimen to be composed solely of them.

Prepared Low-Calorie Meals

An increasingly popular trend in weight loss products for self-initiated efforts is the availability of frozen low-calorie main dishes, now widely available in grocery stores and supermarkets. These items are preportioned so that the dieter can consume a mixed meal with a fixed and known amount of energy, fat, and other nutrients. As noted earlier, such products include Healthy Choice, Ultra SlimFast Frozen Entrees, Weight Watchers (e.g., Smart Ones), Stouffer's Lean Cuisine, and Budget Gourmet Light, among others. These frozen low-calorie products usually provide about 200–300 kcal/serving (Ultra SlimFast Frozen Entrees provide 230–400 kcal) from a variety of recipes. Most of the dishes are low in fat and cholesterol and relatively high in carbohydrate. They vary in their vitamin and mineral contents. Since these meals are convenient and quickly prepared, they can be useful as adjuncts to a total weight management program. However, the potential for abuse is present, as it is with other products for self-initiated weight loss efforts. In addition, these entrees are relatively expensive.

Low-Fat, Low-Sugar, and Low-Calorie Products

Table 12.3 provides a description of some of the many products that are modified to be low in or devoid of calories. Throughout the 1990s, literally thousands of reduced-fat, low-fat, and fat-free foods were introduced to the U.S. market. These foods include cookies, crackers, soups, salad dressings, cheese and meat products, entrees, and many more. Data have

TABLE 12.3. Some Sugar Alternatives and Fat Replacers (Not All Currently Approved in the United States)

Ingredient	Comments
High-intensity noncaloric sweeteners	Noncaloric, sweeter than sugar; vary in bulk.
Acesufame K (acesulfame potassium). Brand names: Sunnet food ingredient and Sweet One, Swiss Sweet, and Twinsweet (acesulfame K–aspartame combination) tabletop sweeteners.	Contains potassium, but content is insufficient to cause concern in persons with diabetes.
Aspartame. Brand name: Nutrasweet.	An alert that the product contains phenylalanine is required in the United States so that persons with phenylketonuria can avoid it.
Sucralose. Brand name: Splenda.	No effect on insulin secretion, glucose, or fructose absorption; bulk and heat stability provide useful functional qualities in baked goods.
Saccharin	Some consumers can detect bitter taste. Saccharin–aspartame blends are sometimes used.
Cyclamate	Not approved currently in the United States. Often used in blends with saccharin.
Altitamme	Not approved in the United States.
Polyols (sugar alcohols): Sorbitol, isomalt, lactitol, mannitol, xylitol, maltitol syrup, polydextrose, specific sugar names, hydrogenated starch hydrolysate mixtures, hydrogenated glucose syrup. Brand names include Lycasin, Hystar, Neosor, Letisse, StaLite.	Occur in certain plants, but are usually manufactured from mono-, di-, or polysaccharides for use as food ingredients. Not as sweet as sugar. Most polyols are incompletely absorbed, providing from 1 to 4 kcal/g. Polyols do not elevate blood glucose and insulin levels. If polyols are used between meals in products such as cough drops, candy, chewing gums, or other between-meal snacks, their glycemic response is less. They may be useful alternatives for handling blood glucose fluctuations between meals. These products do not help restore blood glucose levels in hypoglycemia. When they are consumed as part of a meal, blood glucose effects are less apparent, since other foods buffer or dilute the differences in glycemic response. Consumption of very high amounts of some polyols may cause laxative effects or other gastrointestinal discomfort.
Natural sweeteners	Naturally occurring in plants. Incompletely absorbed and so are lower in calories (2 kcal/g) and have lower glycemic effects than other nutritive sweeteners.
Steviodose	Not presently approved in the United States.
Glycyrrhizen	Used as licorice flavoring, but not approved for use as a low-calorie sweetener in the United States. In very large amounts, may increase blood pressure.
Carbohydrate-based fat replacers	Provide carbohydrate, which varies in its bioavailability.
Carbohydrate polymers: Maltodextrin, corn syrup solids, starch, hydrolyzed cornstarch, modified food starch, polydextrose. Brand names: Maltrin, Lycadex, Paselli Excell, Stelar, N-Oil, Sta-Slim, Oatrim.	Derived from cereals, grains, and starches. They hold up to three times their weight in water, provide 1 kcal/g when hydrated, and vary in amounts of carbohydrate.

(continued)

TABLE 12.3. *continued*

Ingredient	Comments
Carbohydrate-based fat replacers (*cont.*)	
Hydrocolloids (gums, gels, and fibers): Pectin, carrageenan, sugar beet fiber, beet powder, cellulose gel, locust bean gum, xanthan, guar gum, applesauce, pureed prunes, bran fiber. Brand names include Slendid, Viscarin, Sactarin, Gelcarin, Fibrex, Avicel, Novagel, Rohodigel, Uniguar, Pycol, Jaquar.	Provide 0–0.5 kcal/g, depending on hydration.
Protein-based fat replacers	Provide 1.3 kcal/g or more. Not heat-stable.
Microparticulated egg white and milk protein with whey protein concentrate. Brand names include Simplesse, K Blazer, Lite, Dairy Low, Verilo.	
Fat-based fat replacers	
Olestra (sucrose polyester that cannot be hydrolyzed by gastrointestinal enzymes). Brand name: Olean.	Provides 1.3 kcal/g. May produce gastrointestinal discomfort and stool softening—a label alert is currently required in the United States.
Salatrim (contains fatty acids and triglycerides that are poorly absorbed).	Provides 5–9 kcal/g, depending upon fatty acid composition.
Caprenin (contains poorly absorbed fatty acids).	Provides 5 kcal/g.
Trailblazer (contains poorly absorbed fatty acids).	Composed of poorly absorbed fatty acids and provides between 5 and 9 kcal/g, depending on formulation.

shown that individuals who choose these low-fat alternatives are likely to consume less total dietary fat, although in the past few years, a slight trend toward increased dietary fat in the United States has once again been noted.

During this period of low-fat food alternatives, obesity prevalence and severity have continued to rise. Often, in searching for weight loss regimens, people seek a "silver bullet"; perhaps they have viewed low-fat foods as just that, even to such an extent that other important health messages (such as those promoting high fiber and low sugar consumption, as well as increased exercise) are ignored. In addition, many people tend to feel that if they are consuming low-fat foods, they can eat more of them. However, many low-fat foods have the same, and sometimes more, calories than their higher-fat alternatives. Therefore, increased consumption of these products has a synergistic effect on total energy intake. Often sugar is used in place of the fat in these products to improve palatability. Examples include low-fat cookies, muffins, and cakes. Therefore, while these foods may be helpful in reducing overall fat intake, they may not help decrease caloric consumption. As emphasized earlier, it is the total diet that matters, not just one aspect or macronutrient. For example, just as fat replacements did not cure obesity in the 1990s, sugar replacements did not cure obesity in the 1970s and 1980s. However, if these foods are used in the context of a well-balanced energy-restricted diet, then they can be helpful tools for weight loss.

SUMMARY AND CONCLUSIONS

This new century marks the worst of times and the best of times for health professionals wishing to assist individuals who want to control their weights. The pessimists point to the present obesity epidemic (Mokdad et al., 1999), the considerable disease burden associated with it (Must et al., 1999), its effects on quality of life (Han, Tijhuis, Lean, & Seidell, 1998), the proliferation of unsound and ineffective diets (Allara, 2000), environmental forces that foster overconsumption and sedentary lifestyles, and the ineffectiveness of presently available weight control tools to sustain weights at healthy levels over the long run. But there are also reasons for optimism.

A key positive development is that the focus of weight control efforts is changing. There is increasing stress on the need for primary prevention of weight gain and maintenance of weight loss by a combination of moderation in energy intake and increased energy output (Koplan & Dietz, 1999). For those who are already overweight or obese, the new focus on achieving modest and sustained weight losses of 5%–10% may provide hope (NHLBI, 1988; USDA & USDHHS, 2000; Willett, Dietz, & Colditz, 1999). The emphasis has shifted from the aesthetic aspects of body weight to the health aspects. Although the attainment of ideal weights associated with minimal mortality as the goal may be desirable over the long run, they are unattainable for many individuals, and these new targets are more realistic (Metropolitan Life Insurance Company, 1983; NIILBI, 1998). The metabolic effects of different diets are also being clarified. In addition, much has been learned about the prevention of weight gain and of recidivism after successful weight loss from the National Weight Control Registry (Klem, Wing, McGuire, Seagle, & Hill, 1997). Data collected from individuals successful at weight loss and maintenance have provided understanding of strategies that may be most effective. Of particular significance are behavioral and attitude adjustments, careful attention to diet, and high levels of physical activity (McGuire, Wing, Klem, & Hill, 1999). Finally, many excellent books, programs, and World Wide Web sites are now available to help those who wish to maintain or achieve healthy weights on their own. We hope that health professionals using the principles and evidence-based weight control techniques discussed in this chapter will find it easier to separate the wheat from the chaff among the popular diets, and thus will be more effective in advising their patients.

ACKNOWLEDGMENTS

This material is based upon work supported by the U.S. Department of Agriculture, under Agreement No. 58-1950-9-001. Any opinions, findings, conclusions, or recommendations expressed in this publication are our own and do not necessarily reflect the views of the U.S. Department of Agriculture.

REFERENCES

Abbott, W. G. H., Howard, B. E., Christin, L., Freymond, D., Lillioja, S., Boyce, V. L., Anderson, T. E., Bogardus, C., & Ravussin, E. (1988). Short term energy balance: Relationship with protein, carbohydrate, and fat balances. *American Journal of Physiology, 255,* E332–E337.

Acheson, K. J., Schutz, Y., Bessard, T., Anantharaman, K., Flatt, J. P., & Jequier, E. (1988). Glycogen storage capacity and de novo lipogenesis during massive carbohydrate overfeeding in men. *American Journal of Clinical Nutrition, 48,* 240–247.

Allara, L. (2000). The return of the high-protein, low carbohydrate diet: Weighing the risks. *Nutrition in Clinical Practice, 15,* 26–29.

Amatruda, J. M., Biddle, T. L., Patton, M. L., & Lockwood, D. H. (1982). Vigorous supplementation

Kanders, B. S., & Blackburn, G. L. (1994). Very low calorie diets for the treatment of obesity. In G. L. Blackburn & B. S. Kanders (Eds.), *Obesity: Pathophysiology, psychology and treatment* (pp 197–216). New York: Chapman & Hall.

Katahn, M. (1986). *The Rotation diet*. New York: Bantam Books.

Katahn, M. (1989). *The T-factor diet*. New York: Norton.

Katahn, M., with Pope, J. (1999). *The T-factor 2000 diet*. New York: Norton.

Kendall, A., Levitsky, D. A., Strupp, B. J., & Lissner, L. (1991). Weight loss on a low-fat diet: Consequences of the imprecision of the control of food intake in humans. *American Journal of Clinical Nutrition, 53,* 1124–1129.

Kirby, J. (1998). *Dieting for dummies*. Foster City, CA: IDG Books Worldwide.

Kleiner, S. M. (1999). Water: An essential but overlooked nutrient. *Journal of the American Dietetic Association, 99*(2), 200–206.

Klem, M. L., Wing, R. R., McGuire, M. T., Seagle, H. M., & Hill, J. O. (1997). A descriptive study of individuals successful at long-term maintenance of substantial weight loss. *American Journal of Clinical Nutrition, 66,* 239–246.

Koplan, J. P., & Dietz, W. H. (1999). Caloric imbalance and public health policy. *Journal of the American Medical Association, 282,* 1579–1581.

Kovacs, E., Brouns, F., Melanson, K. J., & Westerterp-Plantenga, M. S. (in press). The effects of guar gum on blood glucose dynamics and appetite regulation during and after weight loss in moderately obese men. *American Journal of Physiology.*

Kuczmarski, R. J., Flegal, K., & Campbell, S. M. (1994). Increasing prevalence of overweight among U. S. adults. *Journal of the American Medical Association, 272,* 205–211.

Lands, W. E. M. (1995). Alcohol and energy intake. *American Journal of Clinical Nutrition, 62*(Suppl.), 1101S–1106S.

Leibel, R. L., Rosenbaum, M., & Hirsch, J. (1995). Changes in energy expenditure resulting from altered body weight. *New England Journal of Medicine, 332*(10), 621–628.

Lissner, L., & Heitmann, B. L. (1995). Dietary fat and obesity: Evidence from epidemiology. *European Journal of Clinical Nutrition, 49,* 79–90.

Lissner, L., Levitsky, D. A., Strupp, B. J., Kalkwarf, H. J., & Roe, D. A. (1987). Dietary fat and the regulation of energy intake in human subjects. *American Journal of Clinical Nutrition, 46,* 886–892.

Ludwig, D. S., Majzoub, J. A., Al-Zahrani, A., Dallal, G. E., Blanco, I., & Roberts, S. B. (1999). High glycemic index foods, overeating, and obesity. *Pediatrics, 103*(3), 261–266.

Marks, B. L., Ward, A., Morris, D. H., Castellani, J., & Rippe, J. M. (1995). Fat free mass is maintained in women following a moderate diet and exercise program. *Medicine and Science in Sports and Exercise, 27,* 1243–1251.

Mattes, R. D. (1996). Dietary compensation by humans for supplemental energy provided as ethanol or carbohydrate in fluids. *Physiology and Behavior, 59,* 179–187.

Mazel, J., with Wyatt, M., & Sokol, A. (1996). *The new Beverly Hills diet*. Deerfield Beach, FL: Health Communications.

McCrory, M. A., Fuss, P. J., McCallum, J. E., Yao, M., Vinken, A. G., Hays, N. P., & Roberts, S. B. (1999). Dietary variety within food groups: Association with energy intake and fatness in men and women. *American Journal of Clinical Nutrition, 69*(3), 440–447.

McGuire, M. T., Wing, R. R., Klem, M. L., & Hill, J. O. (1999). Behavioral strategies of individuals who have maintained long-term weight losses. *Obesity Research, 7*(4), 334–341.

McQuillan, S. (1998). *The complete idiot's guide to losing weight*. New York: Alpha Books.

Meillin, L. (1997). *The solution: Never diet again*. New York: HarperCollins.

Melanson, K. J., Saltzman, E., Russell, R., & Roberts, S. B. (1997). Fat oxidation in response to four graded energetic challenges in young and older women. *American Journal of Clinical Nutrition, 66,* 860–866.

Melanson, K. J., Westerterp-Plantenga, M. S., Campfield, L. A., & Saris, W. H. M. (1999). Short term regulation of food intake in humans. In M. S. Westerterp-Plantenga, A. B. Steffens, & A. Tremblay (Eds.), *Regulation of food intake and energy expenditure* (pp. 37–58). Milan, Italy: Edra.

Melanson, K. J., Westerterp-Plantenga, M. S., Saris, W. H. M., Smith, F. J., & Campfield, L. A.

(1999). Blood glucose patterns and appetite in time-blinded humans: Carbohydrate versus fat. *American Journal of Physiology, 277*(2, Pt. 2), R337-R345.

Metropolitan Life Insurance Company. (1983). New weight standards for men and women. *Statistical Bulletin of the Metropolitan Life Insurance Company, 64,* 2–9.

Miller, P. (1989). *The Hilton Head over-35 diet.* New York: Warner Books.

Miller, W. C., Lindeman, A. K., Wallace, J., & Niederpruem, M. (1990). Diet composition, energy intake, and exercise in relation to body fat in men and women. *American Journal of Clinical Nutrition, 52,* 426–430.

Mokdad, A. H., Serdula, M. K., Dietz, W. H., Bowman, B. A., Marks, J. S., & Koplan, J. P. (1999). The spread of the obesity epidemic in the United States, 1991–1998. *Journal of the American Medical Association, 282,* 1519–1522.

Montignac, M. (1999a). *Eat yourself slim.* Frederick, MD: Erica House.

Montignac, M. (1999b). *The Montignac method.* Brentwood, England: Montignac Publishing.

Must, A., Spadano, J., Coakley, E. H., Field, A. E., Colditz, G, & Dietz, W. H. (1999). The disease burden associated with overweight and obesity. *Journal of the American Medical Association, 282,* 1523–1529.

National Heart, Lung, and Blood Institute (NHLBI). (1998). Clinical guidelines on the identification, evaluation, and treatment of overweight and obesity in adults: The evidence report. *Obesity Research, 6*(Suppl.), 51S–210S.

National Task Force on the Prevention and Treatment of Obesity. (1993). Very-low calorie diets. *Journal of the American Medical Association, 270*(8), 967–974.

Natow, A., & Heslin, J. A. (1990). *The fat attack plan.* New York: Pocket Books.

Ornish, D. (1997). *Eat more, weigh less: Dr. Dean Ornish's life choice program for losing weight safely.* San Francisco: Harper.

Pasman, W. J., Saris, W. H. M., & Westerterp-Plantenga, M. S. (1999). Predictors of weight maintenance. *Obesity Research, 7*(1), 43–50.

Poppit, S. D., Eckhardt, J. W., McGonagle, J., Murgatroyd, P. R., & Prentice, A. M. (1996). Short-term effects of alcohol consumption on appetite and energy intake. *Physiology and Behavior, 60,* 1063–1070.

Prentice, A. M., & Poppit, S. D. (1996). Importance of energy density and macronutrients in the regulation of energy intake. *International Journal of Obesity, 20*(Suppl. 2), S18–S23.

Pritikin, R. (1990). *The new Pritikin program.* New York: Simon & Schuster.

Pritikin, R. (1999). *The Pritikin weight loss breakthrough: Five easy steps to outsmart your fat instinct.* New York: Signet Books.

Puhn, A. (1996). *The 5-day miracle diet.* New York: Ballantine Books.

Raben, A., Jensen, M. D., Marckmann, P., Sandstrom, B., & Astrup, A. (1995). Spontaneous weight loss during 11 weeks ad libitum intake of a low-fat/high fiber diet in young, normal weight subjects. *International Journal of Obesity and Related Metabolic Disorders, 19,* 916–922.

Rolls, B. J. (1995). Carbohydrates, fats, and satiety. *American Journal of Clinical Nutrition, 61,* 960S–967S.

Rolls, B. J., & Barnett, R. A. (1999). *Volumetrics: Feel full on fewer calories.* New York: Harper Collins.

Rolls, B. J., Bell, E. A., & Thorwart, M. L. (1999). Water incorporated into a food but not served with a food decreases energy intake in lean women. *American Journal of Clinical Nutrition, 70,* 448–455.

Rolls, B. J., & Hammer, V. A. (1995). Fat, carbohydrate, and the regulation of energy intake. *American Journal of Clinical Nutrition, 62,* 1086S–1095S.

Rolls, B. J., Rowe, E. A., & Rolls, E. T. (1982). How sensory properties of food affect human feeding behavior. *Physiology and Behavior, 29,* 409–417.

Rolls, B. J., & Shide, D. J. (1992). The influence of dietary fat on food intake and body weight. *Nutrition Reviews, 50*(10), 283–290.

Roubenoff, R., & Kehayias, J. J. (1991). The meaning and measurement of lean body mass. *Nutrition Reviews, 49,* 163–175.

Rumpler, W. V., Seale, J. L., Miles, C. W., & Bodwell, C. E. (1991). Energy intake restriction and diet-composition effects on energy expenditure in men. *American Journal of Clinical Nutrition, 53,* 430–436.

Saltzman, E., Dallal, G. E., & Roberts, S. B. (1997). The effect of high-fat and low-fat diets on voluntary energy intake and substrate oxidation: Studies in identical twins using diets matched for energy density, fiber, and palatability. *American Journal of Clinical Nutrition, 66,* 1332–1339.

Schaefer, E. J., Lichtenstein, A. H., Lamon-Fava, S., McNamara, J. R., Schaefer, M. M., & Rasmussen, H. (1995). Body weight and low density lipoprotein cholesterol changes after consumption of a low-fat ad libitum diet. *Journal of the American Medical Association, 274,* 1450–1455.

Schutz, Y., Flatt, J. P., & Jequier, E. (1989). Failure of dietary fat to promote fat oxidation: A factor favoring the development of obesity. *American Journal of Clinical Nutrition, 50,* 307–314.

Schwartz, M. W., & Seeley, R. J. (1997). The new biology of body weight regulation. *Journal of the American Dietetic Association, 97,* 54–58.

Sears, B., with Lawren, B. (1995). *The zone: A dietary road map to lose weight permanently, reset your genetic code, prevent disease, achieve maximum physical performance.* New York: HarperCollins.

Shelmet, J. J., Reichard, G. A., Skutches, C. L., Hoeldtke, R. D., Owen, O. E., & Boden, G. (1998). Ethanol causes acute inhibition of carbohydrate, fat, and protein oxidation and insulin resistance. *Journal of Clinical Investigation, 81,* 1137–1145.

Shetty, P. S., Prentice, A. M., Goldberg, G. R., Murgatroyd, P. R., McKenna, A. P. M., Stubbs, R. J., & Volschenk, P. A. (1994). Alterations in fuel selection and voluntary food intake in response to isoenergetic manipulation of glycogen stores in humans. *American Journal of Clinical Nutrition, 60,* 534–543.

Siggard, R., Raben, A., & Astrup, A. (1996). Weight loss during 12 weeks' ad libitum carbohydrate-rich diet in overweight and normal-weight subjects at a Danish work site. *Obesity Research, 4,* 347–356.

Slabber, M., Barnard, H. C., Kuyl, J. M., Dannhauser, A., & Schall, R. (1994). Effects of a low-insulin-response, energy-restricted diet on weight loss and plasma insulin concentrations in hyperinsulinemic obese females. *American Journal of Clinical Nutrition, 60,* 48–53.

Smith-Schneider, L. M., Sigman-Grant, M. J., & Kris-Etherton, P. M. (1992). Dietary fat reduction strategies. *Journal of the American Dietetic Association, 92,* 34–38.

Steward, H. L. (1999). *Sugar busters!* New York: Ballantine Books.

Stubbs, R. J., Harbron, C. G., Murgatroyd, P. R., & Prentice, A. M. (1995). Covert manipulation of dietary fat and energy density: Effect on substrate flux and food intake in men eating ad libitum. *American Journal of Clinical Nutrition, 62,* 316–329.

Stubbs, R. J., Murgatroyd, P. R., Goldberg, G. R., & Prentice, A. M. (1993). Carbohydrate balance and day-to-day regulation of food intake in humans. *American Journal of Clinical Nutrition, 57,* 897–903.

Stunkard, A. J., & Messick, S. (1985). The three-factor Eating Questionnaire to measure dietary restraint, disinhibition and hunger. *Journal of Psychosomatic Research, 29,* 71–83.

Swinburn, B., & Ravussin, E. (1993). Energy balance or fat balance? *American Journal of Clinical Nutrition, 57*(Suppl.), 766S–771S.

Thomas, C. D., Peters, J. C., Reed, G. W., & Hill, J. O. (1992). Nutrient balance and energy expenditure during ad libitum feeding of high-fat and high-carbohydrate diets in humans. *American Journal of Clinical Nutrition, 55,* 934–932.

Tremblay, A., Plourde, G., Despres, J. P., & Bouchard, C. (1989). Impact of dietary fat content and fat oxidation on energy intake in humans. *American Journal of Clinical Nutrition, 49,* 824–831.

Tremblay, A., & St.-Pierre, S. (1996). The hyperphagic effect of a high-fat diet and alcohol intake persists after control for energy density. *American Journal of Clinical Nutrition, 63,* 479–482.

Tremblay, A., Wouters, E., Wenker, M., St.-Pierre, S., Bouchard, C., & Despres, J. P. (1995). Alcohol and a high-fat diet: A combination favoring overfeeding. *American Journal of Clinical Nutrition, 62,* 639–644.

Tribole, E., & Resch, E. (1995). *Intuitive eating.* New York: St. Martin's Press.

U.S. Department of Agriculture (USDA) & U.S. Department of Health and Human Services (USDHHS). (2000). *Dietary guidelines for Americans.* Washington, DC: U.S. Government Printing Office.

Van Amelsvoort, J. M., & Weststrate, J. A. (1992). Amylose–amylopectin ratio in a meal affects postprandial variables in male volunteers. *American Journal of Clinical Nutrition, 55*, 712–718.

VanItallie, T. B. (1980). Diets for weight reduction: Mechanisms of action and physiological effects. In G. Bray (Ed.), *Obesity: Comparative methods of weight control* (pp. 15–24). London: John Libby.

VanItallie, T. B., & Yang, M. U. (1977). Current concepts in nutrition: diet and weight loss. *New England Journal of Medicine, 297*, 1158–1160.

Wadden, T. A., & Bartlett, S. J. (1992). Very low calorie diets: An overview and appraisal. In T. A. Wadden & T. B. VanItallie (Eds.), *Treatment of the seriously obese patient* (pp. 44–79). New York: Guiford Press

Westerterp, K. R., Verboeket-van de Venne, W. P., Westerterp-Plantenga, M. S., Velthuis-te Wierik, E. J., de Graaf, C., & Westrate, J. A. (1996). Dietary fat and body fat: An intervention study. *International Journal of Obesity and Related Disorders, 20*, 1022–1026.

Westerterp-Plantenga, M. S., & Verwegen, C. R. T. (1997). Short-term effects of an alcohol, fat, protein, or carbohydrate preload on energy intake. *International Journal of Obesity, 21*, S79.

Westerterp-Plantenga, M. S., & Verwegen, C. R. T. (1999). The appetizing effect of an alcohol aperitif in overweight and normal weight humans. *American Journal of Clinical Nutrition, 69*, 205–212.

Willett, W. C., Dietz, W. H., & Colditz, G. A. (1999). Guidelines for healthy weight. *New England Journal of Medicine, 341*(6), 427–434.

Wolever, T. M. S. (1999). The glycemic index: Methodology and clinical implications. *Nutrition Today, 34*(2), 73–77.

Wolever, T. M. S., Jenkins, D. J. A., Jenkins, A. L., & Josse, R. G. (1991). The glycemic index: methodology and clinical implications. *American Journal of Clinical Nutrition, 54*, 846–854.

World Health Organization. (1998). *Obesity: Preventing and managing the global epidemic* (Publication No. WHO/NUT/NCD/98.1). Geneva: Author.

Zurlo, F., Lillioja, S., Esposito-Del Puente, A., Nyomba, B. L., Raz, I., Saad, M., Swinburn, B., Knowler, W. C., Bogardus, C., & Ravussin, E. (1990). Low ration of fat to carbohydrate oxidation as a predictor of weight gain: A study of 24-h RQ. *American Journal of Physiology, 259*, E650–E657.

bohydrate is not available from the diet, skeletal muscle and other body protein must be metabolized to provide it.

In studies of free-living humans ranging from 11 weeks to 1 year in duration, fat restriction in the absence of other dietary changes produced only modest body weight losses of about 1–3 kg (Boyar et al., 1988; Raben et al., 1995; Siggard, Raben, & Astrup, 1996). As discussed later, this may be related to the fact that overall energy deficit is more important in the hypocaloric state than is macronutrient composition. Some data suggest that energy balance is more strongly defended during energy deprivation than it is during energy surplus, impeding weight loss to a greater extent than weight gain (Blundell, 1991; Caputo & Mattes, 1992; Saltzman et al., 1997). In part, these effects may be due to alterations in resting metabolism and nonobligatory physical activity.

Alcohol

Alcohol (ethanol), though not an essential nutrient, is another source of metabolizable energy for many individuals. With approximately 7 kcal/g, alcohol provides more energy per unit of weight than carbohydrate or protein (each ~4 kcal/g), but less than fat (~9 kcal/g). Since the body has no storage capacity for alcohol, any ingested alcohol is oxidized immediately; the rate at which this occurs will depend on the individual's rate of energy expenditure (Lands, 1995). Excess alcohol awaiting oxidation circulates in the blood and may reach toxic levels, with effects on both physical and mental performance. Therefore, in normal individuals, chronically positive alcohol balance does not occur. It is just positive transiently upon ingestion, and alcohol oxidation eventually becomes equal to alcohol intake. If protein, carbohydrate, and/or fat are consumed at the same time as alcohol is ingested, their oxidation will be suppressed (most notably fat oxidation), since alcohol is preferentially oxidized, and the other macronutrients will be stored (Shelmet et al., 1988). Therefore, consumption of alcohol can lead to a positive fat balance through the sparing effect of alcohol on fat oxidation, leading to increased fat storage. Chronic overconsumption of alcohol can thus lead to fatty liver and dyslipidemia.

Another important consideration for alcohol's influence on energy balance is its effects on energy intake. Alcohol is positioned at the bottom of the hierarchy of satiating efficiency of metabolic fuels consumed by humans. Generally, it is accepted that the fuels satiate from lowest to highest: alcohol, fat, carbohydrate (depending on type), and protein (Westerterp-Plantenga & Verwegen, 1997). Alcohol energy is additive to the diet, producing no compensation in energy intake under most *ad libitum* situations, and in fact it may stimulate appetite (Poppit, Eckhardt, McGonagle, Murgatroyd, & Prentice, 1996; Tremblay et al., 1995). In nonalcoholic individuals, alcohol (as beer or wine) stimulates appetite and food intake to a greater extent than the other metabolic fuels do (Mattes, 1996; Westerterp-Plantenga & Verwegen, 1997, 1999). This appetite-stimulating effect of alcohol is probably dose-dependent within usual levels of alcohol intakes (Mattes, 1996). Alcohol consumption has been associated with higher eating rates, prolonged meal durations, delayed increases in satiation during a meal, and prolonged eating after satiation has reached its maximum in nonalcoholic individuals (Westerterp-Plantenga & Verwegen, 1999). When alcohol is combined with high fat consumption, these two fuels act synergistically to produce a hyperphagic response (Tremblay et al., 1995), which is independent of the energy density of the fuels (Tremblay & St.-Pierre, 1996). For these reasons, alcohol consumption is usually contraindicated in weight loss diets.

Macronutrient Balance

Just as a dynamic equation is more appropriate for expressing energy balance than is a static one in humans, so too are dynamic equations appropriate for expressing macronutrient balances. For example, as an individual accumulates body fat (from a positive fat balance), the rate of fatty acid turnover increases, and thus fat oxidation increases until it becomes commensurate with fat intake. A new fat balance is achieved at this new higher level until it is perturbed again. Fat stored in adipocytes can only significantly be depleted through oxidation, by using it as a metabolic fuel. Increased fat oxidation from exercise and/or decreased fat (or energy) intake from the diet will result in negative fat balance. A positive fat balance results from decreases in oxidation, perhaps from more sedentary behavior and/or further increases in dietary fat (or energy). Overweight and obesity are thus actually conditions of chronically positive fat balance—that is, greater fat retention than oxidation.

Macronutrient balances and imbalances are expressed as the match, or mismatch, of the "food quotient" (ratio of dietary carbohydrate to fat) and the "respiratory quotient" (ratio of carbohydrate to fat oxidation). During periods of stability in body weight and composition, the respiratory quotient reflects the food quotient (Flatt, 1995). When an individual is gaining body fat, the respiratory quotient is higher than the food quotient (reflecting lower fat oxidation than intake). As a person loses fat, the respiratory quotient is lower than the food quotient (reflecting higher fat oxidation than intake). In prospective studies, a high 24-hour respiratory quotient (low ratio of fat to carbohydrate oxidation) has been found to be predictive of weight gain over 6–15 months (Froidevaux, Schutz, Christin, & Jequier, 1993) and up to 3 years (Zurlo et al., 1990).

The corollary to these metabolic considerations is that a high-fat, low-carbohydrate *ad libitum* diet should cause weight gain and a low-fat, high-carbohydrate *ad libitum* diet should cause weight loss, all other factors being equal. This is supported by population studies (Lissner & Heitmann, 1995) and by food intake studies showing that fat intake tends to be positively correlated with body fatness (Dreon et al., 1988; Prentice & Poppit, 1996; Tremblay, Plourde, Despres, & Bouchard, 1989; Westerterp et al., 1996). In clinical studies of free-living individuals, switches from a high- to a low-fat diet have been shown to result in weight loss, at least in the first few months (Kendall et al., 1991; Schaefer et al., 1995). Whether eventual adjustments occur with chronic feeding of such low-fat regimens is not so clear, however. Increases in energy expenditure with overfeeding of fat are not as high as if the overfeeding is in the form of carbohydrate (Horton et al., 1995). On the other hand, at weight maintenance or on hypocaloric intakes, changes in energy expenditure may not be significantly different between high-fat and low-fat diets (Hill et al., 1991).

Data showing that high-fat diets are associated with overweight and obesity (Miller, Lindeman, Wallace, & Niederpruem, 1990; Tremblay et al., 1989) support the hypothesis that both high-energy and high-fat intakes are involved in the etiology of obesity. As mentioned above, carbohydrate balance is more tightly regulated than fat balance, and fat balance may be chronically positive over years. The combination of these data and others has led some to equate fat balance with energy balance (Swinburn & Ravussin, 1993), and to recommend counting fat grams instead of kilocalories in weight reduction and maintenance regimens (Smith-Schneider, Sigman-Grant, & Kris-Etherton, 1992). Although fat gram counting may be appropriate for some individuals, this strategy has not proven effective for all obese persons in their efforts to lose weight.

Over the 1980s, overall fat intake in the United States reportedly decreased, while the prevalence of obesity continued to rise (Ernst, Sempos, Briefel, & Clark, 1997; Kuczmarski, Flegal, & Campbell, 1994). Thus the usefulness of low-fat diets in preventing obesity, in the absence of control over energy intake, is questionable (Ludwig et al., 1999; Willett et al., 1999). Moreover, the causation of the increase in obesity is not well established; it may also be due to declines in energy expenditure. Another explanation of the lack of effect of fat reduction on overweight may be underreporting of fat intakes, which is known to be common (Heymsfield et al., 1995). It is also highly likely that energy intakes have increased even in the presence of reduced fat intake, due to increased dietary carbohydrate intake (and perhaps, in some individuals, increased alcohol intake). If excess energy is taken in and not oxidized, it must be stored. Probably, in many individuals over the long term, energy intake compensation does occur. Therefore, even on a low-fat, high-carbohydrate diet, excess energy intake may result with consequent increases in energy storage preferentially from the remaining dietary fat and excessive accumulation of adipose tissue. However, this needs to be demonstrated experimentally, and the question of the long-term effectiveness of dietary fat reduction in prevention of weight gain and stimulation of weight loss needs to be considered.

vided in adequate amounts, body fat and weight are lost in a more or less linear manner. However, early and/or rapid weight loss may largely be the result of glycogen depletion and water balance shifts. Since glycogen stores in the liver and in muscles amount to approximately 500 g in the average person (about 2,000 kcal), one would expect that this would not be very noticeable. However, since each gram of glycogen holds with it 3 g of water, 0.5 kg of glycogen oxidization may be reflected on the scale as a total weight loss of 2 kg. The reverse holds true if glycogen is synthesized; rapid gains in weight far in excess of calories consumed often occur on refeeding of a glycogen-depleted individual due to such shifts.

Body fat contains about 3,500 kcal/pound (454 g adipose tissue × 9 kcal/g × correction factor for glycerol and adipocyte structural proteins). Thus a negative energy balance of 3,500 kcal is required for each pound of adipose tissue loss. About 1 pound would be lost per week with a daily deficit of 500 kcal (500 kcal × 7 days), and a negative energy balance of 1,000 kcal/day would result in 2 pounds of body fat loss. Weight losses of more than 0.5 to 1 pound per week are not suggested for self-initiated efforts. Even under medical supervision, a loss of no more than 2 pounds per week is usually recommended. When weight losses are more rapid than this, risks of excessive loss of lean body mass increase, as do the risks of nutrient deficiencies, fatigue, and increases in other side effects (discussed in the chapter text). Furthermore, weight loss that occurs rapidly may be more difficult to maintain than gradual weight loss.

13

Exercise and Weight Management

STEVEN N. BLAIR
ELIZABETH A. LEERMAKERS

Much attention has recently been paid to overweight and obesity as public health problems (National Heart, Lung, and Blood Institute [NHLBI], 1998; World Health Organization, 1998). It is clear that the prevalence of overweight and obesity is increasing in many countries around the world, and that the rate of increase may be especially rapid. The prevalence of obesity (body mass index [BMI] $\geq$ 30.0 kg/m^2) in the United States during 1990 to 1998 increased from 12% to 18% in adults—a remarkable increase of 50% in just 8 years (Mokdad et al., 1999). There was a comparable increase in women and men, and increases occurred in all demographic groups. Concern about this rapid increase has generated a call to action for changes in public health policy (Koplan & Dietz, 1999).

We agree that there has been an increase in the prevalence of overweight and obesity in the past few years, and that this represents an important public health problem. However, we are concerned that there is too much emphasis placed solely on markers of obesity such as BMI and diet, with too little attention given to other important issues, such as physical inactivity.

In this chapter, we first address issues related to the possible causes of the increasing prevalence of overweight and obesity in the United States and other countries. We then review the effects of physical activity on weight loss and weight loss maintenance, followed by a discussion of the current consensus public health recommendation for physical activity. Next, we discuss various approaches to physical activity interventions, with an emphasis on lifestyle physical activity. The last major section includes a review of the interrelationships among obesity, physical activity, and health outcomes. This is followed by a summary and conclusion.

CAUSES OF THE INCREASE IN THE PREVALENCE OF OVERWEIGHT AND OBESITY

Most experts and recent guidelines acknowledge a role for physical activity in the etiology and treatment of overweight and obesity (Bouchard & Blair, 1999a, 1999b; Bouchard, De-

up, gained 2.1 kg and 1.9 kg more, respectively, than women whose activity levels were high at both measurements. The relative risk of major weight gain (>13 kg) for people whose activity level was low at both the baseline and follow-up interviews was 2.3 times higher in men and 7.1 times higher in women than in individuals whose activity level was high at baseline and follow-up. These results suggest that individuals who maintain a consistently high level of physical activity experience less weight gain than people who do not exercise regularly.

French and colleagues (1994) examined predictors of weight change over a 2-year period in 1,639 male and 1,913 female employees from area worksites. Body weight was measured at baseline and 2-year follow-up. Physical activity was estimated with a 13-item exercise frequency recall. Participants indicated how often they participated in leisure-time and occupational physical activities of varying intensity. Analyses were conducted on the average weekly frequency of physical activity in each of four categories: (1) high-intensity activities; (2) moderate-intensity activities; (3) group and racquet sports; and (4) occupational activity. Increases in physical activity from baseline to follow-up were associated with weight losses. Among women, an increase of one walking session per week was associated with a decrease in body weight of 0.79 kg, and an increase of one high-intensity training session per week was associated with a decrease in body weight of 0.63 kg, over the 2-year period. For men, an increase of one walking session per week or one high-intensity activity was associated with a decrease of 0.39 or 1.59 kg, respectively, over the 2-year period.

Regular physical activity may delay or prevent the weight gain that often accompanies aging. We (DiPietro, Kohl, Barlow, & Blair, 1997) followed 4,599 men and 724 women who received three examinations at the Cooper Clinic in Dallas, Texas, during the interval 1970 to 1994. This study assessed weight and physical activity or fitness at three time points, allowing us to examine changes in fitness from the first to the second examination as a predictor of weight gain by the third examination. At each examination, weight, cardiorespiratory fitness (determined by a maximal exercise test on a treadmill), and other clinical variables were measured. The interval between the first and second examinations averaged 1.8 years, and the total observation period from the first to the third examination was about 7.5 years.

Results showed that each 1-minute improvement in treadmill time from the first to the second examination was associated with a 9% decrease in the odds of a 5-kg weight gain for women and a 14% decrease for men. There were even stronger reduced odds (21%) of a 10-kg weight gain in both women and men with each additional minute on the treadmill test. These data suggest that a fit and active way of life prevents weight gain.

Physical Activity and Weight Loss

Physical activity alone produces only modest weight loss. A meta-analysis of weight loss studies found that 21-week aerobic exercise programs produce weight losses of 2.9 kg, compared with losses of 11 kg from 15-week programs of caloric restriction (Miller, Koceja, & Hamilton, 1997). Adding 30–60 minutes of physical activity, three times a week, to a caloric restriction program increases the amount of weight lost by approximately 2 kg (NHLBI, 1998).

It is very difficult for people to lose large amounts of weight, or at least to lose weight quickly, by exercise alone. A general guideline is that a pound of body fat yields about 3,500 kilocalories (kcal) when oxidized. Given that a 75-kg person burns approximately 100 kcal by walking 1 mile, one would have to walk about 35 miles to expend the energy contained in 1 pound of fat. For individuals who may be 50 or 100 pounds overweight, losing that much weight by exercise alone is a formidable challenge. Furthermore, given that many overweight or obese individuals are quite sedentary and unfit, they cannot perform large amounts of exercise, at least over the short term. Thus they do not have the capacity to expend large amounts of energy.

Physical Activity and Maintenance of Weight Loss

Even though physical activity is not the most efficient method of losing weight, it appears to be crucial for maintaining weight loss. One study examined self-reported activity levels of obese women who regained weight after successful weight loss ("relapsers"), formerly obese women who maintained their weight loss ("maintainers"), and normal-weight women who maintained their weight (controls) (Kayman, Bruvold, & Stern, 1990). Regular physical activity (at least three times a week for ≥ 30 minutes) was reported by 90% of the maintainers and 82% of the controls, but by only 34% of the relapsers. These results suggest the importance of physical activity in maintaining weight, both among normal-weight individuals and formerly obese individuals who have lost weight.

The National Weight Control Registry, a group of 1,047 women and men who lost at least 30 pounds (13.6 kg) and maintained that loss for at least 1 year, provides even stronger support for the importance of physical activity in maintaining weight loss (McGuire, Wing, Klem, Seagle, & Hill, 1998). The average weight loss in this group was 64 pounds (29.0 kg) over an average 6.9 years of follow-up. Successful weight maintainers averaged 1 hour or more of moderate to vigorous intensity physical activity per day. Schoeller and colleagues (1986), who determined energy expenditure objectively by the doubly labeled water technique, found similarly high levels of physical activity among successful weight loss maintainers. Maintainers had an average daily energy expenditure of 1.9 metabolic equivalents, which requires about 80 minutes of moderate-intensity physical activity or 35 minutes of vigorous activity per day.

Although the immediate effects of exercise are limited, the long-term cumulative effect of small changes in activity level can be beneficial. For example, if a 100-pound person played golf only 2 hours per outing (an additional 350 kcal per outing), for 2 days a week (700 kcal), it would take about 5 weeks, or 10 golfing days, to lose 0.45 kg (1 pound) of fat (3,500 kcal). If the person played golf year-round, golfing 2 days per week (hypothetically) would produce a 4.5-kg loss of fat during the year, provided that food intake remained fairly constant (Katch & McArdle, 1993).

We speculate, based on the epidemiological studies reviewed above, that an individual who is regularly active throughout his or her lifetime would be approximately 13.6 kg (30 pounds) lighter by age 65 than someone who had a consistently sedentary lifestyle over this period. Jeffery and French (1997) found that men and women 20–45 years of age gained an average of 1.9 pounds and 1.4 pounds, respectively, in 1 year. If we assume that people gain 50 pounds over 40 years, how much physical activity would it take to counteract the increased caloric intake? Assuming that people who gain 1–1.5 pounds per year consume an extra 10–15 kcal per day, it would not require very much physical activity to burn those extra kilocalories. For example, a 75-kg person would burn 15 kcal by walking for 2.5 minutes. Physical activity, then, may play a very important role in long-term weight regulation. (For more information on exercise and weight maintenance, see Wing, Chapter 14, and Perri & Corsica, Chapter 17, this volume.)

PUBLIC HEALTH RECOMMENDATIONS FOR PHYSICAL ACTIVITY

It is clear that a sedentary and unfit way of life increases risk of several chronic diseases, premature mortality, loss of physical function, and depressed mood (U.S. Department of

TABLE 13.1 *continued*

Week	Session title	Activity/discussion topic	Home assignment	Behavioral/cognitive processes
20	*Jack Be Nimble, Jill Be Quick, We'll Keep Jumping over the Candlestick*	Cognitive restructuring	*Talking to Yourself*	Substituting alternatives, comprehending benefits
22	*Potluck*	Volleyball and potluck	*Planning Your Potluck*	Enlisting social support, substituting alternatives
24	*Onward*	Review of past sessions and looking ahead—doing things on your own	*The Things I Need to Do to Stay Active*	Increasing knowledge, warning of risks, comprehending benefits, rewarding yourself

During the first 6 months, structured participants (n = 114) were asked to exercise 3–5 days per week for at least 30 minutes per session under supervision. They received a free membership to the Cooper Fitness Center, and a member of our staff was available several hours each day in the fitness center. The exercise counselor talked with the participants about the appropriate intensity and duration of exercise sessions. Structured participants were encouraged to continue their exercise on their own during the maintenance phase.

Participants in both groups had similar improvements in physical activity, cardiorespiratory fitness, blood pressure, and body composition from baseline to 24 months (see Figures 13.1 and 13.2). Both groups significantly reduced their body fat percentage (by 2.39% and 1.85% in the lifestyle and structured groups, respectively), although participants in neither group lost weight. The fact that the Project *Active* intervention did not produce weight loss is not surprising, because the intervention did not focus on changing diet. These results suggest that a lifestyle physical activity program is as effective as a structured exercise program in improving physical activity and health outcomes.

Long-term maintenance of physical activity in Project *Active* was associated with small weight losses. Participants were asked to indicate what percentage of the weeks (between months 6 and 24) they were physically active at least 30 minutes per day, at least 5 days per week. Participants in both groups who reported being active at least 70% of the time had greater decreases in weight and body fat than participants who were active less than 70% of the time. Participants who maintained their activity at least 70% of the time lost 1 kg, whereas participants who maintained their activity less than 30% of the time gained 2.5 kg. This very large difference of 3.5 kg, which occurred over a relatively short period of 18 months, is a good example of the cumulative effect of modest amounts of daily physical activity.

Lifestyle Activity Plus Diet

The effectiveness of lifestyle activity, compared with structured activity, on weight loss was evaluated among 40 obese women (mean BMI = 32.9 kg/m^2) who participated in a 16-week cognitive-behavioral weight loss program, including a low-calorie, low-fat diet of approximately 1,200 kcal/day (Andersen et al., 1999). Lifestyle activity participants were asked to increase their physical activity by 30 minutes per day on most days of the week by building several short bouts of activity into their day (e.g., taking the stairs instead of the elevator). Structured activity participants were instructed to attend three step aerobics classes per

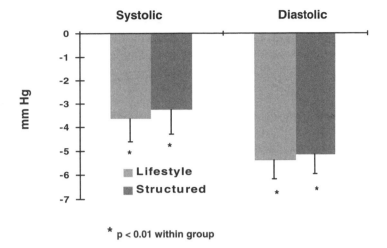

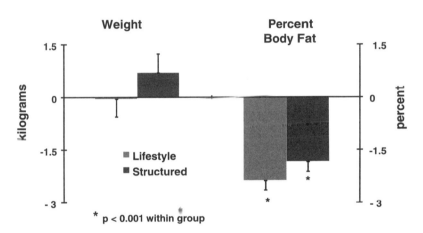

FIGURE 13.1. The 24-month changes in blood pressure (upper panel) and weight and body composition (lower panel) for Project *Active* participants. Data from Dunn et al. (1999).

week. Participants in both groups were asked to exercise on their own during the 1-year follow-up period.

During the 16-week treatment phase, participants in both groups lost similar amounts of weight (8.3 ± 3.8 kg in the structured group vs. 7.9 ± 4.2 kg in the lifestyle group), but during the 1-year follow-up, lifestyle participants regained significantly less weight (0.08 ± 4.6 kg) than structured participants (1.6 ± 5.5 kg). These results suggest that a lifestyle physical activity program is as effective in promoting weight loss, and is potentially more effective in maintaining weight loss, compared with a structured exercise program.

Short Bouts of Activity

One hundred and forty-eight sedentary, overweight women participated in an 18-month behavioral weight loss program with three treatment groups: (1) long-bout exercise; (2) multiple short-bout exercise; or (3) multiple short-bout exercise with exercise equipment (a treadmill) in the home (Jakicic, Winters, Lang, & Wing, 1999). All participants received a

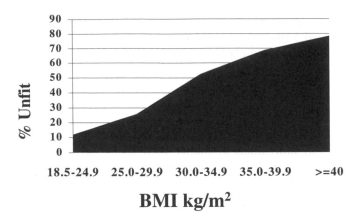

FIGURE 13.3. The association between body mass index (BMI) and the prevalence of low cardiorespiratory fitness (dark area of the figure) in 6,840 women (upper panel) and 23,190 men (lower panel) who were free of coronary heart disease, cancer, and abnormal electrocardiograms. The number of individuals across the BMI strata of 18.5–24.9, 25.0–29.9, 30.0–34.9, 35.0–39.9, and ≥ 40 were 5,499, 959, 262, 83, and 37 for women, and 9,838, 10,544, 2,308, 361, and 139 for men. Data from Barlow, Kohl, Gibbons, and Blair (1995).

men for an average of 8.5 years after their baseline examination at the Cooper Clinic (Barlow et al., 1995). We classified the least fit 20% of the men as "unfit" and the remainder as "fit," and also assigned them to normal, overweight, or obese categories based on their BMI. A summary of the results is presented in Table 13.2. Mortality rates were not elevated in men in the higher BMI categories if they were fit, and obese men who were fit had much lower death rates than normal-weight men who were unfit.

A concern with the results of this first study was that the obese men who were fit might have been muscular rather than fat, and this could have led to misinterpretation of the data. We addressed this issue in a follow-up investigation in which body fatness rather than BMI was measured (Lee, Blair, & Jackson, 1999). Body composition was determined by hydrostatic weighing, seven skinfold measurements, or both. We classified the men as lean (body fat < 16.7%), normal (body fat = 16.7%–24.9%), or obese (body fat ≥ 25.0%), and further stratified the data by fitness group. Results of the analyses are shown in Figure 13.4. The findings are similar to those from the earlier report on BMI, fitness, and mortality. Fit men in each fatness stratum had substantially lower risk of cardiovascular disease and all-cause mortality than unfit men in the same fatness stratum. Fit but obese men had lower mortali-

TABLE 13.2. Age-Adjusted Relative Risks for All-Cause Mortality by Fitness and Body Mass Index (BMI) Strata, 25,389 Men, Aerobics Center Longitudinal Study

Fitness level	Number of deaths	Age-adjusted relative risks	95% confidence interval
	17,178 men with BMI < 27 kg/m^2		
Low	133	1.0	
Moderate	180	0.49	0.31–0.76
High	119	0.34	0.21–0.57
	5,277 men with BMI = 27–30 kg/m^2		
Low	63	1.0	
Moderate	67	0.61	0.38–0.96
High	17	0.40	0.24–0.68
	2,934 men with BMI ≥ 30 kg/m^2		
Low	75	1.0	
Moderate–high	19	0.29	0.17–0.49

Note. The data are from Barlow, Kohl, Gibbons, and Blair (1995).

ty risk than lean men who were unfit. A similar pattern of results was observed for a cross-tabulation of fitness and waist circumference in the 14,043 men with this measurement.

We also compared low cardiorespiratory fitness to other established risk factors, such as baseline cardiovascular disease or diabetes, elevated blood pressure or cholesterol, and smoking, as predictors of cardiovascular disease and all-cause mortality in normal-weight, overweight, and obese men (Wei et al., 1999). With extended mortality surveillance, we now have more than 1,025 deaths in 25,714 men followed for an average of about 10 years. We calculated mortality risks in each weight group for men with each of the risk factors mentioned above. In each analysis, normal-weight men without the risk factor comprised the reference group, and risk of mortality for men with the risk factor was calculated in each of the weight groups.

Not surprisingly, baseline cardiovascular disease was the strongest predictor of mortality of the various predictors considered in this study. A summary of mortality risks for each of the other predictors is presented in Figure 13.5. For each of the predictors, there was a gradient of risk from the reference group across normal-weight, overweight, and obese men. The relative risk for mortality in obese men was similar for each of the risk predictors. Low cardiorespiratory fitness was as strongly associated with mortality as was having diabetes at baseline, and this was observed in both overweight and obese men.

Summary of Findings

Overweight and obesity do not appear to increase risk of cardiovascular disease and all-cause mortality in men who are fit. Although the prevalence of acceptable levels of fitness is progressively lower with higher levels of BMI, there are many overweight and obese individuals who are fit. Our studies have limitations in that the published data are from men, although we now have data from preliminary analyses, as well as a review of the literature, that show similar results in women (Blair & Brodney, 1999). In addition, our cohort includes few members of minority groups and is drawn from middle to upper socioeconomic strata. We do not know whether similar results will be found in other demographic groups.

viduals should be encouraged to be physically active, whether it makes them slim or not. Available data strongly support the conclusion that activity enhances health and delays mortality in overweight and obese individuals.

ACKNOWLEDGMENTS

We thank Ming Wei, MD, MPH, for analyses on the prevalence of low fitness by BMI strata; Melba Morrow for editorial review; and Stephanie Parker for assistance with figure preparation. The work reported here is supported in part by grants from the National Institutes of Health (Nos. HL48597, HL58608, and AG06945) and Polar Electro Oy.

REFERENCES

American College of Sports Medicine (ACSM). (1998). The recommended quantity and quality of exercise for developing and maintaining cardiorespiratory and muscular fitness, and flexibility in healthy adults. *Medicine and Science in Sports and Exercise, 30*(6), 975–991.

Andersen, R. E., Wadden, T. A., Bartlett, S. J., Zemel, B., Verde, T. J., & Franckowiak, S. C. (1999). Effects of lifestyle activity vs structured aerobic exercise in obese women: A randomized trial. *Journal of the American Medical Association, 281*(4), 335–340.

Bandura, A. (1986). *Social foundations of thought and action: A social cognitive theory.* Englewood Cliffs, NJ: Prentice-Hall.

Barlow, C. E., Kohl, H. W., III, Gibbons, L. W., & Blair, S. N. (1995). Physical fitness, mortality and obesity. *International Journal of Obesity, 19*(Suppl. 4), S41–S44.

Blair, S. N., & Brodney, S. (1999). Effects of physical inactivity and obesity on morbidity and mortality: Current evidence and research issues. *Medicine and Science in Sports and Exercise, 31*(11, Suppl.), S646–S662.

Bouchard, C., & Blair, S. N. (1992a). Physical activity in the prevention and treatment of obesity and its co-morbidities [Abstract]. *Medicine and Science in Sports and Exercise, 31*(11, Suppl.), S39.

Bouchard, C., & Blair, S. N. (1999b). Roundtable introduction: Introductory comments for the consensus on physical activity and obesity. *Medicine and Science in Sports and Exercise, 31*(11, Suppl.), S498–S501.

Bouchard, C., Despres, J.-P., & Tremblay, A. (1993). Exercise and obesity. *Obesity Research, 1*(2), 133–147.

Briefel, R. R., Sempos, C. T., McDowell, M. A., Chien, S., & Alaimo, K. (1997). Dietary methods research in the third National Health and Nutrition Examination Survey: Underreporting of energy intake. *American Journal of Clinical Nutrition, 65*(4, Suppl), 1203S–1209S.

Centers for Disease Control and Prevention. (1994). Daily dietary fat and total food-energy intakes—NHANES III, Phase 1, 1988–91. *Journal of the American Medical Association, 271*(17), 1309.

Cooper, K. H., Pollock, M. L., Martin, R. P., White, S. R., Linnerud, A. C., & Jackson, A. (1976). Physical fitness levels vs. selected coronary risk factors: A cross-sectional study. *Journal of the American Medical Association, 236,* 166–169.

DiPietro, L., Kohl, H. W., III, Barlow, C. E., & Blair, S. N. (1997). Physical fitness and risk of weight gain in men and women: The Aerobics Center Longitudinal Study [Abstract]. *Medicine and Science in Sports and Exercise, 29,* S115.

Drucker, E. (1999). Drug prohibition and public health: 25 years of evidence. *Public Health Reports, 114*(1), 14–29.

Dunn, A. L., Marcus, B. H., Kampert, J. B., Garcia, M. E., Kohl, H. W., III, & Blair, S. N. (1999). Comparison of lifestyle and structured interventions to increase physical activity and cardiorespiratory fitness: A randomized trial. *Journal of the American Medical Association, 281*(4), 327–334.

Fletcher, G. F., Blair, S. N., Blumenthal, J., Caspersen, C., Chaitman, B., Epstein, S., Falls, H.,

Froelicher, E. S. S., Froelicher, V. F., & Pina, I. L. (1992). Position statement: Statement on exercise. Benefits and recommendations for physical activity programs for all Americans: A statement for health professionals by the Committee on Exercise and Cardiac Rehabilitation of the Council on Clinical Cardiology, American Heart Association. *Circulation, 86,* 340–344.

French, S. A., Jeffery, R. W., Forster, J. L., McGovern, P. G., Kelder, S. H., & Baxter, J. E. (1994). Predictors of weight change over two years among a population of working adults: The Healthy Worker Project. *International Journal of Obesity, 18*(3), 145–154.

Gibbons, L. W., Blair, S. N., Cooper, K. H., & Smith, M. (1983). Association between coronary heart disease risk factors and physical fitness in healthy adult women. *Circulation, 67*(5), 977–983.

Jakicic, J. M., Wing, R. R., Butler, B. A., & Robertson, R. J. (1995). Prescribing exercise in multiple short bouts versus one continuous bout: Effects on adherence, cardiorespiratory fitness, and weight loss in overweight women. *International Journal of Obesity, 19,* 893–901.

Jakicic, J. M., Winters, C., Lang, W., & Wing, R. R. (1999). Effects of intermittent exercise and use of home exercise equipment on adherence, weight loss, and fitness in overweight women: A randomized trial. *Journal of the American Medical Association, 282*(16), 1554–1560.

Jeffery, R. W., & French, S. A. (1997). Preventing weight gain in adults: Design, methods and one year results from the Pound of Prevention Study. *International Journal of Obesity, 21*(6), 457–464.

Katch, F. I., & McArdle, W. D. (1993). *Introduction to nutrition, exercise, and health.* Philadelphia: Lea & Febiger.

Kayman, S., Bruvold, W., & Stern, J. S. (1990). Maintenance and relapse after weight loss in women: Behavioral aspects. *American Journal of Clinical Nutrition, 52*(5), 800–807.

Koplan, J. P., & Dietz, W. H. (1999). Caloric imbalance and public health policy. *Journal of the American Medical Association, 282*(16), 1579–1581.

Lee, C. D., Blair, S. N., & Jackson, A. S. (1999). Cardiorespiratory fitness, body composition, and all-cause and cardiovascular disease mortality in men. *American Journal of Clinical Nutrition, 69*(3), 373–380.

Levy, A. S. (1993). Weight control practices of U.S. adults trying to lose weight. *Annals of Internal Medicine, 119,* 661–666.

McGuire, M. T., Wing, R. R., Klem, M. L., Seagle, H. M., & Hill, J. O. (1998). Long-term maintenance of weight loss: Do people who lose weight through various weight loss methods use different behaviors to maintain their weight? *International Journal of Obesity, 22*(6), 572–577.

Miller, W. C., Koceja, D. M., & Hamilton, E. J. (1997). A meta-analysis of the past 25 years of weight loss research using diet, exercise or diet plus exercise intervention. *International Journal of Obesity, 21*(10), 941–947.

Mokdad, A. H., Serdula, M. K., Dietz, W. H., Bowman, B. A., Marks, J. S., & Koplan, J. P. (1999). The spread of the obesity epidemic in the United States, 1991–1998. *Journal of the American Medical Association, 282*(16), 1519–1522.

National Heart, Lung, and Blood Institute (NHLBI). (1998). Clinical guidelines on the identification, evaluation, and treatment of overweight and obesity in adults: The evidence report. *Obesity Research, 6*(Suppl.), 51S–210S.

National Institutes of Health (NIH) Consensus Development Panel on Physical Activity and Cardiovascular Health. (1996). NIH Consensus Conference: Physical activity and cardiovascular health. *Journal of the American Medical Association, 276*(3), 241–246.

Paffenbarger, R. S., Jr., Blair, S. N., Lee, I.-M., & Hyde, R. T. (1993). Measurement of physical activity to assess health effects in free-living populations. *Medicine and Science in Sports and Exercise, 25,* 60–70.

Pate, R. R., Pratt, M., Blair, S. N., Haskell, W. L., Macera, C. A., Bouchard, C., Buchner, D., Ettinger, W., Heath, G. W., King, A. C., Kriska, A., Leon, A. S., Marcus, B. H., Morris, J., Paffenbarger, R. S., Jr., Patrick, K., Pollock, M. L., Rippe, J. M., Sallis, J., & Wilmore, J. H. (1995). Physical activity and public health: A recommendation from the Centers for Disease Control and Prevention and the American College of Sports Medicine. *Journal of the American Medical Association, 273,* 402–407.

Pollock, M. L., Bohannon, R. L., Cooper, K. H., Ayres, J. J., Ward, A., White, S. R., & Linnerud, A.

TABLE 14.1. Summary of Behavioral Weight Loss Treatments Using Conventional Low-Calorie Diets, 1970–1995

	1974	1984	1990–1995
No. of studies included	15	15	14
Initial weight (kg)	73.4	88.7	91.6
Length of treatment (wk)	8.4	13.2	26.0
Weight loss (kg)	3.8	6.9	9.0
Length of follow-up (wk)	5.5	58.4	40.0
Loss at follow-up (kg)	4.0	4.4	5.2

Note. Data from Wadden (1993) and Wing (1998).

the initial intensive phase of treatment now typically involves 6 months of weekly meetings. Although the specific entry criteria differ across studies, the average participant entering behavioral programs is middle-aged and weighs approximately 90 kg. Women are more commonly treated in behavioral programs than men, and some studies are specifically restricted to women. The emphasis of the treatment has also shifted to focus explicitly on energy balance. Participants are now given specific goals for calorie intake (typically 1,000–1,500 kilocalories [kcal]/day, depending on body weight), and dietary fat gram goals have recently been prescribed, as well. Similarly, participants are given specific goals for physical activity. These goals are gradually increased until the participant is completing 1,000 kcal/week in activity (equivalent to walking 10 miles/week). Key behavioral components of these programs include self-monitoring, stimulus control strategies, problem solving, preplanning, and relapse prevention.

With these changes in behavioral programs, weight losses have gradually improved. Table 14.1 shows the weight losses achieved in programs from the 1970s to the 1990s (Wadden, 1993; Wing, 1998). As shown, there has been more than a doubling in the initial weight loss achieved. On average, participants in behavioral programs in the 1990s lost 9.0 kg, or approximately 10% of their initial body weight.

Unfortunately, there has been less improvement in the maintenance of weight loss. On average, patients regain more than one-third of their initial weight loss over the first year of follow-up. Thus overall weight loss from entry to a 40-week follow-up averages 5.2 kg.

Tables 14.2 and 14.3 summarize the major behavioral weight loss trials that were published since 1996. (Pilot studies, studies with posttreatment randomization that focused on maintenance, and studies conducted with minimal face-to-face contact are omitted from these tables.) As can be seen, these recent studies have focused largely on comparison of different types of exercise interventions. Participants achieved an average weight loss of 9.6 kg over 21 weeks. These initial weight losses appear comparable to those achieved in 1990–1995. However, the follow-up period is now longer (averaging 18 months), and patients maintained a weight loss of 6.0 kg (62% of their initial weight loss) over this longer follow-up.

The following sections of this chapter describe the behavioral studies published since 1996 that focused on changing eating behavior, changing physical activity, and motivational strategies to improve weight loss.

CHANGING EATING BEHAVIOR

In order to lose weight, it is necessary to modify dietary intake. However, the optimal dietary prescription for weight loss is still unclear. Typically, behavioral weight loss programs

Table 14.2. Behavioral Weight Loss Studies, 1996–1999

Reference	Pretreatment			Treatment			Follow-up			Follow-up		
	n	Wt. (kg)	Characteristics	Duration (mo)	n	Wt. loss (kg)	Duration (mo)	n	Wt. loss (kg)	Duration (mo)	n	Wt. loss (kg)
Andersen et al. (1999)												
Lifestyle activity	20	87	All females; 42.9 yr	4	19	7.9	16	16	7.8			
Structured exercise	20			4	19	8.3	16	17	6.7			
Jakicic et al. (1999)												
Long bout	49	90	All females; 36.7 yr	6	37	8.2	18	37	5.8			
Short bout	51			6	36	7.5	18	36	3.7			
Short bout–Equipment	48			6	42	9.3	18	42	7.4*			
Jeffery et al. (1998)												
SBT	40	86	29 males, 167 females; 25–55 yr	6	86%	8.3	18	78%	7.6*			
SBT + walks	41			6	comp.	6.0	18	comp.	3.8			
SBT + walks + trainer	42			6		3.6	18		2.9			
SBT + walks + $	37			6		6.7	18		4.5			
SBT + walks + trainer + $	36			6		7.9	18		5.1			
Perri et al. (1997)												
Home-based exercise	24	88	All females; 48.7 yr	6	23	10.4	15	23	11.6*			
Group-based exercise	25			6	25	9.3	15	25	7.0			

(continued)

303

TABLE 14.2. *continued*

Reference	Pretreatment			Treatment			Follow-up			Follow-up		
	n	Wt. (kg)	Characteristic	Duration (mo)	*n*	Wt. loss (kg)	Duration (mo)	*n*	Wt. loss (kg)	Duration (mo)	*n*	Wt. loss (kg)
Skender et al. (1996)												
Control	127		Males + females	3	38							
Diet				3	42	6.8*	12	29	6.8	24	15	+0.9
Exercise				3	43	0.7	12	30	2.9	24	25	2.7
Diet + exercise				3	42	6.5*	12	27	8.9	24	21	2.2
Wadden et al. (1997)												
Diet	29	96	All females;	6	27	16.7	12	24	14.4	24	21	6.9
Diet + aerobic	31		41.1 yr	6	30	16.2	12	28	13.7	24	21	8.5
Diet + resistance	31			6	29	16.8	12	24	17.2	24	18	10.1
Diet + aerobic + resistance	29			6	27	16.3	12	23	15.2	24	17	8.6
Wing et al. (1996)												
SBT	40	86	All females;	6	35	8.0	18	32	3.3			
SBT + menu	41		41.3 yr	6	37	12.0*	18	37	6.9*			
SBT + buy food	41			6	36	11.7*	18	37	7.5*			
SBT + free food	41			6	40	11.4*	18	38	6.6*			
Wing et al. (1998)												
Control	40	99	21 males,	6	32	1.5	12	29	0.3	24	31	0.3
Diet	37		78 females;	6	35	9.1*	12	33	5.5*	24	35	2.1
Exercise	37		45.7 yr	6	33	2.1	12	28	0.4	24	31	+1.0
Diet + exercise	40			6	31	10.3*	12	30	7.4*	24	32	2.5

Note. SBT, standard behavioral treatment.

*Treatment groups differ in weight loss at *p* < 0.05.

304

TABLE 14.3. Summary of Behavioral Weight Loss Studies, 1996–1999

No. of studies	9
Number of treatment conditions[a]	28
Length of treatment (wk/mo)	21/5.25
Weight loss (kg)	9.61[b]
Length of final follow-up (wk/mo)	74.2/18.5
Weight loss (kg)	5.97[b]

[a]Excluding control groups and exercise-only groups.

[b]If the study by Wadden et al. (1998) is omitted, the average weight loss during treatment is 8.45 kg, and the average weight loss at follow-up is 5.54 kg.

encourage participants to consume 1,000–1,500 kcal/day. Often dietary fat intake is restricted to 20%–30% of calories. Several studies conducted in the 1980s and early 1990s examined the effectiveness of much more stringent dietary restriction, in the form of very-low-calorie diets (VLCDs) (Wadden, Foster, & Letizia, 1994; Wadden & Stunkard, 1986; Wing, Blair, Marcus, Epstein, & Harvey, 1994; Wing et al., 1991). VLCDs provide 400–800 kcal/day and are consumed as a liquid formula or as lean meat, fish, and fowl. These diets were shown to be effective for initial weight loss, with patients losing an average of 20 kg over 12 weeks (Wadden, Stunkard, & Brownell, 1983). However, two major problems were identified. First, these dietary regimens were expensive, because they necessitated ongoing medical monitoring to ensure their safety. Second, even when a VLCD was used in combination with behavioral training, participants tended to regain weight rapidly after termination of the VLCD. Wadden and colleagues (1994) attempted to curtail this weight regain by providing a full year of weekly behavioral treatment. Wing, Blair, Marcus, Epstein, and Harvey (1994) utilized an intermittent VLCD approach, with 12 weeks of VLCD followed by 12 weeks of refeeding, and then another 12 weeks of VLCD followed by 12 weeks of refeeding. At the end of both the Wadden and colleagues (1994) and Wing and colleagues (1994) studies, no significant benefits of the VLCD compared to a more balanced, less restricted diet of 1,000–1,500 kcal/day were observed.

Structured Meal Plans

Behaviorists have recently been experimenting with several new approaches to the diet. One approach is to provide participants with more structured meal plans and grocery lists, which may serve as models of how to achieve a low-calorie, low-fat intake. Wing and colleagues (1996) analyzed the effectiveness of such an approach in a study of 163 women. These women were randomly assigned to one of four groups. The first group was given a standard behavioral treatment program, with a goal of consuming no more than 1,000–1,500 kcal/day, goals for physical activity, and standard behavioral strategies. The second group received the identical behavioral program with the same calorie goal; in addition, participants were given structured meal plans that told them exactly what they should consume for five breakfasts and five dinners each week, and a shopping list to guide them in purchasing the required foods. The third and fourth groups received the same behavioral program and the same meal plan, but at each weekly meeting they were also given a box of food that contained exactly what they should eat for five breakfasts and five dinners during the next week. Group 3 participants shared the cost of the food with the study, and those in group 4 received the food free of charge.

As seen in Table 14.2, weight losses both at the end of the 6-month intervention and at 12-month follow up were significantly better in groups 2–4 than in group 1. Groups 2–4 also reported more regular meal patterns and changes in the types of foods available in the home.

Meal Replacements

Another approach to strengthening the diet component of behavioral weight loss programs has been to use prepared meals or liquid meal replacements. These diets differ from the earlier VLCDs in that the calorie level of these diets is at least 900 kcal/day, reducing the need for medical monitoring, and at least some meals each day are consumed as regular food. Wadden and his colleagues (Wadden et al., 1997; Wadden, Vogt, Foster, & Anderson, 1998), in their study of exercise strategies, used a 900- to 925-kcal/day diet that consisted of four servings/day of a liquid meal replacement (150 kcal/meal) and a dinner meal of a shelf-stable entree (280–300 kcal/day) plus 2 cups of salad. After 16 weeks on this diet, the liquid meals were reduced, and calories were increased to 1,250 kcal/day; at week 22, the calories were further increased to 1,500 kcal/day, and participants selected their own foods. The diet-only group in this study was seen weekly for 28 weeks and then biweekly during weeks 29–48. Subjects in the diet-only condition lost 16.7 kg at 6 months, and maintained a weight loss of 14.4 kg at 12 months. In the 72% of participants who completed the 2-year follow-up, the average weight loss was 6.9 kg.

A similar regimen involving a combination of liquid formula (SlimFast) and regular food was used by Ditschuneit, Flechtner-Mors, Johnson, and Adler (1999). Participants who were randomly assigned to the SlimFast condition were instructed to consume two SlimFast meal replacements each day and to have a healthy dinner meal. These participants lost 7 kg over the first 3 months of the program, compared to 1 kg in subjects prescribed the same number of calories with a free-choice diet. Both groups were then maintained on a diet of 1,200–1,500 kcal/day, which included one meal and one snack each day of SlimFast products. Both groups were seen monthly over the next 24 months. Weight losses at the end of 24 months averaged 10.2 kg for the group that was prescribed SlimFast throughout, and 7.7 kg for the group that started on regular food and was then switched to SlimFast. Although such weight losses at 2 years are excellent, the fact that weight data were available for only 63% of the sample limits the conclusions that can be drawn. However, these studies all suggest the benefit of simplifying dietary adherence by providing at least some of the food to participants.

CHANGING PHYSICAL ACTIVITY

Physical activity is the component of behavioral treatment that has received the greatest attention since 1995. This emphasis is based on the fact that physical activity level has been the most consistent predictor of the long-term maintenance of weight loss (Pronk & Wing, 1994).

Randomized studies have likewise supported the benefit of diet plus exercise versus diet alone, although the differences between these conditions are often not statistically significant. This literature on the effect of exercise on weight loss and maintenance has been examined in two reviews (NHLBI Expert Panel, 1998; Wing, 1999). Both reviews concluded that exercise alone (without diet) produces a small weight loss of approximately 2 kg; in 6 of 10 studies comparing exercise alone to a no-exercise control condition, the exercise group experienced significantly greater weight loss than the control group. In contrast, only 2 of 13 studies that compared diet only to diet plus exercise found a significant effect of exercise on initial weight loss (4 months to 1 year), although the direction of the difference consistently favored the combination of diet plus exercise. Finally, most important is the issue of whether diet plus exercise improves long-term maintenance of weight loss. The NHLBI Expert Panel (1998) discussed three studies related to this issue and noted that in all three, the combination condition produced a long-term weight loss 1.5–3 kg greater than that produced by diet or exercise alone. Wing (1999) identified six studies with a 1-year or longer follow-up interval that compared diet only to diet-plus-exercise. Although all six studies showed greater long-term weight loss in the diet-plus-exercise condition, only two of the six studies indicated a statistically significant difference in weight loss for the diet-plus-exercise condition versus the diet-only condition.

Long-Term Weight Loss

Results of three of the studies comparing the long-term effects of diet plus exercise versus diet alone have been reported since 1995 (Table 14.2). Skender and colleagues (1996) reported 2-year results of a study comparing diet, exercise, and the combination of diet plus exercise. At 2 years, the diet-plus-exercise group maintained a weight loss of 2.2 kg, and the diet-only group was 0.9 kg over baseline weight. This difference between groups was not significant. The fact that only 36% of the diet-only group and 50%–58% of the other groups attended this follow-up limits these conclusions. Similarly, Wing and colleagues presented the 2-year results of our study with individuals who had a family history of diabetes (Wing, Venditti, Jakicic, Polley, & Lang, 1998). In this study, the behavioral treatment program included 6 months of weekly meetings, 6 months of biweekly meetings, and then two 6-week refresher courses in year 2. The diet-only group and the diet-plus-exercise condition started their programs with 8 weeks of a structured 800- to 1,000-kcal/day diet, which was then made more flexible and gradually increased in calories to 1,200–1,500 kcal/day. Participants in the exercise condition exercised together as a group during each of their treatment sessions; they were instructed to also exercise on their own and to achieve a goal of 1,500 kcal/week of physical activity. The diet-only group and the diet-plus-exercise condition experienced similar excellent initial weight losses (9.1 kg and 10.3 kg, respectively). These groups maintained 60% and 72%, respectively, of this initial weight loss at 12 months. However, both groups regained a great deal over the 1- to 2-year follow-up. At the end of the 2-year study, there were no significant differences in weight loss between groups, and only the diet-plus-exercise group was significantly below baseline levels. Although attendance at the annual assessments was good in this study, many participants ceased to attend the treatment sessions after the initial 6 months. This poor participation in the treatment may have led to the poor long-term outcome in this study. Finally, the third post-1995 study that compared diet only to diet plus exercise also found no significant long-term differences in weight loss for these two interventions (Wadden et al., 1997, 1998). Wadden and colleagues (1997) randomly assigned 128 overweight women to diet alone, diet plus aerobic exercise, diet plus strength training, or diet plus aerobic and strength training. All groups received the same 48-week program with weekly sessions for 28 weeks and then biweekly sessions, and all groups consumed the same diet of 900–925 kcal/day (see above) for weeks 2–17. The exercise conditions participated in three supervised exercise sessions/week for the first 6 months and then two sessions/week for the second half of the study. Of the 128 participants, 99 completed the 12-month study. Weight losses at both 6 months (16 kg) and 12 months (13.7–17.2 kg) were outstanding in this study, but there were no statistically significant differences between treatment conditions. Moreover, the 2-year follow-up completed on 77 of the initial 128 subjects (60%) again showed no benefit of diet plus any type of exercise versus diet alone (Wadden et al., 1998). The authors noted that participants who continued exercising at 2 years had better weight losses than those who stopped exercising. However, by 2 years, there were an equal proportion of participants in each group who reported exercising.

These three recent studies, thus, all raise questions about the widely held belief that treatments that focus on diet plus exercise produce better long-term weight losses than diet only. They suggest, however, that the failure to confirm the benefits of the combination intervention may be due primarily to the difficulty of getting participants to maintain their physical activity over the long term. Several other recent studies have focused specifically on this issue and tried to determine how best to promote long-term adherence to physical activity.

Improving Exercise Adherence

Studies by Andersen and colleagues (Andersen, Frankowiak, Snyder, Bartlett, & Fontaine, 1999) and Perri and colleagues (Perri, Martin, Leermakers, Sears, & Notelovitz, 1997) addressed the question of whether a supervised group exercise program, conducted at a designated location, was more or less effective than a home-based or lifestyle approach to physical activity. Group approaches allow for greater social support from peers and more guidance and reinforcement from the group leader. However, the extra time commitment of having to travel to the exercise location, as well as the fact that the exercise sessions are held at a designated time or times may limit the long-term appeal of this approach.

Perri and colleagues (1997) recruited 49 overweight women (mean age = 49 years, mean baseline weight = 88 kg) and randomly assigned them to behavioral treatments that included group-based or home-based exercise. Both groups attended weekly 2-hour meetings for the first 26 weeks and then biweekly sessions during weeks 27–52. Both were prescribed a diet of 1,200 kcal/day, with 25% of calories from fat. Participants in the group exercise condition were asked to exercise at a clinical facility three times/week for the first 6 months and then two times/week. Exercise classes were also held before each weekly or biweekly behavioral treatment session. The home-based group was instructed to complete 30 minutes of exercise 5 days/week. These participants completed no group exercise at any time during the study. Number of minutes of exercise per week was similar in the two conditions for months 1–6 (104 minutes/week in both groups); however, subjects in the home-exercise condition completed more minutes of activity during months 7–12. The two groups experienced similar weight loss during the first 6 months of the program, but the home-based group had better maintenance of this weight loss from 6 to 15 months. Overall weight loss from months 0 to 15 was significantly greater in the home exercise condition than in the group exercise condition (11.7 kg vs. 7.0 kg; $p < .05$). The dropout rate was also greater in the group program, and was frequently noted to be due to the difficulty of traveling to exercise classes.

Andersen and colleagues (1999) tested a similar hypothesis in a study of 40 overweight women (mean age = 43 years, mean weight at entry = 87 kg). Participants in this study attended weekly group behavioral sessions for 16 weeks and were prescribed a 1,200-kcal/day low-fat diet. The diet-plus-structured-exercise group participated in three aerobics classes a week (estimated expenditure of 450–500 kcal/session) for the first 16 weeks. They were then given tapes of their exercise sessions and instructed to continue exercising on their own at home. The diet-plus-lifestyle-activity group was instructed to complete 30 minutes of moderate-intensity activity on most days of the week. Accelerometers were used to document physical activity level, and participants were given a graph of their activity at the end of each weekly group meeting. At week 16, the average weight loss of the lifestyle group was 7.9 kg, and that of the aerobic group was 8.3 kg. Participants in the lifestyle group regained 0.08 kg from month 6 to 1-year follow-up (week 68), and the aerobics group regained 1.6 kg ($p = .06$).

Considering these two studies together, the most appropriate conclusion seems to be that either a home-based or a clinic-based activity program can be utilized during the initial phase of treatment, but that the home-based program may have some long-term advantage. The weight losses of the home-based condition in the Perri and colleagues (1997) study stand out as the best long-term outcome across these two studies. This observation may suggest the importance of using a home-based exercise prescription in combination with on-going biweekly group behavioral treatment sessions for maintenance of weight loss.

Short-Bout Activity

Several other approaches to improving long-term adherence to physical activity have also been investigated. We (Jakicic, Wing, Butler, & Robertson, 1995) reported that prescribing exercise in multiple short bouts may help overweight individuals initiate an exercise program. This study found that participants who were instructed to complete four 10-minute bouts of activity had better adherence to exercise and better weight losses than individuals who were instructed to exercise in one 40-minute bout. Since this initial study lasted only 6 months, Jakicic, Wing, and Winters (1999) replicated this intervention more recently but continued the treatment for 18 months. In addition, a third treatment was examined, in which subjects were instructed to complete their activity in four 10-minute bouts, but were given a home treadmill to facilitate this activity. This study confirmed the benefits of initially prescribing exercise in multiple bouts, but showed that after the initial weeks of the program, this benefit was no longer observed. By 18 months, there were no differences between the short-bout and long-bout conditions for adherence to physical activity or for weight loss. However, providing exercise equipment to participants did have a positive long-term effect. The short-bout group that was given home exercise equipment reported the best maintenance of physical activity during months 12–18, as well as the best overall weight loss.

Personal Trainer

Physical activity equipment may modify the home environment and serve as a cue to exercise. Another approach to modifying the antecedents for exercise is to use a personal trainer or coach who calls participants to remind them to exercise and exercises with the participants, thus modeling and supporting the activity. Jeffery, Wing, Thorson, and Burton (1998) examined this antecedent-control approach and compared its effectiveness to that of changing the consequences for activity by paying participants small incentives for exercise. The participants were 196 overweight individuals (29 men and 167 women), with a mean baseline weight of 86 kg, who were randomly assigned to one of five conditions. All five groups received a standard behavioral weight loss program, with weekly meetings for 6 months, biweekly meetings for 6 months, and then monthly meetings for the final 6 months. The exercise prescription for all groups was to gradually increase physical activity to a goal of 1,000 kcal/week. Group 1 participants were given this goal and instructed to complete their exercise on their own at home. Group 2 was invited to three exercise sessions per week; these sessions were conducted at a local track, and participants walked 3 miles at each session. Group 3 participants were given "personal trainers" to help increase their adherence to the exercise sessions. These trainers called the participants to remind them to participate in the exercise session and met them at the track to walk with them; makeup sessions were also arranged. Participants in group 4 were paid $1–$5 per session for attending the scheduled activity sessions. Group 5 received the combination of the personal trainers and the incentives for attending the exercise sessions.

The study suggested that the antecedent control (trainers) and the consequent control (payment) were equally effective approaches for increasing attendance at exercise sessions. Either approach used alone doubled attendance at these sessions, and the combination of the two resulted in a tripling of exercise attendance. However, despite the benefits for attendance, these procedures had no effect on overall physical activity level. All five groups reported comparable levels of activity, all approximating the 1,000-kcal goal that was assigned. The most unexpected finding from this study was that group 1—the group given the standard behavioral treatment with no supervised exercise sessions—had the best long-term weight loss. This finding supports the studies described above that showed benefits of home-based physical activity interventions. The fact, however, that all groups reported similar levels of activity raises questions about this interpretation. Another possibility is that the increased emphasis on exercise in groups 2–4 decreased the focus on weight loss in these conditions.

Amount of Exercise

The Jeffery and colleagues (1998) study also raised the possibility that the exercise level recommended in behavioral weight loss programs (namely, 1,000 kcal/week) is lower than what should be prescribed. In post hoc analyses, we (Jeffery et al., 1998) divided subjects into quartiles according to their self-reported physical activity level at 18 months. The top quartile, which reported a mean activity level of 2,500 kcal/week, had the best long-term weight loss. Weight losses of the other three quartiles, which reported activity levels of approximately 1,000 kcal/week, did not differ significantly from each other. Similarly, the Jakicic and colleagues (1999) study found that the best weight losses occurred in individuals who spent at least 200 minutes/week in physical activity. In the National Weight Control Registry, a registry of individuals who have lost at least 13.6 kg (i.e., 30 pounds) and kept it off at least 1 year, successful weight loss maintainers report an average of 2,800 kcal/week of physical activity (Klem, Wing, McGuire, Seagle, & Hill, 1997). Thus a new direction being pursued by several investigators is the use of higher exercise goals (2,000–2,500 kcal/week) as a means to promote long-term maintenance of weight loss. The topic of exercise and weight management is further addressed by Blair and Leermakers in Chapter 13 of this volume.

MOTIVATIONAL STRATEGIES TO IMPROVE WEIGHT LOSS

The fact that participants lose weight successfully for approximately 6 months and then begin to experience weight regain has led investigators to begin to focus on ways to help maintain motivation over the long term. In a pilot study on this topic, Smith, Heckemeyer, Kratt, and Mason (1997) applied motivational interviewing techniques at three individual sessions during a 16-session behavioral weight control program for patients with Type 2 diabetes. Motivational interviews explored the participants' personal goals, examined the discrepancy between these goals and the participants' current behavior, and acknowledged the ambivalence participants felt about behavior change. The group given motivational interviewing ($n = 6$) had better adherence to the treatment program (i.e., better attendance, self-monitoring, exercise, and blood sugar monitoring) than those who received the standard behavioral program (n = 10). Although weight losses were comparable in the two conditions, the motivational interviewing group had better glycemic control following the program. Smith and colleagues are currently conducting a longer study with a larger number of participants to further examine the benefits of motivational interviewing.

Weight Loss Satisfaction

Another approach to increasing motivation is to try to increase satisfaction with the weight loss that participants attain during treatment. Unfortunately, most individuals who enter weight loss programs desire to lose more weight than typically occurs in these programs, and thus finish treatment feeling dissatisfied. Since most individuals who enter weight loss programs are motivated by a desire to improve their health and/or their appearance, Smith, Burke, and Wing (1999) hypothesized that if treatments were modified to help participants achieve these goals (i.e., better health and/or appearance), participants might be more satisfied with their weight losses. As reported in an abstract presented at a recent meeting (Smith et al., 1999) found support for this hypothesis. Women (n = 49) were randomly assigned to either a standard behavioral program, a program that stressed physical appearance changes accompaning weight loss, or a program that stressed health changes with weight loss. Persons in the appearance-focused condition lost more weight at 6 months than the standard group (10.4 kg vs. 6.2 kg) and reported greater satisfaction with their overall appearance. Participants in the health-focused condition lost 8.2 kg and reported greater satisfaction with their health improvements than did the standard-condition participants. The effect of these approaches on long-term maintenance of weight loss is currently being studied.

Social Support

Wing and Jeffery (1999) have tried to improve motivation for long-term weight loss by increasing social support. Two types of social support were investigated: natural support and experimentally manipulated support. Participants (n = 166) who expressed interest in the study were asked to identify three other individuals who would like to participate in the study with them. Participants who identified three friends were treated together as a "team" and were compared to persons who signed up for the program alone (thus this component of the study was not randomized). Within both the group of participants recruited with friends and those recruited alone, half of the subjects were then randomly assigned to a standard behavioral treatment program, while the other half were assigned to a weight loss program with social support strategies. These social support strategies included both intragroup team-building activities and intergroup competitions, in which financial incentives were awarded to the team(s) with the best maintenance of weight loss from month 4 to month 10.

At both month 4 and month 10, participants who were recruited with friends had better weight losses than those who were recruited alone. However, both the recruitment condition and the social support intervention affected the maintenance of weight loss from month 4 to month 10. In the group recruited alone and given the standard behavioral treatment (which would represent what is typically done in behavioral weight loss programs), only 24% maintained their weight loss in full over this 6-month follow-up. In contrast, 66% of subjects who were recruited with friends and given the social support intervention maintained their weight loss in full. These findings suggest that further attention to social support may improve long-term maintenance of weight loss.

INCREASING THE AUDIENCE FOR WEIGHT CONTROL INTERVENTIONS

The studies reviewed above have all utilized a clinical treatment model in which overweight participants are treated in group behavioral weight loss classes. Such approaches have produced the largest weight losses to date. However, an alternative strategy is to try to increase the audience served by weight loss programs, rather than trying to increase the number of kilograms lost by a small number of individuals. The use of various types of media, including telephone, television, and Internet, may provide greater convenience and anonymity for participants and thereby increase the number of individuals who are willing to embark on such weight loss efforts.

Hellerstedt and Jeffery (1997) examined the effects of a telephone-based intervention. Sixty-four participants were recruited and randomly assigned to a minimal-contact control group or to one of two telephone-based interventions. All three groups attended two initial group meetings and were given basic information about diet, exercise, and self-monitoring, as well as a 6-month supply of food diaries. The control group received no further contact, whereas participants in the phone conditions were called every week for the next 24 weeks and asked to report either their weight or their eating and exercise behavior. Interestingly, the control group lost 5.8 kg over 12 weeks, compared to 3.7 kg for the weight-focused phone group and 3.4 kg for the behaviorally focused phone group. Another surprising finding from this study was that the participants who signed up for this study appeared similar to those usually seen in face-to-face group programs. Thus it was unclear whether this minimal intervention really accomplished the goal of broadening the population served.

Another media approach is to use television broadcasting to deliver the weight loss program. Meyers, Graves, Whelan, and Barclay (1996) compared a standard face-to-face treatment group, a group receiving a face-to-face program that was videotaped for subsequent use, a group that was shown the videotape via television as its treatment contact, and a waiting-list control. The three treatment groups all achieved similar weight losses (4.1–4.5 kg over 8 weeks), and differed from the waiting-list control (0.9 kg). The maintenance of weight loss through 15 months also appeared comparable in the group receiving the face-to-face program and the group viewing the TV broadcast. The fact that the group that was shown the TV broadcast was weighed before and after the 8 weeks and was asked to send self-monitoring records to the therapist may have influenced these outcomes. Similarly, Harvey-Berino (1998) found that weight losses achieved by participants who viewed an interactive television program were comparable to those achieved by participants in a face-to-face program (7.6 kg vs. 7.9 kg over 12 weeks). Based on these two studies, it appears that further examination of televised programs is warranted. It would be interesting to evaluate the effectiveness of a televised version of a 24-week behavioral program, which is now considered the standard length of such programs, and to compare these results to those for a state-of-the-art face-to-face program.

Finally, the most recent approach to mediated intervention is the use of Internet interventions and e-mail. Currently there are many weight loss Web sites that provide valuable information about diet and/or exercise, but most do not include the use of standard behavioral procedures, such as self-monitoring or feedback. Tate, Wing, and Winett (2000) developed an Internet-based behavioral weight loss program, which included weekly lessons, prompting for submission of weekly self-monitoring data, personalized feedback on these data, and an online bulletin board for social support. To test the effectiveness of this Internet intervention, a total of 90 participants (with computer access) were recruited and randomly assigned to Internet Behavior Therapy or Internet Education. Both groups attended an initial start-up meeting in which they were taught basic weight control strategies. Those who were randomly assigned to Internet Behavior Therapy were then given a 12-week intervention delivered entirely via Web site and e-mail, with contact only for 3- and 6-month weigh-ins. These participants were sent a new behavioral lesson each week; they self-monitored their diet and exercise, and sent these records in weekly via e-mail. Personalized feedback was then provided based on these reports. The Internet Education group was given access to a Web site that catalogued and organized available weight-related Web sites related to diet, exercise, or body weight. However, these participants received none of the behavioral strategies described above. At the end of the 12-week intervention, Internet Behavior Therapy had a mean weight loss of 4.1 kg, versus 1.3 kg in Internet Education control group. Thus these low-contact approaches may be quite effective for producing initial weight loss.

IMPLICATIONS FOR PRACTICE AND RESEARCH

The most effective weight loss programs appear to be those that combine diet, exercise, and behavior modification. This review of the recent literature on such programs suggests that weight loss may be improved in the following ways:

1. Use of structured meal plans or portion-controlled diets during initial weeks of the program.
2. Use of home-based or supervised exercise during the initial 6 months of intervention, followed by home-based exercise with continued biweekly therapy contact for months 7–12, and provision of home exercise equipment for long-term maintenance of exercise and weight loss.
3. Use of motivational strategies, such as recruitment with friends and intergroup competition.
4. Development of media-based programs (using telephone, television, or Internet) to increase access to behavioral weight control interventions.

Although behaviorists have made tremendous progress in developing weight control programs, a large number of very basic questions remain unanswered. For example, we still know little about the ideal diet recommendation in terms of either calorie level or macronutrient content. Although the field has typically utilized balanced low-calorie, low-fat diets, there has been little empirical investigation comparing such diets with more extreme low-fat diets (e.g., the Ornish 10% fat diet), vegetarian diets, or other popular diets (e.g., the Atkins diet). A recent study (Smith, Burke, & Wing, 2000) showed that individuals embarking on a vegetarian diet remained on this diet far longer than individuals starting a diet for weight loss. This difference in duration was seen even in subjects who had tried both types of diets and was not due to participants' reaching their desired weight loss goal. Interestingly, participants were far more likely to cite boredom as the explanation for stopping their weight loss regimen than for discontinuing the vegetarian diet. These data suggest that teaching patients to maintain variety while on a weight loss diet may be helpful (although the positive results of VLCDs might suggest the opposite).

Similar basic issues remain on the activity side of the energy balance equation. As noted above, weight loss programs typically recommend 1,000 kcal/week of activity, whereas studies of individuals who successfully lose weight suggest that these individuals are completing 2,500–2,800 kcal/week of activity. The benefits of these higher levels of physical activity, and of including some higher-intensity activity within the prescription, remain untested.

Probably the most consistent finding in the behavioral weight loss literature is the fact that maximal weight loss occurs at about 6 months. This seems to be true in diets of differing calorie levels (and thus appears to be due more to length of time on the diet than to the magnitude of weight loss achieved). The reason for this phenomenon remains unclear. Researchers have attempted to improve long-term weight loss outcomes by increasing initial weight loss, extending treatment contact, using stronger behavioral techniques, and teaching specific skills related to maintenance (Jeffery et al., 2000). All these approaches have had only modest effects. Further research, examining new approaches to the long-term maintenance of weight loss, is clearly needed. For further information on behavioral treatment and weight maintenance, see Perri and Corsica, Chapter 17, this volume.

Finally, it is important to explore new ways to increase the number of participants in weight loss interventions. Strategies for maintaining the advantages of therapist-led group treatment programs (including accountability, feedback, and group support), while reducing the "costs" of such programs (the need to travel to a given location at a set time during the week, the potential embarrassment), should be examined.

REFERENCES

Andersen, R., Frankowiak, S., Snyder, J., Bartlett, S., & Fontaine, K. (1999). Effects of lifestyle activity vs. structured aerobic exercise in obese women: A randomized trial. *Journal of the American Medical Association, 281*(4), 335–340.

Ditschuneit, H. H., Flechtner-Mors, M., Johnson, T. D., & Adler, G. (1999). Metabolic and weight-loss effects of a long-term dietary intervention in obese patients. *American Journal of Clinical Nutrition, 69,* 198–204.

Ferster, C. B, Nurnberger, J. I., & Levitt, E. B. (1962). The control of eating. *Journal of Mathematics, 1,* 87–109.

Harvey-Berino, J. (1998). Changing health behavior via telecommunications technology: Using interactive television to treat obesity. *Behavior Therapy, 29,* 505–519.

Hellerstedt, W., & Jeffery, R. (1997). The effects of a telephone-based intervention on weight loss. *American Journal of Health Promotion, 11,* 177–182.

Jakicic, J., Wing, R. R., & Winters, C. (1999). Effects of intermittent exercise and use of home exercise equipment on adherence, weight loss, and fitness in overweight women. *Journal of the American Medical Association, 282*(16), 1554–1560.

Jakicic, J. M., Wing, R. R., Butler, B. A., & Robertson, R. J. (1995). Prescribing exercise in multiple short bouts versus one continuous bout: Effects on adherence, cardiorespiratory fitness, and weight loss in overweight women. *International Journal of Obesity, 19,* 893–901.

Jeffery, R. W., Drewnowski, A., Epstein, L., Stunkard, A. J., Willson, G., Wing, R. R., & Hill, R. (2000). Long-term maintenance of weight loss: Current status. *Health Psychology, 19*(1), 5–16.

Jeffery, R W., Wing, R. R., Thorson, C., & Burton, L. C. (1998). Use of personal trainers and financial incentives to increase exercise in a behavioral weight-loss program. *Journal of Consulting and Clinical Psychology, 66,* 777–783.

Klem, M. L., Wing, R. R., McGuire, M. T., Seagle, H. M., & Hill, J. O. (1997). A descriptive study of individuals successful at long-term maintenance of substantial weight loss. *American Journal of Clinical Nutrition, 66,* 239–246.

Meyers, A., Graves, T., Whelan, J., & Barclay, D. (1996). An evaluation of a television-delivered behavioral weight loss program: Are the ratings acceptable? *Journal of Consulting and Clinical Psychology, 64,* 172–178.

National Heart, Lung, and Blood Institute (NHLBI). (1998). Clinical guidelines on the identification, evaluation, and treatment of overweight and obesity in adults: The evidence report. *Obesity Research, 6*(Suppl.), 51S–210S.

Perri, M. G., Martin, A. D., Leermakers, E. A., Sears, S. F., & Notelovitz, M. (1997). Effects of group- versus home-based exercise in the treatment of obesity. *Journal of Consulting and Clinical Psychology, 65,* 278–285.

Pronk, N. P., & Wing, R. R. (1994). Physical activity and long-term maintenance of weight loss. *Obesity Research, 2,* 587–599.

Skender, M. S., Goodrick, G. K., DelJungo, D. J., Reeves, R. S., Darnell, L., Gotto, A. M., & Foreyt, J. P. (1996). Comparison of 2-year weight loss trends in behavioral treatments of obesity: Diet, exercise, and combination interventions. *Journal of the American Dietetic Association, 96,* 342–346.

Smith, C., Burke, L., & Wing, R. R. (1999). 6-month outcome of two behavioral weight loss treatments focusing on primary motivations for weight loss [Abstract]. *Obesity Research, 7,* 19S.

Smith, C., Burke, L., & Wing, R. R. (2000). Vegetarian and weight loss diets among young adults. *Obesity Research, 8*(2), 123–129.

Smith, D., Heckemeyer, C., Kratt, P., & Mason, D. (1997). Motivational interviewing to improve adherence to a behavioral weight-control program for older obese women with NIDDM. *Diabetes Care, 20*(1), 52–58.

Stuart, R. B. (1967). Behavioural control of overeating. *Behavioural Research and Therapy, 5,* 357–365.

Tate, D., Wing, R. R., & Winett, R. (2001). Development and evaluation of an Internet behavior therapy program for weight loss. *Journal of the American Medical Association, 285,* 1172–1177.

Wadden, T. A. (1993). The treatment of obesity: An overview. In A. J. Stunkard & T. A. Wadden (Eds.), *Obesity: Theory and therapy* (2nd ed., pp. 197–218). New York: Raven Press.

Wadden, T. A., Foster, G. D., & Letizia, K. A. (1994). One-year behavioral treatment of obesity: Comparison of moderate and severe caloric restriction and the effects of weight maintenance therapy. *Journal of Consulting and Clinical Psychology, 62,* 165–171.

Wadden, T. A., & Stunkard, A. J. (1986). Controlled trial of very low calorie diet, behavior therapy, and their combination in the treatment of obesity. *Journal of Consulting and Clinical Psychology, 54,* 482–488.

Wadden, T. A., Stunkard, A. J., & Brownell, K. D. (1983). Very low calorie diets: Their efficacy, safety, and future. *Annals of Internal Medicine, 99,* 675–684.

Wadden, T. A., Vogt, R. A., Andersen, R. E., Bartlett, S. J., Foster, G. D., Kuehnel, R. H., Wilk, J., Weinstock, R., Buckenmeyer, P., Berkowitz, R. I., & Steen, S. N. (1997). Exercise in the treatment of obesity: Effects of four interventions on body composition, resting energy expenditure, appetite, and mood. *Journal of Consulting and Clinical Psychology, 65,* 269–277.

Wadden, T. A., Vogt, R. A., Foster, G. D., & Anderson, D. A. (1998). Exercise and maintenance of weight loss: 1-year follow-up of a controlled clinic trial. *Journal of Consulting and Clinical Psychology, 66*(2), 429–433.

Wing, R. R. (1998). Behavioral approaches to the treatment of obesity. In G. Bray, C. Bouchard, & W. P. T. James (Eds.), *Handbook of obesity* (pp. 855–873). New York: Marcel Dekker.

Wing, R. R. (1999). Physical activity in the treatment of the adulthood overweight and obesity: Current evidence and research issues. *Medicine and Science in Sports and Exercise, 31*(11), S547–S552.

Wing, R. R., Blair, E., Marcus, M., Epstein, L. H., & Harvey, J. (1994). Year-long weight loss treatment for obese patients with Type II diabetes: Does inclusion of an intermittent very low calorie diet improve outcome? *American Journal of Medicine, 97,* 354–362.

Wing, R. R., & Jeffery, R. W. (1979). Outpatient treatments of obesity: A comparison of methodology and clinical results. *International Journal of Obesity, 3,* 261–279.

Wing, R. R., & Jeffery, R. W. (1999). Benefits of recruiting participants with friends and increasing social support for weight loss maintenance. *Journal of Consulting and Clinical Psychology, 67*(1), 132–138.

Wing, R. R., Jeffery, R. W., Burton, L. R., Thorson, C., Sperber Nissinoff, K., & Baxter, J. E. (1996).

Food provision vs. structured meal plans in the behavioral treatment of obesity. *International Journal of Obesity, 20,* 56–62.

Wing, R. R., Marcus, M. D., Salata, R., Epstein, L. H., Miaskiewicz, S., & Blair, E. H. (1991). Effects of a very-low-calorie diet on long-term glycemic control in obese Type 2 diabetic subjects. *Archives of Internal Medicine, 151,* 1334–1340.

Wing, R. R., Venditti, E. M., Jakicic, J. M., Polley, B. A., & Lang, W. (1998). Lifestyle intervention in overweight individuals with a family history of diabetes. *Diabetes Care, 21*(3), 350–359.

15

Drug Treatment of Obesity

GEORGE A. BRAY

Drug treatment for obesity has been tarnished by a number of disasters (Bray, 1998a). Since 1893, almost any drug treatment that has been used in obese patients has generated undesirable outcomes that have resulted in their termination. Table 15.1 is a historical presentation of drug treatments for obesity and the disasters that befell them.

An additional serious negative impact on the use of drug treatment for obesity is the negative halo spread by the addictive properties of amphetamine (Bray, 1993, 1998b; Bray, Atkinson, & Inoue, 1995; Bray & Greenway, 1999; Bray & Inoue, 1992). Amphetamine, or α-methyl-β-phenethylamine, is an addictive β-phenethylamine that reduces food intake. The addictiveness of dextroamphetamine is probably related to its effects on dopaminergic neurotransmission. Its anorectic effects, on the other hand, are probably due to its modulation of noradrenergic neurotransmission. Because this β-phenethylamine was addictive, other β-phenethylamine derivatives were presumed to be addictive. Whether actually addictive or not, they were presumed guilty by association. This has led to restrictions on the use of this entire class of drugs by the U.S. Drug Enforcement Agency (DEA) (Bray, 1993, 1998a; Bray & Greenway, 1999).

Appetite-suppressing drugs such as phentermine, diethylpropion, fenfluramine, and sibutramine, and the antidepressant venlafaxine, are all β-phenethylamines (Bray & Greenway, 1999). Phentermine and diethylpropion are sympathomimetic amines like amphetamine, but differ from amphetamine in having little or no effect on dopamine release at the synapse. Abuse of either phentermine or diethylpropion is rare. Fenfluramine, on the other hand, has no effect on reuptake or release of either norepinephrine (NE) or dopamine in the brain, but increases serotonin release and partially inhibits serotonin reuptake. Thus the derivatives of β-phenethylamine have a wide range of pharmacological effects. However, if examined uncritically, they could all be lumped with amphetamine and carry its negative halo (Bray et al., 1995). It is thus misleading to use "amphetamine-like" in reference to appetite-suppressant β-phenethylamine drugs except amphetamine and methamphetamine, because of the negative linguistic images.

A third issue in drug treatment of obesity is the perception that because patients regain weight when drugs are stopped, the drugs are ineffective (Bray, 1998b; Bray et al., 1995).

TABLE 15.1. Disasters with Drug Treatments for Obesity

Date	Drug	Outcome
1893	Thyroid	Hyperthyroidism
1934	Dinitrophenol	Cataracts, neuropathy
1937	Amphetamine	Addiction
1967	Rainbow pills (digitalis, diuretics)	Deaths
1971	Aminorex	Pulmonary hypertension
1997	Fenfluramine ± phentermine Dexfenfluramine ± phentermine	Valvular insufficiency

Quite the contrary is true. Overweight is a chronic disease that has many causes. Cure is rare, however, and treatment is thus aimed at palliation. As clinicians, we do not expect to cure with medications such diseases as hypertension or hypercholesterolemia. Rather, we expect to palliate them. When the medications for any of these diseases are discontinued, we expect the disease to recur. This means that medications only work when used. The same arguments go for medications used to treat overweight: It is a chronic, incurable disease for which drugs only work when used.

Recent reports of valvular heart disease associated with the use of fenfluramine, dexfenfluramine, and phentermine have provided the most recent problem for drug treatment of obesity (Connolly et al., 1997; Ryan et al., 1999). This is an example of the "law of unintended consequences." The report of valvulopathy in up to 35% of patients treated with the combination of fenfluramine and phentermine was totally unexpected. The finding, however, will add caution to the marketing of any future drugs to treat obesity, and will provide support for those who believe that drug treatment of obesity is inappropriate.

MECHANISMS FOR DRUG EFFECTS IN TREATMENT OF OBESITY

Corpulence results from an imbalance between energy intake and energy expenditure (Bray, 1998b). This relationship can be described with a nutrient balance–feedback model (Figure 15.1). The targets in this model where drugs might be used are shown as shaded boxes in Figure 15.1. The nutrient balance–feedback model provides the framework for this approach to drug treatment. Drugs can reduce food intake, alter metabolism, and/or increase energy expenditure. This framework is used in discussing the available and potential drug leads for treatment of obesity.

Reduction of Food Intake

Noradrenergic Receptors

A number of monoamines and neuropeptides are known to modulate food intake (Bray, 1993; Bray & Greenway, 1999). Both noradrenergic receptors and serotonergic receptors have served as the sites for clinically useful drugs to decrease food intake (Table 15.2).

Activation of the α_1 or β_2 adrenoceptors decreases food intake. Stimulation of the α_2 adrenoceptor in experimental animals, on the other hand, increases food intake. Direct agonists and drugs that release NE or block NE reuptake can activate one or more of these receptors, depending on where the NE is released. Phenylpropanolamine (PPA) is an α_1 agonist that decreases food intake by acting on α_1-adrenergic receptors in the paraventricular

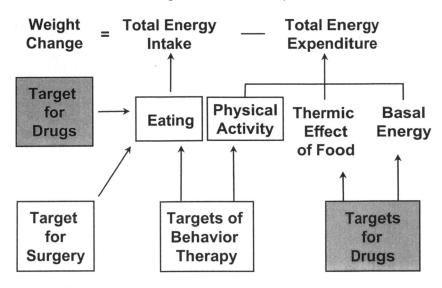

FIGURE 15.1. Targets for drug treatment in an energy balance model.

nucleus. The weight gain seen in patients treated for hypertension or prostatic hypertrophy with α_1-adrenergic antagonists indicates that the α_1 adrenoceptor is clinically important in regulation of body weight in human beings. Stimulation of the β_2 adrenoceptor by NE or agonists like terbutaline, clenbuterol, or salbutamol reduces food intake. The small weight gain in patients treated with some β_2-adrenergic antagonists also indicates that this is a clinically important receptor for regulation of body weight.

Serotonergic Receptors

The serotonin receptor system, which consists of seven families of receptors, is also involved in modulating food intake (Baez, Kursar, Helton, Wainscott, & Nelson, 1995). Stimulation of receptors in the 5-HT$_1$ and 5-HT$_2$ families have the major effects on feeding. Activation of 5-HT$_{1A}$ receptors increases food intake, but this acute effect is rapidly down-regulated and is not clinically significant in regulation of body weight. Activation of the 5-HT$_{2C}$ and

TABLE 15.2. Monoamine Mechanisms that Reduce Food Intake

Neurotransmitter system	Mechanism of action	Examples
Noradrenergic	α_1 agonist	Phenylpropanolamine (PPA)
	β_2 agonist	Clenbuterol
	Stimulates NE release	Phentermine
	Blocks NE reuptake	Mazindol
Serotonergic	5-HT$_{1B}$ or 5-HT$_{2C}$ agonists	Quipazine
	Stimulates 5-HT release	Fenfluramine
	Blocks 5-HT reuptake	Fluoxetine
Dopaminergic	D$_1$ agonist	Bromocriptine
Histaminergic	H$_1$ antagonist	Chlorpheniramine

possibly 5-HT$_{1B}$ receptors decreases food intake (Bray & Greenway, 1999). Direct agonists (quipazine) or drugs that block serotonin reuptake will reduce food intake by acting on these receptors or by providing the serotonin that modulates these receptors.

Altered Metabolism

Excess fat is the visible sign of obesity. Metabolic strategies have been directed to preabsorptive and postabsorptive mechanisms (Bray, 1998b). Preabsorptive mechanisms that influence digestion and absorption of macronutrients are used by orlistat, which inhibits intestinal digestion of fat and lowers body weight.

The second strategy is to affect intermediary metabolism. Enhancing lipolysis, inhibiting lipogenesis, and affecting fat distribution between subcutaneous and visceral sites are strategies that can be developed.

Increased Energy Expenditure

Increased energy expenditure through exercise would be an ideal approach to treating obesity. Drugs with the same physiological consequences as exercise would provide useful ways of treating obesity.

DRUGS THAT REDUCE FOOD INTAKE

Table 15.3 summarizes the effects of a number of drugs that treat obesity by reducing food intake. They are discussed in more detail below.

Noradrenergic Drugs Approved for Short-Term Treatment of Obesity

The noradrenergic drugs are grouped together because they can increase blood pressure and, in part, act like the neurotransmitter NE. Drugs in this group work by a variety of mechanisms, including the release of NE from synaptic granules (benzphetamine, phendimetrazine, phentermine, and diethylpropion); blockade of NE reuptake (mazindol); blockade of reuptake of both NE and serotonin (sibutramine); or direct action on adrenoceptors (PPA) (Table 15.2).

All of these drugs are absorbed orally and reach peak blood concentrations within 1–2 hours (Bray & Greenway, 1999). The half-life in blood is short for all except the metabolites of sibutramine, which have a long half-life. Both metabolites of sibutramine are active, but this is not true of the other drugs in this group. Liver metabolism inactivates a large fraction of these drugs before excretion. Side effects include dry mouth, constipation, and insomnia. Food intake is suppressed either by delaying the onset of a meal or by producing early satiety. Sibutramine and mazindol have both been shown to increase thermogenesis experimentally.

The efficacy of an appetite-suppressing drug can be established by showing in double-blind randomized clinical trials that it produces a significantly greater weight loss than a placebo drug (Bray & Greenway, 1999), and that this weight loss is more than 5% below baseline weight. An alternative criterion is that a significantly greater proportion of drug-treated patients than placebo-treated patients lose more than 5% or more than 10% of baseline weight (Bray et al., 1995). Clinical trials of sympathomimetic drugs done before 1975 were generally short term, because it was widely believed that short-term treatment would "cure obesity" (Bray, 1993; Bray & Greenway, 1999). This was unfounded opti-

TABLE 15.3. Drugs That Reduce Food Intake

Drug group	FDA approval	Approved duration of treatment	DEA schedule	Trade names	Dosage form (mg)	Administration
Sympathomimetic drugs approved for short-term use						
Diethylpropion	Yes	Few weeks	IV	Tenuate	25	25 mg, three times daily
				Tenuate, Dospan	75	75 mg, once daily
Phentermine	Yes	Few weeks	IV	Standard:	37.5	37.5 mg, in A.M.
				Adipex-P	30	30 mg/day, 2 hr after breakfast
				Duromine	37.5	37.5 mg/day, 9 A.M.
				Fastin	30	30 mg/day, 2 hr after breakfast
				Obenix	30	30 mg/day, 2 hr after breakfast
				Oby-Cap	30	30 mg/day, 2 hr after breakfast
				Oby-Trim		
				Zantryl	15, 30	15 mg/day, before breakfast (30 mg for less responsive patients)
				Slow-release Ioamin		
Sympathomimetic drug approved for long-term use						
Serotonin–norepinephrine reuptake inhibitor						
Sibutramine	Yes	Long-term	IV	Meridia	5, 10, 15	Initial dose: 10 mg/day Maximum dose: 15 mg/day

mism, but because the trials were of short duration and were often crossover in design, they provided few long-term data. This discussion focuses on longer-term trials lasting over 24 weeks, and on those trials in which there was an adequate control group.

Phentermine and Diethylpropion

A 36-week trial comparing continuous administration of phentermine with intermittent phentermine and placebo is shown in Figure 15.2 (Munro, MacCuish, Wilson, & Duncan, 1968). Both continuous and intermittent phentermine therapy produced more weight loss than the placebo. In the drug-free periods, weight loss slowed only for the intermittently treated patients; then the patients would lose weight more rapidly when the drug was reinitiated. A small trial with diethylpropion showed greater weight loss than with placebo (Bray & Greenway, 1999). Phentermine and diethylpropion are Schedule IV drugs in the DEA regulatory classification, indicating the potential for abuse, although the potential appears to be very low. Phentermine and diethylpropion are only approved for a few weeks, which is widely interpreted as up to 12 weeks in any calendar year. Weight loss with phentermine and diethylpropion persists for the duration of treatment, suggesting that tolerance does not develop to these drugs. If tolerance does develop, the drugs would be expected to lose their effectiveness or require increased amounts of drug for patients to maintain weight loss. This does not seem to occur.

Mazindol

There are no long-term, double-blind, placebo-controlled, parallel-arm studies with mazindol, but there are two open-label studies that deserve comment. Enzi, Baritussio, Marchiori, and Crepaldi (1976) studied 102 patients on mazindol (2 mg/day) and 102 patients on

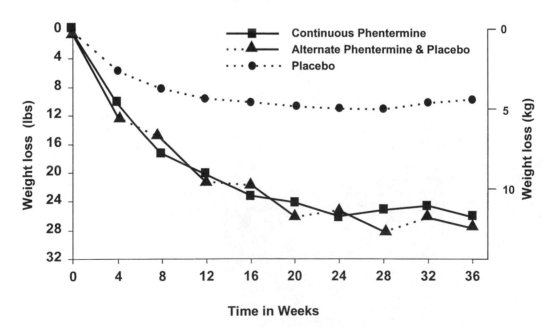

FIGURE 15.2. Comparison of weight loss with continuous and intermittent therapy with phentermine. From Mason and Ito (1969). Copyright 1969 by Annals of Surgery. Adapted by permission.

placebo in a 15-week trial using a crossover design, with an additional 12 months of treatment with mazindol. There was no significant difference between the drug and placebo conditions during the 15-week controlled trial, but mazindol produced significantly more weight loss during the long-term (15-month) period of treatment.

In a 12-month open-label study of mazindol in Japan, Inoue (1995) enrolled 32 subjects, half of whom dropped out prior to 1 year of treatment. In a last-observation-carried-forward analysis, there was a 9% loss of initial body weight, which is comparable to that produced by several other weight loss medications. Blood pressure, glucose, insulin, cholesterol, triglycerides, and alanine transaminase levels declined during treatment.

Phenylpropanolamine

PPA is an α_1-adrenergic agonist of the propanolamine group. It is an over-the-counter preparation with a provisional FDA approval for weight loss. In reviews by Weintraub (1985) and Greenway (1992), including published and unpublished studies obtained from the manufacturer, 1,439 subjects were on active medication and 1,086 on placebo. At the end of the studies, which were up to 12 weeks in length and performed before 1985, subjects on PPA lost about 0.27 kg/week more than the subjects on placebo.

To date, there is only one controlled trial of PPA that has lasted 20 weeks. In this double-blind placebo-controlled trial, 101 subjects were treated with placebo or PPA for 6 weeks, with an optional double-blind extension to week 20 (Schteingart, 1992). At 6 weeks, the PPA-treated group had lost 2.4 kg (0.43 kg/week), compared to 1.1 kg (0.18 kg/week) in the placebo group. In the optional extension, 24 subjects on PPA lost 5.1 kg (6.5%), compared to 12 subjects treated with placebo who lost 0.4 kg/week (0.5%) of initial body weight ($p < .05$).

Sympathomimetic Drugs Approved for Long-Term Use

Sibutramine

In experimental animals, the inhibition of food intake by sibutramine is duplicated by combining a noradrenergic reuptake inhibitor (nisoxetine) with a serotonin reuptake inhibitor (fluoxetine) (Ryan, Kaiser, & Bray, 1995). Sibutramine produces the behavioral sequence of satiety (Halford, Heal, & Blundell, 1994). Sibutramine does not bind to any of a wide variety of receptors on which it has been tested. In addition to the inhibition of food intake (Rolls, Shide, Thorwart, & Ulbrecht, 1998), sibutramine stimulates thermogenesis in experimental animals (Stock, 1997). The human data on thermogenesis are contradictory (Hansen, Toubro, Stock, Macdonald, & Astrup, 1998; Seagle, Bessesen, & Hill, 1998).

Both short-term (Hanotin, Thomas, Jones, Leutenegger, & Drouin, 1998; Lean, 1997; Weintraub, Rubio, Golik, Byrne, & Scheinbaum, 1991) and long-term (Apfelbaum et al., 1999; Bray et al., 1996, 1999; Jones, Smith, Kelly, & Gray, 1995) clinical trials have been reported with sibutramine. In an 8-week trial comparing placebo with 5 and 20 mg/day of sibutramine, Weintraub and colleagues (1991) noted a weight loss of 1.4 ± 2.1 kg in the placebo group, 2.9 ± 2.3 kg in the group treated with 5 mg/day and 5.0 ± 2.7 kg in the group treated with 20 mg/day.

In a multicenter dose-ranging trial (Bray et al., 1996, 1999), sibutramine produced a dose-related weight loss lasting up to 6 months (Figure 15.3). A total of 1,043 patients were randomly assigned to receive placebo or 1, 5, 10, 15, 20, or 30 mg/day of sibutramine. There was a clear dose response, with the placebo group losing 1% and the 30-mg/day group losing 9.5% of initial body weight. By the end of the 6 months, patients receiving the

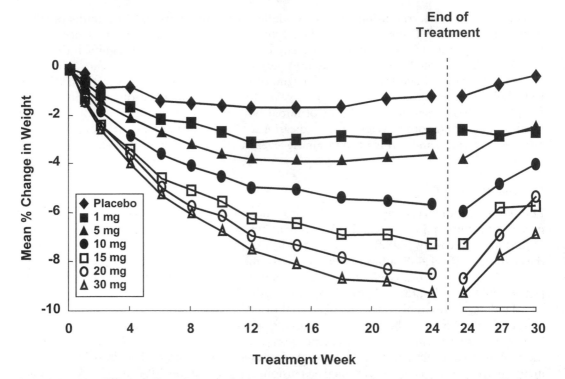

FIGURE 15.3. Effect of sibutramine on body weight. There was a dose-dependent reduction in body weight over the 24 weeks of the trial. From Bray et al. (1999). Copyright 1999 by *Obesity Research*. Adapted by permission.

lower doses had plateaued in their weight loss, but the groups receiving 15, 20, and 30 mg/day were still losing weight.

There have been two 1-year trials with sibutramine (Apfelbaum et al., 1999; Jones et al., 1995). In one trial, reported only in abstract form, doses of 10 and 15 mg/day of sibutramine were compared with placebo (Jones et al., 1995). A total of 463 patients began the trial, and 259 completed it. Among those completing the trial, those in the placebo group lost 2.4 kg, compared with 6.2 kg, in those receiving 10 mg/day and 6.9 kg in the group receiving 15 mg/day (Jones et al., 1995). In the second study, patients who lost at least 6 kg during a 4-week period on a very-low-energy diet were randomly assigned to a double-blind controlled trial comparing placebo and 10 mg/day of sibutramine (Apfelbaum et al., 1999). Of the 78 patients in the placebo group, 48 completed 1 year of treatment and essentially maintained their weight loss, weighing 7.6 kg less than at baseline. In the group treated with sibutramine (10 mg/day), weight loss was further increased to 13.5 kg below baseline (Apfelbaum et al., 1999).

The Sibutramine Trial of Obesity Reduction Maintenance was a double-blind randomized comparison of sibutramine (10 mg/day) versus placebo following 6 months of weight loss induced by sibutramine. During the initial weight loss period, the diet assignment was based on estimates of resting energy expenditure, and was readjusted at the third month. At the end of 6 months, the body weight was reduced by nearly 15%. During the next 18 months of treatment in the randomized trial, the subjects in the sibutramine treatment group maintained most of their body weight loss, whereas the group assigned to placebo showed a steady regain in weight (James et al., 2000). Thus sibutramine appears to be useful for both weight loss and maintenance of weight loss, or secondary prevention.

An analysis of the effect of sibutramine on changes in lipids was done by combining data from 11 trials. There were significant dose-related reductions in triglycerides, total cholesterol, and low-density lipoprotein (LDL) cholesterol (Bray et al., 1999). Sibutramine raises blood pressure slightly (as discussed below).

Initial weight loss in patients treated with sibutramine predicts long-term response. Of those losing >2 kg in 4 weeks, only 20% of those on placebo versus 49% of those on sibutramine lost more than 10% of initial body weight in 12 months (Bray et al., 1996). Sibutramine is approved for weight loss and the maintenance of weight loss in the United States. It has not been associated with valvulopathy.

Safety of Noradrenergic/Sympathomimetic Drugs

The side effect profile for sympathomimetic drugs is similar. They mainly produce insomnia, dry mouth, asthenia, and constipation. The safety of older sympathomimetic appetite-suppressant drugs has been the subject of considerable controversy, because dextro-amphetamine is addictive (Bray & Greenway, 1999). The other sympathomimetic drugs—phentermine, diethylpropion, and mazindol—have very little abuse potential, as assessed by the low rate of reinforcement when the drugs are available intravenously to test animals. In this same paradigm, neither PPA nor fenfluramine showed any reinforcing effects, and no clinical data revealed any abuse potential for either of these drugs. Sibutramine likewise has no abuse potential in this paradigm, but it is nonetheless a Schedule IV drug (Heal et al., 1992).

Sympathomimetic drugs can affect blood pressure (Bray & Greenway, 1999). PPA is an α_1 agonist and, at doses of 75 mg or more, can increase blood pressure. Phenylpropanolamine has been associated with stroke and it should not be used above 75 mg/day. PPA has also been reported in association with cardiomyopathy.

In the placebo-controlled studies with sibutramine, systolic and diastolic blood pressure increased by 1–3 mm Hg, and pulse increased by approximately 4–5 beats per minute (Bray et al., 1999). Caution should be used in combining sibutramine with other drugs that may increase blood pressure. Sibutramine should not be used in patients with a history of coronary artery disease, congestive heart failure, cardiac arrhythmias, or stroke. There should be a 2-week interval between terminating monoamine oxidase inhibitors (MAOIs) and beginning sibutramine, and sibutramine should not be used with MAOIs or selective serotonin reuptake inhibitors. Because sibutramine is metabolized by the cytochrome P_{450} enzyme system (isozyme CYP3A4), it may interfere with metabolism of erythromycin and ketoconazole.

Peptides That Reduce Food Intake

Leptin

Leptin is a peptide produced primarily in adipose tissue (Mantazoros, 1999). Absence of leptin produces massive obesity in mice (*ob/ob*) and in humans (Montague et al., 1997). Treatment with the peptide decreases food intake in the *ob/ob* mouse and in leptin-deficient human beings. The diabetes mouse (*db/db*) and the fatty rat (*fa/fa*) that have genetic defects in the leptin receptor are also obese, but they do not respond to leptin. Humans with defects in the leptin receptor are also obese (Bray & Tartaglia, 2000). Leptin levels in the blood are highly correlated with body fat levels, yet obesity persists, suggesting that there may be "leptin resistance." An initial clinical trial with leptin showed that it reduced food intake in

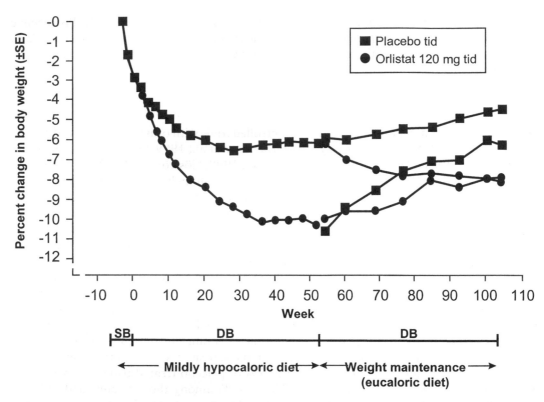

FIGURE 15.4. Orlistat and body weight. From Sjöström et al. (1998). Copyright 1998 by *The Lancet* Ltd. Adapted by permission.

weight-maintaining diet in an 8-week, double-blind, randomized trial. Total cholesterol and LDL cholesterol were reduced 4%–11% and 5%–10%, respectively, in the orlistat groups compared to the placebo group (Tonstad et al., 1994). This reduction in cholesterol is probably related to the solubility of cholesterol in the fat lost in the feces as a result of taking orlistat. This fecal loss may necessitate supplementation with fat-soluble vitamins during treatment, because they may also be lost. During the weight loss period, there was a decline in total cholesterol, LDL cholesterol, high-density lipoprotein (HDL) cholesterol, fasting glucose, and blood pressure. Reitsma and colleagues (1994) reported that postprandial lipemia was reduced. Orlistat appears to reduce cholesterol, but not glucose or blood pressure, by more than can be accounted for by the decrease in body weight.

Changes in Glycemic Control

In a 1-year trial in patients with diabetes (Hollander et al., 1998), the orlistat-treated patients lost 6.2% and the placebo-treated patients 4.3% of their initial weight. There was also a reduction in the need for hypoglycemic medication.

Side Effects

The side effects of orlistat are to be expected from its mechanism of action on pancreatic lipase (Canovatchel, 1997; Zhi, Melia, Eggers, Joly, & Patel, 1995). These include intestinal borborygmi, flatus, and abdominal cramps. The most troubling effects were fecal incontinence, oily spotting, and flatus with discharge. In a comparison of pooled data on 1,740 placebo-treated and 2,038 orlistat-treated patients, orlistat appeared to be well tolerated, with the principal complaints being gastrointestinal symptoms. Most were mild and occurred within the first few weeks (Canovatchel, 1997). More placebo-treated patients (35%) withdrew prematurely than orlistat-treated patients (29%). There was no evidence for gallstones, renal stones, or cardiovascular or central nervous system events. Orlistat has been approved worldwide for weight loss and the maintenance of weight loss.

Postabsorptive Drugs

Metformin

Metformin is a biguanide that is approved for the treatment of diabetes mellitus, a disease that is exacerbated by obesity and weight gain. Metformin has been associated with significant weight loss when compared to sulfonylureas or placebo (Bray & Greenway, 1999). Campbell, Menzies, Chalmers, McBain, and Brown (1994) compared metformin and glipizide in a randomized double-blind study of individuals with Type 2 diabetes who had not achieved control of their disease on diet. The 24 subjects on metformin lost weight and had better control of fasting glucose and glycohemoglobin than the glipizide group. The glipizide group gained weight, and the difference in weight between the two groups at the end of the study was highly significant. In a double-blind placebo-controlled trial in subjects with the insulin resistance syndrome, metformin also increased weight loss.

Fontbonne and colleagues (1996) reported the results from the BIGPRO study, a 1-year French multicenter study that compared metformin with placebo in 324 middle-aged subjects with upper-body obesity and the insulin resistance syndrome. The subjects on metformin lost significantly more weight (1–2 kg) than the placebo group, and the study concluded that metformin may have a role in the primary prevention of Type 2 diabetes. The package insert for metformin describes a 29-week double-blind study comparing glyburide (20 mg/day) with metformin (2.5 g/day) and their combination in 632 subjects with Type 2 diabetes who had inadequate glucose control. The metformin group lost 3.8 kg, compared to a loss of 0.3 kg in the glyburide group and a gain of 0.4 kg in the combined group. The package insert also described a double-blind controlled study in subjects with poorly controlled Type 2 diabetes, comparing metformin (2.5 g/day) to placebo. Weight loss in the placebo group was 1.1 kg, compared to 0.6 kg in the metformin group (Scheen, Letiexhe, & Lefebvre, 1995).

Lee and Morley (1998), however, compared 48 women with Type 2 diabetes in a double-blind controlled trial, randomly assigning subjects to metformin (i.e., 850 mg twice daily) or placebo. Subjects on metformin lost 8.8 kg over 24 weeks, compared to only 1.0 kg in the placebo group ($p < .001$). Although metformin may not produce enough weight loss to receive an indication from the U.S. Food and Drug Administration for treating obesity, it certainly deserves consideration in obese individuals with Type 2 diabetes who have not achieved control of their disease with diet and exercise treatment. This medication has been used in children (Lutjens & Smit, 1977).

Hydroxycitrate

The –(–)hydroxycitrate isomer is an inhibitor of ATP-citrate lyase, the rate-limiting enzyme in lipogenesis. In experimental animals, Sullivan, Trscari, Hamilton, and Miller (1974) showed that this drug reduced food intake and body weight. Clinical data have been disap-

stomach after 90 minutes was 70.3% ± 5.1% after placebo and 80.9% ± 3% in the ephedrine group ($p < .02$), which may represent a mechanism for decreased hunger.

In a 6-month trial, Astrup, Breum, Toubro, Hein, and Quaade (1992) compared placebo, caffeine (600 mg/day), ephedrine (60 mg/day), and the combination of caffeine with ephedrine in 180 obese subjects (Figure 15.5). Withdrawals were equal in all groups, and 141 subjects completed the trial. Weight loss was significantly greater in the group receiving both caffeine and ephedrine (16.6 ± 8.6 kg vs. 13.2 ± 6.6 kg; $p < .0015$). Weight loss in the caffeine-only group and the ephedrine-only group was not different from that in the placebo group. Side effects of tremor, insomnia, and dizziness were transient, and by 8 weeks were no different from those in the placebo group. Blood pressure fell equally in all four groups. After 6 months, the medication was stopped for 2 weeks to assess withdrawal symptoms. One hundred twenty-seven subjects then entered a 6-month open-label study of caffeine (600 mg/day) with ephedrine (60 mg/day) (Toubro, Astrup, Breum, & Quaade, 1993). The 99 subjects who completed the study lost an additional 1.1 kg ($p < .02$), and no clinically significant withdrawal symptoms were observed (Figure 15.5).

Caffeine and ephedrine, in the one other long-term controlled trial that combined two medications for weight loss (Weintraub, 1992), gave 16% loss of initial body weight over 6 months, which was maintained for the remainder of the year of treatment.

β₃-Adrenergic Receptor Agonists

The sympathetic nervous system has a tonic role in maintaining energy expenditure and blood pressure. Blockade of the thermogenic part of this system will reduce the thermic response to a meal. NE, the neurotransmitter of the sympathetic nervous system, may also decrease food intake by acting on β_2- or β_3-adrenergic receptors. Several synthetic β_3 agonists

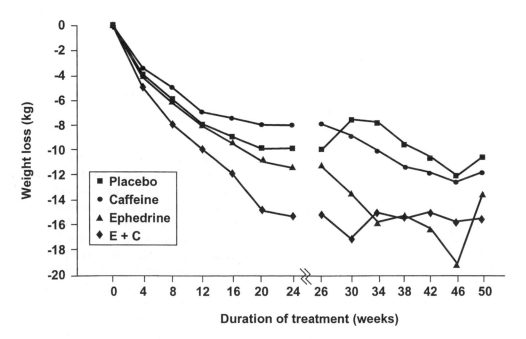

FIGURE 15.5. Effect of ephedrine and caffeine on weight loss and weight maintenance for 1 year. From Astrup et al. (1992) and Toubro et al. (1993). Copyright 1992 and 1993 by Nature Publishing Group. Adapted by permission.

have been developed against the animal β_3 receptor, but the clinical responses have been disappointing (Arch & Wilson, 1996; Bray & Greenway, 1999; Connacher, Bennett, & Jung, 1992). After cloning of the human β_3 receptor, several new compounds are being synthesized. Results of clinical trials are awaited.

PATIENT SELECTION FOR DRUG TREATMENT

The BMI can serve as a guide to the risk–benefit evaluation of an overweight patient (Bray, 1998b). Those patients who have a BMI above 30 kg/m^2 are potential candidates for drug therapy. The presence of comorbidities such as dyslipidemia, hypertension, diabetes or impaired glucose tolerance, symptomatic osteoarthritis, or sleep apnea increases the rationale for treatment by shifting the BMI to 27–30 kg/m^2 from a risk-adjusted BMI above 30 kg/m^2.

The currently available noradrenergic sympathomimetic drugs can reduce body weight, but only sibutramine is approved for long-term use. However, this drug should not be used in patients with stroke, congestive failure, or myocardial infarction. Orlistat is also approved for long-term use and for weight maintenance.

Weight loss of 10%–15% can improve health risks. However, failure to lose weight or failure to improve comorbid conditions during treatment with a drug indicates either noncompliance with the drug or lack of response to the drug. Either situation requires reevaluation of therapy and addition of other medications or other modalities of treatment. As a guideline, patients being treated with drugs should lose more than 2 kg (4 pounds) in the first month, and should achieve and maintain more than a 5% weight loss by 6 months. As long as weight loss is more than 5% and/or the patient's comorbidities have improved, the drug may be continued. The data with phentermine (Figure 15.2) suggests that intermittent use may be beneficial.

At least two groups of patients merit long-term drug therapy. The first group consists of patients who are considered for surgical treatment of their obesity. Individuals with a BMI above 35 kg/m^2 should first be treated with antiobesity drugs. If they respond with more than a 15% weight loss, drugs should be continued as long as they respond and their comorbidities improve. The second group of patients who deserve vigorous treatment consists of individuals with sleep apnea. A modest weight loss is often sufficient to alleviate their problem.

REFERENCES

Apfelbaum, M., Vague, P., Ziegler, O., Hanotin, C., Thomas, F., & Leutenegger, E. (1999). Long-term maintenance of weight loss after a VLCD: Sibutramine vs. placebo. *American Journal of Medicine, 106,* 179–194.

Arch, J. R., & Wilson, S. (1996). Prospects for beta 3-adrenoceptor agonists in the treatment of obesity and diabetes [Review]. *International Journal of Obesity, 20,* 191–199.

Astrup, A., Breum, L., Toubro, S., Hein, P., & Quaade, F. (1992). The effect and satiety of an ephedrine/caffeine compound compared to ephedrine, caffeine and placebo in obese subjects on an energy restricted diet: A double blind trial. *International Journal of Obesity, 16,* 269–277.

Astrup, A., Lundsgaard, C., Madsen, J., & Christensen, N. J. (1985). Enhanced thermogenic responsiveness during chronic ephedrine treatment in man. *American Journal of Clinical Nutrition, 42,* 83–94.

Baez, M., Kursar, J. D., Helton, L. A., Wainscott, D. B., & Nelson, D. L. (1995). Molecular biology of serotonin receptors [Review]. *Obesity Research, 3*(Suppl. 4), 441–447.

Lardy, H. E., Kneer, N., Wei, Y., Partridge, B., & Marwah, P. (1998). Ergosteroids: II. Biologically-active metabolites and synthetic derivatives of dehydroepiandrosterone. *Steroids, 63,* 158–165.

Lean, M. E. J. (1997). Sibutramine: A review of clinical efficacy. *International Journal of Obesity, 21,* S30–S36.

Lee, A., & Morley, J. E. (1998). Metformin decreases food-consumption and induces weight-loss in subjects with obesity with Type-II non-insulin-dependent diabetes. *Obesity Research, 6,* 47–53.

Lockene, A., Skottova, N., & Olivecrona, G. (1994). Interactions of lipoprotein lipase with the active-site inhibitor tetrahydrolipstatin (orlistat). *European Journal of Biochemistry, 222,* 395–403.

Lovejoy, J. C., Bray, G. A., Bourgeois, M. O., Macchiavelli, R., Rood, J. C., Greeson, C., & Partington, C. (1996). Exogenous androgens influence body composition and regional body fat distribution in obese postmenopausal women: A clinical research center study. *Journal of Clinical Endocrinology and Metabolism, 81,* 2198–2203.

Lovejoy, J. C., Bray, G. A., Greeson, C. S., Klemperer, M., Morris, J., Partington, C., & Tulley, R. (1995). Oral anabolic steroid treatment, but not parenteral androgen treatment, decreases abdominal fat in obese, older men. *International Journal of Obesity, 19,* 614–624.

Lovejoy, J. C., Smith, S. R., Bray, G. A., DeLany, J. P., Rood, J. C., Gouvier, D., Windhauser, M., Ryan, D. H., Macchiavelli, R., & Tulley, R. A. (1997). Paradigm of experimentally induced mild hyperthyroidism: Effects on nitrogen balance, body composition, and energy expenditure in healthy young men. *Journal of Clinical Endocrinology and Metabolism, 82,* 765–770.

Lustig, R. H., Rose, S. R., Burghen, G. A., Velasquez-Mieyer, P., Broome, D. C., Smith, K., Li, H., Hudson, M. M., Heideman, R. L., & Kun, L. E. (1999). Hypothalamic obesity caused by cranial insult in children: Altered glucose and insulin dynamics and reversal by a somatostatin agonist. *Journal of Pediatrics, 135,* 162–168.

Lutjens, A., & Smit, J. L. (1977). Effect of biguanide treatment in obese children. *Helvetica Paediatrica Acta, 31,* 473–480.

Mantazoros, C. S. (1999). The role of leptin in human obesity and disease: A review of current evidence. *Annals of Internal Medicine, 130,* 671–680.

Marin, P., Holmang, S., Gustafsson, C., Jonsson, L., Kvist, H., Elander, A., Eldh, J., Sjöström, L., Holm, G., & Bjorntorp, P. (1993). Androgen treatment of abdominally obese men. *Obesity Research, 1,* 245–251.

Marin, P., Holmang, S., Jonsson, L., Sjöström, L., Kvist, H., Holm, G., Lindstedt, G., & Bjorntorp, P. (1992). The effects of testosterone treatment on body composition and metabolism in middle-aged obese men. *International Journal of Obesity, 16,* 991–997.

Melia, A. T., Zhi, J., Koss-Twardy, S. G., Min, B. H., Smith, B. L., Freundlich, N. L., Arora, S., & Passe, S. M. (1995). The influence of reduced dietary fat absorption induced by orlistat on the pharmacokinetics of digoxin in healthy volunteers. *Journal of Clinical Pharmacology, 35,* 840–843.

Montague, C. T., Farooqi, S., Whitehead, J. P., Soos, M. A., Rau, H., Wareham, N. J., Sewter, C. P., Digby, J. E., Mohammed, S. N., Hurst, J. A., Cheetham, C. H., Earley, A. R., Barnett, A. H., Prins, J. B., & O'Rahilly, S. (1997). Congenital leptin deficiency is associated with severe early-onset obesity in humans. *Nature, 387,* 903–908.

Mortola, J. F., & Yen, S. S. C. (1990). The effects of oral dehydroepiandrosterone on endocrine–metabolic parameters in postmenopausal women. *Journal of Clinical Endocrinology and Metabolism, 71,* 696–704.

Munro, J. F., MacCuish, A. C., Wilson, E. M., & Duncan, L. J. P. (1968). Comparison of continuous and intermittent anorectic therapy in obesity. *British Medical Journal, i,* 352–356.

Nestler, J. E., Barlascini, C. O., Clore, J. N., & Blackard, W. G. (1988). Dehydroepiandrosterone reduces serum low density lipoprotein levels and body fat but does not alter insulin sensitivity in normal men. *Journal of Clinical Endocrinology and Metabolism, 66,* 57–61.

Nielsen, B., Astrup, A., Samuelsen, P., Wengholt, H., & Christensen, N. J. (1993). Effect of physical training on thermogenic responses to cold and ephedrine in obesity. *International Journal of Obesity, 17,* 383–390.

Reitsma, J. B., Castro Cabezas, M., de Bruin, T. W., & Erkelens, D. W. (1994). Relationship between improved postprandial lipemia and low-density lipoprotein metabolism during treatment with tetrahydrolipstatin, a pancreatic lipase inhibitor. *Metabolism, 43,* 293–298.

Rolls, B. J., Shide, D. J., Thorwart, M. L., & Ulbrecht, J. S. (1998). Sibutramine reduces food intake in non-dieting women with obesity. *Obesity Research, 6,* 1–11.

Ryan, D. H., Bray, G. A., Helmcke, F., Sander, G., Volaufova, J., Greenway, F., Subramaniam, P., & Glancy, D. L. (1999). Serial echocardiographic and clinical evaluation of valvular regurgitation before, during, and after treatment with fenfluramine or dexfenfluramine and mazindol or phentermine. *Obesity Research, 7,* 313–322.

Ryan, D. H., Kaiser, P., & Bray, G. A. (1995). Sibutramine: A novel new agent for obesity treatment. *Obesity Research, 3*(Suppl. 4), 553–559.

Scheen, A. J., Letiexhe, M. R., & Lefebvre, P. J. (1995). Short administration of metformin improves insulin sensitivity in android obese subjects with impaired glucose tolerance. *Diabetic Medicine, 12,* 985–989.

Schteingart, D. E. (1992). Effectiveness of phenylpropanolamine in the management of moderate obesity. *International Journal of Obesity, 16,* 487–493.

Seagle, H. M., Bessesen, D. H., & Hill, J. O. (1998). Effects of sibutramine on resting metabolic rate and weight loss in overweight women. *Obesity Research, 6,* 115–121.

Sjöström, L., Rissanen, A., Andersen, T., Boldrin, M., Golay, A., Koppeschaar, H. P., & Krempf, M. (1998). Randomized placebo-controlled trial of orlistat for weight loss and prevention of weight regain in obese patients: European Multicentre Orlistat Study Group. *Lancet, 352,* 167–172.

Smith, G. P. (Ed.). (1998). *Satiation: From gut to brain.* New York: Oxford University Press.

Stock, M. J. (1997). Sibutramine: A review of the pharmacology of a novel anti-obesity agent. *International Journal of Obesity, 21,* S25–S29.

Sullivan, A. C., Triscari, J., Hamilton, J. G., & Miller, O. N. (1974). Effect of (–)-hydroxycitrate upon the accumulation of lipid in the rat: II. Appetite. *Lipids, 9,* 129–134.

Svec, F., & Porter, J. R. (1998). The actions of exogenous dehydroepiandrosterone in experimental animals and humans. *Proceedings of the Society of Experimental Biology and Medicine, 218,* 174–191.

Tonstad, S., Pometta, D., Erkelens, D. W., Ose, L., Moccetti, T., Schouten, J. A., Golay, A., Reitsma, J., Del Bufalo, A., & Pasotti E. (1994). The effects of gastrointestinal lipase inhibitor, orlistat, on serum lipids and lipoproteins in patients with primary hyperlipidaemia. *European Journal of Clinical Pharmacology, 46,* 405–410.

Toubro, S., Astrup, A., Breum, L., & Quaade, F. (1993). The acute and chronic effects of ephedrine/caffeine mixtures on energy expenditure and glucose metabolism in humans. *International Journal of Obesity, 17*(Suppl. 3), 73–77.

U.K. Prospective Diabetes Study Group. (1998). Intensive blood-glucose control with sulphonylureas or insulin compared with conventional treatment and risk of complications in patients with Type 2 diabetes (UKPDS 33). *Lancet, 352,* 837–853.

Usiskin, K. S., Butterworth, S., Clore, J. N., Arad, Y., Ginsberg, H. N., Blackard, W. G., & Nestler, J. E. (1990). Lack of effect of dehydroepiandrosterone in obese men. *International Journal of Obesity, 14,* 457–463.

Weber, C., Tam, Y. K., Schmidtke-Schrezenmeier, G., Jonkmann, J. H., & van Brummelen, P. (1996). Effect of the lipase inhibitor orlistat on the pharmacokinetics of four different antihypertensive drugs in the healthy volunteers. *European Journal of Clinical Pharmacology, 51,* 87–90.

Weintraub, M. (1985). Phenylpropanolamine as an anorexiant agent in weight control: A review of published and unpublished studies. In J. P. Morgan, D. V. Kagan, & J. S. Brody (Eds.), *Clinical pharmacology and therapeutics series: Vol. 5. Phenylpropanolamine: Risks, benefits and controversies* (pp. 53–79). New York: Praeger.

Weintraub, M. (1992). Long-term weight control: The National Heart, Lung, and Blood Institute funded multimodal intervention study. *Clinical Pharmacology and Therapeutics, 51,* 581–585.

Weintraub, M., Rubio, A., Golik, A., Byrne, L., & Scheinbaum, M. L. (1991). Sibutramine in weight control: A dose-ranging, efficacy study. *Clinical Pharmacology and Therapeutics, 50,* 330–337.

Welle, S., Jozefowicz, R., & Statt, M. (1990). Failure of dehydroepiandrosterone to influence energy and protein metabolism in humans. *Journal of Clinical Endocrinology and Metabolism, 71,* 1259–1264.

Zhi, J., Melia, A. T., Eggers, H., Joly, R., & Patel, I. H. (1995). Review of limited systemic absorption of orlistat, a lipase inhibitor, in healthy human volunteers. *Journal of Clinical Pharmacology, 35,* 1103–1108.

Zhi, J., Melia, A. T., Funk, C., Viger-Chougnet, A., Hopfgartner, G., Lausecker, B., Wang, K., Fulton, J. S., Gabriel, L., & Mulligan, T. E. (1996). Metabolic profiles of minimally absorbed orlistat in obese/overweight volunteers. *Journal of Clinical Pharmacology, 36,* 1006–1011.

Zhi, J., Melia, A. T., Guerciolini, R., Chung, J., Kinberg, J., Hauptman, J. B., & Patel, I. H. (1994). Retrospective population-based analysis of the dose–response (fecal fat excretion) relationship of orlistat in normal and obese volunteers. *Clinical Pharmacology and Therapeutics, 56,* 82–85.

Zhi, J., Melia, A. T., Koss-Twardy, S. G., Min, B., Guerciolini, R., Freundlich, N. L., Milla, G., & Patel, I. H. (1995). The influence of orlistat on the pharmacokinetics and pharmacodynamics of glyburide in healthy volunteers. *Journal of Clinical Pharmacology, 35,* 521–525.

Zumoff, B., Strain, G. W., Heymsfield, S. B., & Lichtman, S. (1994). A randomized double-blind crossover study of the antiobesity effects of etiocholanedione. *Obesity Research, 2,* 13–18.

16

Surgical Treatment of Obesity

RIFAT LATIFI
JOHN M. KELLUM
ERIC J. DE MARIA
HARVEY J. SUGERMAN

An estimated 97 million adults in the United States are overweight or obese. Thirty-two percent of the population is overweight, defined as having a body mass index (BMI) of 25–29.9 kg/m², while 22.5% are obese, with a BMI ≥ 30 kg/m² (National Heart, Lung, and Blood Institute [NHLBI], 1998). "Extreme obesity" is classified as a BMI ≥ 40 kg/m² and is associated with an extremely high risk of disease, especially cardiovascular disease (NHLBI, 1998). As the BMI increases, so does the mortality rate from all causes, which is 100% or more above that of persons who have a BMI of 20–25 kg/m² (National Institutes of Health [NIH], 1992).

Extreme obesity (previously referred to as "morbid obesity") is associated with several predictable significant clinical syndromes: (1) cardiovascular-related problems, such as coronary artery disease, heart failure, and increased complications following coronary artery bypass; (2) respiratory insufficiency due to obesity hypoventilation syndrome and obstructive sleep apnea syndrome (multiple nocturnal awakenings, loud snoring, falling asleep while driving, and daytime somnolence); (3) metabolic complications, such as diabetes mellitus, hypertension, elevated triglycerides, cholesterol, and gallstones; (4) increased intra-abdominal pressure, which is manifested as stress overflow urinary incontinence, gastroesophageal reflux, nephrotic syndrome, hernias, venous stasis, pre-eclampsia, or nephrotic syndrome; (5) hypercoagulapathy; (6) increased intracranial pressure, leading to pseudotumor cerebri; (7) sexual hormone dysfunction, such as amenorrhea, hypermenorrhea, and Stein–Leventhal syndrome; (8) increased incidence of breast, uterine, colon, prostate, and other cancers; and (9) debilitating joint disease (NHLBI, 1998; NIH, 1992). Furthermore, there are significant difficulties in diagnosing obese patients with such surgical conditions as peritonitis, necrotizing panniculitis, necrotizing fasciitis, diverticulitis, necrotizing pancreatitis, and other intra-abdominal infections. In addition, psychosocial impairment and work-related difficulties are integral parts of the pathology of extreme obesity (Wadden, Sarwer, Arnold, Gruen, & O'Neil, 2000).

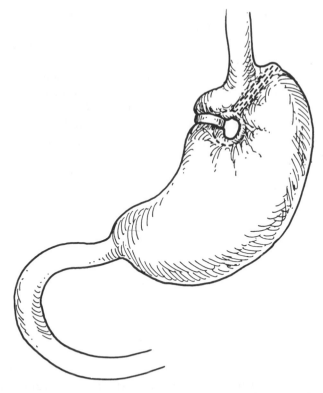

FIGURE 16.1. Vertical banded gastroplasty. From Sugerman, Starkey, & Birkenhauer (1987). Copyright 1987 by Lippincott Williams & Wilkins. Reprinted by permission.

CURRENT BARIATRIC OPERATIONS

Over the last decade, the safety and effectiveness of many surgical weight loss procedures have evolved. Currently, most bariatric surgical centers in North America and Europe perform VBG, adjusted gastric banding, or RYGBP.

Gastroplasty

In gastroplasty, the upper stomach is stapled near the gastroesophageal junction; this creates a small upper gastric pouch, which communicates with the rest of the stomach and gastrointestinal (GI) tract through a small outlet. The concept and the technique of gastroplasty were originally suggested as a safer and relatively easier method for restricting food intake. Gastroplasties are performed with either horizontal or vertical placement of the staples. Horizontal gastroplasty, which usually requires ligation and division of the short gastric vessels between the stomach and spleen, carries the risk of devascularization of the gastric pouch or splenic injury. Moreover, it has been associated with very high failure rates (42%–70%).

VBG, on the other hand, is a procedure in which a stapled opening is made in the stomach with an end-to-end anastomosing (EEA) stapling device 5 cm from the cardioesophageal junction (see Figure 16.1). The pouch is constructed with a 90-mm stapling device made between this opening and the angle of His, and a 1.5-cm × 5-cm strip of polypropylene mesh is wrapped around the stoma on the lesser curvature and sutured to itself but not to the stomach. VBG can be associated with severe gastroesophageal reflux. VBG is more effective than horizontal gastroplasty, but significantly less effective then RYGBP, as demonstrated in randomized prospective trials in which several centers have reported inferior weight reduction with this operation as compared with standard RYGBP (Bø & Modalsi, 1983; Hall et al., 1990; MacLean, Rhode, Sampalis, & Forse, 1993; Sugerman, Starkey, & Birkenhauer, 1987).

Gastric Banding

Bø and Modalsli (1983) introduced gastric banding as a treatment for morbid obesity. In this technique, a Dacron tube or silicone band is used to compartmentalize the stomach into small proximal and large distal segments. This approach has the advantage of producing a pure restrictive operation using a very simple, reversible technique, in which stapling, with its inherent risk of staple line disruption, is avoided. More recent developments include the introduction of an adjustable silicone gastric banding device, originally described by Kuzmak (1992), which can be placed laparoscopically (see Figure 16.2). This band has a subcutaneous or subfascial reservoir. If weight loss is meager, or if vomiting is excessive, the outlet diameter of the upper gastric segment can be adjusted.

Gastric Bypass

In recent years RYGBP has become favored by most American bariatric surgeons as the procedure of choice in extremely obese patients, mainly because of superior long-term weight loss effects when compared with VBG (see Figure 16.3). In randomized prospective trials, as well as retrospective studies, RYGBP has been found to induce significantly greater weight loss than VBG. This is particularly true for patients who overconsume sweets. Such

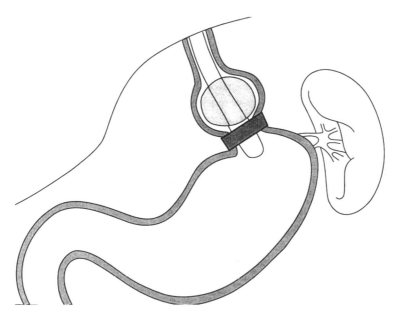

FIGURE 16.2. Illustration of adjustable gastric banding.

scopically; however, these operations are technically challenging due to adhesions from the previous operation.

Gastric Bypass

The initial experience with 75 patients who underwent laparoscopic RYGBP (LRYGBP), using a 21-mm EEA, was reported to be comparable to that with open RYGBP. Furthermore, follow-up from 3 to 60 months on 500 patients who underwent LRYGBP has been reported, with major complications in 11% of patients, anastomotic leak in 5%, and no mortality (Witgrove & Clark, 1999).

As experience is gained with LRYGBP, complications related to the complex technical nature of the procedure will probably decrease. As of this writing, most surgeons perform LRYGBP in patients with BMI < 50 kg/m², although a few groups have reported successful LRYGBP in patients with a BMI up to 70 kg/m². For the most part, the results are comparable to the open technique. However, the laparoscopic operation still takes significantly longer then the open technique, and mastering this procedure is difficult and the learning curve very steep.

PARTIAL BILIOPANCREATIC DIVERSION AND DUODENAL SWITCH OPERATIONS

The partial biliopancreatic diversion has been developed as both a gastric-restrictive and a malabsorptive procedure that does not have a "blind" intestinal limb where bacterial overgrowth can occur. This operation involves a subtotal gastrectomy, leaving a 400-cc gastric pouch for the average obese patient and a 200-cc gastric pouch for the superobese patient. The distal small bowel is transected 250 cm proximal to the ileocecal valve, and the proximal, bypassed bowel is anastomosed to the ileum 50 cm proximal to the ileocecal valve. This leaves a 200-cm "alimentary tract"; a 300- to 400-cm "biliary tract" of bypassed intestine; and a 50-cm "common absorptive alimentary tract," where the ingested food mixes with bile and pancreatic juices for digestion and absorption (see Figure 16.4). This operation has demonstrated excellent weight loss and does not appear to be associated with the high incidence of bacterial overgrowth and bacterial translocation problems of JIB, because bile and pancreatic juices wash out the bypassed small intestine. However, the biliopancreatic diversion may be associated with severe protein calorie malnutrition, necessitating hospitalization and total parenteral nutrition. It may also be associated with frequent, foul-smelling steatorrheic stools that float, leading to fat-soluble vitamin deficiencies and calcium loss secondary to chelation with fat, producing severe osteoporosis.

Our group at the Medical College of Virginia (Liska, Sugerman, & Kellum, 1988) has described a modification of biliopancreatic diversion in which the stomach is merely stapled, as in gastric bypass, and the enteroenterostomy is placed 50-150 cm proximal to the ileocecal valve. This modification, which has been termed "distal gastric bypass," has been associated with better weight loss in superobese patients than standard gastric bypass has been. In a randomized prospective trial using a much smaller proximal stomach pouch (50 cc), without gastric resection and a longer common absorptive intestinal tract (150 cm), distal gastric bypass was associated with a much greater weight loss than standard gastric bypass, but had a 25% incidence of severe malnutrition (Liska et al., 1988). Four of 14 patients required conversion to a standard GBP due to protein calorie malnutrition. We currently reserve distal gastric bypass for superobese patients who have had unsuccessful standard gastric bypass and have persistent obesity-related comorbidities (e.g., diabetes,

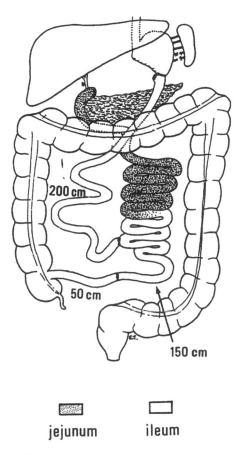

jejunum   **ileum**

FIGURE 16.4. Biliopancreatic diversion. From Scopinaro, Gianetti, Adami, et al. (1996). Copyright 1996 by Mosby. Reprinted by permission.

pickwickian syndrome, etc.). These patients require fat-soluble vitamin supplementation and may develop severe malnutrition.

A modified surgical procedure combining restriction and malabsorption, known as the "biliopancreatic diversion with a duodenal switch" operation, has been developed with the hope that there will be less protein and fat-soluble vitamin malabsorption (Lagace et al., 1995). In an effort to avoid bypass of the pylorus, Hess and Hess (1998) introduced the concept of wedge resection of the greater curvature of the stomach, combined with a "duodenal switch." This operation divides the duodenum in the distal bulb and the ileum 250 cm proximal to the ileocecal valve, with anastomosis of the proximal duodenal segment to the distal ileal segment. The distal end of the transected duodenum is oversewn as a duodenal stump. The proximal ileal segment, which carries the biliary and pancreatic secretions, is anastomosed from end to side for an enteroenterostomy 50–100 cm proximal to the ileocecal valve. The segment that carries the biliary and pancreatic secretions is anastomosed to the ileum 100 cm proximal to the ileocecal valve (see Figure 16.5). It is not yet clear whether this operation will prevent the protein malnutrition, calcium deficiency, and fat-soluble vitamin deficiencies associated with the partial biliopancreatic bypass procedure.

This operation was performed in 440 patients as the initial bariatric procedure, and it was associated with weight loss of 70% of excess weight 8 years after surgery (Hess & Hess, 1998). Seventeen of these patients underwent reoperations for excessive weight loss to

the retrocolic Roux-en-Y limb is brought; and third, through the mesenteric defect located under the Roux-en-Y limb before it passes through the mesocolon, known as a Petersen hernia. These hernias may manifest principally with periumbilical abdominal pain, and their diagnosis may be difficult. A computed tomography scan of the abdomen may be more helpful than upper-GI contrast studies in establishing the diagnosis. When the diagnosis is uncertain and the radiological studies are not helpful, the safest course of action is to reoperate in a patient with recurrent pain attacks, since massive intestinal infarction has been seen with these internal hernias.

Another significant complication of bariatric surgery is incisional hernia, which in open surgery has an incidence of about 20%. Furthermore, many superobese patients require abdominoplasty following weight loss. Although abdominoplasty may be followed with complications in as many as 55% of patients (Vastine et al., 1999), previous bariatric surgery does not influence the rate of complications following this operation, and these patients should be offered body-contouring surgery when indicated. The most important factor that will influence the complications following abdominoplasty is the degree of obesity at the time of the surgery, which has profound influence on wound complications.

Nutritional Complications

Following any gastric surgery for extreme obesity, significant nutritional complications such as protein calorie malnutrition may develop. Specifically, a very rare syndrome of polyneuropathy has been reported after these operations. This usually occurs in association with intractable vomiting and severe protein calorie malnutrition with subsequent acute thiamin deficiency. The risk of vitamin B_{12} deficiency mandates long-term follow-up with annual measurement of the vitamin B_{12} level. B_{12} deficiency is probably due to decreased acid digestion of vitamin B_{12} from food, with subsequent failure of coupling to intrinsic factor. Postoperatively patients should need to take 500 μg of oral vitamin B_{12} daily or 1 mg of vitamin B_{12} intramuscularly per month.

Iron deficiency anemia most commonly occurs in menstruating women following gastric bypass. This can be refractory to supplemental ferrous sulfate because iron absorption takes place primarily in the duodenum and upper jejunum. Occasionally, iron dextran injections may be necessary. All menstruating women should take two iron sulfate tablets (325 mg/day) by mouth after gastric bypass as long as they continue to menstruate. Magnesium deficiency may also occur and require supplementation. Calcium supplementation is often necessary after any gastric bypass procedure. Patients with either a long-limb gastric or partial biliopancreatic bypass can develop calcium and fat-soluble vitamin deficiencies that need to be monitored and treated.

OUTCOMES OF OBESITY SURGERY

Positive Outcomes

Gastric procedures for extreme obesity can yield dramatic and long-term weight reduction, with an average loss of two-thirds of excess weight within 1–2 years. Weight becomes stable at this level and is well maintained at long-term follow-up. The patients must be followed carefully to ensure adequate protein, vitamin, and other micronutrient levels.

Weight loss corrects non-insulin-dependent diabetes mellitus in almost all cases. No other therapy has produced more durable and complete control of Type 2 diabetes (Pories et al., 1995). Hypertension is cured in two-thirds to three-fourths of patients, as well as the headaches that are associated with cerebrospinal fluid pressure elevation in almost all patients with pseudotumor cerebri (Kellum et al., 1998; Sugerman et al., 1999). The obstructive sleep apnea syndrome, which poses the greatest immediate risk to life of any extreme obesity complications, resolves with weight loss. The hypoventilation and hypercarbia seen in the obesity hypoventilation syndrome return toward normal with weight loss (Sugerman, Baron, Fairman, Evans, & Vetrovec, 1988). Elevated pulmonary artery and pulmonary capillary wedge pressures also improve significantly following weight loss, with correction of abnormal arterial blood gases (Sugerman et al., 1988). Postsurgery weight loss is associated with significant improvement of left ventricular ejection fraction, and to some extent with improvements in cardiac chamber size and ventricular wall thickness (Alpert, Terry, & Kelly, 1985). Improvement in the lipid profile of extemely obese patients has been documented (Brolin al., 1990). A decrease in levels of cytokines following gastric surgery for obesity has also been reported (Kyzer, Binyamini, Chaimoff, & Fishman, 1999).

In addition, the loss of weight usually corrects female sexual hormone abnormalities; permits healing of chronic venous stasis ulcers associated with venous insufficiency; prevents reflux esophagitis; relieves stress overflow urinary incontinence; and improves low back pain, as well as joint-related pain. Furthermore, weight loss may permit successful total artificial joint replacement. Finally, patients' self-image and quality of life often improve dramatically following weight loss with bariatric surgery. The Swedish Obese Subjects study has documented significant decreases in depression and anxiety, as well as improvement in patients' social functioning (Sjöström, Lissner, & Sjöström, 1997). As would be expected after weight loss, the Swedish patients reported far greater comfort in shopping for clothes, swimming in public, and even eating at restaurants.

Failed Gastric Surgery and Reoperation

We believe that a patient's inability to lose at least 40% of excess weight should be considered a failure of obesity surgery. About 10%–15% of patients regain lost weight or fail to achieve an acceptable weight loss. Although some patients can overcome a gastric bypass and regain weight by expanding either the stoma or pouch, this finding is not common. The cause for this failure appears to be excessive, constant nibbling on foods with a high caloric density and/or failure to maintain regular exercise.

Reoperation for failed gastric surgery for morbid obesity can be extremely challenging and can herald significantly higher risk for morbidity and possible mortality. Attempts to revise a failed gastroplasty are often unsuccessful because of recurrence of stomal dilatation and problems with gastric emptying. Reoperation in these patients is extremely difficult because of extensive adhesions to the liver and spleen. Results appear to be significantly better when these patients are converted to RYGBP. Because of the technical difficulties, these patients must understand that the risks of serious complications are far higher after a secondary than after a primary gastric bypass procedure. It is probably inappropriate and dangerous to convert a failed gastric bypass to VBG. Furthermore, revision of a dilated gastrojejunal stoma has not been effective (Schwartz, Strodel, Simpson, & Griffen, 1988). In most cases, a failed gastric bypass is a consequence of excessive fat ingestion. If a patient has significant obesity comorbidity that has failed to resolve or has returned with weight regain, conversion to a malabsorptive distal gastric bypass (modified partial biliopancreatic diversion) can be performed. This, however, can be associated with protein calorie malnutrition, steatorrhea, fat-soluble vitamin deficiencies, and osteoporosis.

Sugerman, H. J., Brewer, W. H., Shiffman, M. L., Brolin, R. E., Fobi, M. A., Linner, J. H., MacDonald, K. G., MacGregor, A. M., Martin, L. F., & Oram-Smith, J. C. (1995b). Prophylactic ursodeoxycholic acid prevents gallstone formation following gastric bypass induced rapid weight loss: A multicenter, placebo-controlled randomized, double-blind, prospective trial of prophylactic ursodiol for prevention of gallstone formation following gastric-bypass induced rapid weight loss. *American Journal of Surgery, 169,* 91–97.

Sugerman, H. J., Felton, W. L., III, Sismasis, A., Kullum, J. M., De Maria, E. J., & Sugerman, E. L. (1999). Gastric surgery for pseudotumor cerebri associated with severe obesity. *Annals of Surgery, 229,* 634–642.

Sugerman, H. J., Starkey, J. V., & Birkenhauer, R. A. (1987). A randomized prospective trial of gastric bypass versus vertical banded gastroplasty for morbid obesity and their effects on sweets versus non-sweet eaters. *Annals of Surgery, 205,* 613–624.

Toppino, M., Morino, M., Bonnet, G., Nigra, I., & Siliquini, R. (1999). Laparoscopic surgery for morbid obesity: Preliminary results from SICE Registry (Italian Society of Endoscopic and Minimally Invasive Surgery). *Obesity and Surgery, 9,* 62–65.

Vastine, V. L., Morgan, R. F., Williams, G. S., Gampper, T. J., Drake, D. B., Knox, L. K., & Lin, K. Y. (1999). Wound complications of abdominoplasty in obese patients. *Annals of Plastic Surgery, 42,* 34–39.

Wadden. T. A., Sarwer, D. B., Arnold, M. E., Gruen, D., & O'Neil, P. M. (2000). Psychosocial status of severely obese patients before and after bariatric surgery. *Problems in General Surgery, 17,* 13–22.

Wisser, M., Bouter, M., McQuillan, G. M., Wener, M. H., & Harris, T. B. (1999). Elevated C-reactive protein levels in overweight and obese adults. *Journal of the American Medical Association, 282,* 2131–2135.

Witgrove, A. C., & Clark, G. W. (1999). Laparoscopic gastric bypass: A five-year prospective study of 500 followed from 3 to 60 months. *Obesity and Surgery, 9,* 124.

APPENDIX 16.1. OPERATIVE TECHNIQUE OF OPEN GASTRIC BYPASS

The abdomen is entered through a midline incision carried superiorly alongside the xiphoid process and inferiorly to the umbilicus, or inferior enough to obtain adequate access (Sugerman, 1997). Upon entering the peritoneal cavity, the surgeon performs a complete exploration to exclude unanticipated pathology before the gastric bypass is begun. If gallstones, sludge, or polyps are present on palpation or found on intraoperative ultrasound, then cholecystectomy is performed (Sugerman et al., 1995a). The distal esophagus is mobilized and encircled with a soft rubber drain. The gastrohepatic omentum is entered overlying the caudate lobe. An aberrant left hepatic artery may be present and should be avoided (see Figure 16.6). The phrenoesophageal ligament overlying the anterior and lateral distal esophagus is sharply incised. This will facilitate blunt mobilization of the distal esophagus. Laterally, the dissection must be at the level of the esophagus. Low lateral dissection may lead to injury of the short gastric vessels or spleen, or to creation of a large proximal pouch. An opening is made in the mesentery alongside the stomach between the first and a second branch of the left gastric artery, large enough to admit a right-angled clamp.

Following blunt dissection of the avascular space on the posterior stomach wall, between the opening in the gastrohepatic omentum and the lateral angle of His, a rubber tube is placed that will serve as a guide for introduction of the stapling device (see Figure 16.6). Before staplers are applied, all intraluminal tubes (the nasogastric tube, the esophageal stethoscope) must be removed by the anesthesiologist. The ligament of Treitz is identified; 45 cm distally, the jejunum is divided with a GIA stapling device, and the Roux-en-Y limb is created. A side-to-side jejunojejunostomy is created at 45 cm for standard bypass or at 150 cm for superobese patients. With blunt dissection, an opening is created in the transverse colon mesentery, and the Roux-en-Y limb is brought through to the proximal stomach without tension. At this point a 55-mm or 90-mm stapling device is placed across the stomach, using the rubber tube as a guide. Once the surgeon is assured that the staple line is across the stomach, and that the stomach is not folded on itself, the stomach is stapled three times with superimposed staple applications.

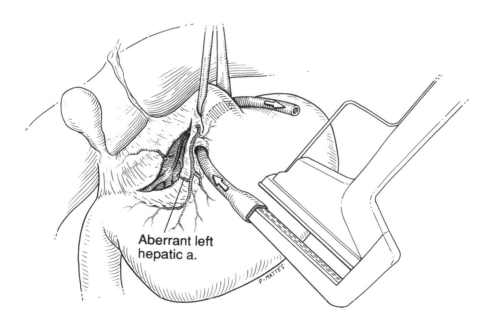

FIGURE 16.6. Illustration of atraumatic compartmentalization of the stomach for GBP. From Kellum, De Maria, & Sugerman (1998). Copyright 1998 by Mosby. Reprinted by permission.

ditional key consideration is whether the degree of weight change is sufficient to improve health. Modest reductions in body weight (e.g., 5%–10% of body weight), maintained for sufficient periods of time, can confer health improvements such as reductions in blood pressure, blood glucose, and hyperlipidemia (Pi-Sunyer, 1996). Thus the Institute of Medicine (IOM, 1995), in its report on criteria for assessing the outcome of weight management programs, has defined "success" as a weight loss of ≥5% of body weight maintained for 1 or more years. We use the IOM definition, along with the other indicators noted above, in reviewing long-term outcome.

Numerous studies have examined the short-term effects of behavioral treatment and outcome at 1-year follow-up. Reviews (Brownell & Wadden, 1992; National Heart, Lung, and Blood Institute [NHLBI], 1998; Perri, 1998; Perri & Fuller, 1995; Wadden, Sarwer, & Berkowitz, 1999) of randomized trials conducted during the 1990s show that behavioral treatments, typically delivered in 15–26 weekly group sessions, produced mean losses of approximately 0.4 kg/week of treatment and mean posttreatment losses of approximately 8.5 kg. (For more information on behavioral treatment, see Wing, Chapter 14, this volume.) Significant improvements in blood pressure, blood glucose, and psychological well-being have been associated with weight losses of this magnitude (NHLBI, 1998; Pi-Sunyer, 1996). Nonetheless, the clinical utility of an 8.5-kg loss is determined by how well the lost weight is maintained. The IOM (1995) succinctly summarized the longer-term findings, stating that "those who complete weight-loss programs lose approximately 10 percent of their body weight, only to regain two thirds of it back within one year and almost all of it back within 5 years" (p. 1).

In Table 17.1, we summarize the results of nine behavioral treatment studies with follow-ups of 2 or more years (Björvell & Rössner, 1985, 1992; Elmer et al., 1995; Graham, Taylor, Hovell, & Siegel, 1983; Hypertension Prevention Trial Research Group, 1990; Kramer, Jeffery, Forster, & Snell, 1989; Stalonas, Perri, & Kerzner, 1984; Wadden, Sternberg, Letizia, Stunkard, & Foster, 1989; Wadden, Stunkard, & Liebschutz, 1988; Whelton et al., 1998). Three of the studies included behavioral weight loss treatment as part of a hypertension reduction intervention (Elmer et al., 1995; Hypertension Prevention Trial Research Group, 1990; Whelton et al., 1998). The initial weight losses in these three trials were somewhat smaller than those usually observed in behavioral treatments with healthy adults, but their large sample sizes and long follow-up periods provide additional documentation about long-term outcome following behavioral treatment.

Initial weight changes for the studies in Table 17.1 ranged from 4.5 to 14.3 kg (M across studies = 8.3 kg, unadjusted for study n). The magnitude of initial losses appears to reflect the length of treatment and the pretreatment weight of the samples. Studies with longer treatment periods and/or heavier subjects showed larger posttreatment losses. In each study, the mean reductions at 1-year follow-up met or exceeded the IOM criterion for successful maintenance (i.e., ≥5% reduction in body weight). Final follow-up evaluations, conducted 2–12 years after initial treatment, showed a mean net loss of 3.0 kg (unadjusted for study n) across all studies. However, only two of the nine studies met the IOM criterion for successful maintenance at final follow-up. The exceptions were one of the hypertension studies (Whelton et al., 1998), which had the shortest follow-up period (2 years), and the study by Björvell and Rössner (1985, 1992), which showed a maintenance of a 10.6-kg loss 10–12 years after initial treatment. The obvious distinguishing feature of the Björvell and Rössner study was its inclusion of an intensive 4-year maintenance program that incorporated ongoing behavioral treatment, exercise, dietary counseling, and relapse prevention training, along with admission of relapsed patients to a day hospital unit for intensive treatment. If the Björvell and Rössner study is omitted from consideration because of its unusually intensive nature, the follow-up data in Table 17.1 suggest a reliable pattern of gradual

TABLE 17.1. Studies of Behavioral Weight Loss Treatment with 2 Years or More of Follow-Up

Study	n	Tx. & length (wk)	Pre-tx. wt. (kg)	Initial wt. loss (kg)	Net loss at 1 yr	IOMC[a] met at 1 yr	Time to final f/u (yr)	Net loss (kg) at final f/u	% initial loss maintained	IOMC[a] met at final f/u?
Graham et al. (1983)	60	BT (NA)	NA	4.5	NA	NA	4.5	3.3	74%	NA
Stalonas et al. (1984)	36	BT (10)	82	4.8	4.1	Yes	5.0	+0.7	−14%	No
Kramer et al. (1989)	152	BT (15)	98	11.5	6.5	Yes	4/5	2.7	23%	No
Björvell & Rössner (1985)	74	Multicomponent[b]	125	11.1	23.3	Yes	4.0	15.0	100%	Yes
Björvell & Rössner (1992)	49	Same	125	12.6	23.0	Yes	10–12	10.6	89%	Yes
Wadden et al. (1988)	16	BT (26)	122	14.3	9.5	Yes	3.0	4.8	33%	No
Wadden et al. (1989)	22	BT (26)	106	13.0	4.7	Yes	5.0	+2.7	−21%	No
Hypertension Prevention Trial[c] Research Group (1990)	254	BT[d] (14)	87	5.8	NA	Yes	3.0	1.6	29%	No
Elmer et al.[c] (1995)	902	BT[d] (26)	85	5.0	4.8	Yes	3.5	2.6	52%	No
Whelton et al.[c] (1998)	147	BT (32)	87	4.8	4.6	Yes	2.0	4.7	98%	Yes

Note. BT, behavior therapy; NA, not available; f/u, follow-up.

[a] Institute of Medicine (1995) criterion for successful long-term loss—that is, ≥5% body weight lost and maintained for >1 year.

[b] Data presented for multicomponent behavioral program, which included a 6-week inpatient stay, relapse prevention, exercise, nutritional counseling, and ongoing maintenance sessions for 4 years.

[c] Interventions designed to reduce hypertension included a weight loss component. Initial weight and weight losses are therefore lower.

[d] Interventions consisted of dietary counseling, behavior modification, support, cooking demonstrations, and nonsupervised exercise (walking).

TABLE 17.2. Response to Behavior Therapy for Obesity with Extended Contact (Weekly or Biweekly Sessions beyond 6 Months)

Study	n	Initial tx. length (wk)	Mean initial wt. (kg)	Mean initial wt. loss (kg)	Type & no. of extended-contact sessions	Length of extended-contact period (wk)	Net loss after extended contact (kg)	% initial loss maintained	Add'l f/u without contact (wk)	Net loss at f/u (kg)	% initial loss maintained	IOMC met at final f/u?
Perri et al. (1987)	16	20	88.1	10.3	0	30	7.8[a]	76%	48	3.1[a]	30%	No
	27	20	89.8	10.7	15 bw		11.5[b]	107%	48	6.4[b]	60%	Yes
Perri et al. (1988)	16	20	89.0	10.8	0	52	5.7[a]	53%	26	3.6[a]	33%	No
	19	20	96.5	13.2	26 bw		12.9[b]	98%	26	11.4[b]	86%	Yes
Perri et al. (1989)	16	20	96.6	8.9	0	20	6.4[a]	71%	32	4.6[a]	52%	No
	16	20	100.4	10.1	20 wk		13.6[b]	135%	32	9.9[b]	98%	Yes
Viegener et al. (1990)	32	26	98.7	8.9	13 bw	26	9.0	101%	None	—	—	—
Wadden et al. (1994)	16	26	105.4	11.9	26 wk + 13 bw	52	12.2	103%	None	—	—	—
Wing et al. (1994)	41	26	107.7	13.5	26 wk	26	10.5	78%	52	5.7	42%	Yes
Perri et al. (1997)	24	26 H	87.1	10.4	13 bw	26	12.1[a]	116%	13	11.7[a]	113%	Yes
	25	26 G	89.8	9.4	13 bw	26	8.1[b]	86%	13	7.01[b]	75%	Yes

Study												
Wadden et al. (1997)	77	26[c]	96	17.4	22 wk	22	15.6	90%	52	8.5	49%	Yes
Wadden et al. (1998)	38	20[d]	97.1	11.0	10 bw	20	12.4	113%	None	—	—	—
Wing et al. (1998)	37	26 D	99.6	9.1	13 bw	26	5.5	56%	52	2.1	23%	No
	40	26 DE	98.7	10.3	13 bw	26	7.4	72%	52	2.5	24%	No
Weinstock et al. (1998)	45	28[c]	96.9	13.8	10 bw	20	15.2	110%	48	10.0	72%	Yes
Jakicic et al. (1999)	148	26 Lb	90	8.2	13 bw	26	7.0	85%	26	5.8	71%	Yes
		26 Sb	92	7.5	13 bw	26	5.7	76%	26	3.7^a	49%	No
		26 SbE	88.3	9.3	13 bw	26	10.0	108%	26	7.4^b	80%	Yes
Leermakers et al. (1999)	28	26 EF	94	9.6	13 bw	26	7.9	82%	26	5.2	$54\%^a$	Yes
	20	26 WF	94	8.7	13 bw	26	8.5	98%	26	7.9	$91\%^b$	Yes

Note. bw, biweekly; D, diet; E, exercise; WF, weight-focused; EF, exercise-focused; H, home-based exercise; G, group-based exercise; Lb, long-bout exercise; Sb, short-bout exercise; SbE, short-bout exercise with home equipment. Other abbreviations as in Table 17.1.

[a,b]Means with differing superscripts indicate significant between-group differences ($p < .05$).

[c]Included short-term use of a low-calorie liquid diet (925 kcal/day).

[d]Included use of low-calorie (1,000 kcal/day) or balanced-deficit (1,200 kcal/day) diet.

groups had a mean net loss of 6.6 kg, maintaining about two-thirds (66.5%) of their initial weight reduction. Thus judging the effects of the extended treatments by comparison with the standard-length groups suggests a beneficial impact for extended contact (i.e., 96.3% vs. 66.5% of initial loss maintained).

Of the 13 studies listed in Table 17.2, 10 included additional follow-up periods beyond the extended-treatment period. The results of these additional follow-up assessments conducted on average 22 months after initiation of treatment showed that the extended-treatment groups demonstrated mean net loss of 7.0 kg (65.8% of their initial reduction; range = 23%–113%). In contrast, the three groups without extended contact maintained a mean net loss of 3.8 kg (38.3% of their initial reduction; range = 30%–52%). At final follow-up, none of the three groups *without* extended contact met the IOM criterion for successful maintenance, whereas 12 of the 15 extended-treatment groups met or exceeded this criterion. Moreover, two of the three extended-treatment groups that failed to meet the IOM criterion were from one study (Wing et al., 1998). That study, conducted with diabetic patients, suffered from unusually low attendance rates (29%), perhaps because of the large initial therapy group sizes ($n \cong 20$) and the requirement in the exercise condition that subjects complete a 50- to 60-minute walk as part of the treatment session. Collectively, the data in Table 17.2 strongly suggest that extended treatment improves the maintenance of weight loss.

Table 17.3 presents the results of randomized trials that evaluated various other strategies designed to enhance the long-term effect of behavioral weight loss treatment. Included in the table are studies with posttreatment follow-up evaluations of 12 months or longer that tested maintenance procedures implemented (or continued) during the period following initial treatment.

Relapse Prevention Training

Two studies have tested relapse prevention training (RPT), in which participants are taught how to avoid or cope with slips and relapses. Perri, Shapiro, Ludwig, Twentyman, and McAdoo (1984) found that including RPT during the course of initial treatment was not effective, but that combining RPT with a multicomponent program of client–therapist contacts by mail and telephone significantly improved the maintenance of weight loss. Similarly, Baum, Clark, and Sandler (1991) showed that following behavioral treatment, clients in a minimal-contact condition experienced significant weight regain, while participants who received RPT combined with posttreatment therapist contacts maintained their end-of-treatment losses.

Food Provision/Monetary Incentives

Jeffery and colleagues (1993) have evaluated, both during initial treatment and during the year following initial treatment, the effectiveness of providing participants with prepackaged, portion-controlled, low-calorie meals (10 meals/week at no cost) or with monetary incentives for weight loss or with both. No significant effects were observed for monetary incentives, but participants in the food provision groups showed significantly greater weight losses than those without food provision, both during initial treatment and during the 12-month maintenance period. However, the results of an additional 12-month follow-up (24 months after the initiation of treatment) showed poor maintenance of weight loss in all conditions (Jeffery & Wing, 1995).

Wing, Jeffery, Hellerstedt, and Burton (1996) also tested the effectiveness of food provision as a maintenance strategy, but in this study food provision was optional. Over the

TABLE 17.3. Results of Randomized Trials of Other Maintenance Strategies Implemented or Continued after Initial Behavioral Treatment

Study	Initial tx. & length (wk)	n	Pre-tx. wt (kg)	Mean initial wt. loss (kg)	Maint. strategies	Length of maint. (wk)	Net loss after maint.	% initial loss maintained	Add'l f/u (wk)	Net loss at f/u (kg)	% initial loss maintained	IOMC met at final f/u?
Perri, McAdoo, et al. (1984)	B	17	90.9	5.6	None	65	2.1	38%	26	0.4[a]	7%	No
	B (14)	26	84.1	6.1	TC (mail/phone) + peer mtg.	65	5.8[c]	95%	26	4.6[b]	75%	Yes
Perri, Shapiro, et al. (1984)	B	21	88.6	7.5	None	26	7.6	98%	26	6.3	84%	Yes
	B + C	15	88.6	8.7	TC (mail/phone)	26	8.7	100%	26	5.8	66%	Yes
	B + RP	15	88.6	8.5	None	26	4.9[a]	58%	26	3.0[a]	35%	No
	B + RP + C (15)	17	88.6	9.7	TC (mail/phone)	26	10.8[b]	111%	26	10.3[b]	106%	Yes
Perri et al. (1986)	B	16	92.1	7.5[a]	None	52	0.3[a]	4%	26	0.7[a]	9%	No
	B	17	92.1	8.3[a]	TC (mail/phone)	52	6.5[b]	78%	26	5.2[b]	63%	Yes
	B + A	16	92.1	10.3[b]	None	52	5.2[b]	50%	26	3.1[b]	30%	No
	B + A (20)	18	92.1	11.0[b]	TC (mail/phone) + peer mtg.	52	9.7[c]	88%	26	7.6[c]	69%	Yes
Perri et al. (1987)	B	16	88.1	10.3	None	30	7.8[a]	76%	48	3.1[a]	30%	No
	B	32	94.2	10.9	Peer mtg.	30	9.3[a]	85%	48	6.5[b]	60%	Yes
	B (20)	27	89.8	10.7	TC	30	11.5[b]	107%	48	6.4[b]	60%	Yes
Perri et al. (1988)	B	16	89.0	10.8	None	52	5.7[a]	52%	26	3.6[a]	33%	No
	B	19	97.4	13.2	TC	52	12.9[b]	97%	26	9.9[b]	98%	Yes
	B	19	95.2	11.3	TC + increased AE	52	13.4[b]	117%	26	8.4[b]	74%	Yes
	B	18	96.9	13.1	TC + social influence	52	13.0[b]	99%	26	9.1[b]	70%	Yes
	B (20)	19	97.4	13.7	TC + increased AE + social influence	52	15.7[b]	114%	26	13.5[b]	99%	Yes
Baum et al. (1991)	B	16	81.5	4.0	None	12	3.5	87%	39	1.5[a]	38%	No
	B (26)	16	81.5	3.9	TC + RPT	12	5.4	138%	39	3.6[b]	92%	No

(continued)

TABLE 17.3. *continued*

Study	Initial tx. & length (wk)	n	Pre-tx. wt (kg)	Mean initial wt. loss (kg)	Maint. strategies	Length of maint. (wk)	Net loss after maint.	% initial loss maintained	Add'l f/u (wk)	Net loss at f/u (kg)	% initial loss maintained	IOMC met at final f/u?
Jeffery et al. (1993, 1995)	B	40	89.4	7.5[a]	TC (monthly)	52	4.4	58.6%	52	1.4	19%	No
	B + I	41	92.3	7.9[a]	TC + incentives	52	3.8	48.1%	52	1.6	20%	No
	B + F	40	88.1	10.0[b]	TC + food	52	6.7[b]	67.0%	52	2.2	22%	No
	B + I + F (20)	41	91.1	10.2[b]	TC + incentives + food	52	6.2[b]	60.8%	52	1.6	16%	No
Wing et al. (1996)	B	27	NA	14.2	None	52	8.6	60.6%	—	—	—	Yes
	B	26		12.8	Phone prompts (1/wk)	52	9.3	72.7%	—	—	—	Yes
	B	22		13.4	None	52	9.2	68.7%	—	—	—	Yes
	B (26)	26		13.2	Optional food provision	52	9.0	68.2%	—	—	—	Yes
Wadden et al. (1997, 1998)	B + D	29	96.3	16.7	bw mtg.	20	14.4	86%	52	6.9	41%	Yes
	B + D + A	31	98.7	16.2	S aerobics (2/wk)	20	13.7	85%	52	8.5	52%	Yes
	B + D + S	31	96.8	16.8	S strength (2/wk)	20	17.2	102%	52	10.1	60%	Yes
	B + D + AS (26)	29	92.4	16.3	S aerobics & strength (2/wk)	20	15.2	93%	52	8.6	53%	Yes
Jeffery et al. (1998)	B	40	86	8.3	None	52	7.6[a]	92%	—	—	—	Yes
	B	41	87	6.0	S walks (3/wk)	52	3.8[b]	63%	—	—	—	No
	B	42	85	5.6	PT walks (3/wk)	52	2.9[b]	52%	—	—	—	No
	B	37	88	6.7	S walks + I	52	4.5[b]	67%	—	—	—	Yes
	B (24)	36	86	7.9	PT walks + I	52	5.1[b]	65%	—	—	—	Yes
Jakicic et al. (1999)	B + Lb	49	90	8.2	Lb (13 bw)	26	7.0	85%	26	5.8	71%	Yes
	B + Sb	51	92	7.5	Sb (13 bw)	26	5.7[a]	76%	26	3.7[a]	49%	No
	B + SbE (26)	48	88.3	9.3	SbE (13 bw)	26	10.0[b]	108%	26	7.4[b]	80%	Yes
Leermakers et al. (1999)	B	28	94	9.6	EF (13 bw)	26	7.9	82%	26	5.2	54%[a]	Yes
	B (26)	20	94	8.7	WF (13 bw)	26	8.5	98%	26	7.9	91%[b]	Yes

Note. B, behavior therapy; AE, aerobic exercise; TC, therapist contact; PT, personal trainer; RPT, relapse prevention training; S, supervised; I, incentives; F, food provision; E, exercise equipment. Other abbreviations, as in Tables 17.1 and 17.2.
[a,b,c] Different superscripts denote significant between-group differences ($p < .05$).

366

course of a 12-month posttreatment period, participants were provided with the opportunity to purchase prepackaged, portion-controlled, low-calorie meals as a means of sustaining the weight losses they accomplished during initial treatment. The optional food provision strategy was not effective, largely because participants did not purchase the prepackaged meals.

Telephone Prompts

Wing and colleagues (1996) also evaluated the effects of frequent contact with participants through telephone calls designed to prompt adherence to self-monitoring. Over the course of a 12-month posttreatment period, interviewers contacted participants on a weekly basis to inquire about their monitoring of body weight and food intake. The interviewers, who were not the participants' therapists and who were previously unknown to the participants, offered no counseling or guidance. Although participation in the telephone prompt condition was negatively related to weight regain ($r = -.52$), it did not enhance maintenance of weight loss compared to a no-contact control condition. In contrast, Perri, Shapiro, and colleagues (1984), found that client–therapist contacts by telephone and mail significantly improved the maintenance of weight loss. In the Perri, Shapiro, and colleagues study, the clients' therapists actually made the contacts and offered advice, whereas in the Wing and colleagues (1996) study, the contacts were made by callers who were unknown to the clients and who did not offer advice. These procedural differences may account for the better outcome observed in the Perri, Shapiro, and colleagues study.

Peer Support

Perri and colleagues (1987) examined the effects of a peer support maintenance program. Following an initial treatment period, participants were taught how to run their own peer group support meetings. They were provided with a meeting place equipped with a scale, and biweekly meetings were scheduled over a 7-month period following initial treatment. Attendance at the peer group meetings was relatively high (67%), but no advantage was observed in terms of adherence or weight change during the maintenance period, compared to a no-maintenance-program condition. The follow-up results revealed a significant regaining of weight in both conditions, but the peer support group had a greater mean net loss than the control condition (6.5 vs. 3.1 kg, respectively).

In a partially randomized study with a brief follow-up period, Wing and Jeffery (1999) recently evaluated the effects of recruiting participants alone or with three friends or family members. Participants were assigned to receive either standard behavior therapy or behavior therapy with social support training. At a 6-month follow-up, those individuals who were recruited with friends and received social support training maintained 66% of their initial weight losses, whereas subjects who entered the study alone and received standard treatment maintained only 24% of their initial losses. The promising findings from this study await replication in a fully randomized design with a longer follow-up period.

Exercise/Physical Activity

Correlational studies generally indicate that long-term weight loss is associated with increased physical activity (e.g., Harris, French, Jeffery, McGovern, & Wing, 1994; Kayman, Bruvold, & Stern, 1990; McGuire, Wing, Klem, Lang, & Hill, 1999; Sherwood, Jeffery, & Wing, 1999). Several controlled trials have shown that the combination of diet plus exercise produces greater weight loss than does diet alone (Pavlou, Krey, & Steffee, 1989; Perri,

McAdoo, McAllister, Lauer, & Yancey, 1986; Wing et al., 1988). In a recent review, Wing (1999) evaluated evidence regarding the short- and long-term effects of exercise in the treatment of obesity. Wing found that only 2 of 13 studies showed significantly greater initial weight losses for the combination of diet plus exercise versus diet alone. Similarly, only 2 of 6 studies with follow-ups of 1 year or longer showed significantly better maintenance for diet plus exercise versus diet alone. Wing noted, however, that in every study reviewed, the direction of the between-group difference favored the groups with exercise. She suggested that this modest effect of exercise on weight loss might have been due to the short duration of treatments and the relatively low levels of exercise prescribed. Wing also noted that inconsistencies in subject adherence to assigned treatments might have contributed to the modest effects of exercise on weight change.

Subjects in exercise conditions often show great variability in their long-term adherence to prescribed exercise, and individuals assigned to "diet-only" conditions often initiate exercise regimens on their own. As a consequence, the long-term effects of exercise manipulations may be obscured. This pattern was observed in a study by Wadden and colleagues (1997), who tested the additions of aerobic exercise, strength training, and their combination to a 48-week behavioral treatment program. Compared to behavior therapy with diet only, none of the exercise additions produced an incremental benefit in weight loss or weight loss maintenance (Wadden et al., 1998). The authors found that adherence to exercise assignments was highly variable across all conditions, particularly during the course of follow-up. Nonetheless, exercise was positively associated with the long-term maintenance of weight loss. At follow-up, those individuals who reported that they "exercised regularly" maintained a weight loss of 12.1 kg, whereas those who indicated that they were "nonexercisers" had maintained a mean loss of only 6.1 kg.

Findings such as those of Wadden and colleagues (1997, 1998) highlight the need to develop strategies for improving exercise adherence. Several approaches have been tested that may improve exercise adherence in obesity treatment, including home-based exercise; the use of personal trainers and monetary incentives for exercise; the use of short bouts of exercise and the provision of home exercise equipment; and posttreatment programs focused exclusively on exercise.

Home-Based Exercise

Perri and colleagues (1997) investigated the use of home-based versus supervised group-based exercise programs in the treatment of obesity. After 6 months of treatment, both conditions displayed significant improvements from baseline in exercise participation, cardiorespiratory fitness, eating patterns, and weight loss. At 12 months, however, the home-based program showed better performance than the group condition in exercise participation and treatment adherence. Participants in the home-based condition completed a significantly higher percentage of prescribed exercise sessions than subjects in the group condition (83.3% vs. 62.1%, respectively). Moreover, attrition in the home-based program was significantly lower than in the group program, and the long-term superiority of the home-based program was evident both for exercise adherence and for weight loss at follow-up.

Personal Trainers and Monetary Incentives

Jeffery, Wing, Thorson, and Burton (1998) evaluated the use of personal trainers and financial incentives as strategies to improve exercise adherence and long-term weight loss. Personal trainers walked with participants and made phone call reminders for exercise. Financial incentives ranged from $1 to $3 per bout of walking. The use of personal trainers and financial incentives both increased attendance at supervised exercise sessions. However, neither manipulation improved weight loss. In fact, consistent with the findings of Perri and colleagues (1997), the control condition, which received a home-based exercise regimen, showed better maintenance of weight loss at follow-up than all other conditions.

Short Exercise Bouts and Home Exercise Equipment

Recently Jakicic and colleagues (1999) evaluated the effects of intermittent exercise (i.e., four 10-minute bouts per day versus one 40-minute bout per day) and the use of home exercise equipment on adherence, weight loss, and fitness. Among the short-bout subjects, half were provided with a motorized treadmill for home use and half were not. The results showed equivalent benefits from exercising in short or long bouts. However, subjects in the short-bout condition *with* the home exercise equipment maintained significantly higher levels of long-term exercise adherence and weight loss than did subjects in the short-bout condition *without* exercise equipment.

Programs Focused Exclusively on Exercise

Can a posttreatment program focused exclusively on exercise improve long-term outcome in obesity treatment? Leermakers and colleagues (1999) tested this proposition by comparing the effects of exercise-focused and weight-focused posttreatment programs. The exercise-focused program included supervised group walking sessions, incentives for exercise completion, and RPT aimed at the maintenance of exercise. The weight-focused maintenance program entailed problem solving of obstacles to maintaining weight loss. At follow-up, participants in the weight-focused program demonstrated significantly greater reductions in fat consumption and significantly better maintenance of weight loss than subjects in the exercise-focused program. The findings from this study suggest the importance of an emphasis on dietary intake as well as physical activity in the long-term management of obesity. (See Blair & Leermakers, Chapter 13, this volume, for more information on physical activity.)

Multicomponent Posttreatment Programs

Several studies have examined the effects of posttreatment programs with multiple components. Perri, Shapiro, and colleagues (1984) tested the effects of a multicomponent maintenance program (conducted over a 65-week period) consisting of peer group meetings combined with ongoing client–therapist contacts by mail and telephone. Clients were taught to run their own peer group meetings and were provided with preprinted sets of postcards designed for simplified self-monitoring of food intake and the use of key weight loss strategies. The therapists, in turn, made phone calls to provide support and guidance during the maintenance phase. Compared to a comparison condition that received initial treatment plus 6 biweekly booster sessions, the multicomponent program demonstrated significantly better maintenance of weight loss both at the end of the maintenance phase and at additional follow-up 6 months later. These findings were replicated by Perri and colleagues (1986), who used a longer initial treatment period (20 rather than 14 weeks), included a group-based aerobic exercise program, and obtained larger weight losses at posttreatment and at follow-ups.

Perri and colleagues (1988) tested the effects of adding increased exercise and a social influence program (or both) to a posttreatment therapist contact program consisting of 26 biweekly group sessions. At the conclusion of the posttreatment phase, all four programs produced significantly greater maintenance of weight losses than a comparison condition that consisted of behavior therapy without posttreatment contact. The study showed no significant between-group effects for the exercise and social influence manipulations. However, the group that received therapist contacts, combined with both increased exercise and the social influence program, was the only one to demonstrate a significant additional weight loss (4.1 kg—observed during the first 6 months of the maintenance period). Indeed, the effectiveness of the therapist contact programs was most pronounced during the first half of the year-long maintenance phase. During the second half of the maintenance phase (which corresponded to months 11–17 of continuous treatment), adherence diminished in all maintenance groups, and all experienced some (albeit a nonsignificant) amount of weight regain. Six months after the posttreatment programs ended, the four maintenance groups succeeded in sustaining 70%–99% (M = 83%) of their initial weight losses, compared to 33% for the group without posttreatment therapist contact.

IMPLICATIONS

Long-Term Effects of Behavioral Treatment

The findings in our review of studies with posttreatment follow-up evaluations of 2 years or more suggest a pattern of gradual regaining of weight with maintenance of a small weight loss ($\cong 1.8$ kg, or 23% of initial loss) 4 years after initial behavioral treatment (see Table 17.1). When considered in the context of secular trends showing a steady pattern of weight gain in untreated obese adults, these findings suggest a modestly beneficial long-term impact of behavioral treatment. However, the presentation of outcome in terms of group means obscures the fact that only a subset of individuals (perhaps 20%) successfully sustains long-term weight losses of 5 kg or more.

Can large weight losses be successfully maintained? Support for the possibility of successful long-term maintenance of large weight losses can be found in the study by Björvell and Rössner (1985, 1992). These researchers argued that successful long-term management of obesity would require an intensive, multifaceted approach to maintenance. Following initial treatment, their subjects received an intensive 4-year maintenance program. Each individual was expected to attend one of two group sessions that were offered each week. Therapists made vigorous efforts to contact any participant who missed a scheduled appointment. Posttreatment contacts by both telephone and mail were used to keep patients actively involved in the maintenance sessions. Finally, whenever a subject relapsed, the investigators initiated a "refresher course" of treatment. Almost all of the participants returned for at least one refresher course of treatment. The study sample achieved a mean loss of 14.5 kg at year 1. After 4 years of continuous care, the participants had maintained 77% of their peak losses (M = 11.2 kg). Even more impressive were the 10-year results, showing that 6 years after treatment ended the participants had maintained a mean loss of 9.0 kg.

These findings strongly suggest that providing patients with an intensive program of continuous care can result in successful long-term management of obesity. Moreover, the investigation may serve as a model of the type of continuous-care program that should be tested in future studies. We note, however, that the Björvell and Rössner research was conducted in Sweden, where the medical system treats obesity seriously. In the United States, the costs of obesity treatment are rarely covered by health insurance, except in cases of extreme obesity (BMI $\geq$ 40 kg/m^2) or obesity complicated by the presence of a comorbid disease condition.

Effective Maintenance Strategies

Our review suggests that strategies such as peer group meetings, RPT without continued therapist contact, telephone prompts by nontherapists, monetary incentives for weight loss, supervised group exercise, the use of personal trainers, and the availability of portion-controlled meals do not appear effective in enhancing the maintenance of weight loss. However, home-based exercise programs and the use of home exercise equipment seem to enhance exercise adherence and also appear to improve the maintenance of lost weight.

Our review also very clearly documents that continuing treatment beyond 6 months, through the use of weekly or biweekly sessions, improves the maintenance of weight loss. Follow-up assessments conducted on average 22 months after initiation of treatment showed that extended-treatment groups demonstrated mean net losses of 7.0 kg (65.8% of their initial reduction). Moreover, 12 of the 15 extended-treatment groups considered in our review met or exceeded the IOM criterion for successful maintenance of weight loss. Similarly, multicomponent approaches that combine ongoing client–therapist contacts (whether in person or by telephone and mail) with RPT or social support programs have shown improved maintenance, compared to behavioral treatment without such programs.

Continued adherence to the changes in eating and exercise patterns induced during the initial treatment phase appears to be the mechanism responsible for the better outcomes observed in extended treatments. In the studies that directly tested behavior therapy with and without extended contact, significantly better maintenance of *behavior change* was observed in the groups with continuing contact than in those without it. Weekly or biweekly therapy sessions provide ongoing prompts for appropriate eating and exercise behaviors, combined with opportunities for therapists to reinforce adherence and to assist participants in problem solving to overcome obstacles to continued maintenance.

Despite encouraging findings regarding long-term behavior therapy for obesity, several factors require consideration in the evaluation of extended treatment. For example, a key issue concerns the decreased "motivation" of clients during extended therapy. As treatment duration approaches 1 year, session attendance becomes sporadic, adherence falls off, and participants often begin to regain weight. When weight loss plateaus during the course of long-term treatment, many become disheartened, and their participation in treatment flounders. Therefore, educating clients about realistic weight loss expectations is essential to successful treatment (IOM, 1995).

Certain tactics may enhance motivation for participation in extended therapy. For example, Perri and colleagues (1988) utilized an array of social influence procedures that increased adherence (but not weight loss) in maintenance sessions. The tactics included group contingencies with monetary incentives based on adherence, "learning by teaching" (i.e., client participation in preparing and delivering lectures on weight loss maintenance strategies), and "telephone networking" (i.e., planned peer support phone calls between sessions). Alternatively, incorporating the perspective and techniques of "motivational interviewing" (i.e., a participant-centered approach to dealing with problems of ambivalence and decreased motivation for change; Miller & Rollnick, 1991) may hold benefits in extended treatment. Smith, Heckemeyer, Kratt, and Mason (1997) have demonstrated the effectiveness of motivational interviewing strategies in improving dietary adherence among obese diabetic patients.

Does extending treatment simply forestall the regaining of lost weight? Wilson (1994) has argued that when treatment ends, the biological mechanisms that regulate body weight undermine an obese person's ability to sustain the behaviors needed for lasting weight control. However, as a chronic condition similar to hypertension or diabetes, obesity may require ongoing, lifelong care (Perri et al., 1992). Alternatively, as seen in the Björvell and

Rössner (1985, 1992) study, long periods of intensive treatment may be required before clients fully incorporate the skills needed to sustain the eating and exercise habits required for successful weight maintenance.

FUTURE CLINICAL DIRECTIONS

Comprehensive Assessment

A comprehensive assessment of the effects of obesity on the individual's health and emotional well-being may enhance the effectiveness of treatment (Beliard, Kirschenbaum, & Fitzgibbon, 1992). The impact of obesity on risk factors for disease (e.g., hypertension, glucose tolerance, dyslipidemia, etc.) and quality of life (e.g., emotional state, body image, binge eating, etc.) should be assessed (Kushner & Weinsier, 2000). A careful individualized assessment will often reveal important behavioral and emotional targets for intervention, such as binge eating, body image disparagement, and anxiety or depression—problems that need to be addressed whether or not weight loss itself becomes an objective of treatment (Perri et al., 1992; Wadden & Foster, 1992). Individuals who have failed to lose weight using a particular treatment modality should be counseled that they are unlikely to lose weight in a repeated effort using the same approach (Smith & Wing, 1991). Finally, self-acceptance, independent of weight loss, may be an important treatment objective for many obese individuals (Wilson, 1996).

Focus on Maintenance of Behavior Change

Obese persons do not have direct control over how much weight they lose. Therefore, treatment goals should be framed in terms of behaviors that they can control, such as the quantity and quality of food they consume and the amounts and types of physical activity they perform. Moreover, obese persons should be informed that significant health benefits can be derived from even modest weight losses of 5%–10% (NHLBI, 1998; Pi-Sunyer, 1996). The maintenance of stable weight and the prevention of weight gain should be recognized as legitimate treatment options for some obese persons, particularly since the natural course of obesity entails weight gain.

Redefining Success

Successful outcome in the care of obese persons should not be viewed solely in terms of weight change. Beneficial changes in risk factors for disease and improvements in quality of life (Atkinson, 1993) represent important indicators of success. Improvements in the quality of diet should be a component of care, independent of whether weight reduction is an identified objective of care (Hill, Drougas, & Peters, 1993). Reductions in amounts of dietary fats, particularly saturated fats, can improve health as well as assist in weight loss (Astrup et al., 2000; Insull et al., 1990). Similarly, increased physical activity and a decrease in sedentary lifestyle can represent beneficial components of long-term care, irrespective of the impact of exercise on weight loss (Lee, Blair, & Jackson, 1999; Paffenbarger & Lee, 1996).

FUTURE RESEARCH DIRECTIONS

More research is needed on the development of interventions for the long-term management of obesity. Successful long-term management of obesity may require maintenance programs involving years rather than months of follow-up care. Few studies have examined the effects of maintenance programs that extend beyond 1 year.

Frequency of Follow-Up Care

Future research should address the frequency and timing of professional contacts needed to sustain progress during follow-up care. The Björvell and Rössner (1985, 1992) study included a very high frequency of contacts (i.e., a minimum of once per week plus occasional refresher courses) to help patients overcome relapses and sustain long-term weight losses. Effective regimens of extended therapy in other studies (see Table 17.2) have typically included client–therapist contacts on a weekly or biweekly basis, and quantitative reviews have shown that amount of therapist contact is the most important factor positively correlated with weight loss. Thus one might conclude that the more contact, the better. However, if the burden of session attendance is too high, clients may experience therapy "burnout" and discontinue their involvement in follow-up care (see, e.g., Wing et al., 1994). Furthermore, in research studies, extended treatment is almost always provided on an interval schedule, determined in advance by the experimenters. Such an approach may not provide clients with assistance at the particular times when they need it most (e.g., when facing a significant stressor or after experiencing a weight gain).

The effects of various schedules of follow-up care represents an area worth researching. It will be important to determine (1) the extent to which a "dose–response" relationship exists between therapist contact and client progress; (2) the minimal and optimal frequency of contacts needed for maintenance of treatment effects; and (3) whether follow-up care should be tailored to clients' progress rather than a fixed-interval schedule. In addition, more research is needed on methods to increase long-term attendance during follow-up care. For example, initial behavioral treatment typically entails a closed-group format, but open groups are often used by self-help groups such as Overeaters Anonymous and commercial programs such as Weight Watchers to encourage easy access to assistance. Research on the benefits of open versus closed groups during follow-up is worth pursuing.

Treating Faulty Weight Loss Expectations

Virtually all obese clients begin weight loss therapy with unrealistically high expectations about the amount of weight loss they can achieve (Foster, Wadden, Vogt, & Brewer, 1997). These faulty expectations may lead clients to discount the beneficial impact of modest weight losses. Foster and colleagues (1997) propose that the mismatch between clients' expectations and actual performance may lead to demoralization and consequently to poor maintenance of the behavior changes needed to sustain weight loss. A corollary of this hypothesis suggests that treatment of faulty weight loss expectations may improve clients' satisfaction with the outcome of weight loss therapy and thereby foster better maintenance of weight loss. Furthermore, Foster and Kendall (1994) have outlined a treatment for countering the internalized aesthetic standards that produce faulty weight loss expectations, including resisting social pressure to achieve an "ideal" body, adopting nonderogatory self-statements about large body size, and uncoupling the association between body weight and self-esteem. A controlled study is needed to examine the effects of such an intervention on clients' expectations, self-esteem, mood, and maintenance of weight loss.

Matching Treatments to Clients

The development of an empirical database is needed for matching long-term care to the specific needs of particular subgroups of obese persons (Brownell & Wadden, 1991). The development of such a database might begin with the identification of clinical markers associated with poor response to treatment. For example, binge eating, depression, significant life stress, and minimal weight loss in the first month of treatment are behavioral factors associated with poor outcome in standard behavioral interventions (Wadden & Letizia, 1992). Whether an alternative treatment, such as behavior therapy combined with pharmacotherapy, would produce better outcomes for such individuals has yet to be determined. Similarly, we need to identify those persons for whom combined behavioral plus pharmacological treatment is necessary for maintenance of weight loss, as opposed to individuals for whom behavioral management alone provides a satisfactory outcome.

As progress continues on the identification of the biological disposition to obesity (Campfield, Smith, Guisez, Devos, & Burn, 1995), more research is needed on the interaction of genetic and environmental contributors to success and failure in the long-term management of obesity. For example, leptin, the protein product of the ob gene, is responsible for the regulation of fat storage, and recent research has suggested that leptin resistance may be involved in weight gain and the maintenance of excess weight (Folsom et al., 1999). The use of leptin as an obesity treatment is a promising area, and clinical trials of the effects of leptin administered as a treatment for obesity have yielded a positive dose–response effect on weight loss in both obese and normal-weight subjects (Heymsfield et al., 1999). These findings may contribute significantly to treatment matching in patients with a potential biological disposition for obesity.

Testing Alternative Models

Finally, Cooper and Fairburn (2001) have recently suggested that innovative cognitive-behavioral interventions based on a newer conceptualization of the "maintenance problem" may produce improved long-term results. They have observed that most treatment strategies have been dictated by clinical pragmatism, rather than by an accurate conceptual understanding of the cognitive and behavioral skills required for the maintenance of lost weight. Specifically, Cooper and Fairburn note that existing programs focus on the maintenance of "weight loss" rather than the maintenance of "weight lost." Consequently, they believe that clients never learn the key skills required to maintain a stable weight. Cooper and Fairburn have proposed that after an active period of weight loss, it is essential to provide subjects with training in the maintenance of a stable body weight. At the current time, Cooper and Fairburn are conducting a randomized clinical trial to test the effects of this innovative cognitive-behavioral model of maintenance.

CONCLUSIONS

As the prevalence of obesity in the United States reaches epidemic proportions, the need for effective methods to enhance the maintenance of treatment effects has become increasingly apparent. Compared to the vast literature on methods to initiate weight loss, relatively few studies have addressed the problem of poor maintenance following therapy of obesity. Over the past decade, an increasing number of studies have evaluated methods to improve the long-term effects of treatment. No simple solution to the maintenance problem has been discovered, but progress has been made. Support for the efficacy of extended treatment for obesity has been well documented. Compared to behavior therapy without additional therapist contacts, extended treatment in the form of weekly or biweekly therapy sessions improves the maintenance of treatment effects for as long as 1 year following initial therapy. Continued adherence to the changes in eating and exercise patterns induced during the initial treatment phase appears to be the mechanism responsible for the better outcomes observed in extended behavioral treatments.

We believe that obesity should be viewed as a chronic condition requiring long-term, if not lifelong, care. The research challenge entails the development of effective programs for the ongoing management of obesity. The clinical challenge is to convince health care professionals, obese persons, and the general public that obesity is a complex, chronic condition that can be managed effectively through intensive programs of ongoing care.

REFERENCES

Allison, D. B., Fontaine, K. R., Manson, J. E., Stevens, J., & VanItallie, T. B. (1999). Annual deaths attributable to obesity in the United States. *Journal of the American Medical Association, 282,* 1530–1538.

Astrup, A., Ryan, L., Grunwald, G. K., Storgaard, M., Saris, W., Melanson, E., & Hill, J. O. (2000). The role of dietary fat in body fatness: Evidence from a preliminary meta-analysis of ad libitum low-fat dietary intervention studies. *British Journal of Nutrition, 83*(Suppl. 1), S25–S32.

Atkinson, R. L. (1993). Proposed standards for judging the success of the treatment of obesity. *Annals of Internal Medicine, 119,* 677–680.

Baum, J. G., Clark, H. B., & Sandler, J. (1991). Preventing relapse in obesity through posttreatment maintenance systems: Comparing the relative efficacy of two levels of therapist support. *Journal of Behavioral Medicine, 14,* 287–302.

Beliard, D., Kirschenbaum, D. S., & Fitzgibbon, M. L. (1992). Evaluation of an intensive weight control program using a priori criteria to determine outcome. *International Journal of Obesity, 16,* 505–517.

Bennett, G. A. (1986). Behavior therapy for obesity: A quantitative review of the effects of selected treatment characteristics on outcome. *Behavior Therapy, 17,* 554–562.

Björvell, H., & Rössner, S. (1985). Long-term treatment of severe obesity: Four-year follow-up of a combined behavioural modification programme. *British Medical Journal, 291,* 379–382.

Björvell, H., & Rössner, S. (1992). A ten year follow-up of weight change in severely obese subjects treated in a behavioural modification programme. *International Journal of Obesity, 16,* 623–625.

Brownell, K. D., & Jeffery, R. W. (1987). Improving long-term weight loss: Pushing the limits of treatment. *Behavior Therapy, 18,* 353–374.

Brownell, K. D., & Wadden, T. A. (1991). The heterogeneity of obesity: Fitting treatments to individuals. *Behavior Therapy, 22,* 153–177.

Brownell, K. D., & Wadden, T. A. (1992). Etiology and treatment of obesity: Understanding a serious, prevalent, and refractory disorder. *Journal of Consulting and Clinical Psychology, 60,* 505–517.

Campfield, L., Smith, F., Guisez, Y., Devos, R., & Burn, P. (1995). Recombinant mouse OB protein: Evidence for peripheral signal linking adiposity and central neural networks. *Science, 269,* 475–476.

Cooper, Z., & Fairburn, C. G. (2001). A new cognitive behavioral approach to the treatment of obesity. *Behavior Research and Therapy, 39,* 499–511.

Dulloo, A. G., & Jacquet, J. (1998). Adaptive reduction in basal metabolic rate in response to food deprivation in humans: A role for feedback signals from fat stores. *American Journal of Clinical Nutrition, 68*(3), 599–606.

Elmer, P. J., Grimm, R., Laing, B., Grandits, G., Svendsen, K., Van Heel, N., Betz, E., Raines, J., Link, M., & Stamler, J. (1995). Lifestyle intervention: Results of the Treatment of Mild Hypertension Study (TOMHS). *Preventive Medicine, 24,* 378–388.

Folsom, A. R., Jensen, M. D., Jacobs, D. R., Hilner, J. E., Tsai, A. W., & Schreiner, P. J. (1999). Serum leptin and weight gain over eight years in African American and Caucasian young adults. *Obesity Research, 7*(1), 1–8.

Foster, G. D., & Kendall, P. C. (1994). The realistic treatment of obesity: Changing the scales of success. *Clinical Psychology Review, 14,* 701–736.

Foster, G. D., Wadden, T. A., Vogt, R. A., & Brewer, G. (1997). What is a reasonable weight loss?: Patients' expectations and evaluations of obesity treatment outcomes. *Journal of Consulting and Clinical Psychology, 65,* 79–85.

Goodrick, G. K., Raynaud, A. S., Pace, P. W., & Foreyt, J. P. (1992). Outcome attribution in a very low calorie diet program. *International Journal of Eating Disorders, 12,* 117–120.

Graham, L. E., Taylor, C. B., Hovell, M. F., & Siegel, W. (1983). Five-year follow-up to a behavioral weight-loss program. *Journal of Consulting and Clinical Psychology, 51,* 322–323.

Harris, J. K., French, S. A., Jeffery, R. W., McGovern, P. G., & Wing, R. R. (1994). Dietary and physical activity correlates of long-term weight loss. *Obesity Research, 2,* 307–313.

Heymsfield, S. B., Greenberg, A. S., Fujioka, K., Dixon, R. M., Kushner, R., Hunt, T., Lubina, J. A., Patane, J., Self, B., Hunt, P., & McCamish, M. (1999). Recombinant leptin for weight loss in obese and lean adults. *Journal of the American Medical Association, 282*(16), 1568–1575.

Hill, J. O., Drougas, H., & Peters, J. C. (1993). Obesity treatment: Can diet composition play a role? *Annals of Internal Medicine, 119,* 694–697.

Hill, J. O., & Peters, J. C. (1998). Environmental contributions to the obesity epidemic. *Science, 280,* 1371–1374.

Hypertension Prevention Trial Research Group. (1990). The Hypertension Prevention Trial: three-year effects of dietary changes on blood pressure. *Archives of Internal Medicine, 150,* 153–162.

Institute of Medicine (IOM). (1995). *Weighing the options: Criteria for evaluating weight-management programs.* Washington, DC: National Academy Press.

Insull, W., Henderson, M., Prentice, R., Thompson, D. J., Moskowitz, M., & Gorbach, S. (1990). Results of a feasibility study of a low-fat diet. *Archives of Internal Medicine, 150,* 421–427.

Jakicic, J. M., Winters, C., Lang, W., & Wing R. R. (1999). Effects of intermittent exercise and use of home exercise equipment on adherence, weight loss, and fitness in overweight women: A randomized trial. *Journal of the American Medical Association, 282*(16), 1554–1560.

Jeffery, R. W., French, S. A., & Schmid, T. L. (1990). Attributions for dietary failures: Problems reported by participants in the Hypertension Prevention Trial. *Health Psychology, 9,* 315–329.

Jeffery, R. W., & Wing, R. R. (1995). Long-term effects of interventions for weight loss using food provision and monetary incentives. *Journal of Consulting and Clinical Psychology, 63,* 793–796.

Jeffery, R. W., Wing, R. R., Thorson, C., & Burton, L. R. (1998). Use of personal trainers and financial incentives to increase exercise in a behavioral weight-loss program. *Journal of Consulting and Clinical Psychology, 66*(5), 777–783.

Jeffery, R. W., Wing, R. R., Thorson, C., Burton, L. R., Raether, C., Harvey, J., & Mullen, M. (1993). Strengthening behavioral interventions for weight loss: A randomized trial of food provision and monetary incentives. *Journal of Consulting and Clinical Psychology, 61,* 1038–1045.

Kayman, S., Bruvold, W., & Stern, J. S. (1990). Maintenance and relapse after weight loss in women: Behavioral aspects. *American Journal of Clinical Nutrition, 52,* 800–807.

Kern, P. A. (1997). Potential role of TNFalpha and lipoprotein lipase as candidate genes for obesity. *Journal of Nutrition, 127*(9), 1917S–1922S.

Kern, P. A., Ong, J. M., Saffari, B., & Carty, J. (1990). The effects of weight loss on the activity and expression of adipose-tissue lipoprotein lipase in very obese humans. *New England Journal of Medicine, 322,* 1053–1059.

Kramer, F. M., Jeffery, R. W., Forster, J. L., & Snell, M. K. (1989). Long-term follow-up of behavioral treatment for obesity: Patterns of weight gain among men and women. *International Journal of Obesity, 13,* 124–136.

Kushner, R. F., & Weinsier, R. L. (2000). Evaluation of the obese patient. *Medical Clinics of North America, 84,* 387–399.

Lee, C. D., Blair, S. N., & Jackson, A. S. (1999). Cardiorespiratory fitness, body composition, and all-cause and cardiovascular mortality in men. *American Journal of Clinical Nutrition, 69,* 373–380.

Leermakers, E. A., Perri, M. G., Shigaki, C. L., & Fuller, P. R. (1999). Effects of exercise-focused versus weight-focused maintenance programs on the management of obesity. *Addictive Behaviors, 24*(2), 219–227.

Leibel, R. L., Rosenbaum, M., & Hirsch, J. (1995). Changes in energy expenditure resulting from altered body weight. *New England Journal of Medicine, 332*(10), 673–674.

McGuire, M., Wing, R., Klem, M., Lang, W., & Hill, J. (1999). What predicts weight regain in a group of successful weight losers? *Journal of Consulting and Clinical Psychology, 67*(2), 177–185.

Miller, W. R., & Rollnick, S. (1991). *Motivational interviewing.* New York: Guilford Press.

Mokdad, A. H., Serdula, M. K., Dietz, W. H., Bowman, B. A., Marks, J. S., & Koplan, J. P. (1999). The spread of the obesity epidemic in the United States. *Journal of the American Medical Association, 282,* 1519–1522.

National Heart, Lung, and Blood Institute (NHLBI). (1998). Clinical guidelines on the identification, evaluation, and treatment of overweight and obesity in adults: The evidence report. *Obesity Research, 6*(Suppl. 2), 51S–210S.

Paffenbarger, R. S., & Lee, I. M. (1996). Physical activity and fitness for health and longevity. *Research Quarterly for Exercise and Sport, 67,* 11–28.

Pavlou, K. N., Krey, S., & Steffee, W. P. (1989). Exercise as an adjunct to weight loss and maintenance in moderately obese subjects. *American Journal of Clinical Nutrition, 49,* 1115–1123.

Perri, M. G. (1998). The maintenance of treatment effects in the long-term management of obesity. *Clinical Psychology: Science and Practice, 5*(4), 526–543.

Perri, M. G., & Fuller, P. R. (1995). Success and failure in the treatment of obesity: Where do we go from here? *Medicine, Exercise, Nutrition, and Health, 4,* 255–272.

Perri, M. G., Martin, A. D., Leermakers, E. A., Sears, S. F., & Notelovitz, M. (1997). Effects of group- versus home-based exercise in the treatment of obesity. *Journal of Consulting and Clinical Psychology, 65,* 278–285.

Perri, M. G., McAdoo, W. G., McAllister, D. A., Lauer, J. B., Jordan, R. C., Yancey, D. Z., & Nezu, A. M. (1987). Effects of peer support and therapist contact on long-term weight loss. *Journal of Consulting and Clinical Psychology, 55,* 615–617.

Perri, M. G., McAdoo, W. G., McAllister, D. A., Lauer, J. B., & Yancey, D. Z. (1986). Enhancing the efficacy of behavior therapy for obesity: Effects of aerobic exercise and a multicomponent maintenance program. *Journal of Consulting and Clinical Psychology, 54,* 670–675.

Perri, M. G., McAdoo, W. G., Spevak, P. A., & Newlin, D. B. (1984). Effect of a multi-component maintenance program on long-term weight loss. *Journal of Consulting and Clinical Psychology, 52,* 480–481.

Perri, M. G., McAllister, D. A., Gange, J. J., Jordan, R. C., McAdoo, W. G., & Nezu, A. M. (1988). Effects of four maintenance programs on the long-term management of obesity. *Journal of Consulting and Clinical Psychology, 56,* 529–534.

Perri, M. G., Nezu, A. M., Patti, E. T., & McCann, K. L. (1989). Effect of length of treatment on weight loss. *Journal of Consulting and Clinical Psychology, 57,* 450–452.

Perri, M. G., Nezu, A. M., & Viegener, B. J. (1992). *Improving the long-term management of obesity: Theory, research, and clinical guidelines.* New York: Wiley.

Perri, M. G., Shapiro, R. M., Ludwig, W. W., Twentyman, C. T., & McAdoo, W. G. (1984). Maintenance strategies for the treatment of obesity: An evaluation of relapse prevention training and posttreatment contact by mail and telephone. *Journal of Consulting and Clinical Psychology, 52,* 404–413.

Pi-Sunyer, F. X. (1996). A review of long-term studies evaluating the efficacy of weight loss in ameliorating disorders associated with obesity. *Clinical Therapeutics, 18*(6), 1006–1035.

Ravussin, E., & Swinburn, B. A. (1993). Energy metabolism. In A. J. Stunkard & T. A. Wadden (Eds.), *Obesity: Theory and therapy* (2nd ed., pp. 97–124). New York: Raven Press.

Rodin, J., Schank, D., & Striegel-Moore, R. (1989). Psychological features of obesity. *Medical Clinics of North America, 73,* 47–66.

Shah, M., Hannan, P. J., & Jeffery, R. W. (1991). Secular trends in body mass index in the adult population of three communities from the upper mid-western part of the USA: The Minnesota Heart Health Program. *International Journal of Obesity, 15,* 499–503.

Sherwood, N. E., Jeffery, R. W., & Wing, R. R. (1999). Binge status as a predictor of weight loss treatment outcome. *International Journal of Obesity, 23*(5), 485–493.

Smith, D. E., Heckemeyer, C. M., Kratt, P. P., & Mason, D. A. (1997). Motivational interviewing to improve adherence to a behavioral weight-control program for older obese women with NIDDM: A pilot study. *Diabetes Care, 20*(1), 52–54.

PART V

TREATMENT OF ADULT OBESITY: ADDITIONAL APPROACHES AND RESOURCES

common disorders, has caught the attention of several national health organizations. The American Heart Association, for example, has ranked obesity as a major, modifiable risk factor for coronary heart disease, and thus as deserving of treatment by physicians. In 1998, an expert panel convened by the National Heart, Lung, and Blood Institute (NHLBI) published "Clinical Guidelines on the Identification, Evaluation, and Treatment of Overweight and Obesity in Adults: The Evidence Report," to assist health care providers and medical organizations to develop appropriate management strategies. In 2000, the *Practical Guide to the Identification, Evaluation, and Treatment of Overweight and Obesity in Adults* was published by the NHLBI and the North American Association for the Study of Obesity (NAASO), to assist the health care practitioner in the office setting. This document provides education about obesity and its treatment, along with a set of patient education and treatment materials. Most of this chapter is based on material contained in the *Practical Guide*.

ASSESSMENT OF THE OBESE PATIENT

The clinical approach to the obese patient follows two steps used in the care of any patient with a multifactorial, chronic disease: assessment and management. Assessment includes determining the degree of obesity and evaluating the overall health status of the patient. Based on the results of the assessment, decisions about management can then be made. Management includes treatment of obesity and maintenance of weight loss, as well as management of comorbid conditions. An obesity-specific approach is outlined in Table 18.1.

History and Physical Examination

The history is important for evaluating risk and deciding upon treatment. The general risk of health complications can be estimated with the information provided in Table 18.2. Risks of morbidity and mortality increase as the body mass index (BMI) increases, particularly above a value of 30 kg/m^2. Risk is increased further (in patients with a BMI of 25.0–34.9 kg/m^2) by the presence of upper-body fat patterning, which is indicative of intraabdominal (i.e., visceral) obesity. Fat patterning may be estimated by measuring the waist

TABLE 18.1. Assessment and Management of Overweight and Obese Patients

---

1. Measure height and weight. Estimate body mass index (BMI).
2. Measure waist circumference.
3. Review the patient's medical condition. Assess comorbidities:
   How many are present, and how severe are they?
   Do they need to be treated, in addition to the effort at weight loss?
4. Look for causes of obesity, including the use of medications known to cause weight gain.
5. Assess the risk of this patient's obesity, as described in Table 18.2.
6. Is the patient ready and motivated to lose weight?
7. If the patient is not ready to lose weight, urge weight maintenance and manage the complications.
8. If the patient is ready, agree with the patient on reasonable weight and activity goals and write them down.
9. Use the information gathered to develop a treatment plan based on Table 18.4.
10. Involve other professionals if necessary.
11. Do not forget that a supportive, empathic approach is necessary throughout treatment.

Note. Adapted from National Heart, Lung, and Blood Institute (NHLBI) and North American Association for the Study of Obesity (NAASO) (2000).

TABLE 18.2. Classification of Overweight and Obesity by BMI, Waist Circumference, and Associated Disease Risk

	BMI (kg/m²)	Obesity class	Disease risk[a] relative to normal weight and waist circumference	
			Men: ≤40 in (≤102 cm) Women: ≤35 in (≤88 cm)	Men: >40 in (>102 cm) Women: >35 in (<88 cm)
Underweight	<18.5		—	—
Normal[b]	18.5–24.9		—	—
Overweight	25.0–29.9		Increased	High
Obesity	30.0–34.9	I	High	Very high
	35.0–39.9	II	Very high	Very high
Extreme obesity	≥40	III	Extremely high	Extremely high

Note. Adapted from World Health Organization (1998).

[a]Disease risk for Type 2 diabetes mellitus, hypertension, and cardiovascular disease.

[b]Increased waist circumference can also be a marker for increased risk even in persons of normal weight.

circumference. Upper-body obesity is indicated by a waist over 35 inches in women and by a waist over 40 inches in men.[1]

Atkinson (Chapter 9, this volume) has provided a thorough description of the history, physical examination, and laboratory tests that should be obtained in evaluating an obese individual. The reader is referred to that chapter. I wish to underscore the importance, noted by Atkinson, of assessing a patient's medication regimen. As noted in Table 18.3, several classes of medications are associated with weight gain. Patients taking such drugs should be switched to alternative medications whenever possible.

Contraindications to Weight Reduction

In addition to identifying the etiology and complications of the patient's obesity, the history and physical examination may reveal contraindications to weight loss. A history of eating disorders, including bingeing and purging (by vomiting or laxative abuse), is a relative con-

TABLE 18.3. Drugs That May Promote Weight Gain (and Alternatives to Them)

Category	Drugs that may promote weight gain	Alternatives
Neurology and psychiatry	Antipsychotics Antidepressants Lithium Anti-epileptics	Ziprasidone Buproprion, nefazodone Topiramate, lamotrigine
Steroid hormones	Hormonal contraceptives Corticosteroids Progestational steroids	Barrier methods of contraception Nonsteroidal anti-inflammatory agents Weight loss for menometrorrhagia
Diabetes treatments	Insulin Sulfonylureas Thiazolidinediones	Metformin Acarbose, miglitol Orlistat, sibutramine
Antihistamines	Diphenhydramine, cyproheptadine, others	Newer agents, inhaled steroids
α- and β-adrenergic blockers	Propranolol, others	Angiotensin-converting enzyme inhibitors, calcium-channel blockers

WEIGHT REDUCTION OPTIONS

Behavior and Lifestyle Change

Behavioral techniques are not used alone, but in conjunction with many other approaches, including diet and exercise, medication, or surgery (NHLBI, 1998). The goal of behavior therapy is to facilitate adherence to a diet and physical activity regimen (Brownell & Wadden, 1998). Behavior therapy assumes that patterns of eating and physical activity are learned behaviors that can be changed, and that to change these patterns over the long term, the environment must be changed. In some cases lifestyle modification is administered on an individual basis, though usually it is provided in group sessions. The *Practical Guide* (NHLBI & NAASO, 2000) contains a section on the behavioral techniques that have been shown to assist with weight loss, and describes how to implement them in a primary care practice.

Exercise

Physical activity is a key component of any weight management program because of its role in increasing energy expenditure, which is reduced markedly with weight loss (Leibel, Rosenbaum, & Hirsch, 1995). Clinical studies suggest that the benefit of exercise appears to be greater in preventing weight regain than in facilitating weight loss (Pavlou, Krey & Steffe, 1989). Aerobic exercise is usually recommended for weight management because of the large number of calories burned, as well as the health benefits achieved. Strength training may also be of benefit to build lean body mass and improve body composition (Grilo, Brownell, & Stunkard, 1993). Regular adherence to an exercise program is associated with better outcome because it may also improve dietary compliance or be a marker of better dietary compliance. Exercise may improve quality of life by enhancing self-esteem, reducing stress, and relieving depression.

Any physical activity that a patient enjoys and is willing to perform is recommended. For a patient who is completely sedentary, walking is often the best way to get started. Patients with physical limitations (because of their size or arthritis) may start with water exercises, bedside stretching, seated activities, or a program designed by an exercise physiologist or physical therapist. In general, 30–45 minutes of exercise 3–5 days per week are recommended, although more exercise is better, and greater intensity may be better. No maximum amount of activity has been suggested, but generally up to 1 hour daily, with 1 day off, is reasonable. Three 10-minute periods of activity yield about the same benefit as a single 30-minute period, and adherence to such programs is better (Jakicic, Wing, Butler, & Robertson, 1995). Climbing stairs instead of taking an elevator, walking or cycling rather than taking a car, and parking further away from the entrance to a mall are simple ways to increase lifestyle activity, which has been shown to be as effective as structured exercise in maintaining weight loss (Andersen et al., 1999).

Diets

A caloric deficit must be created in order to reduce body weight. This can be achieved by giving general recommendations for healthy eating, such as reducing sugar, starch, alcohol, and saturated fat intake, or by setting calorie guidelines. No single approach to diet works for everyone; the best approach is to try to customize the diet to "solve" a patient's "problems." For example, a businesswoman who eats almost every meal in restaurants when she is on the road may benefit from a different approach than a woman who cooks all of the meals for her family. Recent findings suggest that foods with a lower glycemic index (blood glucose rise per ounce of food) may reduce food consumption later in the day (Ludwig,

2000). Foods with a lower calorie density (i.e., number of calories per ounce), such as vegetables appear to be more filling and may reduce overall food consumption (Rolls & Bell, 2000). As a result, our practice prescribes diets that derive a higher percentage of carbohydrate from vegetables and a lower percentage from starch and sugars. In general, we recommend an adequate amount of lean protein and large quantities of vegetables as the mainstay of the diet, with smaller amounts of whole grains and healthy oil sources.

Formula diets, such as OPTIFAST, can be of value to individuals who have a medical need to lose weight (National Task Force on the Prevention and Treatment of Obesity, 1993). These diets should only be administered in a medical setting by staff members familiar with their use. A minimum intake of 800 kcal/day is recommended.

Fad diets and other methods that promise quick, easy ways to lose weight distract a patient from the real task at hand. Although almost any (unhealthy) diet can reduce weight in the short run, the true test comes over the long term. Diets that are too drastic cannot be followed on a long-term basis. Unfortunately, the patient too often bears the blame for the lack of success, adding to a vicious cycle of failure. High-fat, high-protein diets represent the most recent fad. They induce short-term weight loss, but have not been shown to have long-term value, and in some patients they may induce osteoporosis, dehydration, weight gain, or a worsening of lipids. (For a fuller discussion of popular diets, see Melanson & Dwyer, Chapter 12, this volume.)

Weight Loss Medication

A growing body of evidence indicates that obesity is as much a metabolic/endocrine disorder as is diabetes, and therefore that it is equally deserving of medical and surgical management (Aronne, 1998; Bray, 1998). In general, weight loss medications help patients adhere to a reduced calorie regimen. Not every patient responds to a given medicine. If a patient loses more than 4 pounds during the first month, the prognosis for losing more than 5% of body weight is good. If not, consideration should be given to changing medication after another month of treatment. Orlistat and sibutramine (Table 18.5) are the only two drugs currently approved for long-term use by the U.S. Food and Drug Administration.

Sibutramine

Sibutramine (Meridia, Knoll Pharmaceuticals, Mount Olive, NJ) is a norepinephrine, dopamine, and serotonin reuptake inhibitor that was originally developed as an antidepressant but has been shown to be effective at reducing body weight (Bray et al., 1999). Sibu-

TABLE 18.5. Weight Loss Drugs Approved for Long-Term Use

Drug	Daily dose	Action	Adverse effects
Sibutramine (Meridia)	10 mg orally to start; may be increased to 15 mg or decreased to 5 mg	Norepinephrine, dopamine, and serotonin reuptake inhibitor	Increase in heart rate and blood pressure
Orlistat (Xenical)	120 mg orally, three times a day before meals	Inhibits pancreatic lipase, decreases fat absorption	Decrease in absorption of fat-soluble vitamins; soft stools and anal leakage

Note. Ephedrine and caffeine, mazindol, fluoxetine, and phentermine have also been tested for weight loss, but are not approved for long-term use. Herbal preparations are not recommended as part of a weight loss program; these preparations have unpredictable amounts of active ingredients, and unpredictable and potentially harmful effects. Adapted from NHLBI and NAASO (2000).

Adults (NHLBI & NAASO, 2000). (This information can also be obtained on the NHLBI Web site at http://www.nhlbi.nih.gov/nhlbi/cardio/obes/prof/guidelns/ob_home.htm.)

A comprehensive program for lifestyle modification is provided by *The LEARN Program for Weight Control* (Brownell & Wadden, 1998). It may be used on a group or individual basis, with or without medication. In some cases patients may choose to utilize commercial weight loss programs such as Weight Watchers, or self-help groups such as Overeaters Anonymous. Such care may be used to complement office visits. In cases in which patients have a serious behavioral or metabolic disorder, beyond the scope of the clinician's usual practice, referral to an obesity specialist or endocrinologist with an interest in obesity is appropriate. NAASO lists its members on its Web site, located at http://www.naaso.org.

PREPARING THE OFFICE FOR OBESE PATIENTS

Besides health care providers, office personnel can assist in the management of overweight patients by providing support and encouragement. An empathic, respectful, and positive attitude is of paramount importance. Some staff members may have negative feelings toward obese individuals. Such negative attitudes should be explored, with the goal of having all staffers treating overweight patients with respect and concern. In addition, access for disabled patients, chairs without arms, stepstools next to examination tables, large gowns and blood pressure cuffs, and a scale that can weigh all patients (including those in wheelchairs) are needed in any office in which severely obese patients will be treated.

RESPONDING TO THE OBESITY EPIDEMIC

America is now experiencing an epidemic of overweight and obesity. Public health campaigns directed at changing our toxic food environment are clearly needed to prevent the continued growth of this disorder. Primary care physicians, however, must play a greater role in treating persons who are already obese (Wadden et al., 2000). With the assistance of new treatment guidelines, weight loss medications, and a growing understanding of the etiology of this complex disorder, primary care physicians can make a difference in the prevention and management of obesity.

NOTE

1. To measure waist circumference, place a measuring tape in a horizontal plane at the level of the iliac crest, without compressing the skin. The value is read at the end of a normal expiration. Men with a waist circumference greater than 40 inches and women with a waist circumference greater than 35 inches are at higher risk because of excess abdominal fat and should be considered one risk category above that defined by their BMI (NHLBI, 1998).

REFERENCES

Andersen, R. E., Wadden, T. A., Bartlett, S. J., Zemel, B. S., Verde, T. J., & Franckowiak, S. C. (1999). Effects of lifestyle activity vs. structured aerobic exercise in obese women: A randomized trial. *Journal of the American Medical Association, 281,* 335–340.

Aronne, L. J. (1998). Modern medical management of obesity: The role of pharmaceutical intervention. *Journal of the American Dietetic Association, 98*(10, Suppl. 2), S23–S26.

Blackburn, G. (1995). Effect of degree of weight loss on health benefits. *Obesity Research, 3*(Suppl. 2), 211S–216S.

Boozer, C. N., Leibel, R., Love, R. J., Cha, M. C., & Aronne, L. J. (2001). Synergy of leptin and sibutramine in treatment of dietary obesity in rats. *Metabolism, 50*(8), 889–893.

Bray, G. A. (1998). *Contemporary diagnosis and management of obesity.* Newton, PA: Handbooks in Health Care.

Bray, G. A., Blackburn, G. L., Ferguson, J. M., Greenway, F. L., Jain, A. K., Mendel, C. M., Mendels, J., Ryan, D. H., Schwartz, S. L., Scheinbaum, M. L., & Seaton, T. B. (1999). Sibutramine produces dose-related weight loss. *Obesity Research, 7*(2), 189–198.

Bray, G. A., & Greenway, F. L. (1999). Current and potential drugs for treatment of obesity. *Endocrine Reviews, 20,* 805–875.

Brownell, K. D., & Wadden, T. A. (1998). *The LEARN program for weight control: Special medication addition.* Dallas, TX: American Health.

Campfield, L. A., Smith, F. J., & Burn, P. (1998). Strategies and potential molecular targets for obesity treatment. *Science, 280*(5368), 1383–1387.

Davidson, M. H., Hauptman, J., DiGirolamo, M., Foreyt, J. P., Halsted, C. H., Heber, D., Heimburger, D. C., Lucas, C. P., Robbins, D. C., Chung, J., & Heymsfield, S. B. (1999). Weight control and risk factor reduction in obese subjects treated for 2 years with orlistat: A randomized controlled trial. *Journal of the American Medical Association, 281*(3), 235–242.

Foster, G. D., Wadden, T. A., Vogt, R. A., & Brewer, G. (1997). What is a reasonable weight loss?: Patients' expectations and evaluations of obesity treatment outcomes. *Journal of Consulting and Clinical Psychology, 65,* 79–85.

Frank, A. (1993). Futility and avoidance: Medical professionals in the treatment of obesity. *Journal of the American Medical Association, 269,* 2132–2133.

Grilo, C. M., Brownell, K. D., & Stunkard, A. J. (1993). The metabolic and psychological importance of exercise in weight control. In A. J. Stunkard & T. A. Wadden (Eds.), *Obesity: Theory and therapy* (2nd ed., pp. 253–273). New York: Raven Press.

Jakicic, J. M., Wing, R. R., Butler, B. A., & Robertson, R. J. (1995). Prescribing exercise in multiple short bouts versus one continuous bout: Effects on adherence, cardiorespiratory fitness, and weight loss in overweight women. *International Journal of Obesity, 19,* 893–901.

Kral, J. G. (1998). Surgical treatment of obesity. In G. A. Bray, C. Bouchard, & W. P. T. James (Eds.), *Handbook of obesity* (pp. 977–993). New York: Marcel Dekker.

Leibel, R. L., Rosenbaum, M., & Hirsch, J. (1995). Changes in energy expenditure resulting from altered body weight. *New England Journal of Medicine, 332*(10), 621–628.

Ludwig, D. S. (2000). Dietary glycemic index and obesity. *Journal of Nutrition, 130*(Suppl. 2), 280S–283S.

National Institutes of Health. (1992). Gastrointestinal surgery for severe obesity: NIH Consensus Development Conference consensus statement, 1991, March 25–27. *American Journal of Clinical Nutrition, 55*(2 Suppl), 615S–619S.

National Heart, Lung, and Blood Institute (NHLBI). (1998). Clinical guidelines on the identification, evaluation, and treatment of overweight and obesity in adults: The evidence report. *Obesity Research, 6*(Suppl. 2), 51S–210S.

National Heart, Lung, and Blood Institute (NHLBI) & North American Association for the Study of Obesity (NAASO). (2000). *Practical guide to the identification, evaluation, and treatment of overweight and obesity in adults.* Bethesda, MD: National Institutes of Health.

National Task Force on the Prevention and Treatment of Obesity. (1993). Very low calorie diets. *Journal of the American Medical Association, 270,* 967–974.

Pavlou, K. N., Krey, S., & Steffe, W. P. (1989). Exercise as an adjunct to weight loss and maintenance in moderately obese subjects. *American Journal of Clinical Nutrition, 49*(5, Suppl.), 1115–1123.

Porte, D., Jr., Seeley, R. J., Woods, S. C., Baskin, D. G., Figlewicz, D. P., & Schwartz, M. W. (1998). Obesity, diabetes and the central nervous system. *Diabetologia, 41*(8), 863–881.

tion, we examine self-help approaches such as Overeaters Anonymous (OA), Take Off Pounds Sensibly (TOPS), and the Trevose Behavior Modification Program. Features of supermarket self-help products, such as SlimFast, are distinguished from those of traditional self-help programs. The chapter concludes with a discussion of research needs in this area and likely trends in this field.

WEIGHT LOSS PROGRAMS AND THE FTC

In 1990, Congressman Ron Wyden of Oregon initiated hearings on the purportedly misleading and deceptive advertising practices of the commercial weight loss industry ("Memorandum from Subcommittee Staff to Congressman Ron Wyden," 1990). Industry claims that consumers would lose weight and keep it off were found to be wholly unsubstantiated. Moreover, such claims were contradicted by the results of university-based clinical trials, which found that even with the most successful interventions, obese individuals regained one-third to one-half of their weight loss in the year following treatment (Wadden & Bell, 1990). The hearings revealed that consumers who desperately wanted to lose weight were easy targets for this largely unregulated industry. Testimony of several individuals revealed that, rather than losing weight, they had lost their money and hope.

The congressional hearings led the FTC to step up its monitoring of the weight loss industry's advertising practices (FTC, 1997). Consent decrees (i.e., legally binding settlement agreements) were filed between the FTC and several major commercial weight loss programs (FTC, 1997). Companies agreed to stop airing their questionable advertisements and were required to provide data to support claims of long-term weight loss. In addition, testimonials by successful program participants had to be accompanied by disclaimers that the results reported might not be typical (FTC, 1997). These actions effectively muted the brash advertising claims of the late 1980s.

Believing that these measures did not go far enough, in 1996 the Center for Science in the Public Interest petitioned the FTC to initiate rule making that would legally require commercial programs to disclose data concerning the safety and efficacy (i.e., weight loss) of their interventions (FTC, 1997). Efforts to enact such legislation would have been contentious, costly, and years in the making. Thus, in 1997, as an alternative, the FTC assembled a panel that included members from academia, industry, consumer advocacy groups, the National Institutes of Health, and the FTC to explore the creation of voluntary guidelines for the disclosure of information concerning weight loss programs.

The panel recommended that commercial weight loss programs provide information concerning the safety and costs of their programs, as well as the credentials of program staff (FTC, 1997). The panel could not reach agreement concerning disclosure of program effectiveness, as measured by short- and long-term changes in weight, risk factors, health-related behaviors, and other parameters. Researchers and consumer advocates argued that it was critical for programs to report at least short-term weight losses and the percentage of participants who completed treatment. Industry representatives, however, responded that they did not have the resources or expertise to provide such data.

Based on the recommendations of the panel, the Partnership for Healthy Weight Management was formed, with voluntary membership open to interested parties from industry, academia, consumer groups, and government agencies. In February 1999, the Partnership issued its *Voluntary Guidelines for Providers of Weight Loss Products or Services*. The *Voluntary Guidelines* specify the content of the information that should be provided to prospective patients/clients and the tone of the disclosure, which should encourage consumers to ask questions (Partnership for Healthy Weight Management, 1999). Table 19.1

TABLE 19.1. Voluntary Guidelines for Providers of Weight Loss Products or Services

Criteria	Description
A. Staff qualifications and central components of the program	• Program content and goals • Staff's weight management training, experience, certification, and education
B. Risks associated with overweight and obesity	• Obesity is associated with increased risk of heart disease, diabetes, stroke, etc. • Moderate weight loss (5%–10% of initial body weight) can reduce risks • Weight loss can cause physical changes in the body that are indicative of more serious conditions (e.g., dizziness, interruptions in the menstrual cycle, hair loss), and patients experiencing such changes should talk to their primary care physician immediately
C. Risks associated with the provider's product or program	• Risks associated with any drugs, devices, dietary supplements, exercise plans provided in the course of the program or treatment • Rapid weight loss (>3 pounds/week or >0.5% body weight/week) may cause increased risk of developing gallbladder disease • Very-low-calorie diets (<800 kcal/day) are designed for rapid weight loss in morbidly obese individuals and are medically supervised to minimize risks associated with rapid weight loss
D. Program costs	• Fixed costs (administrative, entry, or renewal fees, etc.) • Periodic costs (weekly attendance fees, mandatory food purchases, etc.) • Optional costs (optional maintenance program, fees for reentering program) • Any refundable costs

Note. Adapted from Partnership for Healthy Weight Management (1999).

summarizes the information that providers should make available to help consumers identify the program that best meets their needs.

NONMEDICAL COMMERCIAL WEIGHT LOSS PROGRAMS

Nonmedical commercial weight loss programs are very popular with consumers. They vary widely in their approaches, but generally focus on diet, exercise, and lifestyle modification. Materials used in the programs are often designed by physicians, psychologists, nutritionists, or exercise physiologists, but treatment is usually conducted by laypeople trained by these companies. Medical care is not provided by these programs, which makes them less attractive to persons with Type 2 diabetes mellitus or other conditions that require physician supervision during weight loss. Although medical care can be coordinated with a patient's physician, nonmedical commercial programs are usually most appropriate for overweight or obese individuals who do not have significant health problems. With the exception of Weight Watchers, there are few empirical data on the short- or long-term effectiveness of nonmedical commercial programs. Thus most of what follows is a description of the programs' treatment components.

Weight Watchers

Weight Watchers International is the world's largest commercial weight loss program and is a member of the Partnership for Healthy Weight Management. Since its establishment in

During the initial weight loss phase, clients meet with a counselor at least three times a week. They are prescribed a meal plan by the company's registered dietitian. The plan provides 1,100–1,900 kcal/day, depending on a client's weight, age, sex, and medical conditions. Clients are told to focus on serving and portion sizes in six different food categories (i.e., protein, vegetables, starches, fruits, fat, and dairy) and are told to eat specific foods in each category (e.g., they can eat pears but not grapes). L.A. Weight Loss recommends that clients consume two 200-kcal supplements per day with meals. These soy-based supplements are called L.A. Lites. No specific exercise program is recommended by the program. Clients follow their meal plan until they reach their goal weight. After reaching this weight, they enter the 6-week "stabilization" period, in which calories and foods are adjusted for weight maintenance. During this phase, clients are also told to expand the variety of foods they eat.

Outcome Data

Similar to Jenny Craig, L.A. Weight Loss has no published data to demonstrate its safety or efficacy.

Nutrisystem.com

Nutri/System, Inc., was established in 1972 as a comprehensive commercial weight loss center. The company has used a number of weight loss methods over the years, including very-low-calorie diets (VLCDs), prepackaged conventional foods, and medication (i.e., fenfluramine–phentermine). The company filed for bankruptcy in 1993 and reemerged as nutrisystem.com in 1999, an entirely online weight management service (Key, 2000). Since that time, reportedly over 150,000 people have joined nutrisystem.com. The only costs associated with the program are those for the food. For $49.95, members can purchase a week's supply of food on-line that will be delivered to their home (nutrisystem.com, 2000). These portion-controlled meal packages contain 1,200–1,500 kcal/day (three meals per day, 7 days per week).

The program offers free, online, real-time counseling sessions with a company-trained counselor. A registered dietitian is on call during counseling visits to answer any nutrition questions. Clients can request that a health and fitness instructor design a personal exercise program. It appears that nutrisystem.com may be a precursor to what will become a deluge of Internet sites that offer weight management services (as discussed later).

Outcome Data

An early study by Pavlou and colleagues (1989) randomly assigned 49 overweight women to either exercise or no-exercise conditions. Participants were instructed to follow a 1,000-kcal/day diet using foods provided by Nutri/System. After 8 weeks, participants who exercised lost 10.9% of initial body weight, compared to 7.9% those who did not exercise. The difference between groups was not significantly different.

Interpretation of Findings

Consumption of the portion-controlled Nutri/System diet was associated with weight loss regardless of exercise condition. It is not clear, however, whether dieters who consumed the foods now sold by nutrisystem.com would achieve the same results, particularly in the absence of participating in a structured weight loss trial.

MEDICALLY BASED PROPRIETARY WEIGHT LOSS PROGRAMS

Medically based proprietary weight loss programs reached the height of their popularity in the late 1980s and have traditionally combined the use of a VLCD, providing 400–800 kcal/day, with a multidisciplinary program of lifestyle modification. These programs, which are supervised by physicians, require patients to undergo a thorough medical evaluation before treatment and usually biweekly examinations during the period of rapid weight loss (National Task Force on the Prevention and Treatment of Obesity, 1993).

VLCDs are recommended for patients with a BMI $\geq$ 30 kg/m^2 who are free of medical contraindications, as described elsewhere (National Task Force, 1993; Wadden & Bartlett, 1992). These diets usually provide 70–100 g/day of protein, 50–100 g/day of carbohydrate, and small amounts of fat. The diets may be consumed as either lean meat, fish, and fowl (in which case they are known as a "protein-sparing modified fast") or as powdered protein mixed with water. The liquid diets include the recommended daily allowance for vitamins and minerals, and may be consumed in lieu of all meals and snacks. VLCDs are generally safe when used by appropriate persons under medical supervision for periods up to 16 weeks (National Task Force, 1993). The diets are, however, associated with an increased risk of gallstones—a complication that can be prevented by the use of ursodeoxycholic acid (Broomfield et al., 1988).

Several randomized trials found that patients treated with a VLCD lost approximately 15%–20% of their initial weight during 8–12 weeks of treatment (Wadden, Foster, & Letizia, 1994; Wadden & Stunkard, 1986; Wing, Blair, Marcus, Epstein, & Harvey, 1994; Wing et al., 1991). This loss was approximately twice that produced during the same period by a diet providing 1,200–1,500 kcal/day. Patients treated by VLCDs regained approximately 35%–50% of their weight loss in the year following treatment. Short-term weight loss was accompanied by reductions in blood pressure, serum cholesterol levels, and blood glucose levels. These improvements, however, tended to dissipate with weight regain, with the possible exception of glycemic control in diabetic women (Wing et al., 1991).

OPTIFAST Program

OPTIFAST has reportedly been used by over 700,000 patients since its introduction in 1974. It is manufactured by Novartis Nutrition Corporation, which is a member of the Partnership for Healthy Weight Management. The costs of the program vary, depending on the type of diet and length of treatment, but typically range from approximately $1,500 to $3,000 (Novartis Nutrition Corporation, 2000).

For the initial phase of treatment (8–16 weeks), patients are prescribed approximately 800 kcal/day to be consumed as a liquid diet, with the optional use of food bars. Each serving of the liquid diet provides 14 g of protein, 20 g of carbohydrate, and 3 g of fat. Patients attend weekly group lifestyle modification classes of 60–90 minutes. During the second phase, conventional foods are gradually reintroduced, after which patients enter the third phase—weight maintenance. This last phase is not time-limited.

Outcome Data

The safety and efficacy of the OPTIFAST Program have been extensively assessed (Barrows & Snook, 1987; Doherty et al., 1991; Wadden, Foster, Letizia, & Stunkard, 1992). We focus here on short- and long-term change in weight. An 18-site evaluation of 517 participants who enrolled in the 26-week OPTIFAST Core Program showed that 54% of men and 56% of women completed the full program. Men and women who completed treatment lost an average of 32.1 and 22.0 kg, respectively, compared with 20.0 and 14.3 kg, respectively, for men and women who did not complete the program. A 1-year follow-up evaluation of 118 patients showed that they maintained 15.3 kg of their original 24.8-kg weight loss (Wadden et al., 1992).

A separate 3- to 5-year follow-up evaluation of participants treated with the OPTIFAST Core Program revealed a familiar pattern of weight regain (Wadden & Frey, 1997). At 3 years, for example, men had regained 20.2 kg of their original 34.3-kg end-of-treatment weight loss, while women had gained 14.1 kg of their 23.7-kg weight loss. A more encouraging view of the findings resulted when the data were examined in terms of the number of patients who maintained a 5% reduction in initial weight, the criterion for success proposed by the Institute of Medicine (1995) expert panel. At the 3-year follow-up, fully 73.3% of men and 55.1% of women maintained a loss of 5%.

Interpretation of Findings

As with the long-term data reported by Weight Watchers, these findings must be interpreted with caution, because they are likely to represent a "best-case scenario." The 566 patients evaluated at the 3-year follow-up represented only 44% of the 1,283 patients who originally enrolled in the programs. Patients who did not participate in the follow-up probably regained more weight than those who participated.

Health Management Resources

Since its introduction in 1983, HMR, which is also a member of the Partnership for Healthy Weight Management, has reportedly treated over 500,000 patients in medical settings and thousands of employees in corporate settings (HMR, 1999). HMR is a medically supervised weight loss program with three major dietary options, which include a VLCD (520 kcal/day), a low-calorie diet (800 kcal/day), and a Healthy Solutions diet (1,000–1,600 kcal/day). All three diets use shakes and bars; however, the Healthy Solutions diet adds a minimum of five servings of fruits and vegetables per day. All patients attend weekly 90-minute behavioral group sessions that provide lifestyle skills for weight management; they are also encouraged to exercise so as to expend a minimum of 2,000 kcal/week. A long-term maintenance program is also available.

Costs of the HMR program vary, depending upon which program the patient joins, the length of treatment, and the level of medical supervision required. In general, costs range from $150 to $250/week, including induction fees, weekly classes, educational materials, behavioral counseling, supplements, and all weight loss foods. The maintenance program averages $95/month.

Outcome Data

Numerous studies have demonstrated the efficacy and safety of HMR (Anderson, Brinkman, & Hamilton, 1992; Anderson, Hamilton, & Brinkman-Kaplan, 1992; Anderson, Vichitbandra, Qian, & Kryscio, 1999). A study of 154 participants who completed the HMR 12-week standard program, and were encouraged to participate in the maintenance program, revealed an average weight loss of 29.7 kg (Anderson et al., 1999). Participants maintained an average of 26.6% ($n = 76$), 22% ($n = 38$), 19.9% ($n = 15$), 18.5% ($n = 42$), and 17.9% ($n = 32$) of their weight loss after 3, 4, 5, 6, and 7 years, respectively. The percentages of patients who maintained a 5% reduction in initial weight were 50.4%, 61.8%,

40%, 49.2%, and 34.7% at these five assessments, respectively. These percentages were similar for males and females.

Interpretation of Findings

These findings, similar to those for the OPTIFAST Program, must be interpreted with caution because they probably represent a "best-case scenario." The 32 patients who participated in the 7-year follow-up represented only 7.5% of the 426 patients who originally enrolled in the program. Clearly, the long-term weight losses for this small minority of patients are likely to be greater than those for the typical participant.

RESIDENTIAL PROGRAMS

Residential weight loss programs are typically administered by a multidisciplinary team which provides nutrition, exercise, lifestyle, and medical management. Patients can stay in the programs for as brief or as long a period as they like. These programs are typically very expensive.

Duke Diet and Fitness Center

The mission of the Duke Diet and Fitness Center (DFC), which opened in 1969, is to assist people with weight loss, disease management, and lifestyle change. The DFC offers programs of varying length, with costs totaling $3,095 for 1 week of the full program. This fee does not include housing. Each program begins with a full medical evaluation. A registered dietitian meets with each patient to develop a personal nutrition intervention. Staff members also meet with each patient to create a personalized exercise program based on the patient's baseline activity level and performance on a stress test. A typical day at the DFC includes three meals. Meditation, yoga, fitness classes, and lectures (e.g., nutrition, strategies for healthy eating) are interspersed throughout the day. Weight loss medication may be used as an adjunct to treatment (DFC, 2000).

Outcome Data

A literature review did not reveal any published studies that evaluated the safety or efficacy of the Duke DFC. However, a DFC program brochure indicated that research is currently being conducted to study weight loss and weight maintenance.

Pritikin Program

The Pritikin Longevity Center and Spa has served over 70,000 participants since 1976. This center advocates healthy eating by specifically monitoring fat ($\leq$10% of total kilocalories/day), protein (10%–20% of kilocalories/day), carbohydrate (70%–80% of kilocalories/day), cholesterol (<100 mg/day), fiber ($\geq$35 g/day), sodium ($\leq$1,600 mg/day), and refined sweetener (<5% of kilocalories/day) rather than focusing on total calorie intake. As at the DFC, patients receive an initial health evaluation that consists of a physical exam, history, and biochemical profile. Patients also receive a stress test, which is used to create a safe, individualized exercise program. Educational, interactive workshops that cover such topics as planning meals, eating out, shopping for food, and managing stress are also of-

ings at which they are instructed in behavioral techniques for weight loss, such as recording food intake and physical activity. Upon joining the program, members choose an ultimate weight loss goal, and in an initial 5-week trial period they must achieve at least 15% of this goal. Attendance is mandatory during this trial period. If these goals are not met, the member will not be accepted as a Full Member. Members are given very specific weight loss and attendance requirements for the duration of the program. Failure to meet these requirements results in dismissal from the program (Latner et al., 2000).

Outcome Data

A recent study assessed the effectiveness of the Trevose Behavior Modification Program in people who became Full Members (*n* = 171) in 1992–1993 (Latner et al., 2000). At the end of 2 years, 47.4% of members remained in the program, falling to 21.6% at the end of 5 years. Average weight losses at these two times were 17.9 kg and 15.7 kg, respectively.

Interpretation of Findings

Results of the Trevose Program rival those produced by medically supervised VLCDs, and clearly win when it comes to cost. The data, however, must be interpreted with caution because of participant self-selection: Participants had to be highly motivated in order to be admitted to the program. In addition, attrition by 5 years was high. Latner and colleagues (2000) concluded (and we agree) that this approach provides an excellent option for long-term weight management at a very affordable cost. Replication of these results would have important implications for treating obesity in community settings.

Bibliotherapy

Self-help is also available in the form of manuals, such as *The LEARN Program for Weight Management 2000* (Brownell, 2000), and hundreds of diet books. These publications vary widely in the type of diet and amount of exercise prescribed. An early study examined the effectiveness of bibliotherapy in general, and assigned 89 undergraduates to one of four groups: (1) weekly group behavior modification with a weight loss manual; (2) weekly weight loss lessons from the manual mailed to participants; (3) weekly group behavior modification with relaxation training; and (4) a no-treatment control. The three treatment groups lost significantly more weight (6.8, 5.4, and 5.4 kg, respectively) than the control group (0.8 kg) over the 10-week study (Hagen, 1974). The results suggest that manualized self-help treatments may be effective.

The LEARN Program for Weight Management

The LEARN Program is a 16-week weight loss program that is described in a 312-page manual. As described by Brownell (2000), the manual may be used on a self-help or professional basis; in the latter case, the dieter would follow the manual as part of an individual or group treatment program. The LEARN Program suggests that women consume approximately 1,200 kcal/day and men 1,500 kcal/day. Dieters are encouraged to eat what they want, but to do so in moderation and to record their food intake. Readers are instructed to exercise as many days a week as possible. The manual addresses many weight loss topics, such as nutrition, eating in restaurants, slowing the rate of eating, and serving foods; it costs $27.95.

Several studies found that when the LEARN Program was used as part of a weekly group behavior modification program, patients lost approximately 7–10 kg of initial weight in 16–26 weeks (Brownell, Heckerman, Westlake, Hayes, & Monti, 1978; Brownell & Stunkard, 1981; Wadden et al., 1994). These favorable results stand in contrast to those obtained with the LEARN Program when patients were provided with the manual but did not attend weekly lifestyle modification classes. Wing, Vendetti, Jakicic, Polley, and Lang (1998) found that patients lost only 1.5 kg after 6 months when provided with the manual alone. By comparison, participants who were provided with a traditional group behavior modification program lost 10.3 kg. Those findings suggest that weekly group meetings enhance patients' adherence to the diet and exercise regimens prescribed by LEARN and similar programs. Several patients we have treated have indicated that the weekly "weigh-in" is a significant motivator.

Self-Help Diet Books

In addition to self-help manuals, hundreds of diet books are available at bookstores. Authors often make outlandish claims in hopes of creating the next best-seller. They are free to make unsubstantiated claims concerning their programs because of their First Amendment rights (i.e., freedom of speech and of the press). For example, the back cover of *Dr. Atkins' New Diet Revolution* (Atkins, 1999) tells readers that by joining the new diet revolution, they can learn "how the Atkins diet can help you reduce major health problems, how the Atkins diet can protect your heart, and why eating rich, delicious gourmet foods can be your path to permanent weight loss." Data on the safety and efficacy of these programs are rarely provided. It is unfortunate that millions of people who are desperately seeking to lose weight are lured by unsubstantiated weight loss claims. In Chapter 12 of this volume, Melanson and Dwyer discuss bibliotherapy and other popular diets consumers use for weight management.

SUPERMARKET SELF-HELP

Supermarket self-help for weight loss emphasizes reducing calorie intake. Portion-controlled, low-calorie/low-fat meals or liquid meal replacements may be purchased at local supermarkets without joining a weight loss program. Consumers are free to choose the number of portion-controlled meals they eat per day or per week, as well as the number of weeks they choose to diet.

SlimFast

The SlimFast Food Company was founded in the late 1970s and is a member of the Partnership for Healthy Weight Management. SlimFast products provide meal replacements in the form of drinks or bars, which generally contain 220 kcal/serving and are made from fat-free milk. These meal replacements contain no drugs, stimulants, or appetite suppressants. The SlimFast Plan instructs consumers to use SlimFast in place of breakfast and lunch and to eat a balanced dinner. Calorie intake should total at least 1,200 kcal/day and induce a loss of 1–2 pounds (0.5–1 kg) per week. For weight maintenance, SlimFast recommends replacing one meal per day instead of two (Slimfast, 2000).

Outcome Data

In a multicenter study (*n* = 301), women who consumed SlimFast twice a day for 12 weeks lost 6.3 kg and men 8.3 kg (Heber, Ashley, Wang, & Elashoff, 1994). After the initial 12 weeks, participants (*n* = 273) entered the 2-year maintenance phase, in which they used

heartening finding, in view of the call for programs to provide data on their results of treatment. The largest number of studies have been conducted on the use of VLCDs (i.e., the HMR and OPTIFAST programs). Participants in these programs are likely to lose 15%–20% of their initial weight, although they will pay a substantial price and will have difficulty maintaining their full end-of-treatment weight loss. By contrast, there has been little research on the effectiveness of residential programs, despite the high cost of such interventions. We were pleased to find outcome data on two of the nation's most widely used approaches—Weight Watchers and SlimFast. Both would appear to be potentially beneficial to participants, as suggested by findings of a 5%–10% reduction in initial weight. This loss was largely maintained at 51 months in the SlimFast study (Flechtner-Mors et al., 2000).

Selecting a Self-Help or Commercial Weight Loss Program

Table 19.2 provides an algorithm for identifying a self-help or commercial weight loss program. The algorithm is based on our review of the literature and considers such factors as demonstrated efficacy and cost. Recommendations are based on a patient's BMI and risk of health complications. As a general rule, the greater the BMI and attendant health complications, the greater the individual's need to reduce. Patients are encouraged to try the least intensive/expensive intervention first before progressing to the next option. Given the very limited data on self-help and commercial programs, these recommendations must be considered tentative.

Similar to the algorithm developed by the NHLBI (1998) expert panel, the goal for persons with a BMI < 25 kg/m² is prevention of weight gain. Individuals with a BMI of 25–26.9 kg/m² who already have weight-related health complications are encouraged to increase their physical activity and decrease their calorie intake, by as much as 500 kcal/day. Use of a weight loss book or manual, such as *The LEARN Program for Weight Management 2000* (Brownell, 2000), may facilitate this effort. The goal is to lose approximately 5% of initial weight.

Persons with a BMI ≤ 27 kg/m² are advised to consult with their physicians to assess their physical health and review the full range of treatment options available, including pharmacotherapy. Those with a BMI of 27–29 kg/m² who have health complications are

TABLE 19.2. Algorithm for Selecting a Self-Help or Commercial Weight Loss Program

Intervention	Body mass index (BMI) category				
	<25	25–26.9	27–29.9	30–34.9	≥35.0
Prevention of weight gain	+	+	+	+	+
Self-directed exercise and diet (<500-kcal/day deficit)		With comorbidities	+	+	+
Weight loss book or manual		With comorbidities	+	+	+
Self-directed portion-controlled diet (500- to 1,000-kcal/day deficit)			With comorbidities	+	+
Self-help or commercial program			With comorbidities	+	+
Medically supervised low-calorie diet				With comorbidities	+

encouraged to increase their physical activity and to decrease their calorie intake by 500–1,000 kcal/day. Use of a portion-controlled diet, such as SlimFast, may help achieve this dietary goal. Two self-help programs, TOPS and OA, are recommended for persons who seek education and/or social support; the latter program may be better for "emotional eaters." Among commercial programs, Weight Watchers provides a sound program of diet and activity for approximately $12/week. Regardless of the approach selected, the goal is to lose approximately 5%–10% of initial weight.

Persons with a BMI ≤ 30 kg/m^2 who have obesity-related health complications (and have not lost weight via the above-described approaches) may wish to consider a medically supervised program. In place of a VLCD, however, we recommend consumption of a low-calorie diet ($\leq$1,000 kcal/day) that combines three or four servings/day of a liquid diet with an evening meal of food (Wadden et al., 1997). This approach induces a loss of approximately 15% of initial weight in 12 weeks and does not require the same intensity of medical monitoring as a VLCD, thus reducing costs. Nonetheless, such programs are likely to cost at least $1,500, and patients typically regain 35%–40% of their weight in the year following treatment. Thus patients must understand the need for a program of weight loss maintenance, which could include the use of pharmacotherapy (Apfelbaum et al., 1999).

The practitioner should encourage patients to shop around for a program and to select one that is consistent with their needs and preferences. The *Voluntary Guidelines for Providers of Weight Loss Products or Services* (Partnership for Healthy Weight Management, 1999) should be helpful in this regard.

Future Research

Presentation of Data

We strongly encourage all weight loss providers to collect and publicize their results of treatment. We believe, like the Center for Science in the Public Interest, that disclosure should include short- and long-term weight losses. Descriptive data are likely to be the most useful to consumers. For example, commercial weight loss programs could report the average number of sessions that enrollees attended; their weight loss and changes in any other health outcomes (blood pressure, cholesterol, etc.) at the time of discontinuation; and the total costs of goods and services. Such data should be collected on a random national sample of 500–1,000 participants. Table 19.3 provides an example of the type of data that might be published by the fictitious "Easy-Off Weight Loss Program." In addition to presenting the average values (and the range of values), providers could also present the results for the top third of participants. As shown in the example, although participants in the Easy-Off Program typically attended only 4.3 treatment visits and lost only 5.1 pounds, those in the top third had 14.7 visits and lost 16.5 pounds. These findings would alert consumers that they could lose more weight (than the average) if they attended more sessions. Consumers could also determine at the outset whether they could afford to attend 10 or more sessions to achieve a larger loss.

Ecological Validity

In assessing the results of weight loss programs or products, industry providers are encouraged to use an ecologically valid study design that will test programs or products in the same conditions in which the public will use them. Such studies differ from clinical trials, which impose more rigorous control over the study participants and provide more professional contact than participants will receive when they diet on their own. For example, in

Levitz, L. S., & Stunkard, A. J. (1974). A therapeutic coalition for obesity: Behavior modification and patient self-help. *American Journal of Psychiatry, 131*(4), 423–427.

Lowe, M. R., Miller-Kovach, K., Frye, N., & Phelan, S. P. (1999). An initial evaluation of a commercial weight loss program: Short-term effects on weight, eating behavior, and mood. *Obesity Research, 7*(1), 51–59.

Malenbaum, R., Herzog, D., Eisenthal, S., & Wyshak, G. (1988). Overeaters Anonymous: Impact on bulimia. *International Journal of Eating Disorders, 7*(1), 139–143.

Memorandum from Subcommittee Staff to Congressman Ron Wyden, March 1, 1990. (1990, March 22). *News from Congressman Wyden,* pp. 185–194.

Metz, J. A., Kris-Etherton, P. M., Morris, C. D., Mustad, V. A., Stern, J. S., Oparil, S., Chait, A., Haynes, R. B., Resnick, L. M., Clark, S., Hatton, D. C., McMahon, M., Holcomb, S., Snyder, G. W., Pi-Sunyer, F. X., & McCarron, D. A. (1997). Dietary compliance and cardiovascular risk reduction with a prepared meal plan compared with a self-selected diet. *American Journal of Clinical Nutrition, 66,* 373–385.

Morris, R. D., & Rimm, A. A. (1992). Long-term weight fluctuation and non-insulin-dependent diabetes mellitus in white women. *Annals of Epidemiology, 2*(5), 657–664.

National Heart, Lung, and Blood Institute (NHLBI). (1998). Clinical guidlines on the identification, evaluation, and treatment of overweight and obesity in adults: The evidence report. *Obesity Research, 6*(Suppl.), 51S–210S.

National Task Force on the Prevention and Treatment of Obesity. (1993). Very low calorie diets. *Journal of the American Medical Association, 270,* 967–974.

Novartis Nutrition Corporation. (2000). Health care provider information. In *OPTIFAST: A medical weight management program* [Online]. Available: http://www.optifast.com/healthcare/index.html [2000, April 1].

nutrisystem. com. (2000). The nutrisystem.com membership. In *nutrisystem.com* [Online]. Available: http://www.nutrisystem.com/tour/ [2000, April, 10].

Overeaters Anonymous (OA). (1996). *Overeaters Anonymous* [Online]. Available: http://www.oa.org [2000, April 1].

Partnership for Healthy Weight Management. (1999). *Voluntary guidelines for providers of weight loss products or services.* Washington, DC: Federal Trade Commission.

Pavlou, K. N., Whatley, J. E., Jannace, P. W., DiBartolomeo, J. J., Burrows, B. A., Duthie, E. A. M., & Lerman, R. H. (1989). Physical activity as a supplement to a weight-loss dietary regimen. *American Journal of Clinical Nutrition, 49,* 1110–1114.

Pritikin Longevity Center. (2000). *Pritikin Longevity Center homepage* [Online]. Available: http://www.pritikin.com [2000, April 19].

Rippe, J. M., Price, J. M., Hess, S. A., Kline, G., DeMers, K. A., Damitz, S., Kreidieh, I., & Freedson, P. (1998). Improved psychological well-being, quality of life, and health practices in moderately overweight women. *Obesity Research, 6*(3), 208–218.

Shape Up America. (1998). Guidance for treatment of adult obesity. In *Shape Up America! 2000* [Online]. Available: http://www.shapeup.org [2000, April 10].

Slimfast. (2000). *Slimfast homepage* [Online]. Available: http://www.slimfast.com [2000, April 11].

Tate, D. F., Wing, R. R., & Winett, R. A. (2001). Using Internet technology to deliver a behavioral weight loss program. *Journal of the American Medical Association, 285,* 1172–1177.

Take off Pounds Sensibly (TOPS) Club. (2000). General info. In *Take Off Pounds Sensibly* [Online]. Available: http://www.tops.org/html/information.html [2000, April 1].

Volkmar, F. R., Stunkard, A. J., Woolston, J., & Bailey, B. A. (1981). High attrition rates in commercial weight reduction programs. *Archives of Internal Medicine, 141,* 426–428.

Wadden, T. A., & Bartlett, S. J. (1992). Very low calorie diets: An overview and appraisal. In T. A. Wadden & T. B. VanItallie (Eds.), *Treatment of the seriously obese patient* (pp. 44–79). New York: Guilford Press.

Wadden, T. A., & Bell, S. T. (1990). Obesity. In A. S. Bellack, M. Hersen, & A. E. Kazdin (Eds.), *International handbook of behavior modification and therapy* (2nd ed., pp. 449–473). New York: Plenum Press.

Wadden, T. A., Foster, G. D., & Letizia, K. A. (1994). One-year behavioral treatment of obesity:

Comparison of moderate and severe caloric restriction and the effects of weight maintenance therapy. *Journal of Consulting and Clinical Psychology, 62,* 165–171.

Wadden, T. A., Foster, G. D., Letizia, K. A., & Stunkard, A. J. (1992). A multicenter evaluation of a proprietary weight reduction program for the treatment of marked obesity. *Archives of Internal Medicine, 152,* 961–966.

Wadden, T. A., & Frey, D. L. (1997). A multicenter evaluation of a proprietary program for the treatment of marked obesity: A five year follow-up. *International Journal of Eating Disorders, 22,* 203–212.

Wadden, T. A., & Stunkard, A. J. (1986). A controlled trial of very-low-calorie diet, behavior therapy, and their combination in the treatment of obesity. *Journal of Consulting and Clinical Psychology, 4,* 482–488.

Wadden, T. A., Vogt, R. A., Anderson, R. E., Bartlett, S. J., Foster, G. D., Kuehnel, R. H., Wilk, J. E., Weinstock, R. S., Buckenmeyer, P., Berkowitz, R. A., & Steen, S. N. (1997). Exercise in the treatment of obesity: Effects of four interventions on body composition, resting energy expenditure, appetite and mood. *Journal of Consulting and Clinical Psychology, 65,* 269–277.

Weight Watchers International. (2000). About Weight Watchers. In *Weight Watchers.com* [Online]. Available: http://www.weightwatchers.com/wwx [2000, April 5].

Wing, R. R., Blair, E. H., Marcus, M. D., Epstein, L. H., & Harvey, J. (1994). Year-long weight loss treatment for obese patients with Type 2 diabetes: Does including an intermittent very-low-calorie diet improve outcome? *American Journal of Medicine, 97,* 354–362.

Wing, R. R., Marcus, M. D., Salata, R., Epstein, L. H., Miaskiewicz, S., & Blair, E. H. (1991). Effects of a very-low-calorie diet on long-term glycemic control in obese Type 2 diabetic subjects. *Archives of Internal Medicine, 151,* 1334–1340.

Wing, R. R., Venditti, E. M., Jakicic, J. M., Polley, B. A., & Lang, W. (1998). Lifestyle intervention in overweight individuals with a family history of diabetes. *Diabetes Care, 21,* 350–359.

Yalom, I. D. (1970). *The theory and practice of group psychotherapy.* New York: Basic Books.

economic circumstances of minority populations differ, on average, from those of the majority white population (Council on Economic Advisers for the President's Initiative on Race, 1998; Pollard & O'Hare, 1999), aspects of obesity and its treatment that depend on these related contextual factors are also different in minority populations. For example, the average educational attainment, income, and financial assets are lower in African American, Hispanic, American Indian, and some subgroups of Asian and Pacific Islander populations. This may affect literacy, baseline knowledge, and knowledge acquisition in the treatment situation, as well as discretionary income and cash flow factors that relate to food purchasing or activity participation.

Community context is an important variable in obesity treatment, to the extent that it influences the type of foods that can be purchased and access to safe and affordable means to increase physical activity. More of the minority than of the white population lives in low-income inner-city neighborhoods, where access to a variety of goods and services is limited. Area of residence may also influence proximity to obesity treatment programs. Family structure and household composition differentiate minority and nonminority women on such factors as the availability of discretionary time outside of employment, child care, or care of other dependents. For example, the estimated proportion of female-headed households with children is 30% among African Americans and 16% among Hispanics, compared to 7% among white Americans (Pollard & O'Hare, 1999).

Obesity Prevalence

No single data source describes the prevalence of obesity among even the major minority population subgroupings. Estimates from the most recent National Health and Nutrition Examination Survey (NHANES III) (Flegal, Carroll, Kuczmarski, & Johnson, 1998) provide for detailed data on obesity prevalence for non-Hispanic black and for Mexican American adults, including age-adjusted comparisons with white Americans based on the current body mass index (BMI) classifications (Table 20.1). In these data, obesity (BMI ≥ 30 kg/m^2) affects more than a third of black and Mexican American women, compared to about one-fourth of non-Hispanic white women. Two-thirds of black and Mexican American women are either overweight or obese. The disproportionate prevalence of Class III

TABLE 20.1. Age-adjusted Percentage of Adults Aged 20 and Over in Subcategories of Overweight or Obesity: United States, 1988–1994, by Ethnicity and Gender

	BMI (kg/m^2)	Non-Hispanic white (%)	Non-Hispanic black (%)	Mexican American (%)
Men				
Overweight	25–29.9	39.9	36.2	44.3
Class I obesity	30.0–34.9	14.4	14.1	17.8
Class II obesity	35.0–39.9	3.4	4.1	3.6
Class III obesity	≥40	1.7	2.5	1.1
Total overweight or obese		59.4	55.9	66.8
Women				
Overweight	25–29.9	23.7	29.6	33.2
Class I obesity	30.0–34.9	12.8	19.1	21.1
Class II obesity	35.0–39.9	6.2	10.3	7.9
Class III obesity	≥40	3.2	7.4	4.5
Total overweight or obese		45.9	66.4	66.7

Note. Data from Flegal, Carroll, Kuczmarski, and Johnson (1998).

obesity (BMI ≥ 40 kg/m²) can also be noted in Table 20.1. At ages 40–59 years, more than 10% of black women have Class III obesity (not shown). The proportion of men who are obese is similar across ethnicity in Table 20.1, at about 20%, although somewhat higher in Mexican American men. More noteworthy is the large proportion of Mexican American men in the overweight or "preobese" range. NHANES III BMI data also indicate that although BMI declines with increasing education among women, ethnic differences in BMI occur within these broad groupings (Winkleby, Kraemer, Ahn, & Varady, 1998) (Figure 20.1).

Higher prevalence of overweight (using the former definition of BMI ≥ 27.3 kg/m² for women and ≥ 27.8 kg/m² for men) has also been reported in representative samples of Puerto Rican, Cuban American, American Indian or Alaskan Native, and Western Samoan women (32%–48%, compared to 24% in non-Hispanic white women), and to a lesser extent in the men in these ethnic groups compared to non-Hispanic white men (Kumanyika, 1994). Overweight is substantially more prevalent in both men and women in samples of Native Hawaiians and Hawaiian Samoans (Kumanyika, 1994). Although these data are less recent than the NHANES III data, the findings are probably still valid, given the general upward trend in obesity in the U.S. population as a whole.

BMI data for Asian Americans have generally indicated less obesity compared to white Americans and other minority populations, with the caveat that a BMI cutoff of 25 or 30 might seriously underestimate fatness-related risks in populations of Asian descent (Lauderdale & Rathouz, 2000; NHLBI, 1998). Nationally representative prevalence data for 18- to 59-year-old Asian Americans in six ethnic subgroups have been reported, based on the self-reported height and weight data in the 1992–1995 National Health Interview Survey (Lauderdale & Rathouz, 2000). The median BMI is below 25 kg/m² and well below that for

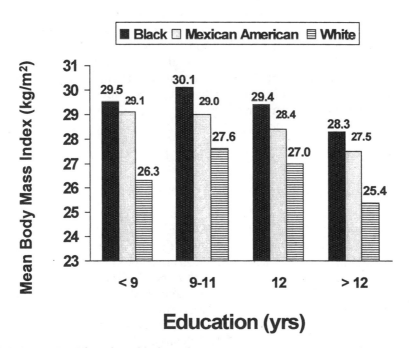

FIGURE 20.1. Mean BMI for white, black, and Mexican American women aged 25–64 years in four education strata, National Health and Nutrition Examination Survey III (NHANES III), 1988–1994. Data from Winkleby, Kraemer, Ahn, and Varady (1998).

whites and blacks in both sexes, particularly among men. Within the Asian American population, mean BMI was highest for Asian Indians and Filipinos among men and for Japanese, Filipinas, and Asian Indians among women. U.S.-born Asian Americans were more likely to be overweight and obese than those who were foreign born. For example, the odds ratio (95% confidence interval in parentheses) for being obese (BMI $\geq$ 30 kg/m^2) in U.S.- versus foreign-born Asian Americans was 4.03 (2.40–6.78) for men and 3.51 (1.74–7.10) for women. Among foreign-born Asian Americans, those with longer duration of U.S. residence were more likely to be obese. Taken together with the observation that obesity-related risks are evident at a lower overall BMI level in Asian-descent than in European-descent populations, the need for effective weight management programs will also apply increasingly to the Asian American population.

Health Implications

Obesity increases the risks of developing several major health problems that lead to disability and premature death—specifically, diabetes, hypertension, coronary heart disease, knee osteoarthritis, and sleep apnea. Increased risk appears to occur in all populations, regardless of race and ethnicity (Kumanyika, 1994; Must et al., 1999; NHLBI, 1998). In particular, Type 2 diabetes has a notably higher incidence and prevalence among essentially all racial/ethnic minority populations and is closely linked to obesity prevalence (Howard et al., 1995; Lee et al., 1995; Lipton, Liao, Cao, Cooper, & McGee, 1993; National Institute of Diabetes and Digestive and Kidney Diseases, 1995). Weight reduction may be a prime strategy for both diabetes control and prevention. The emergence and impact of obesity-related diseases or conditions vary according to the overall health profiles of the population (Kumanyika, 1994; Kumanyika & Golden, 1991), and the relative risks of obesity and various outcomes are therefore not always the same in minority populations as in white populations. For example, there is less coronary heart disease and a lesser overall impact on mortality in some minority populations with a high prevalence of obesity (Howard et al., 1995; NHLBI, 1998; Stevens, 2000). The explanation may lie partly in the lower prevalence of other contributory risk factors (diet, smoking, or alcohol use). Nevertheless, obesity is undoubtedly a direct or indirect contributor to chronic disease in minority populations, and weight reduction is viewed as an important element of the effort to decrease the disproportionate disease burden in minority communities.

RACE AND ETHNICITY AS POTENTIAL INFLUENCES IN OBESITY TREATMENT

Evidence of Ethnic Group Differences in Program Outcomes

The question of whether ethnic considerations should affect the approach to treating obesity was raised by the NHLBI Obesity Education Initiative Expert Panel (NHLBI, 1998, pp. 52–53). The panel concluded that "the possibility that a standard approach to weight loss will work differently in diverse patient populations must be considered when setting expectations about treatment outcomes" (NHLBI, 1998, p. 52). The statement was rated in evidence Category B, signifying a limited amount and quality of relevant supporting data. Findings of smaller weight losses in African American than white participants have been reported in a small number of trials, none of which was designed to study ethnic differences (Kumanyika, Obarzanek, Stevens, Hebert, & Whelton, 1991; Wing & Anglin, 1996; Wylie et al., 1993). These and other relevant trials are highlighted in Table 20.2, along with reports of related observational studies. The clinical trial populations reflected in Table 20.2

TABLE 20.2. Studies Comparing Weight Losses in Black and White Program Participants

Study and objectives	Study design and participants	Results of ethnic comparisons
Wassertheil-Smoller et al. (1985): To compare the success of dietary interventions on body weight and sodium/potassium intake in the Dietary Intervention Study of Hypertension (DISH).	• Multicenter, randomized, controlled trial of dietary interventions as substitutes for drug therapy to control blood pressure. Patients who were 120% above ideal weight with pharmacologically controlled blood pressure were randomly assigned to continue on medication; have medication withdrawn with no dietary intervention; have medication withdrawn and receive counseling to reduce sodium and increase potassium intake; or have medication withdrawn and receive counseling for weight reduction. Ethnicity-specific weight change data are reported for 54 black and 33 white participants at baseline, with follow-up at 8, 32, and 56 weeks. Baseline weight was 86.4 kg. • Dietary interventions used a behavioral approach to facilitate gradual changes in eating patterns.	• Participant numbers decreased over time; at 56 weeks, data were reported for 27 of 33 white participants (82%) and 40 of 54 black participants (74%). • Weight losses of white participants at 8, 36, and 56 weeks postbaseline were 2.5, 4.9, and 4.1 kg, compared to 1.7, 4.4, and 5.0 kg for black participants.
Kumanyika et al. (1991): To compare achieved weight reduction among black and white participants in two hypertension prevention trials: the Hypertension Prevention Trial (HPT) and the Trials of Hypertension Prevention, Phase I (TOHP I).	• Both trials were randomized, controlled, multicenter studies involving overweight men and women aged 25–49 (HPT; 198 white and 38 black participants) or 30–54 (TOHP I; 252 white and 51 black participants) who were not using antihypertensive medications and had diastolic blood pressures between 78 and 89 (HPT) or 80 and 89 (TOHP I) mm Hg at baseline. Follow-up was 18 months (TOHP I) or 36 months (HPT). Mean BMI was 29–30 kg/m². • In both studies, the intervertion was based on a self-selected low-calorie diet with behavioral counseling.	• At 36 months in the HPT, mean weight loss was 2.7 kg less in black than in white women and 1.4 kg less in black than in white men. • At 18 months in the TOHP I, mean weight loss was 2.2 kg less in black than in white women and 2.0 kg less in black than in white men. • Black control participants gained more weight than white controls, but net losses in black participants were still smaller.

(continued)

421

Table 20.2. *continued*

Study and objectives	Study design and participants	Results of ethnic comparisons
Wylie Rosett et al. (1993): To test the efficacy, at 6 months, of a low-sodium/high-potassium diet or of weight reduction alone or in combination with medications, for hypertension management; analysis included a subgroup comparison of blacks and whites.	• Multicenter, randomized, controlled trial of dietary intervention with 582 overweight men and women (324 white and 158 black participants). At enrollment, participants were mildly hypertensive (diastolic blood pressures of 90–100 mm Hg), overweight (110%–160% of weight standards), and not taking antihypertensive medications for at least 2 weeks. • Behavioral intervention approach with self-selected low-calorie diet.	• 13.1% of black vs. 23% of white participants lost more than 10% of initial body weight. • 44% of black vs. 48.6% of white participants lost more than 4.5 kg.
Darga et al. (1994): To compare weight loss and cardiovascular risk factor changes associated with weight loss in a sample of obese black and white men and women.	• Uncontrolled observations in a series of 831 very obese men and women (125 black and 706 white; mean BMI range in race-sex subgroups was 37–42 kg/m²; mean age range was 41–43 years) who entered a clinical research program over a 4-year period and were not taking drug therapy for hypertension. • Very-low-calorie diet intervention with behavior therapy; reintroduction of food occurred after patients came within 5–10 kg of goal weight.	• Weight loss in blacks was 13.3 kg, compared to 18.8 kg in whites. • Fewer black participants had obesity onset before age 18, childhood-onset obesity. • Black women somewhat heavier than white women at entry.
Yanovski et al. (1994): To compare weight loss of obese women with and without binge-eating disorder (BED), including a subgroup analysis to compare black and white participants.	• Uncontrolled observations in 38 women (26 white and 12 black) aged 18–49 who volunteered for a weight loss study; mean initial BMI was 42.3 (BED group) and 38.9 (group without BED); 13 white and 8 black participants had BED. • Very-low-calorie diet program offered for 12 weeks of a 26-week program; behavior therapy also provided.	• Black participants lost 13.7% of initial body weight, whereas whites lost 21.4% of initial body weight; there was no interaction between race and binge status.

Wing and Anglin (1996): To compare weight losses of black and white participants in a 12-month treatment program.

- 30- to 70-year-old men and women (16 black and 59 white); mean BMI 38 kg/m².
- Two behavioral programs over 1 year, one with a self-selected low-calorie diet throughout and one that included two 12-week periods of a very-low-calorie diet.

- Overall weight loss was 7.1 kg in blacks and 13.9 kg in whites, partly explained by greater regain in blacks during the second half of the study. Attendance was lower in blacks during the second 6 months, and the extent of dietary changes appeared to be smaller in blacks. Mood scores, physical activity, and education (at least 12 years vs. less than 12 years), and return to pharmacological therapy were not related to the ethnic differences in weight loss.

Kumanyika et al. (1997): To compare weight losses of black and white men and women participants in two weight reduction programs in the Trials of Nonpharmacologic Interventions in the Elderly (TONE).

- Multicenter, randomized, controlled trial of weight reduction and sodium reduction interventions as substitutes for drug therapy to control blood pressure: TONE participants were 60- to 79-year-old men and women (741 white and 230 black; mean BMI in sex–ethnic subgroups 28–30 kg/m²) with established hypertension that was well controlled on a single antihypertensive drug at the time of enrollment. Follow-up was 15–36 months (median 29 months).
- Behavioral intervention approach with self-selected low-calorie diet or low-calorie and low-sodium diet.

- In the weight-reduction-only program, black men and women lost less weight than whites (~3.4 vs. 4.8 kg, respectively).
- In the combined weight/sodium reduction program, weight loss was 3.2 kg for black men and 4.5 kg for white men; black women lost 3.6 kg, compared to 2.3 kg for white women.

Stevens et al. (2001): To test the efficacy of weight reduction for the prevention of hypertension in the Trials of Hypertension Prevention, Phase II (TOHP II), including a subgroup analysis to compare black and white participants.

- Randomized, controlled, multicenter study involving men and women (595 intervention and 596 controls) aged 30–54 at enrollment who were not using antihypertensive medications, had diastolic blood pressures between 80 and 89 mm Hg at baseline, and were at 110%–165% of weight standards; follow-up was 36–48 months.

- Net weight loss (active intervention minus control) at 6, 18, and 36 months was, respectively, 5.0, 3.1, and 2.0 kg for white and 2.7, 0.9, and 1.5 kg for black participants.
- The differences between blacks and whites were significant at 6 and 18 months, but converged by 36 months.

TABLE 20.3. Environmental Factors of Special Relevance to Obesity Treatment in U.S. Minority Populations

Physical	Economic	Sociocultural
Potential influences on dietary change and maintenance		
• Targeted marketing • Proximity of fast-food restaurants • Proximity of supermarkets • Food choices in neighborhood stores • Food choices at church • Food in house	• Neighborhood demand for low-calorie and low-fat foods • Family income and cash flow • Other household expenses • Home-grown foods	• Traditional cuisine • Fasting and feasting ideology • Food insecurity • Prevalent obesity • Female role expectations • Health profiles • Responsiveness to context • Distrust of or skepticism about "mainstream" information
Potential influences on physical activity change and maintenance		
• Location of fitness facilities • Availability of fitness facilities at work and feasibility of use • Neighborhood recreation facilities • Neighborhood crime	• Local investment in parks and recreational facilities in inner cities • Fees at fitness facilities • Cost of exercise equipment • Employment patterns	• Cultural attitudes about physical activity • Activity lifestyles • Fears about safety

Note. Data from Egger and Swinburn (1997), King et al. (2000), Airhihenbuwa et al. (1995, 1996), Kittler and Sucher (1998), Kumanyika and Morssink (1997), Moore et al. (1996), and Freimuth and Mettger (1990).

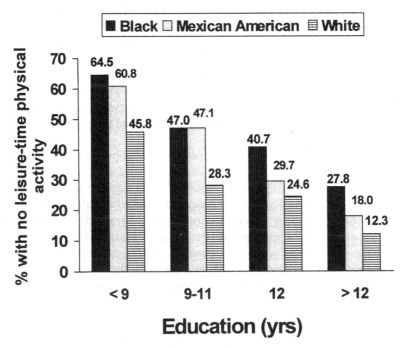

FIGURE 20.3. Percentage of women reporting no leisure-time physical activity by race/ethnicity and education. Data are for 25- to 64-year-old female respondents in NHANES III. Data from Winkleby, Kraemer, Ahn, and Varady (1998).

aged and older women. African American (n = 745), American Indian/Alaskan Native (n = 738), Hispanic (n = 660), and white (n = 769) women aged 40 and over were surveyed by telephone, sampling from zip codes with 20% or more of the ethnic group in question. Logistical problems interfered with completion of an Asian American/Pacific Islander sample. The percentages classified as inactive were highest for black and American Indian women (57% and 59%, respectively), compared to 47% for white women and 53% for Hispanic women. Perceived barriers to exercise were lack of time, caregiving duties, lack of energy, being too tired to exercise, lacking a safe place to exercise, being self-conscious about physical appearance, health problems or impairments, fear of injury, bad weather, and having others discourage exercise. Several of these barriers were mentioned more frequently by minority women than by white women. Neighborhood characteristics assessed included feeling safe while walking or jogging; presence–absence of sidewalks, heavy traffic, hills, streetlights, unattended dogs, enjoyable scenery, and high crime rates; and frequently seeing others exercise.

King and colleagues (2000) reported multivariate analyses of factors that were independently associated with being more or less active within each ethnic group. Variables that were independently associated with being more active in the African American women were frequently observing others exercising in one's neighborhood and the presence of dogs in the neighborhood; caregiving duties were associated with being less active. Analyses for American Indian/Alaskan Native women indicated that education and not being in good health were associated with being less active, and self-consciousness about physical appearance with being more active. For Hispanic women, education, discouragement from others, and being too tired were associated with being less active, and the presence of hills in one's neighborhood with being more active. The model for the white comparison group included age and lack of energy (associated with being less active), and education and presence of hills (associated with being more active).

With respect to food habits, contextual factors may include culturally influenced food preferences (Kittler & Sucher, 1998) and food preparation, as well as food availability variables. These include neighborhood factors—such as the presence of fast-food establishments and supermarkets, and the types of foods offered in supermarkets (Cheadle et al., 1991; Diez-Roux et al., 1999)—for which inner-city neighborhoods are disadvantaged. Targeted advertising of high-calorie foods on black-oriented television is another example (Tirodkar & Jain, 2001). Calorie intakes may not be higher in minority than in white populations (Kumanyika & Krebs-Smith, 2001), although this finding may be due partly to the difficulty of assessing calorie and fat intake or of pinpointing portion sizes of food eaten. Chronic positive energy balance may result from lower physical activity alone. In any case, where there is an established and culturally supported habit of regular consumption of fast foods, fried foods, and other high-fat foods, and where these are the least expensive and most available and most advertised foods, a higher level of motivation may be needed to reduce consumption of these foods sufficiently to create an energy deficit. In addition, the sense of deprivation associated with caloric restriction may be particularly great in ethnic populations where high status is associated with cooking, where food is particularly important as currency in familial and social relationships, where eating large quantities of foods is not only acceptable but sometimes encouraged, and where hunger and food insecurity are present in the community of reference. The extent to which these factors specifically interfere with weight control in minority populations has not been quantified. However, these influences are implicated in qualitative studies to identify potential barriers to dietary adherence in minority populations (Airhihenbuwa et al., 1996; El-Kebbi et al., 1996; Vazquez, Millen, Bissett, Levelnson, & Chipkin, 1998).

TABLE 20.4. Studies of Weight Reduction in U.S. Ethnic Minority Adult Populations in Community Settings

Study population	Participants	Selected program characteristics	Participant retention and weight loss results
Sullivan and Carter (1985): Low-income African American mothers of preschool children at a child development center in New Orleans, Louisiana.	• 10 mothers enrolled; mean age 25 years; mean weight 75.4 kg. • No comparison group.	• 8-week nutrition and aerobic dance program; 1-hour dance classes were held twice per week, followed by a brief nutrition education session. • "Soul variety" dance music was used for aerobic exercise classes; child care was provided.	• 6 of 10 completed the study. • Weight after the program was identical to baseline weight. • Waist, hip, and thigh circumferences also showed no change.
Heath et al. (1987): Zuni Diabetes Project; Zuni Indians with Type 2 diabetes in New Mexico who received health care through the Indian Health Service (IHS).	• Medical record data were analyzed for all persons with Type 2 diabetes in the IHS registry who had attended at least one exercise class ("participants"; $n = 30$); 80% were female; 63% had a BMI of 28 kg/m^2 or more; mean age 42 years. • A matched group of individuals with Type 2 diabetes who had never participated in the exercise program ("nonparticipants"; $n = 56$) was selected from the same registry.	• Community-based exercise program began as two aerobic sessions led by an IHS health educator and two assistants, and grew to 48 sessions offered 5 days per week, several times daily in various locations. Leaders were Zuni Indians trained in exercise and group leadership. • There were also community events such as foot races.	• Average length of participation was 37 weeks, with an average of 1.7 sessions per week. • Average weight loss in participants was 4.1 kg vs. 0.9 kg in nonparticipants. • 25 of the 30 exercise program participants lost weight, compared with only 31 of the 56 nonparticipants. • A dose–response effect was evident with duration of participation: Those who had participated for more than 52 weeks lost 9 kg; less than 8 weeks of participation was associated with a weight loss of 2 kg.
Pleas (1988): African Americans in a Tennessee community.	• 11 women and 1 man enrolled; mean age 44 years; mean weight 80 kg; average 3–4 years of college. • No comparison group.	• 12-week behavioral weight loss program held at a local YMCA. • Weekly 2-hour meetings, with 1 hour devoted to physical activity. • Created a high program expectation through a "program committal form" agreeing to attend; to record eating and activity patterns; to participate in 1 hour of physical activity each meeting and additional activity each week; to have fitness assessments; and to pay $20 to cover the cost of materials. Group leader was experienced in behavioral weight management.	• 8 of 12 attended 9+ sessions and completed all requirements. • Mean weight loss was 3.4 kg (counting all 12). The 8 who completed lost 5.0 kg on average, and 5 lost between 4.5 and 9.1 kg.

Lasco et al. (1989): African American residents of an Atlanta, Georgia, community.

- 70 women participated; age range was 18–59 years; two-thirds were aged 30–49 years; mean weight 91.3 kg; 41% had hypertension.
- No comparison group.

- Leader provided individualized attention, reinforcement, and instruction during group walking times; a Saturday morning walking session was included.
- 10-week weight reduction program with behavioral strategies, nutrition and exercise sessions—the Community Health Assessment and Promotion Project (CHAPP). The program was designed and directed by a community coalition in response to a needs assessment. Participant suggestions were also elicited and incorporated during the program.
- CHAPP operated out of a community health clinic, a local YWCA, and a local school. Format was twice-weekly classes, with 1 hour of nutrition education followed by 1 hour of exercise. Exercise choices included water aerobics, low-impact aerobic dance, and walking. The program provided free transportation, child care, and home visits by a public health educator; banquet at last session with healthful foods prepared by participants. Special interest sessions included classes on makeup, injury control, wardrobe and fashion analysis, and low back pain.

- 72 women started the program; 2 dropped out. 40 others enrolled but dropped out before the end of the second week.
- Weight change results at 3 months: 11 gained weight; 28 were within 0.9 kg of initial weight; 22 lost 1.4–4.5 kg; 9 lost >4.5 kg.
- Of those who lost more than 0.9 kg, the average lost was 4.1 kg.
- 3-month postprogram follow-up data were available for 62 women; 55% weighed less than baseline; average weight loss was 1.3 kg.

Domel et al. (1992a): African American women enrolled at one of four literacy program sites or a recreation center in low-income areas of Dallas, Texas.

- 14 women at a literacy site where the weight loss program was not offered formed the comparison group; each was paid $25.

- Door prizes to encourage attendance; other prizes and recognitions; "buddy system" for social support; traffic light system for calorie control.

- 12 women dropped out.
- Average weight loss of program participants ($n = 31$) was 1.4 kg vs. a loss of 0.1 kg in the comparison group. Among the program participants, 12 lost 2.3 kg or more; 9 lost 0–2.3 kg; 10 gained weight.

Domel et al. (1992b): Hispanic women at two churches in low-income areas of Dallas, Texas.

- 14 women for a comparison group were recruited from a recreation center in another part of Dallas; each was paid $25.

- Modifications included adding ethnic foods and recipes, stressing overall family health, and reformatting pamphlets to comic book format and changing audio programs from a radio show to one involving conversations between two *comadres*.

- 24 women dropped out.
- Average weight loss for the 20 participants was 3.9 kg, compared to a gain of 0.4 kg in the comparison group. Among the program participants, 11 lost 2.3 kg or more; 7 lost less than 2.3 kg; 2 gained weight. *(continued)*

TABLE 20.4. *continued*

Study population	Selected program characteristics	Participant retention and weight loss results
Kumanyika and Charleston (1992): Members of African American churches in Baltimore, Maryland, where a high blood pressure control program was being conducted. • 187 women, of whom 184 were African American, attended at least the first and last sessions; mean age 51 years; mean BMI 31 kg/m². • No comparison group for weight change.	• The program was based within the context of an established church program for blood pressure control, to provide for peer support and sustainability. In response to participant requests, an "alumni program," with longer exercise sessions and held at a central location, was subsequently developed.	• 8-week weight loss was 2.7 kg, with a median loss of 2%–3% of body weight. • Complete follow-up data at 6 months after the end of the program for 74 women. Net weight loss at 8 months was as follows: >4.5 kg for 27%; 2.3–4.1 kg for 17%; 0.5–1.8 kg for 37%; no change for 19%.
Cousins et al. (1992): Mexican American women in Houston, Texas, who were married and had at least one school-age child. • 168 overweight women enrolled; mean age 33 years; mean BMI ~31 kg/m²; mean education 10.1 years; 24% had incomes less than $10,000/year. Women with hypertension, diabetes, and other chronic illnesses were excluded. Mean acculturation score was 2.9 on a scale of 1 (Mexican culture) to 5 (Anglo culture). • Randomized three-group comparison.	• The *Cuidando el Corazon* program was 24 weeks, followed by 6 monthly classes. Classes were taught by bilingual registered dietitians. Teaching methods were specifically geared for low literacy (e.g., personal approach, group support, experiential teaching). • Spanish and English versions of a manual and cookbook were developed and evaluated for cultural appropriateness by bilingual health educators and community members. • Randomization groups were (1) a family-oriented program in which spouses were encouraged to attend classes, and separate classes were held for preschool children; (2) a program oriented to the individual woman; and (3) a control condition in which only the program manual was provided.	• Data are presented for the 86 women who had complete data at all follow-up visits. • Mean weight loss at 12 months was 3.8 kg for the family group, 2.1 kg for the individual condition, and 1 kg for the manual-only condition. The difference between the family and individual conditions was not statistically significant. • Fewer than 50% of husbands attended any classes.
Kanders et al. (1994): African American women in Boston, New York, Houston, and Los Angeles. • 67 women; mean age 49 years; mean BMI 34 kg/m²; 95% had at least high school education; incomes were $1,000–$5,000 per month; women with high blood pressure, high cholesterol, or diabetes were excluded. • No comparison group.	• Pilot study of the Black American Lifestyle Intervention (BALI). The program was a 10-week behavioral weight loss program; the nutrition component involved a 1,200-kcal/day diet program in which two meals were to be consumed as liquid meal replacement shakes, provided free of charge, that were 99% lactose-free; Lactaid was also provided. Group	• 61 women completed the program. • Weight loss was 2.9 kg, or 3.5% of total body weight in the 10 weeks. • 35 of the women lost more than 2.3 kg.

432

- Participants were paid $30 at weeks 5 and 10 for completing evaluations.

Avila and Hovell (1990): Latinas in a low-income community served by a San Diego, California, medical clinic.

- 44 women enrolled; mean age 44 years; mean BMI 31 kg/m^2; 90% had at least a 6th-grade education; 35% had a 12th-grade education or more; more than two-thirds were married; acculturation was minimal; women taking any medications were excluded.
- Participants were randomly assigned to the intervention or to a waiting-list control group.

- sessions were 1 hour and were highly interactive. Participants were advised to exercise several times per week.
- BALI program content was developed with the assistance of minority health professionals, building on a process that began with interviews with African American women to identify obstacles, attitudes, and issues. Group leaders were female African American nutritionists. All program materials were reviewed for cultural appropriateness by minority advisors.

- Intervention program was a 10-week behavioral nutrition and exercise program, with a 1-hour class each week. The program was led by a bicultural, bilingual physician who also participated in all activities. "Buddy system" for social support. A peer leader emerged spontaneously; she encouraged at-home exercise and dietary adherence. The investigators contacted each woman by telephone during the midweek prior to each class. A group car pool was also organized.
- Comparison group received weekly cancer screening education and was invited to join the weight reduction program after the study.

- 39 women completed the program.
- Net 8-week weight change (mean) was a loss of 2.6 kg in the intervention group vs. a gain of 0.6 kg in controls.
- Follow-up data at 3 months after the program were available for 8 control and 10 intervention participants. The overall 5-month weight loss in this subgroup was 6.4 kg in the intervention group vs. 0.7 kg for the control group.

McNabb et al. (1997): African American women who were members of three participating churches.

- 39 obese women participated; average BMI 33.9 kg/m^2 at baseline; mean age 57 years; most had high school education or more.
- 19 women were randomly assigned to receive the program, and the other 20 were assigned to be in a waiting-list comparison group.

- The church-based PATHWAYS program was a 14-week program with a 1.5-hour small group session each week. It was based on an adaptation of the clinic-based PATHWAYS program. As in the original program, the principles of "active learning" and "discovery learning," in which participants identified their own dietary problems and developed alternatives, was followed. Churches were chosen as a venue to promote access and potential sustainability by lay health educators.

- 33 women provided posttreatment data.
- Weight change was a loss of 4.5 kg in PATHWAYS vs. a gain of 0.9 kg in controls, for a net difference of 5.4 kg.
- Note: Results of a pilot study of this church-based version of the program were also noted in the article; that version was led by a registered dietitian, assisted by a lay facilitator. 9 women enrolled; the 7 who provided posttreatment data lost 4.1 kg.

(continued)

433

TABLE 20.4. *continued*

Study population	Participants	Selected program characteristics	Participant retention and weight loss results
McNabb et al. (*cont.*)		• Lay church members were trained to facilitate the program. The format used guided learning activities with minimal lecturing. To be sensitive to culturally based attitudes, the program "encouraged weight loss but not slenderizing" (i.e., health vs. appearance motivation); made extensive use of ethnic foods and food combinations; and stressed inner-city lifestyle issues. A walking program was integral to the program.	
Narayan et al. (1997): Pima Indians in an Arizona community.	• Participants were 95 normoglycemic men (*n* = 23) and women (*n* = 72); median age ~34 years; mean BMI was 36.5 and 33.2 kg/m², respectively, in the intervention and comparison groups. • Participants were randomly assigned to the intervention program (*n* = 48) or comparison program (*n* = 47); 35 eligible individuals who declined randomization were followed as an observational control group.	• The intervention program was "Pima Action"—a 12-month relatively structured weight reduction program focusing on behavioral change, nutrition, and physical activity. Weekly group meetings were reinforced with home visits if needed. Activity choices included walking, water aerobics, softball, volleyball, and paid activities such as community gardening and cleaning the local cemetery. • The comparison program was "Pima Pride." This program was coordinated by a community member and emphasized self-directed learning facilitated by an appreciation of Pima culture. Discussion groups met once per month to talk about current lifestyles and listen to invited speakers talk about culture and history; basic printed information on healthy eating and exercise was provided; a newsletter with cultural content was used to facilitate communication; each member also gave a detailed interview on perceptions of health and lifestyle.	• 6- and 12-month follow-up data were obtained from 97% and 98% of participants, respectively. • Weight increased by 1.0 and 2.5 kg at 6 and 12 months, respectively, in Pima Action, compared to 0.5 and 0.8 kg in Pima Pride. In other words, all gained weight, but Pima Pride participants gained less weight; 7 of the 8 people who lost 4+ kg were in Pima Pride. • Mean 12-month weight change in the observational group was a gain of 1.9 kg.

by 6 additional weekly reinforcement sessions focusing on nutrition and regular exercise. The content was based on qualitative data collected from interviews with women from the proposed study population, with additional expert review by local minority health professionals. The counseling approach and supporting materials were also designed to minimize literacy demands (to an eighth-grade reading level), to have a high personal relevance for participants, and to provide ample opportunities for active discovery learning. Patients (13 low-income black women; mean age 57 years; mean BMI 36 kg/m^2) who had been treated for Type 2 diabetes for at least 3 years were recruited at a Chicago university medical center. Of the 10 women who completed the program, 9 lost weight, and half lost more than 4.5 kg. Average weight loss immediately after the 18-week program was 4.1 kg, which was maintained at a 1-year follow-up. Ten women in a comparison group randomly selected from patients receiving usual care (individual nutrition counseling) gained 1.4 kg over the same 1-year period.

We (Agurs-Collins, Kumanyika, Ten Have, & Adams-Campbell, 1997) conducted a randomized controlled trial of a weight reduction program for older African Americans with Type 2 diabetes at a historically black university hospital in Washington, D.C. The 64 patients enrolled (49 women and 15 men; mean age 62 years; mean BMI 34 kg/m^2) were recruited primarily through medical referrals. Treatment group participants, who received 12 weekly, 1 individual, and 6 biweekly sessions over a 6-month period, were compared with usual-care participants who received a general diabetes education class and periodic mailings. Group meetings involved nutrition counseling and a 30-minute exercise session, and were conducted by a registered dietitian and an exercise physiologist (both African American). Cultural adaptations included the use of cooperative learning strategies, with encouragement of interactive discussions focusing on participants' personal issues and social contexts. In addition, program content emphasized ethnic foods and recipes (obtained from participants) and audiovisual and printed materials depicting older adults and African Americans. Net weight loss (treatment minus control) was 2 kg and 2.4 kg, respectively, at 3 and 6 months.

Kaul and Nidiry (1999) reported weight loss data from the bariatrics clinic at the same university where the Agurs-Collins and colleagues (1997) study was conducted, although the two studies and patient populations were unrelated. Kaul and Nidiry's program is an individualized intervention that includes nutrition education, exercise, and behavior modification, and takes into account individuals' literacy skills, economic status, and food preferences. The dropout rate for the period reported was 10%. Patients lost an average of 0.9 kg per week, with a 6.4-kg loss over a 7-week period.

Although these studies cannot be directly compared, the PATHWAYS study (McNabb et al., 1993) stands out as being the most effective of the group treatment programs with respect to the amount of weight lost. A comparison of the culturally adapted program with a more standard group treatment approach would be needed in order to attribute weight loss outcomes in PATHWAYS to the cultural adaptations as such. However, the adaptations described are logical approaches exemplary of the general strategy of cultural adaptation (Kumanyika & Morssink, 1997; NHBLI, 1998). Such adaptations do not necessarily guarantee success, however. Similar adaptations were made in the Agurs-Collins and colleagues (1997) study, but with less impressive results. Most of the studies report relatively small weight losses and would appear to offer a relatively low return on investment.

Studies in Community Settings

Studies conducted with minority populations in community settings are summarized in Table 20.4. These studies include examples in which participants were recruited through community agencies and the community at large, and in which programs were delivered in venues such as the YMCA, day care centers, adult literacy program sites, and churches. Except for the Black American Lifestyle Intervention (BALI) pilot study (Kanders et al., 1994), in which liquid meal replacements were used, and the Zuni Diabetes Project (Heath, Leonard, Wilson, Kendrick, & Powell, 1987), which did not include a nutrition component, all of these studies were based on helping participants to select balanced reduced-calorie diets (using standard behavioral techniques) and on the promotion of regular physical activity. Studies varied in whether a formal activity component was provided and what it involved. Unlike the programs conducted in clinical settings, most of the community-based programs included explicit measures designed to increase the relevance of the program language, literacy level, and content to participants, and to adapt the counseling approaches to perceived participant motivations and learning preferences.

Some of the adaptations reflected in Table 20.4 were similar to those previously described for culturally adapted clinical studies (e.g., Agurs-Collins et al., 1997; McNabb et al., 1993): conducting preliminary formative assessments of participant needs and preferences through interviews with potential participants, community leaders, or both; directly incorporating participant suggestions into the program; incorporating explicit cultural content related to food, activity, or weight issues; formulating or revising written materials to minimize literacy demands; and emphasizing interactive learning strategies. However, in several of the studies listed in Table 20.4, the adaptations and accommodations to participant needs were more extensive than those reported in the clinical studies and put the clients in even more of a proactive role. For example, in the Community Health Assessment and Promotion Project (CHAPP) study (Lasco et al., 1989), a group theater outing and a fashion show were arranged at the participants' request.

Community-based studies are generally more likely to include outreach or community programming activities that either reduce barriers to or expand opportunities for adherence. An example is the home visit component in the CHAPP study (Lasco et al., 1989). The church-based version of the PATHWAYS study (McNabb, Quinn, Kerver, Cook, & Karrison, 1997) was intended to take a program that was already culturally adapted and further adapt it for broader application in a community context, including implementation by trained lay educators. Although the church-based version was not designed for direct comparison to the clinic program, the weight losses achieved in the two versions were comparable and are among the best weight losses observed in any of the studies in Table 20.4. Auslander, Haire-Joshu, Houston, Williams, and Krebill (2000) reported no weight loss among African American women (n = 112 assigned to the treatment condition; mean age 40 years; mean BMI 36.5 kg/m^2) who were involved in a community-based program led by peer educators (not shown in Table 20.4). However, healthy eating centered around low-fat intake was the primary focus of that study, and a significant reduction in fat intake was reported. We (Kumanyika et al., 1999) have also reported that successful counseling for reduced fat intake does not necessarily promote weight reduction in African American women and men.

The Narayan and colleagues (1998) study of Pima Indians and the Cousins and colleagues (1992) study of Mexican American women are the only ones in which a traditional and a nontraditional approach have been directly compared within the same population. In the Pima Indian study, the findings suggest that the less traditional, more culturally grounded approach would be more effective in weight gain prevention, if not weight reduction, over the long term. The Cousins and colleagues (1992) findings were not clear as to whether the family-based approach was superior to a more traditional approach directed toward the individual woman. However, the low participation by husbands might indicate that the family approach was not fully implemented.

The studies in Table 20.4 can be considered "best-case scenarios" with respect to the weight loss that can be achieved with participants who are retained in programs designed to accommodate their needs and to reduce barriers. Participant age, mean BMI levels, and health status, along with the specifics of program design and implementation, varied across studies. Systematic comparisons adjusting for these variables were not feasible. However, taking into account the varying lengths of the studies and focusing particularly on the shorter term results, one can see that the average weight reduction was best in the studies by Pleas (1988), McNabb and colleagues (1997), and Domel, Alford, Cattlett, Rodriguez, and Gench (1992b). It approximated 0.4 kg per week over 11–14 weeks. Weight reductions in the Lasco and colleagues (1989), Kumanyika and Charleston (1992), Avila and Hovell (1994), and Kanders and colleagues (1994) studies were 0.30–0.35 kg per week over 8–10 weeks. The other programs in which any weight loss was observed, on average, were associated with a weight reduction of less than 0.2 kg per week.

Two issues deserve further mention. One is the extent to which the mean weight changes are affected by participants who gain weight while enrolled in these programs. For example, in the Domel and colleagues (1992a, 1992b) studies, the larger mean weight loss for Hispanic women appears to be related to the fact that fewer women gained weight in the study of Hispanic women than in the study of black women. In addition, as noted by these authors, recruiting at literacy sites might have yielded a participant group with very low motivations for weight reduction. Perhaps there is a qualitative distinction to be made between participants who gain versus lose (or maintain) weight during a weight reduction program. The other issue relates to the short-term nature of many of these programs. If weight loss is slower in minority populations, longer-term studies may be needed to identify the full potential of culturally adapted approaches even with respect to initial weight reduction.

The studies in Table 20.4 constitute most or all of the reports published to date of formal weight reduction studies in minority populations lasting at least 8 weeks. Although these studies were motivated by an interest in improving weight loss outcomes over those that might be observed in standard programs, the weight losses observed have been relatively modest in comparison to those achieved in the primarily white populations reflected in the general obesity treatment literature. Thus, while these studies illustrate the types of approaches that have been attempted, and many suggest approaches that are worthy of further development and evaluation, much more research is needed to determine how these approaches can be used to facilitate better weight losses over a longer term. As reviewed by Taylor, Baranowski, and Young (1998), there is a similar need for research on culturally adapted approaches to physical activity interventions in minority populations.

IMPLICATIONS

The NHLBI (1998) noted that "standard obesity treatment approaches should be tailored to the needs of patients" (p. 89), while also noting that the literature on specially adapted programs was scant and difficult to interpret. Caution was advised in attempting to standardize ethnicity-specific approaches, both because of the large individual variability within ethnic groups and because of the "substantial overlap among subcultures within the larger society" (p. 89). In the absence of sufficient grounding to develop an evidence-based approach related to minority populations, theoretically based general guidelines were provided for tailoring programs with respect to setting, staff, and underlying assumptions about the personal characteristics, lifestyle context, and health status of participants in weight loss programs.

Table 20.5 summarizes the guidance offered by the NHLBI panel. This guidance was based on a more detailed consideration of cultural appropriateness issues in weight manage-

TABLE 20.6. Typology of Possible Adherence Problems in Minority Participants

1. Poor quality of participation
    1.1 Attendance at group or individual sessions
        • Low intention to attend
        • Discomfort level in treatment venue
        • Low perceived benefits of attending
        • High perceived barriers to attending
        • Logistical issues limiting attendance (time, transportation, child care)
    1.2 Insufficient weight loss motivations
        • Ambivalence about net benefits of weight reduction
        • Ambivalence regarding body image
        • Countervailing health beliefs
        • Expressed beliefs or preferences of others in social network
        • Identity and connectedness issues (e.g., deviation from community norms)
        • Competing priorities

2. Problems in adopting or maintaining reduced fat and caloric intake
    2.1 Limited understanding of concepts or specifics
    2.2 Entrenched misconceptions and contrary beliefs
    2.3 Lack of "how to" skills, including self-monitoring
    2.4 Inability to adopt or maintain new behaviors in context
        • Characteristics of high-fat foods consumed
        • Level of involvement in food preparation too high or too low
        • Primary sources of calories (e.g., beverages, large portions?)
        • Numerous food dislikes or intolerances, or inflexible preferences
        • Psychosocial factors (e.g., motivations to change eating habits, motivations to continue eating habits, use of food for coping)
        • Difficulty in following advice because of time or social pressures
        • Self-image, status, and role identity issues
        • Limited food access or flexibility in choice
        • Low purchasing power

3. Problems in adopting or maintaining increased physical activity
    3.1 Limited understanding of concepts or specifics due to literacy issues
    3.2 Entrenched misconceptions and contrary beliefs
    3.3 Lack of "how to" skills, including self-monitoring
    3.4 Inability to adopt or maintain new behaviors in context
        • Characteristics of daily routine (time and place)
        • Limited range of preferred activities
        • Psychosocial factors (e.g., motivation to exercise, motivations to be sedentary)
        • Self-image, status, and role identity issues
        • Countervailing social pressures
        • Lack of options because of limited access or flexibility in choice
        • Functional status limitations

evant contextual cues will favor the prior behaviors—those that are targeted to be unlearned through obesity treatment. It is therefore essential that the new behaviors also be strongly anchored in contextual cues, resources, and constraints within the participants' environments and day-to-day living circumstances. Detailed consideration of what these cues, resources, and constraints are, and where there is the most congruency with desirable behaviors, may help with the adoption of sustainable weight control behaviors. The possibility that the home environment provides strong cues to problematic eating and activity behaviors is also a rationale for encouraging take-home learning approaches.

SUMMARY AND CONCLUSIONS

Development and implementation of effective strategies for treating obesity in minority populations has become both a clinical challenge and a public health priority. In most U.S. racial/ethnic minority populations, the prevalence of obesity is higher than in the non-Hispanic white population. As noted by Ritenbaugh (1982), "the fact that biomedicine does not include culture in its basic explanatory model leads to a) a failure to recognize culture-bound syndromes within Western cultures and within the biomedical system and b) a redefinition of syndromes from other cultures into biomedical terms so that potentially important cultural patterns (may) become irrelevant to diagnosis or treatment" (p. 351). The tendency to view obesity as a biomedical entity has limited the relevance of the obesity treatment literature to minority health. Thus the objective of this chapter has been to describe ways in which the context for obesity treatment in ethnic minority populations depends on social and environmental factors that are in many ways unique, in comparison to those that affect the population at large.

Comparisons of weight losses attained by African American and white participants have usually indicated that African Americans lose less weight or lose weight more slowly. Explanatory factors may include sociocultural and socioeconomic variations in the underlying motivations for weight loss, in the attitudes and behaviors addressed in treatment programs, in the environmental context in which food and eating occur, and in the ways in which members of ethnic minority populations interact with the health care system. Relatively modest weight losses are observed even in those studies designed to explore the effectiveness of culturally adapted weight management approaches in minority populations.

The available literature, although provocative with respect to what might be missing from standard approaches or why the adapted approaches do not yield more impressive results, does not form a sufficient evidence base to support any conclusions about how to proceed beyond a call for more research. Given the nature of the issues raised, research that involves theory, practice, and qualitative data from a variety of disciplines is needed. In the interim, the incorporation of current guidelines for enhancing the effectiveness of obesity treatment in diverse populations (NHLBI, 1998) should be considered.

REFERENCES

Agurs-Collins, T. D., Kumanyika, S. K., Ten Have, T. R., & Adams-Campbell, L. L. (1997). A randomized controlled trial of weight reduction and exercise for diabetes management in older African American subjects. *Diabetes Care, 20,* 1503–1511.

Airhihenbuwa, C. O., Kumanyika, S., Agurs, T. D., & Lowe, A. (1995). Perceptions and beliefs about exercise, rest, and health among African-Americans. *American Journal of Health Promotion, 9*(6), 426–429.

Airhihenbuwa, C. O., Kumanyika, S., Agurs, T. D., Lowe, A., Saunders, D., & Morssink, C. B. (1996). Cultural aspects of African-American eating patterns. *Ethnicity and Health, 1,* 245–260.

Allan, J. D., Mayo, K., & Michel, Y. (1993). Body size values of white and black women. *Research in Nursing and Health, 16,* 323–333.

Allison, D. B., Nezin, L. E., & Clay-Williams, G. (1997). Obesity among African American women: Prevalence, consequences, causes, and developing research. *Women's Health Research, 2*(3–4), 243–274.

Auslander, W., Haire-Joshu, D., Houston, C., Williams, J. H., & Krebill, H. (2000). The short-term impact of a health promotion program for low-income African American women. *Research on Social Work Practice, 10*(1), 78–97.

Kumanyika, S. K., & Krebs-Smith, S. M. (2001) Preventive nutrition issues in ethnic and socioeconomic groups in the United States. In A. Bendich & R. J. Deckelbaum (Eds.), *Preventive nutrition* (Vol. 2, pp. 325–356). Totowa, NJ: Humana Press.

Kumanyika, S. K., & Morssink, C. B. (1997). Cultural appropriateness of weight management programs. In S. Dalton (Ed.), *Overweight and weight management* (pp. 69–106). Gaithersburg, MD: Aspen.

Kumanyika, S. K., Obarzanek, E., Stevens, V. J., Hebert, P. R., & Whelton, P. K. (1991). Weight-loss experience of black and white participants in NHBLI-sponsored clinical trials. *American Journal of Clinical Nutrition, 53,* 1631S–1638S.

Lasco, R. A., Curry, R. H., Dickson, V. J., Powers, J., Menes, S., & Merritt, R. K. (1989). Participation rates, weight loss, and blood pressure changes among obese women in a nutrition–exercise program. *Public Health Reports, 104,* 640–646.

Lauderdale, D. S., & Rathouz, P. J. (2000). Body mass index in a U. S. national sample of Asian Americans: Effects of nativity, years since immigration, and socioeconomic status. *International Journal of Obesity, 24,* 1188–1194.

Lee, E. T., Howard, B. V., Davage, P. J., Cowan, I. D., Fabsitz, R. R., Oopik, A. J., Yeh, J., Go, O., Robbins, D. C., & Welty, T. K. (1995). Diabetes and impaired glucose tolerance in three American Indian populations aged 45–74 years. *Diabetes Care, 18,* 599–610.

Leininger, M. (1991). Becoming aware of types of health practitioners and cultural imposition. *Journal of Transcultural Nursing, 2*(2), 32–39.

Lipton, R. B., Liao, Y., Cao, G., Cooper, R. S., & McGee, D. (1993). Determinants of incident non-insulin-dependent diabetes mellitus among blacks and whites in a national sample. *American Journal of Epidemiology, 138,* 826–839.

Mazzuca, S. A., Moorman, N. H., Wheeler, M. L., Norton, J. A., Fienberg, N. S., Vinicor, F., Cohen, S. J., & Clark, C. M., Jr. (1986). The Diabetes Education Study: A controlled trial of the effects of diabetes patient education. *Diabetes Care, 9,* 1–10.

McNabb, W., Quinn, M., Kerver, J., Cook, S., & Karrison, T. (1997). The PATHWAYS church-based weight loss program for urban African American women at risk for diabetes. *Diabetes Care, 20,* 1518–1523.

McNabb, W. L., Quinn, M. T., & Rosing, L. (1993). Weight loss program for inner-city black women with non-insulin dependent diabetes mellitus. *Journal of the American Dietetic Association, 93,* 75–77.

Moore, D. J., Williams, J. D., & Qualls, W. J. (1996). Target marketing of tobacco and alcohol-related products to ethnic minority groups in the United States. *Ethnicity and Disease, 6*(1–2), 83–98.

Mount, M. A., Kendrick, O. W., Draughon, M., Stitt, K. R., Head, D., & Mount, R. (1991). Group participation as a method to achieve weight loss and blood glucose control. *Journal of Nutrition Education, 23,* 25–29.

Must, A., Spadano, J., Coakley, E. H., Field, A. E., Colditz, G., & Dietz, W. H. (1999). The disease burden associated with overweight and obesity. *Journal of the American Medical Association, 282*(16), 1523–1529.

Narayan, K. M., Hoskin, M., Kozak, D., Kriska, A. M., Hanson, R. L., Pettitt, D. J., Nagi, D. K., Bennett, P. H., & Knowler, W. C. (1998). Randomized clinical trial of lifestyle interventions in Pima Indians: A pilot study. *Diabetic Medicine, 15*(1), 66–72.

National Heart, Lung, and Blood Institute (NHLBI). (1998). Clinical guidelines on the identification, evaluation, and treatment of overweight and obesity in adults: The evidence report. *Obesity Research, 6*(Suppl. 2), 51S–210S.

National Heart, Lung, and Blood Institute (NHLBI) Obesity Education Initiative. (1994). *Strategy development workshop for public education on weight and obesity: Summary report* (NIH Publication No. 94–3314). Washington, DC: U. S. Department of Health and Human Services.

National Institute of Diabetes and Digestive and Kidney Diseases. (1995). *Diabetes in America/National Diabetes Data Group* (2nd ed.) (NIH Publication No. 95–1468). Bethesda, MD: National Institutes of Health.

Neel, J. V. (1999). Diabetes mellitus: A "thrifty" genotype rendered detrimental by "progress"? *Bulletin of the World Health Organization, 77*(8), 694–703. (Original work published 1962)

Pleas, J. (1988). Long-term effects of a lifestyle-change obesity treatment program with minorities. *Journal of the National Medical Association, 8,* 747–752.

Pollard, K., & O'Hare, W. (1999). America's racial and ethnic minorities. *Population Bulletin, 54,* 1–34.

Ravussin, E., Valencia, M. E., Esparza, J., Bennett, P. H., & Schulz, L. O. (1994). Effects of a traditional lifestyle on obesity in Pima Indians. *Diabetes Care, 17,* 1067–1074.

Ritenbaugh C. (1982). Obesity as a culture-bound syndrome. *Culture, Medicine, and Psychiatry, 6,* 347–361.

Rollnick, S., Mason, P., & Butler, C. (1999). *Health behavior change: A guide for practitioners.* New York: Churchill Livingstone.

Serdula, M. K., Mokdad, A. H., Williamson, D. F., Galuska, D. A., Mendlein, J. M., & Heath, G. W. (1999). Prevalence of attempting weight loss and strategies for controlling weight. *Journal of the American Medical Association, 13*(14), 1353–1358.

Serdula, M. K., Williamson, D. F., Anda, R. F., & Levy, A. (1994). Weight control practices in adults: Results of a multistate telephone survey. *American Journal of Public Health, 84*(11), 1821–1824.

Smith, D. E., Heckemeyer, C. M., Kratt, P. P., & Mason, D. A. (1997). Motivational interviewing to improve adherence to a behavioral weight-control program for older obese women with NIDDM: A pilot study. *Diabetes Care, 20,* 52–54.

Stevens, J. (2000). Obesity and mortality in African Americans. *Nutrition Reviews, 58*(11), 346–353.

Stevens, V. J., Obarzanek, E., Cook, N. R., Lee, I. M., Appel, L. J., Smith, D., Milas, N. C., Mattfeldt-Beman, M., Belden, L., Bragg, C., Millstone, M., Raczynski, J., Brewer, A., Singh, B, & Cohen, J. (2001). Long-term weight loss and changes in blood pressure: Results of the Trials of Hypertension Prevention—Phase II. *Annals of Internal Medicine, 134*(1), 1–11.

Story, M., Evans, M., Fabsitz, R. R., Clay, T. E., Rock, B. H., & Broussard, B. (1999). The epidemic of obesity in American Indian communities and the need for childhood obesity-prevention programs. *American Journal of Clinical Nutrition, 69*(Suppl.), 747S–754S.

Striegel-Moore R. H., Wilfley, D. E., Caldwell, M. B., Needham, M. L., & Brownell, K. D. (1996). Weight-related attitudes and behaviors of women who diet to lose weight: A comparison of black dieters and white dieters. *Obesity Research, 4,* 109–116.

Sullivan, J., & Carter, J. P. (1985). A nutrition–physical fitness intervention program for low-income black parents. *Journal of the National Medical Association, 77*(1), 39–43.

Swanson, C. A., Gridley, C., Greenberg, R. S., Schoenberg, J. B., Swanson, G. M., Broan, L. M., Hayes, R., Silverman, D., & Pottern, L. (1993). A comparison of diets of blacks and whites in three areas of the United States. *Nutrition and Cancer, 20,* 153–160.

Taylor, W. C., Baranowski, T., & Young, D. R. (1998). Physical activity interventions in low-income ethnic minority, and populations with disability. *American Journal of Preventive Medicine, 15*(4), 334–343.

Tirodhar, M. A., & Jain, A. (2001). Food messages on African-American television shows. *Pediatric Research, 49*(4, Pt. 2), 19A.

Troiano, R. P., Flegal, K. M., Kuczmarski, R. J., Campbell, S. M., & Johnson, C. L. (1995). Overweight prevalence and trends for children and adolescents. The National Health and Nutrition Examination Surveys, 1963–1991. *Archives of Pediatric and Adolescent Medicine, 149,* 1085–1091.

Vazquez, I. M., Millen, B., Bissett, L., Levelnson, S. M., & Chipkin, S. R. (1998). A preventive nutrition intervention in Caribbean Latinos with Type 2 diabetes. *American Journal of Health Promotion, 13,* 116–119.

Wassertheil-Smoller, S., Langford, H. G., Blaufox, M. D., Oberman, A., Hawkins, M., Levine, B., Cameron, M., Babacock, C., Pressel, S., & Caggiula, A. (1985). Effective dietary intervention in hypertensives: Sodium restriction and weight reduction. *Journal of the American Dietetic Association, 85*(4), 423–430.

Weyer, C., Snitker, S., Bogardus, C, & Ravussin, E. (1999). Energy metabolism in African Americans: Potential risk factors for obesity. *American Journal of Clinical Nutrition, 70*(1), 1–2.

White, S. L., & Maloney, S. K. (1990). Promoting healthy diets and active lives to hard-to-reach groups: Market research study. *Public Health Reports, 105*(3), 224–231.

Williamson, D. F., Serdula, M. K., Anda, R. F., Levy, A., & Byers, T. (1992). Weight loss attempts in

Today magazine, the percentage of American women who are dissatisfied with their overall appearance more than doubled in the 25 years between the first survey in 1972 and the most recent survey in 1997 (see Table 21.1). The percentage of men dissatisfied with their overall appearance almost tripled during that time.

The validity of findings from surveys like this is frequently called into question. Magazine surveys are often subject to sample biases; it is unknown how representative the readers of *Psychology Today* who responded to this survey are of the population at large. Nevertheless, studies that have used strategies to ensure a more representative sample of the American population have found levels of body image dissatisfaction in women similar to those of the 1997 *Psychology Today* survey (Cash & Henry, 1995). Thus the results from the Body Image Survey may accurately reflect Americans' increasing dissatisfaction with their appearance. These more recent findings also suggest that Rodin, Silberstein, and Striegel-Moore's (1985) characterization of body image dissatisfaction as a "normative discontent" appears more true today than ever before.

In a society that puts such a premium on thinness, it is not surprising that overweight and obese individuals report heightened body image dissatisfaction. Furthermore, given society's overemphasis on female physical appearance relative to male appearance, it is not surprising that more research has focused on female than on male body image dissatisfaction. Body image dissatisfaction in overweight and obese individuals frequently varies across different groups of individuals. For example, although African American women are often concerned about the health consequences of their weight, they report a relatively positive body image and an absence of negative societal pressure to be thin (Kumanyika, Wilson, & Guilford-Davenport, 1993). Body image dissatisfaction is not only an American phenomenon; numerous studies in the last 10 years have found high rates of concern about body image and body weight in such countries as England, Australia, Norway, China, Italy, and Argentina (Button, Loan, Davies, & Sonuga-Barke, 1997; Davis & Katzman, 1997; Martinez & Spinetta, 1997; Maude, Wertheim, Paxton, Gibbons, & Szmukler, 1993; Santonastaso, Favaro, Ferrara, Sala, & Zanetti, 1995; Wichstrom, 1995).

Specificity

One question, however, that has not been answered satisfactorily concerns the exact source of the dissatisfaction. Clearly, obese persons may be distressed by particular parts of their bodies, such as their abdomens, hips, or thighs. Alternatively, clinicians often hear a more global complaint: "I just can't stand my body." In the 1997 *Psychology Today* survey, 71%

TABLE 21.1. Percentage of Persons Reporting Body Image Dissatisfaction in the *Psychology Today* Magazine Surveys

	1972		1985		1997	
	Women	Men	Women	Men	Women	Men
Overall appearance	25%	15%	38%	34%	56%	43%
Weight	48%	35%	55%	41%	66%	52%
Height	13%	13%	17%	20%	16%	16%
Muscle tone	30%	25%	45%	32%	57%	45%
Breasts/chest	26%	18%	32%	28%	34%	38%
Abdomen	50%	36%	57%	50%	71%	63%
Hips/upper thighs	49%	12%	50%	21%	61%	29%

Note. From Garner (1997). Copyright 1997 by Sussex Publishers. Reprinted by permission.

of women and 63% of men reported dissatisfaction with their abdomens, while 66% of women and 52% of men reported dissatisfaction with their body weight (Garner, 1997). Thus body weight, or features commonly associated with excess weight, are the focus of body image dissatisfaction for the majority of obese individuals. A more recent study suggested that obese women who sought weight loss had specific rather than more global body image concerns (Sarwer, Wadden, & Foster, 1998). In a sample of 79 obese women, almost half (47%) reported that they were most dissatisfied with their waists and abdomens, whereas only 10% reported dissatisfaction with their overall bodies. Interestingly, 42% of normal-weight controls also indicated that they were most dissatisfied with their waists and abdomens, suggesting that dissatisfaction with the waistline may be independent of actual body weight for American women. Perhaps this finding is not all that surprising, given the current fashion trends celebrating thin and toned waistlines, which are often displayed in form-fitting or midriff-baring fashions.

Severity

Another issue is the severity of the body image dissatisfaction. Although the term "normative discontent" illustrates the prevalence of body image dissatisfaction, it does not convey the degree of severity of the dissatisfaction. In a study of overweight women who sought body image therapy (Rosen, Orosan, & Reiter, 1995), more than 80% of women scored greater than one standard deviation above the norms on two measures of body image dissatisfaction—the Body Dysmorphic Disorder Examination (Rosen & Reiter, 1996) and the Body Shape Questionnaire (Cooper, Taylor, Cooper & Fairburn, 1987). Sarwer, Wadden, and Foster (1998) found that obese women, as compared to normal-weight controls, also scored significantly higher on the Body Dysmorphic Disorder Examination—Self-Report version. Thus, it appears that obese women experience greater body image dissatisfaction than nonobese women do.

Interestingly, the degree of body image dissatisfaction appears to be unrelated to degree of obesity. At least two studies found no correlation between BMI and body image dissatisfaction in obese women with a mean BMI of approximately 35 kg/m^2 (Foster, Wadden, & Vogt, 1997; Sarwer, Wadden, & Foster, 1998). Similarly, no relationship between BMI and body image dissatisfaction was found in a sample of bariatric surgery patients with a mean BMI of 54 kg/m^2 (Sarwer, Wadden, Didie, & Steinberg, 2000). This lack of relationship between the degree of body image dissatisfaction and severity of obesity is consistent with theories of body image, which have suggested that there may be little relationship between what one thinks about the body and the objective reality of one's appearance (Cash, 1990; Sarwer, Wadden, Pertschuk, & Whitaker, 1998). Furthermore, these findings suggest that there may be a "threshold effect," such that as individuals become obese (or perhaps even overweight), they report an increase in body image dissatisfaction. This dissatisfaction, however, does not appear to increase with an increase in the degree of obesity.

This interpretation must be made cautiously. The study by Sarwer, Wadden, and Foster (1998) used a truncated distribution. Normal-weight controls had a mean BMI of 23.8 ± 3.2 kg/m^2 while obese participants had a mean BMI of 35.6 ± 4.3 kg/m^2, with no women having a BMI ≥ 40 kg/m^2. Studies investigating large samples of women with a wide range of BMIs are needed to clarify the relationship between body mass and body image dissatisfaction.

Regardless of its relation to BMI, body image dissatisfaction appears to have a negative influence on behavior. A significantly greater percentage of obese women than nonobese women reported, on more than half of the days of the month, camouflaging their obesity with clothing, changing their posture or body movements, avoiding looking at their bodies,

es on those instruments most relevant for the particular appearance concerns of obese individuals (i.e., body weight and shape). In addition, we review some of the general psychometric and clinical issues to be considered in the selection of a particular measure.

The assessment of body image has an apt maxim: All measures do not assess the same thing. That is, the fact that a measure has "body image," "body dissatisfaction," or some similar word or phrase in its title does not mean that the measure assesses the same aspect of body image as a different scale with a similar name. Table 21.2 contains a list of frequently used words or phrases used to describe assessment tools. In theory, these phrases and their accompanying definitions might provide a useful guide for clinicians and researchers in this area, particularly if investigators consistently used and applied these terms. Unfortunately, this is not the case. These terms, more often than not, are not interchangeable, and are often used to define discrete elements of "body image." As a result, we suggest that clinicians and investigators scan the items of a measure to ensure that the name of the measure adequately captures the content of the instrument.

TABLE 21.2. Definitions of Body Image

Weight satisfaction: Satisfaction with current weight, which may be assessed by measuring discrepancy between current and desired weight.

Size perception accuracy: Accuracy of estimation of the size of body sites; inaccurate estimation is commonly referred to as "body image distortion." (We hope that use of "size perception accuracy" will be discontinued.)

Body satisfaction: Satisfaction with an aspect of one's body; usually measures define which sites are rated (e. g., waist, hips, thighs, breasts, hair, etc.).

Appearance satisfaction: Satisfaction with overall appearance; usually measures contain items that address such issues as facial features, weight-related areas, and hair; items may also address broader features such as sex appeal.

Appearance evaluation: Rather than asking for a satisfaction rating, these scales may ask for a range of agreement (agree–disagree) with statements about broad appearance features.

Appearance orientation: A measure of cognitive-behavioral investment in one's appearance, reflected by items that assess the frequency of appearance-related thoughts and behaviors.

Body esteem: Probably most similar to body satisfaction, these items reflect agreement with positive versus negative features about one's body; they may capture broader concepts (i. e., "I am proud of my body").

Body concern: This term may reflect dissatisfaction, or it may mean a simple focus on one's body (see "appearance orientation"); one must examine the specific study and measure to be sure.

Body dysphoria: This term may mean dissatisfaction, or it might mean distress as a function of dissatisfaction; each actual study and measure must be evaluated.

Body dysmorphia: Typically refers specifically to the *Diagnostic and Statistical Manual of Mental Disorders* definition of body dysmorphic disorder (BDD), which reflects an extreme disparagement of appearance that may be excessive or even imagined.

Body schema: A construct tied closely to cognitive processing theories and models; this generally means a hypothesized preexisting cognitive framework for interpreting appearance-related information; evidence is indirectly inferred from experiments that typically consist of a priming manipulation.

Body percept: See "body schema," above.

Body distortion: Typically used to refer to size estimation accuracy; however, it has been used to describe bizarre perceptual experiences (e. g., schizophrenia).

Body image, body image disturbance, and body image disorder: These global constructs are almost useless without a specification of which particular subjective, affective, cognitive, behavioral, or perceptual processes are intended, and whether the foci are specific body sites or a global aspect of overall appearance.

Note. Definitions are presented in relative order of precision. From Thompson, Heinberg, Altabe, and Tantleff-Dunn (1999). Copyright 1999 by the American Psychological Association. Reprinted by permission.

Measures of Weight Satisfaction

With measures that purport to assess body or weight satisfaction, it is generally easy to review the specific items and determine if the scale has content validity. Table 21.3 describes some of the more commonly used measures that index this aspect of body image. These measures include such scales as the Eating Disorder Inventory's Body Dissatisfaction subscale (Garner, Olmsted, & Polivy, 1983), the Body Satisfaction Scale (Slade, Dewey, Newton, Brodie, & Kiemle, 1990), and the Body Shape Questionnaire (Cooper et al., 1987). These scales appear to be ideal for use with obese samples, because the focus is clearly on the subjective rating of weight-related aspects of the body.

Another method to assess body image dissatisfaction involves the use of schematic-figure-rating methodologies. These consist of a range of figures varying in size from thin/underweight to obese, which are shown to the study participant or patient. Generally, individuals rate the figures using an instructional protocol designed to determine *their* "ideal" body size and their "current" or "actual" body size. The discrepancy between the two ratings is then used as the index of dissatisfaction. These measures include the Figure Rating Scale (Stunkard, Sorenson, & Schulsinger, 1983), the Contour Rating Scale (Thompson & Gray, 1995), and the Body Image Assessment (Williamson, Davis, Bennett, Goreczny, & Gleaves, 1989) (see Table 21.3). Such discrepancies are highly correlated with questionnaire measures of satisfaction (Thompson, 1996).

Measures of Appearance Satisfaction

It is also possible to capture a broader notion of body image disturbance by including measures that assess overall appearance satisfaction. These measures may focus on non-weight-related features, such as discrete body parts or muscularity, or may include items that attempt to assess an individual's conception of how he or she looks in clothes or appears to other people. Such measures include the Multidimensional Body–Self Relations Questionnaire's Appearance Evaluation subscale (Cash, 1995, 1996, 1997) and the Physical Appearance State and Trait Anxiety Scale's Nonweight subscale (Reed, Thompson, Brannick, & Sacco, 1991) (see Table 21.3). Such measures may be useful because they provide information regarding the generality of the obese individual's appearance concerns. For instance, it may be clinically useful to determine whether dissatisfaction is specific to certain body areas, or generalized to other aspects of the body image. Similarly, it may be relevant to examine the specific cognitions or behavioral characteristics of someone with high levels of subjective weight dissatisfaction. The Body Image Automatic Thoughts Questionnaire (Cash, Lewis, & Keeton, 1987), the Body Image Avoidance Questionnaire (Rosen, Srebnik, Saltzberg, & Wendt, 1991), and the Situational Inventory of Body Image Dysphoria (Cash, 1994b) are examples of measures that focus on the cognitive and behavioral dimensions.

Measures of Size Perception

Finally, no discussion of body image assessment is complete without some reference to "perceptual" aspects of disturbance. This is perhaps the most controversial area in body image assessment. Many of the early studies of persons with eating disorders noted that patients with anorexia nervosa actually tended to overestimate the size of their bodies. As a result, the field of body image was somewhat dominated by interest in this phenomenon until the late 1980s (Thompson, 1990). More recent work has questioned the specificity of overestimation to any diagnostic group (eating-disordered or obese), and contemporary work has demonstrated convincingly that "perceptual" ratings are affected by attitudinal and af-

toring form designed to allow for self-recording of body-image-related experiences outside the clinical setting. Rosen and Cash (1995) developed the Body Image Diary, which may be an excellent tool for collecting information that could corroborate interview and/or questionnaire data. In some cases, there may be signs of extreme body image dissatisfaction; if such is the case, further testing with the Body Dysmorphic Disorder Examination should be considered (Rosen & Reiter, 1996).

When a clinician is considering the inclusion of a body image measure, it is important that the measure be appropriate for the individual in question. Both the gender and ethnicity of the person should always be considered when one is choosing a psychological test, as the instrument may have been developed/validated on a sample with different characteristics. This may be particularly true for the assessment of body size. Many of the measures currently available, including those listed in Table 21.3, were developed, normed, and validated on college students. Certainly these samples contained some proportion of overweight or obese individuals; however, studies have often failed to evaluate the psychometric characteristics of scales of body weight. Similarly, it is often not known whether the psychometric qualities of a scale developed on nonpatient samples can be generalized to patient samples. For these reasons, we recommend contacting the authors of specific scales and requesting any normative and psychometric data for obese samples, by gender and ethnicity. Given these caveats, it is encouraging that recent investigations of body image dissatisfaction in obese persons have found acceptable reliabilities with these samples (Foster, Wadden, & Vogt, 1997; Sarwer, Wadden & Foster, 1998; Smith, Thompson, Raczynski, & Hilner, 1999).

TREATMENT OF BODY IMAGE DISSATISFACTION IN OBESE PERSONS

The treatment of body image dissatisfaction in obese persons (much like the treatment of such dissatisfaction in nonobese persons) is still in its infancy. Through 1990, no study in the obesity treatment literature had included psychological interventions specifically designed to address body image concerns (Brownell & Wadden, 1986; Rosen, 1996). On the one hand, this is surprising, given that almost 25 years earlier Stunkard and Mendelson (1967) had noted the occurrence of body image dissatisfaction in obese persons. On the other hand, it may not be so surprising, as body image is commonly considered a psychological issue. Obesity, by contrast, is often seen as a physical condition with psychological components. The last decade, however, has witnessed the blending of these two perspectives, such that the treatment of body image dissatisfaction is becoming a more important part of comprehensive behavioral obesity treatment.

The role of body image treatment in obesity treatment, however, has not been fully determined. Studies have shown that improvements in the body image of obese persons occur with weight loss. Other studies have shown that body image improvements can occur without weight reduction. The importance of body image in both satisfaction with weight loss treatment and long-term weight maintenance, however, is unknown.

Improvements in Body Image with Weight Reduction

Several studies have assessed changes in body image in obese persons during weight loss. Cash (1994a) reported significant improvements in the body image of obese women who lost an average of 22 kg with a very-low-calorie diet. These findings, however, were limited by a 59% attrition rate. Foster, Wadden, and Vogt (1997) assessed changes in body image in women following 48 weeks of weight loss treatment by calorie reduction and exercise. At the midpoint of treatment (24 weeks and a 19-kg weight loss), women reported significant improvements in body image. A weight regain of approximately 3 kg from weeks 24 to 48 was associated with a slight but significant worsening in body image. Nevertheless, at the end of treatment patients reported significant improvements in body image as compared to baseline. Improvements, however, were only modestly related to the magnitude of weight loss.

At least two studies have investigated changes in body image following bariatric surgery for severe obesity. Halmi, Long, Stunkard, and Mason (1980) found that 70% of patients reported body image dissatisfaction before surgery, but only 4% reported dissatisfaction postoperatively. Adami and colleagues (1994) also reported significant improvements in body image after a mean weight loss of 60 kg.

In some respects, these findings confirm intuitive thought. Bariatric surgery patients are frequently distressed about their physical appearance and are subjected to extreme social disparagement as a result of their size (Rand & Macgregor, 1990). A recent study of body size evaluations of postoperative bariatric surgery patients, however, suggests that such patients may be more critical of the range of "socially acceptable" body types (Rand, Liss-Resnick, & Macgregor, 1999). As compared to a sample of adults from the general population, postoperative surgery patients identified a narrower range of body sizes as "socially acceptable." This finding suggests that some bariatric surgery patients may struggle to reach a desired level of body image satisfaction postoperatively. This is consistent with the idea of a "vestigial body image" proposed by Cash (1990), which suggests that some individuals who have lost weight still experience heightened body image dissatisfaction similar to that of overweight individuals. This term appears to have been initially applied to persons who still saw themselves as "fat" following weight loss. In the case of bariatric surgery patients, it may refer to a different type of body image dissatisfaction, perhaps related to body frame size, hip circumference, or other non-weight-related concerns (Bailey, Goldberg, Swap, Chomitz, & Houser, 1990; Davis, Durnin, Dionne, & O'Conner, 1994; Rosen et al., 1995). One of us (Sarwer), in working with bariatric surgery patients postoperatively, has been struck by the relatively common body image complaint of excessive and redundant skin following significant weight loss.

Improvements in Body Image without Weight Reduction

Beginning in 1990, several groups of investigators have studied the efficacy of improving body image without weight loss in overweight and obese persons. In one of the first such studies, Roughan, Seddon, and Vernon-Roberts (1990) reported significant improvements in body image, as well as improvements in self-esteem and depression, following a program designed to promote weight acceptance and decrease overeating and dietary restraint. Polivy and Herman (1992) found that after a 10-week "undieting" program, obese women also reported improvements in self-esteem and depression, but did not report improvements in body image. One possible explanation for the difference in body image findings for the two studies may be that Roughan and colleagues' (1990) participants lost 3 kg, while those treated by Polivy and Herman (1992) gained approximately 6 kg.

More recently, Rosen and colleagues (1995) have developed an extensive cognitive-behavioral body image therapy program specifically tailored for overweight and obese individuals. The program is typically administered in a group format (although it can be conducted individually), with one 2-hour meeting per week for 8 weeks. At the outset of treatment, participants are taught about the origins of body image development and are shown how negative body image attitudes are both learned and maintained through sociocultural influences and personal experiences. A key component throughout treatment is self-

faction and significant depression may not be good candidates for a group treatment approach. Future studies should strive not only to further understand these relationships in treatment-seeking patients, but also to investigate them in persons not seeking treatment as well.

The next generation of studies should also include a wider range of assessment measures. The majority of body image studies to date have relied heavily on paper-and-pencil measures of body image. As a result, the perceptual component of body image has been relatively neglected. Recently developed computer programs that allow for the "morphing" of body features may provide interesting opportunities to assess body image in obese persons.

Much remains to be learned about the role of body image in the treatment of obesity. Given that obese persons seeking weight reduction have unrealistic expectations about the magnitude of weight loss typically achieved in obesity treatment (Foster, Wadden, Vogt, & Brewer, 1997; Wadden, Berkowitz, Sarwer, Prus-Wisniewski, & Steinberg, 2001), it is likely that they may have equally unrealistic expectation about changes in both body image (and body shape) following weight loss. This hypothesis, however, has yet to be empirically evaluated. Furthermore, changes in body image for different groups of obese persons, including persons with binge-eating disorder and those who undergo bariatric surgery, have yet to be investigated.

Treatment for body image dissatisfaction in obese persons has drawn heavily from cognitive-behavioral models of psychotherapy. Although there is growing evidence for the effectiveness of such approaches, there has been little study of the components of treatment that are most critical to treatment success. It is unclear whether the behaviorally based strategies (such as exposure to avoided situations) or the cognitive elements of treatment (such as cognitive restructuring) play a more central role in treatment outcome. Ultimately, studies of the differential effectiveness of these strategies may provide important information on the treatment of body image dissatisfaction.

Although the study of the complex relationship between obesity and body image remains in its infancy, it appears that two separate camps of research are developing. The first group is looking primarily at changes in body image that accompany weight loss. These investigators are focusing more on how changes to the physical body influence the body image. The second group is looking more specifically at changes in body image through the use of psychotherapy, independent of weight loss. The focus of this group is changing the body image without changing weight or shape. Though both approaches have evidence to support their effectiveness, it may turn out that the combination of both approaches—changing the body and the body image simultaneously—may lead to the most successful outcomes.

Alternatively, given the struggles of many obese persons with long-term weight control, it may be that body image interventions play their most important role in weight maintenance. Cognitive-behavioral therapy for body image following weight loss may help patients change their beliefs about what constitutes successful long-term weight control. Rather than giving up efforts to maintain their weight loss because they are unhappy with the way they look, persons who receive body image therapy may enjoy greater satisfaction with their appearance and may be more motivated to continue weight control efforts. This hypothesis, however, awaits further study. Regardless, it is likely that body image will play a significant role in the treatment of obesity in years to come.

ACKNOWLEDGMENTS

We would like to acknowledge Elizabeth R. Didie, MA, and Gretchen Haselhahn for their assistance with the preparation of the chapter.

REFERENCES

Adami, G. F., Gandolfo, P., Campostano, A., Bauer, B., Cocchi, F., & Scopinaro, N. (1994). Eating Disorder Inventory in the assessment of psychosocial status in the obese patient prior to and at long-term following biliopancreatic diversion for obesity. *International Journal of Eating Disorders, 15,* 265–274.

Alfonso, V. C., Allicon, D. B., Rader, D. E., & Gorman, B. S. (1996). The Extended Satisfaction with Life Scale: Development and psychometric properties. *Social Indicators Research, 38,* 275–301.

American Psychiatric Association. (1994). *Diagnostic and statistical manual of mental disorders* (4th ed.). Washington, DC: Author.

Bailey, S. M., Goldberg, J. P., Swap, W. C., Chomitz, V. R., & Houser, R. F. (1990). Relationships between body dissatisfaction and physical measurements. *International Journal of Eating Disorders, 9,* 457–461.

Beck, A. T., & Steer, R. A. (1987). *Manual for the Beck Depression Inventory.* New York: Psychological Corporation.

Brown, T. A., Cash, T. F., & Mikulka, P. J. (1990). Attitudinal body image assessment: Factor analysis of the Body–Self Relations Questionnaire. *Journal of Personality Assessment, 55,* 135–144.

Brownell, K. D., & Wadden, T. A. (1986). Behavioral therapy for obesity: Modern approaches and better results. In K. D. Brownell & J. P. Foreyt (Eds.), *Handbook of eating disorders: Physiology, psychology, and treatment of obesity, anorexia, and bulimia* (pp. 180–199). New York: Basic Books.

Butters, J. W., & Cash, T. F. (1987). Cognitive-behavioral treatment of women's body image dissatisfaction. *Journal of Consulting and Clinical Psychology, 55,* 889–897.

Button, E. J., Loan, P., Davies, J., & Sonuga-Barke, E. J. S. (1997). Self-esteem, eating problems, and psychological well-being in a cohort of schoolgirls aged 15–16: A questionnaire and interview study. *International Journal of Eating Disorders, 21,* 39–47.

Cash, T. F. (1990). The psychology of physical appearance: Aesthetics, attributes, and images. In T. F. Cash & T. Pruzinsky (Eds.), *Body images: Development, deviance, and change* (pp. 51–79). New York: Guilford Press.

Cash, T. F. (1994a). Body image and weight changes in a multisite comprehensive very-low calorie diet program. *Behavior Therapy, 25,* 239–254.

Cash, T. F. (1994b). The Situational Inventory of Body Image Dysphoria: Contextual assessment of a negative body image. *The Behavior Therapist, 17,* 133–134.

Cash, T. F. (1995). *What do you see when you look in the mirror?: Helping yourself to a positive body image.* New York: Bantam Books.

Cash, T. F. (1996). The treatment of body image disturbances. In J. K. Thompson (Ed.), *Body image, eating disorders, and obesity: An integrative guide for assessment and treatment* (pp. 83–107). Washington, DC: American Psychological Association.

Cash, T. F. (1997). *The body image workbook: An 8-step program for learning to like your looks.* Oakland, CA: New Harbinger.

Cash, T. F., & Henry, P. (1995). Women's body images: The results of a national survey in the U.S.A. *Sex Roles, 33,* 19–28.

Cash, T. F., Lewis, R. J., & Keeton, W. P. (1987, March). *The Body Image Automatic Thoughts Questionnaire: A measure of body-related cognitions.* Paper presented at the annual meeting of the Southeastern Psychological Association, Atlanta, GA.

Collins, M. E. (1991). Body figure perceptions and preferences among preadolescent children. *International Journal of Eating Disorders, 10,* 199–208.

Cooper, P. J., Taylor, M. J., Cooper, Z., & Fairburn, C. G. (1987). The development and validation of the Body Shape Questionnaire. *International Journal of Eating Disorders, 6,* 485–494.

Davis, C., Durnin, J. V. G. A., Dionne, M., & O'Conner, M. (1994). The influence of body fat content and bone diameter measurements on body dissatisfaction in adult women. *International Journal of Eating Disorders, 15,* 257–263.

Davis, C., & Katzman, M. (1997). Charting new territory: Body esteem, weight satisfaction, depression, and self-esteem among Chinese males and females in Hong Kong. *Sex Roles, 36,* 449–459.

and figure in obese girls: Discontent but not depression. *International Journal of Obesity, 13,* 89–97.

Wadden, T. A., Sarwer, D. B., Arnold, M. E., Gruen, D., & O'Neil, P. M. (2000). Psychosocial status of severely obese patients before and after bariatric surgery. *Problems in General Surgery, 17,* 13–22.

Wichstrom, L. (1995). Social, psychological and physical correlates of eating problems: A study of the general adolescent population in Norway. *Psychological Medicine, 25,* 567–579.

Williamson, D. A., Davis, C. J., Bennett, S. M., Goreczny, A. J., & Gleaves, D. H. (1989). Development of a simple procedure for assessing body image disturbances. *Behavioral Assessment, 11,* 433–446.

22

Cognitive-Behavioral Treatment of Obesity

ZAFRA COOPER
CHRISTOPHER G. FAIRBURN

This chapter is concerned with the use of cognitive-behavioral therapy in the treatment of obesity. It begins with a description of the defining features of cognitive-behavioral therapy and of how this treatment differs from behavior therapy. After a brief review of the literature on the cognitive-behavioral treatment of obesity, a new cognitive-behavioral treatment is described. This focuses primarily on the problem of posttreatment weight regain, which is arguably the most pressing issue in the treatment of obesity.

THE CHARACTERISTICS OF COGNITIVE-BEHAVIORAL THERAPY

Cognitive-behavioral treatments have three features that together distinguish them from behavior therapy and from other forms of psychological treatment.

1. *Cognitive-behavioral treatments are based on a cognitive conceptualization of the processes that maintain the problem in question.* In other words, they are derived from a theory concerning the maintenance of the problem that places central importance on the contribution of cognitive processes. For example, in the case of depression, it is proposed that the disorder is maintained to a large extent by the presence of certain characteristic depressive thoughts and assumptions regarding the self, the world, and the future (Beck, 1976); in bulimia nervosa, it is proposed that a central maintaining mechanism is the judging of self-worth largely in terms of shape or weight (Fairburn, 1985); and in panic disorder, it is proposed that the key psychopathological feature is the interpretation of bodily sensations as being highly threatening (Clark, 1986). In each of these disorders, the particular cognitive theory of maintenance provides the basis for a specific cognitive-behavioral treatment.

2. *Cognitive-behavioral treatments are designed to modify the postulated cognitive maintaining mechanisms, the prediction being that this is necessary for there to be lasting change.* The primary aim of cognitive-behavioral treatments is to produce cognitive change, although other features are also directly addressed. Examples of these other features include the social withdrawal seen in depression, the avoidance of fear-engendering situations found in anxiety disorders, and the characteristically rigid and extreme dieting of many patients with eating disorders.

3. *Cognitive-behavioral treatments use a combination of cognitive and behavioral procedures to help the patient identify and change the targeted maintaining mechanisms.* Commonly used treatment procedures include the presentation and personalization of the relevant cognitive theory of maintenance; the use of behavioral "experiments" to help patients try new ways of behaving, and to test their expectations regarding the consequences of behavior change; and the systematic identification and evaluation of dysfunctional thoughts and assumptions.

In many other respects, cognitive-behavioral therapy is similar to behavior therapy. Many therapeutic techniques are common to both treatments. Both are short-term, problem-oriented treatments, and both are primarily focused on the present and future rather than on the past. Both involve the presentation of an explicit model of the maintenance of the problem in question; both use a similar collaborative therapeutic style; and both require patients to be active participants in the change process. Lastly, both are committed to seeking empirical evidence to evaluate their effectiveness and to evolving in response to clinical and research findings. Despite these similarities, behavior therapy, unlike cognitive-behavioral therapy, does not stress cognitive processes; the primary aim of behavioral treatments is not to produce cognitive change; and behavioral experiments and cognitive restructuring are not central characteristics of behavior therapy.

COGNITIVE-BEHAVIORAL THERAPY AND OBESITY

There is a substantial body of evidence supporting the use of behavior therapy in the treatment of obesity (Wing, 1998). It reliably results in an average weight loss of about 10% of initial weight (among treatment completers)—a weight loss that is thought to result in clinically significant health benefits (Goldstein, 1992; Kanders & Blackburn, 1992; Tremblay et al., 1999; Wing & Jeffery, 1995). Equally reliably, however, the lost weight is regained over the following 3 years (Perri, 1998; Perri & Corsica, Chapter 17, this volume).

Behavioral treatments for obesity have evolved since the 1960s when they were first developed. Among the developments has been the addition of cognitive procedures, and sometimes this has resulted in the relabeling of the treatment as "cognitive-behavioral therapy" (see, e.g., DeLucia & Kalodner, 1990; Foreyt & Poston, 1998; Kalodner & DeLucia, 1991; Kirsch, Montgomery, & Sapirstein, 1995). Nowadays many behavioral programs include sessions on such topics as negative thinking and relapse prevention (see, e.g., Wardle & Rapoport, 1998), but this change must be put in the context of the general characteristics of a typical behavioral treatment for obesity (see Wing, 1998, pp. 860–862).

- It is delivered to groups of 10–20 patients.
- The program is presented as a series of preplanned "lessons" (the entire group receives lesson 1 on week 1, lesson 2 on week 2, etc.).
- There is no assessment of whether the lessons relate to individual participants' particular problems or whether participants have mastered the contents of any one lesson be-

fore moving on to the next. (On the other hand, many of these programs include training in problem solving, which does provide participants with a general strategy for addressing their particular difficulties.)

• Many programs use a team of therapists (e.g., a behavior therapist, an exercise physiologist, and a nutritionist) and rotate therapists by topic.

• Treatment usually involves weekly meetings for 16–24 weeks, with a series of less frequent meetings thereafter.

• The principal components of such programs are as follows: the self-monitoring of eating; the setting of specific behavioral goals regarding eating and exercise; lessons on nutrition; emphasis on increasing both lifestyle activity and formal exercising; the use of stimulus control techniques; training in problem solving; simple cognitive restructuring; and relapse prevention. (See Wadden & Osei, Chapter 11, this volume.)

Such programs bear almost no resemblance to cognitive-behavioral therapy in their theoretical basis (which, if present, places little weight on the contribution of cognitive processes), aims (which are to change eating and exercise habits rather than to achieve cognitive change), or treatment procedures (which are almost exclusively behavioral). Indeed, their highly structured prescriptive format bears only a limited resemblance to behavior therapy as commonly practiced outside the treatment of obesity. Rather, these programs might be better characterized as behaviorally oriented group psychoeducational interventions. However, it must be acknowledged that there is no evidence that a more flexible and individualized form of behavior therapy would be any more effective.

To our knowledge, no cognitive-behavioral theories or treatments for obesity (as defined above) have been described or evaluated. A possible exception is the "behavioral choice treatment" of Sbrocco, Nedegaard, Stone, and Lewis (1999).[1] Specific cognitive-behavioral treatments have been developed for problems associated with obesity, such as binge eating (Fairburn, Marcus, & Wilson, 1993) and body image disturbance (Rosen, 1997), and there are cognitive-behavioral "nondieting" treatments that aim to improve participants' well-being (see, e.g., Tanco, Linden, & Earle, 1998). In none of these treatments is the primary emphasis on achieving weight loss.

THE PROBLEM OF WEIGHT REGAIN

Perri (1998) has written that "The maintenance of treatment effects represents the single greatest challenge in the long-term management of obesity" (p. 526). This widely held view is based on the substantial body of evidence indicating that 5%–10% percent weight loss can be achieved with both behavioral and pharmacological treatments for obesity, and that it is probably worth achieving from the standpoint of physical health. The problem is that once treatment is stopped, the lost weight is regained.

Two approaches to the prevention of weight regain have been advocated. The first is long-term drug treatment. For a number of reasons, this is never likely to be a complete answer. First, many patients would prefer not to be treated with drugs at all; moreover, as treatment is extended in duration, there are likely to be increasing problems with the acceptability of drug treatment and therefore with compliance. Second, there is the ever-present possibility that long-term drug use will be associated with adverse physical effects. Third, there are situations in which drug treatment is inappropriate—for example, during pregnancy.

The second approach advocated is long-term, or even indefinite, treatment. This is supported by the evidence suggesting that extending treatment delays weight regain (Perri,

are trained to count calories. Patients are also taught to plot their weight each week on a graph. This is followed by Module II ("Establishing and Maintaining Weight Loss"), in which the emphasis is on helping patients restrict their energy intake to about 1,500 kilocalories (kcal) daily. We have found that this level of dietary restriction is sufficient to achieve, on average, a weight loss of 0.5–1.0 kg per week. Patients are encouraged to devise their own flexible dietary regimen, taking into account their circumstances and food preferences.

Module III ("Addressing Barriers to Weight Loss") runs in parallel with Module II. It focuses on identifying and addressing the various problems that may interfere with patients' adherence to the energy-restricted diet. These include motivational issues, inaccurate monitoring of energy intake, poor food choice (particularly the consumption of a highly restricted range of food or a high-fat diet), excessive alcohol intake, frequent snacking, and eating either as a reward or in response to adverse mood states. In our experience, true binge eating (as defined in DSM-IV, American Psychiatric Association, 1994) is not common among people with obesity and often resolves itself without requiring direct attention. (For further information on binge eating and its management, see Stunkard, Chapter 6, this volume.)

Module IV on nutrition ("Eating Well") is also introduced at this stage. At this point in treatment, it is concerned with healthy eating while losing weight. The module is reintroduced in Phase Two when the focus is on healthy eating as part of long-term weight control. It follows standard contemporary nutritional guidelines (U.S. Department of Agriculture, 1995; see Melanson & Dwyer, Chapter 12, this volume).

Module V, on activity and exercise ("Increasing Activity"), may also form part of Phase One, although it is primarily concerned with establishing a more active lifestyle as part of weight maintenance. Thus it is of more relevance in Phase Two. However, this notion is referred to earlier in treatment to help those patients who would like to incorporate lifestyle activity and exercise in their weight loss efforts. The emphasis is on increasing activity level in general (which necessarily includes decreasing sedentariness), rather than on exclusively increasing formal exercising.

Addressing Obstacles to Acceptance of Weight Maintenance (Modules VI–VIII)

The other three modules that constitute Phase One (Modules VI, VII, and VIII) are not designed to produce weight loss; rather, they address potential obstacles to the acceptance of weight maintenance (i.e., weight stability) as a goal in Phase Two. They are employed flexibly with respect both to their timing and the degree of emphasis that is placed on them. They are described here in rather more detail than the previous modules, since their content and style overlaps less with that of existing behavioral programs for obesity. Similar considerations apply to Module IX, which is concerned with weight maintenance.

Body Image (Module VI)

Concerns about appearance—in particular, a desire to change shape—are a major reason why patients want to lose weight. These concerns contribute to their adopting weight goals that are significantly lower than the ones they are likely to achieve. We suggest that these goals, and the concerns they reflect, are major obstacles to patients' recognition and positive acceptance of what they can achieve in treatment.

Module VI ("Body Image") is designed to identify and address body image concerns. It consists of six partially independent sections, incorporating a number of strategies and techniques developed by others for addressing these problems (see especially Cash, 1996; Rosen, 1997). The first and second sections, which are concerned with education and assessment, are relevant to all patients. The remaining sections, which address factors maintaining a poor body image, are used as needed in whatever order seems appropriate for individual patients. The addressing of body image, which often needs to be continued over a number of weeks, is always integrated with other aspects of ongoing treatment. It is not introduced in the very early stages of treatment, but once weight loss is well underway at any point between week 8 and week 20 (see Figure 22.1).

The first educational section concentrates on explaining what is meant by "body image"; conveying to the patient that dissatisfaction with appearance, or some aspect of it, is very common; and emphasizing that it is only when this dissatisfaction affects everyday functioning and overall self-evaluation that it becomes a problem. On the basis of this discussion, and information obtained from a checklist that each patient completes, the therapist assesses the nature and extent of the patient's body image concerns and decides which maintaining factors (if any) need to be specifically addressed. For those patients with significant body image concerns, the therapist explains that the focus on improving their body image will take place in parallel with their attempts to lose weight and will not be a substitute for these. The therapist also explains that a negative body image is likely to interfere with the acquisition of weight maintenance strategies (in Phase Two) and therefore to make them vulnerable to weight regain.

Before introducing any of the specific cognitive or behavioral interventions designed to improve patients' body image, the therapist discusses the development and, more importantly, the maintenance of body image problems. The aim is to identify and discuss with patients the relative contribution of the following factors to the persistence of their concerns: social pressures to be thin; their own body-checking and avoidance behavior; and negatively biased thoughts and attributions about their appearance. To assist assessment and change, patients are requested to keep a body image diary. The material from this diary provides a means of identifying the most important problems, as well as examples of the operation of maintaining factors.

For most obese patients, living in a society that values thinness tends to perpetuate a negative body image, as may certain patient-specific social pressures such as critical family attitudes or a working environment in which these pressures are intensified (e.g., through having to wear a uniform). Of course, there is often nothing a patient or therapist can do to alter such influences. Patients are therefore helped to identify them and to question society's ideals and stereotypes; this assists them in distancing and protecting themselves from these pressures.

The next two sections of the module are concerned with excessive body checking and avoidance, respectively. The therapist first ensures that patients understand the rationale for tackling these forms of behavior, and then makes plans with patients for reducing and eliminating checking behavior and for progressive exposure to avoided situations. In both cases, patients are encouraged to predict the likely consequences of performing the agreed-upon tasks. Once they have been attempted, the consequences are discussed with particular reference to the difference between predicted and actual outcomes and what has been learned as a result.

The fifth section of the module addresses negative thoughts and attributions about body shape and the beliefs that they express. The therapist explains that this way of thinking plays an important role in maintaining a poor body image because, despite its excessively self-critical nature, it tends to be accepted as true. Furthermore, it encourages avoidance and checking behavior and leads to further biases in the interpretation of information. Various standard cognitive restructuring techniques are used to examine these thoughts, including reality or hypothesis testing, the identification of biased thinking, and the consideration of the advantages and disadvantages of holding a particular view. Addressing this way of

loss and weight regain is described in a way that invites them to speculate on what is likely to happen.

Once the process of reevaluating weight loss goals has begun, patients are encouraged to consider any benefits that they have already achieved in treatment. Attention is drawn to possible areas in which changes may have occurred, such as an increase in energy and sense of well-being, improved fitness and ease of daily life, and more choice in clothes. The therapist supplements this discussion by pointing out (in some detail) the health benefits of moderate weight loss, and by helping patients to see that through recognizing their achievements they are more likely to continue to be successful. In addition, patients' attention is drawn to the possibility of simultaneously achieving their primary goals (which are addressed in Module VIII).

The final step in the guided argument involves reemphazing the importance of both acceptance and change. To be successful at long-term weight control, patients need to make those changes that it is possible to make and to accept what cannot be changed (Wilson, 1996). Particular emphasis is placed on the fact that patients are able to achieve many of their primary goals, regardless of the degree of weight loss they have achieved, and that they should not have unreasonable expectations of themselves.

Primary Goals (Module VIII)

"Primary goals" are objectives that patients hope to achieve as a result of weight loss. They include changing appearance, improving self-confidence, enhancing interpersonal functioning, and increasing fitness. The aim of Module VIII ("Primary Goals") is to help patients directly address these goals. We suggest that this is an essential element in treatment, since it is likely to result in greater satisfaction with what has been accomplished in treatment (regardless of whether patients' initial weight loss goal has been reached), and therefore the acceptance of weight maintenance as an objective in Phase Two. Although primary goals are discussed in outline as part of the initial assessment process, they are not formally addressed until weight loss is well underway. Thus this module is usually introduced in the course of discussing weight goals (between weeks 12 and 20), and runs concurrently with it (see Figure 22.1).

Once a patient's primary goals have been identified, they become additional treatment goals in their own right, although they never take precedence over achieving weight loss and then weight maintenance. They are addressed via the well-established problem-solving approach used in cognitive-behavioral therapy (Goldfried & Goldfried, 1975), in which patients have already been trained during Module III. As part of this process, patients are encouraged to set themselves specific achievable tasks, implement a plan to realize them, and regularly evaluate their progress. Examples include joining a club (to help form new relationships); going to an exercise class or taking up a sport (to improve fitness); and buying a new outfit to wear on a special occasion or trying a new hairstyle (to change appearance). It will be found that only a minority of primary goals, such as buying some types of clothes, actually require weight loss. Such goals may have to be deferred until further weight loss is achieved. In some instances it will not be possible to attain these, in which case the therapist encourages acceptance along the lines discussed earlier.

Weight Maintenance (Module IX)

The most distinctive feature of this cognitive-behavioral treatment is the priority it gives to long-term weight maintenance. The subject is raised at the beginning of treatment when the therapist explains that the treatment has both a weight loss and a weight maintenance phase, and it is addressed during weight loss when potential barriers to long-term weight maintenance are tackled (Modules VI–VIII).

During Phase Two, weight maintenance is the major focus of treatment; patients are strongly discouraged from attempting to lose further weight, whatever their weight loss has been up to this point. The introduction of Module IX ("Weight Maintenance") coincides with entering Phase Two and is unique to it. The module is introduced according to individual need at any point between week 24 and week 30, thus allowing a minimum of 14 weeks before the end of treatment for the acquisition and practice of weight maintenance skills (see Figure 22.1).

Since eating a healthy low-fat diet and establishing and maintaining an active lifestyle are probably important for successful long-term weight control (McGuire, Wing, Klem, & Hill, 1999), Module IV ("Eating Well") and Module V ("Increasing Activity") are also central to Phase Two. Patients are encouraged to continue to eat a low-fat diet and to establish a high level of activity (by increasing walking and other forms of lifestyle activity) if they have not already done so as part of their weight loss efforts. The emphasis with regard to eating is on patients' adopting a flexible diet (with no forbidden foods) within the suggested guidelines. With respect to activity, the focus is on increasing activity levels in a realistic and sustainable way, and not just on increasing formal exercising.

Before embarking on Module IX, the therapist ensures that the patient appreciates the need to devote a substantial amount of time in treatment to acquiring maintenance skills. The therapist explains that although there are many different ways of losing weight, to date none has proved effective at maintaining the weight lost. This treatment aims to address this problem by helping patients develop and practice the skills needed for long-term weight control. In order to do this, weight maintenance needs to be the focus at this stage in treatment, and weight stability rather than weight loss should be the new goal. Despite the therapist's making these points, a minority of patients will be reluctant to stop attempting to lose weight. With such patients, further work is often needed on Modules VI, VII, and VIII.

In preparation for weight maintenance, the differences between losing weight and maintaining a stable weight are highlighted, as are the difficulties commonly encountered with long-term weight control. There are three major differences: First, weight maintenance is less reinforcing than weight loss, in part because there is less encouragement from others; second, the process is indefinite rather than time-limited; and third, it may involve accepting a weight and shape that were previously regarded as unacceptable (Wadden, 1995).

The next step is to define a specific target weight range and establish a weight-monitoring system that provides patients with the information needed to keep their weight within this target range. To allow for natural weight fluctuations, we recommend a range of about 4 kg in magnitude, with the center of the range being the average of a patient's weight over the 6 weeks prior to beginning Phase Two. Once this range has been agreed, its upper and lower limits are highlighted by drawing two parallel lines on the patient's ongoing weight graph, and the patient is asked to maintain weight within these boundaries. In order to monitor their progress in doing so, patients are advised to weigh themselves weekly (on a predetermined day) and record their weight on their weight graph. It is also made clear that this system of weight monitoring will need to continue indefinitely, because without it there will be a risk of inadvertent weight regain. This need for indefinite weight monitoring is stressed again at the very end of treatment by providing patients with a large set of blank weight maintenance graphs for future use.

Once a target weight range has been established, the next step is to help patients distinguish significant changes in their weight from trivial fluctuations and to learn how to take corrective action when necessary. Patients are helped to assess their progress each time they weigh themselves. They are advised that in order to evaluate the significance of

treated in a combined behavioural modification programme. *International Journal of Obesity, 16*, 623–625.

Cash, T. F. (1996). The treatment of body image disturbances. In J. K. Thompson (Ed.), *Body image, eating disorders, and obesity* (pp. 83–107). Washington, DC: American Psychological Association.

Clark, D. M. (1986). A cognitive approach to panic disorder. *Behaviour Research and Therapy, 24*, 461–470.

Cooper, Z., & Fairburn, C. G. (2001). A new cognitive behavioural approach to the treatment of obesity. *Behaviour Research and Therapy, 39*, 499–511.

DeLucia, J. L., & Kalodner, C. R. (1990). An individualized cognitive intervention: Does it increase the efficacy of behavioral interventions for obesity? *Addictive Behaviors, 15*, 473–479.

Fairburn, C. G. (1985). Cognitive-behavioral treatment for bulimia. In D. M. Garner & P. E. Garfinkel (Eds.), *Handbook of psychotherapy for anorexia nervosa and bulimia* (pp. 160–192). New York: Guilford Press.

Fairburn, C. G., Marcus, M. D., & Wilson, G. T. (1993). Cognitive-behavioral therapy for binge eating and bulimia nervosa: A comprehensive treatment manual. In C. G. Fairburn & G. T. Wilson (Eds.), *Binge eating: Nature, assessment, and treatment* (pp. 361–404). New York: Guilford Press.

Foreyt, J. P., & Poston, W. S. C. (1998). What is the role of cognitve-behavior therapy in patient management? *Obesity Research, 6*(Suppl. 1), 18S–22S.

Goldfried, M. R., & Goldfried, A. P. (1975). Cognitive change methods. In F. H. Kanfer & A. P. Goldstein (Eds.), *Helping people change* (pp. 89–116). New York: Pergamon Press.

Goldstein, D. J. (1992). Beneficial health effects of modest weight loss. *International Journal of Obesity, 16*, 397–415.

Kalodner, C. R., & DeLucia, J. L. (1991). The individual and combined effects of cognitive therapy and nutrition education as additions to a behavior modification program for weight loss. *Addictive Behaviors, 16*, 255–263.

Kanders, B. S., & Blackburn, G. L. (1992). Reducing primary risk factors by therapeutic weight loss. In T. A. Wadden & T. B. VanItallie (Eds.), *Treatment of the seriously obese patient* (pp. 213–230). New York: Guilford Press.

Kirsch, I., Montgomery, G., & Sapirstein, G. (1995). Hypnosis as an adjunct to cognitive-behavioral psychotherapy: A meta-analysis. *Journal of Consulting and Clinical Psychology, 63*, 214–220.

Latner, J. D., Stunkard, A. J., Wilson, G. T., Jackson, M. L., Zelitch, D. S. & Labouvie, E. (2000). Effective long-term treatment of obesity: A continuing care model. *International Journal of Obesity and Related Metabolic Disorders, 24*(7), 893–898.

McGuire, M. T., Wing, R. R., Klem, M. L., & Hill, J. O. (1999). Behavioral strategies of individuals who have maintained long-term weight losses. *Obesity Research, 7*, 334–341.

Perri, M. G. (1998). The maintenance of treatment effects in the long-term management of obesity. *Clinical Psychology: Science and Practice, 5*, 526–543.

Rosen, J. C. (1997). Cognitive-behavioral body image therapy. In D. M. Garner & P. E. Garfinkel (Eds.), *Handbook of treatment for eating disorders* (2nd ed., pp. 188–201). New York: Guilford Press.

Sbrocco, T., Nedegaard, R. C., Stone, J. M., & Lewis, E. L. (1999). Behavioral choice treatment promotes continuing weight loss: Preliminary results of a cognitive-behavioral decision-based treatment for obesity. *Journal of Consulting and Clinical Psychology, 67*, 260–266.

Tanco, S., Linden, W., & Earle, T. (1998). Well-being and morbid obesity in women: A controlled therapy evaluation. *International Journal of Eating Disorders, 23*, 325–339.

Tremblay, A., Doucet, E., Imbeault, P., Mauriege, P., Despres, J.-P., & Richard, D. (1999). Metabolic fitness in active reduced-obese individuals. *Obesity Research, 7*, 556–563.

U.S. Department of Agriculture. (1995). *Report of the Dietary Guidelines Advisory Committee on the Dietary Guidelines for Americans.* Washington, DC: Author.

Wadden, T. A. (1995). Characteristics of successful weight loss maintainers. In D. B. Allison & F. X. Pi-Sunyer (Eds.), *Obesity treatment: Establishing goals, improving outcomes and reviewing the research agenda* (pp. 103–111). New York: Plenum Press.

Wardle, J., & Rapoport, L. (1998). Cognitive-behavioural treatment of obesity. In P. G. Kopelman & M. J. Stock (Eds.), *Clinical obesity* (pp. 409–428). Oxford: Blackwell.

Wilson, G. T. (1996). Acceptance and change in the treatment of eating disorders and obesity. *Behavior Therapy, 27,* 417–439.

Wilson, G. T., Fairburn, C. G., & Agras, W. S. (1997). Cognitive-behavioral therapy for bulimia nervosa. In D. M. Garner & P. E. Garfinkel (Eds.), *Handbook of treatment for eating disorders* (2nd ed., pp. 67–93). New York: Guilford Press.

Wing, R. R. (1998). Behavioral approaches to the treatment of obesity. In G. A. Bray, C. Bouchard, & W. P. T. James (Eds.), *Handbook of obesity* (pp. 855–873). New York: Marcel Dekker.

Wing, R. R., & Jeffery, R. W. (1995). Effect of modest weight loss on changes in cardiovascular risk factors: Are there differences between men and women or between weight loss and maintenance? *International Journal of Obesity, 19,* 67–73.

6. *Group hatred.* Perhaps the ultimate sadness for fat people is that they tend not to identify with other fat people. Self-hatred becomes group-hatred. This is borne out by the fact that children as young as 6 years of age were found to label silhouettes of obese youngsters as "lazy, stupid, cheats, lies, and ugly" (Staffieri, 1967). But even more troublesome was that these judgments were made by obese youngsters themselves. People's self-esteem is deeply injured when they regard others like themselves with disgust. Most overweight people do not feel that they will be overweight all of their lives. They think of themselves as "temporarily fat"—a belief that discourages group solidarity and cohesion. One of the reasons why diverse racial or ethnic populations have been able to make major strides toward equality and acceptance is that they do not think of themselves as temporarily "black" or temporarily "Hispanic." More importantly, they do not regard their race or ethnicity as an unacceptable characteristic.

VARIABLES THAT INFLUENCE SELF-ESTEEM

Age at Onset of Obesity

Researchers have found that significant body image disparagement occurs in only a subset of obese individuals (Burt & Stunkard, 1964). Studies have shown that a negative body image is more common in persons with childhood or adolescent onset of obesity, presence of an emotional disturbance, and negative evaluation by significant others (Sarwer, Wadden, & Foster, 1998). Furthermore, when those with adult-onset obesity reach a socially accepted weight, they tend to be satisfied with their appearance. This is not true of persons with early-onset obesity, many of whom appear unsatisfied with their bodies, even if they succeed in maintaining a nearly normal body weight. This is most likely related to the fact that the body image construct develops at an early age and is fairly well entrenched by the time a child enters adolescence (Adami et al., 1998). During evaluations, therefore, it may be important to inquire when patients first became overweight.

Self-Esteem and Binge Eating

It is critical for physicians and other health care professionals to make a distinction between obese individuals with binge-eating disorder and obese persons who do not typically binge. Binge eating involves consuming an objectively large amount of food in a short period of time (i.e., 2 hours or less) and experiencing loss of control during the overeating episode. Approximately 15%–30% of persons who seek weight reduction meet criteria for binge-eating disorder (see Stunkard, Chapter 6, this volume). Research has shown that women who engage in binge eating suffer from higher levels of depression and anxiety and lower levels of self-esteem than those who do not binge, regardless of weight category. Obese individuals who do not binge-eat are indistinguishable on these variables from persons of average weight (Webber, 1994). Once again, it is important when one is evaluating an overweight patient to determine whether there is a problem with binge eating. If so, it may be advisable to refer the patient to a mental health professional for further evaluation of mood and self-esteem.

DO HEALTH CARE PROFESSIONALS CONTRIBUTE TO HEAVIER INDIVIDUALS' POOR SELF-ESTEEM?

In the health care community, it has generally been assumed that all people are meant to be slim and could be if they just ate less and exercised more. Physicians may become exasperated when patients are advised to lose weight and fail to do so. The experience may be equally exasperating for larger individuals who, fearful of being "scolded," may start avoiding doctor visits. This is definitely not a desired outcome, as preventive care may be delayed until problems reach an acute stage. An obese patient may feel that "even my doctor doesn't like me," causing his or her self-esteem to fall further.

Research shows that physicians and other health care professionals often view their heavier patients with disdain and may even make insulting remarks to them. As early as 1969, Maddox and Leiderman found that more than half of physicians described their obese patients as "weak-willed" (60%), "ugly" (54%), or "awkward" (55%). In a more recent study of family physicians, 63% of physicians attributed obesity to a lack of willpower, and more than one-third described their obese patients as "lazy" (Price, Desmond, Krol, Snyder, & O'Connell, 1987). Researchers tend to explain these findings by pointing out that health care professionals have been exposed for years to the same antifat messages as the rest of the population, and have developed many of the same prejudices.

In a study by Rand and Macgregor (1990), extremely obese patients were asked a series of questions about how they had been treated by various members of society. One such item was "I have been treated disrespectfully by the medical profession because of weight." Only 6% of patients responded "never," while 79% responded either "usually" or "always." As stated earlier, such experiences may lead larger people to avoid going to their doctors. In another study, only 47.5% of "very overweight" women said they had received annual pelvic exams in the last 2 years, as compared with 68.1% of the average-weight women (Adams, Smith, Wilbur, & Grady, 1993).

The mental health profession is not immune to this type of prejudice. The discipline of psychology commonly assumes that larger people are emotionally stunted and that they eat to compensate for a variety of problems. However, studies have failed to uncover greater degrees of psychopathology in obese women who are not suffering from binge-eating disorder (Telch & Agras, 1993; Wadden & Stunkard, 1985). Indeed, psychologist Eleanor Webber (1994) cautions her profession: "Psychologists have a responsibility not only to examine our own prejudices but also to communicate this awareness to diminish the unfortunate tendency to stereotype obese people in terms of presumed psychological characteristics. Whereas some obese people do struggle with painful emotions, their obesity is not the problem" (p. 348).

CONSEQUENCES OF POOR SELF-ESTEEM

Poor self-esteem can have significant and harmful consequences for heavier persons. Among these are the following:

1. *Postponement of life*. People who are waiting to be thin postpone all sorts of activities because they feel that they will be much better equipped to handle major life challenges in a slim body. So they avoid social events, career opportunities, travel, relationships—even buying attractive clothes. They literally put their lives "on hold." The danger in this reasoning is that the majority of above-average-weight people are probably not going to achieve the weight they would consider "ideal" for moving ahead with their lives, given the present status of our knowledge about obesity and its treatment. This means that if they continue to put their lives on hold, there is a good chance they will never achieve many of their goals and aspirations.

2. *Poor choices and decisions*. Larger people often feel inferior, and this leads them to make poor choices and decisions in many areas of their lives, especially when it comes to re-

general population. It is important, however, to assess patients for binge-eating disorder, because if it is determined to be present, a patient should be referred to a mental health or eating disorder specialist.

4. *Give the same advice and care to obese patients as to nonobese patients presenting with the same types of problems.* If medication is warranted for a medical condition, and would be prescribed for a thin person with the same problem, write a prescription. Weight management can still be part of the overall treatment plan for hypertension or hypercholesterolemia, but an above-average-weight patient, like an average-weight one, should have the benefits of medication immediately.

5. *Buy a scale that can weigh all patients, and provide larger gowns when needed.* Nothing is more humiliating to larger patients than to be given gowns that don't cover them. In addition, use a large blood pressure cuff when appropriate, and provide armless chairs in waiting rooms.

6. *Do not set a goal weight for the next visit.* Patients who are told to lose a specified amount of weight and are not able to achieve it are often afraid to come back. Rather than focusing on "ideal" weights, talk to such patients about "healthy" weights and the fact that even a 5%–10% weight loss can confer significant health benefits.

7. *Focus on overall health and nonweight outcomes.* Examples include improvement in blood pressure, glycemic control, or lipid values.

8. *Encourage exercise.* Too often the emphasis is on eating less rather than being more physically active. Studies continue to show that people who incorporate regular exercise into their weight management programs have better results. But remember that exercise programs for average-weight people may be unsuitable or even impossible for larger patients. The fitness industry has not extended the welcome mat to larger people, who often feel embarrassed exercising in public. Be sensitive to this and suggest that consultation with an exercise physiologist or personal trainer may be the best way to start developing an individualized exercise program.

9. *Stay up to date on the latest research about obesity and its treatment.* Larger individuals need and deserve to have the latest information about this condition. (Once I myself became knowledgeable about obesity research, I could not understand why my physicians had not communicated any of this information to me over years and years of doctor visits. It actually made me angry that professionals who should have known about—and told me about—this body of research never did, leaving me to blame myself for my above-average weight.)

10. *Do not blame a patient for a less-than-desired outcome.* There is still a great deal to be learned about obesity, and the patient cannot be blamed for that.

11. *Tell patients that they do not need to lose even 1 pound to be worthwhile people deserving of love, respect, and self-esteem.*

HELPING LARGER INDIVIDUALS ACHIEVE BETTER SELF-ESTEEM: RESEARCH FINDINGS

There has been very little scientific research on how to improve the self-esteem of heavier people. The popular prejudices cited earlier are probably contributing factors and lead to the question "Why bother?" If the only way larger people can truly improve their self-esteem is by losing weight, why bother investing resources in research that will teach them how to feel better about themselves while they still occupy larger bodies?

The ideal solution would be to eliminate size prejudice. As Quinn and Crocker (1998, p. 141) point out, however, "Research on the stigmatized may be criticized for focusing too much on what to change about the stigmatized and not enough on how to change the culture. Although we would like to see the culture changed such that being overweight and feeling overweight is no longer stigmatizing, there is little evidence that our culture is moving in that direction."

For now, overweight individuals will probably have to take responsibility for their own self-esteem, but how do they do that? There is a small body of research directed at identifying what characteristics distinguish heavier people with good self-esteem from those with poor self-esteem. Some researchers have tried to identify and define what makes some larger people more "resilient" to psychological distress caused by the stigma of being overweight. They have sought to answer the question "Who are 'the resilient'?" The following findings incorporate the research of Quinn and Crocker (1998), Crandall (1994), Heatherton, Kiwan, and Hebl (1995), Parker and colleagues (1995), Kumanyika, Wilson, and Guildford-Davenport (1993), Pierce and Wardle (1997), Crocker, Cornwell, and Major (1993), and Miller (1998). "Resilient" larger people tend to exhibit the following characteristics:

1. *They do not view other overweight individuals with dislike or disgust.* They have not internalized the negative stereotypes about obesity. Research by Crandall (1994) on "antifat attitudes" found that average-weight and above-average-weight people were equally high in dislike of the "fat" population. Disliking overweight people when one is a member of the group seems risky for self-esteem, especially given the difficulty of ever leaving the group.

2. *They do not base their self-regard on others' approval to feel good about themselves.* Individuals whose self-esteem is highly dependent on receiving praise and approval from others are vulnerable to low self-esteem when they fail to receive positive evaluations. Basing one's self-esteem on these "reflected appraisals" is especially risky; it leads to self-esteem that is transient and fluctuates, depending on what sort of feedback one is receiving from others. Those who can tune all this out and build their self-esteem on self-appraisal and self-knowledge will rest on more solid ground.

3. *They realize that not all outcomes are deserved and not all things (including weight) are under personal control.* The idea that personal responsibility governs all aspects of people's lives can be harmful when applied to weight, because it leads people to believe (as mentioned earlier) that diet failures are personal failures. This is not to suggest that personal responsibility should be abdicated. It simply means this: There comes a point when some people realize that despite their very best efforts, the desired outcome may not be achievable and that this is not their "fault." Many diseases cannot be cured, not because the patients did anything wrong, but because we do not fully understand some diseases and how best to treat them.

4. *They are able to reject or ignore society's dictates about acceptable body weight.* Some racial/ethnic groups have been successful at doing this. Recent research has shown that African American and European American women have very different evaluations of larger-size figures (Heatherton et al., 1995). When shown photographs of both average-weight and above-average-weight women, African American women did not denigrate the heavier figure; however, the European American women did. Black women frequently consider themselves attractive even though they feel dissatisfied with their body size. In another study, Parker and colleagues (1995) observed that black girls focused on factors such as personal style and presentation, in addition to body size/weight, when evaluating their attractiveness. This multifaceted definition of beauty may promote both a greater investment in appearance and greater satisfaction with overall appearance regardless of body weight (Heatherton et al., 1995).

5. *They are able to blame the bias and prejudice of critics rather than themselves.* In

they rejected the notion that their figures are flawed, and concluded that everyone is simply shaped differently. Larger women should also learn to reject rules for dressing to look thinner. Clothes should be comfortable and fit well, but the idea that larger women must dress in black and avoid bright colors is silly.

16. *Indulge in body pleasures.* Get a massage, use lotions, or have manicures or pedicures. Larger people sometimes ignore what lies below their necks. They will feel much better if they pamper their bodies, not just their heads.

17. *Use positive self-talk.* Each time you catch yourself making critical comments, fight back by immediately complimenting yourself or mentally hollering "Stop!" to eject the negative "tapes," which are difficult to stop once they start playing.

18. *Make a list of people you admire who have had successful careers and lives in less-than-svelte bodies.* It may also be useful to think of ultraslim people who have had not-so-happy lives. There are many examples of both.

19. *Look for size acceptance support groups and size-positive literature.* There are currently a variety of Web sites and organizations devoted to size acceptance. For a current list, write to Largely Positive Inc., P.O. Box 170223, Glendale, WI 53217.

20. *Become an advocate.* It is very empowering and gratifying to know that you are fighting for a cause you believe in and fighting to eradicate prejudice and discrimination. Whenever you see or hear anything that smacks of size discrimination, express your displeasure by writing, calling, or e-mailing. Do whatever it takes! Your self-esteem will thank you.

ADVICE TO PARENTS

Loss of self-esteem in overweight children starts very early. Health care professionals should advise parents of larger children that their attitudes toward their own bodies and their children's weight will have a direct and major impact on whether these children grow up with their self-esteem intact. Following are lists of "dos" and "don'ts" for parents of heavier children.

"Dos"

1. *Love and accept your children unconditionally.* This will help them to love and accept themselves.

2. *Treat size and weight as characteristics that contribute to their uniqueness.* Teach them that diversity is what makes the world so interesting. Nature provides many examples. Flowers, for instance, come in all shapes, colors, and sizes—and yet all are beautiful.

3. *Examine your own biases and ask yourself whether your concern is for yourself or your child.* An above-average-weight child may make some parents feel embarrassed, and some may feel that having such a child is a banner for a family's lack of self-discipline. As with most forms of prejudice, these feelings stem from myths and misinformation.

4. *Educate yourself about what causes some people to be larger than others, so you can separate myths from facts for your children.* Then educate your children. Have a discussion about heredity. Explain that body size is an inherited characteristic much the same as height.

5. *Emphasize your children's positive attributes and talents.* Teach them that these are the things that count. Help them to develop the things they're good at.

6. *Make an extra effort to help them find clothes similar to those their friends wear.* It is important at this age to blend in.

7. *Arm your children for dealing with the outside world and our culture's obsession with thinness.* Tell them that many groups of people have suffered discrimination and prejudice, and that larger people are one of these groups. Help them plan how they would react to negative comments about their weight. Do some role playing.

8. *Make your home and family a safe haven for them, where they can always count on your support and encouragement.* They'll have enough to deal with outside the home in our "fat-phobic" society.

9. *Be a good role model.* Do not criticize your own body. You are the most important person in your children's lives. If they see that you like your own body, they will find it easier to like theirs. In particular, how a mother feels about her own body has a significant impact on her daughter's body image.

10. *Provide examples for children of attractive and successful larger people, both current and historical.* Also give them an anthropology lesson and inform them that many other cultures value and desire bodies of ample proportions.

11. *Help your larger child to unravel the "thin is in" media hype.* There are about 400 top fashion models, and less than 1% of the female population has the genetic potential to look like them. Attractive people come in assorted shapes, sizes, and colors. One mother I know took her daughter to a mall and a nursing home, where she pointed out various types and shapes of women. She told her daughter that every one of them was a unique and worthwhile individual. She followed this up with a talk about self-worth.

"Don'ts"

1. *Do not ever say or imply that your child's weight makes him or her less attractive or less acceptable in any way.* This can cause lifelong damage to self-esteem. There is no connection between weight and self-worth, and you are responsible for helping your child realize this. For example, do not tell your daughter she has "such a pretty face"—if only she would lose weight. Shaming or teasing children about their weight or bodies will make them hate their bodies even more.

2. *Do not tell your children that no one will want to date them unless they are thin.* It is not true. Plenty of plus-size teenagers have boyfriends or girlfriends. Tell your child that lasting affection looks beneath the surface and is not bound by narrow definitions of attractiveness.

3. *Do not put children on a traditional "diet."* Most dietitians now agree that this is not the way to help them manage their weight. Continual dieting may cause them to be heavier in the long run. Focus instead on development of a healthy lifestyle—for the whole family. Make physical activity a family affair—go for walks together, buy family swimming passes to a community pool, have a family dance party, or go biking.

4. *Do not become the "food police."* Continually nagging children about what they are eating will surely backfire. Children can always find ways of getting forbidden foods. In the worst-case scenario, you could be contributing to development of an eating disorder such as anorexia nervosa or bulimia nervosa. Besides, foods should not be categorized as "good" or "bad." All food has a place in normal eating.

A FINAL WORD FOR PARENTS

Despite his or her very best efforts, your child may never be thin. This is not the worst thing that could happen. Many heavy children become heavy adults—and still live satisfying, fulfilling lives. Researchers will tell you that there is much to learn yet about obesity and what

24

Nondieting Approaches: Principles, Practices, and Evidence

GARY D. FOSTER
BRIAN G. McGUCKIN

During the last decade, dieting has come under attack by a growing movement whose contention is that "diets don't work" and that their physical and psychological ill effects far outweigh any fleeting benefits (Berg, 1999; Garner & Wooley, 1991; Goodrick & Foreyt, 1991; McFarlane, Polivy, & McCabe, 1999; Robison, 1997). This movement—often referred to as "nondieting," "antidieting," or "undieting"—has gained support from professionals and nonprofessionals alike (Kassirer & Angell, 1998; McFarlane et al., 1999; Ross, 1999; Young, 1995). As a result, various nondieting programs targeted for overweight persons, especially women, have been developed (Hirschmann & Munter, 1988; Kano, 1989; Kratina, King, & Hayes, 1996; Polivy & Herman, 1983; Tribole & Resch, 1995). In general, these approaches suggest that overweight persons give up dieting and accept themselves as they are (Foster, 2001; Parham, 1996; Robison, Hoerr, Petersmarck, & Anderson, 1995).

This paradigm shift has left both practitioners and their patients in a quandary about how to manage weight and health. A traditional view argues that excess weight is associated with an increased risk of morbidity and mortality; therefore, weight loss (through diet and exercise) is a principal method for obese patients to improve their health (National Heart, Lung, and Blood Insititute [NHLBI], 1998). A nondieting view questions the relationship between excess weight and mortality; moreover, it contends that dieting is both ineffective and harmful (Berg, 1999; Ernsberger & Koletsky, 1999; McFarlane et al., 1999; Miller, 1999a). If improved health is the desired endpoint, should health care professionals encourage their overweight patients "to diet or not to diet"? In an attempt to shed light on this question, this chapter reviews the assumptions of the nondieting movement, the goals and methods of nondieting programs, and the research evaluating their efficacy.

ASSUMPTIONS

The growing discontent with dieting and the search for alternative approaches are based on three premises: (1) dieting is ineffective; (2) dieting is harmful; and (3) long-standing beliefs about the causes and consequences of overweight are incorrect. Nondieting programs have been developed to address these concerns and offer alternatives to those who have been disappointed, or even harmed, by traditional dieting attempts.

Dieting Is Ineffective

A principal driving force of the nondieting movement is the well-established finding that diets fail to produce their most desired outcome—long-term weight loss (Garner & Wooley, 1991; Kassirer & Angell, 1998; Miller, 1999b; Wadden, 1993; see also Wing, Chapter 14, and Perri & Corsica, Chapter 17, this volume). Any weight that is lost during dieting is promptly regained. It is argued that in the long term, dieters usually end up weighing more, not less, after a diet. Miller (1999a) states that all "review articles on the effectiveness of diet and exercise for weight control over the past 40 years have concluded that diet and exercise are ineffective in producing substantial long-term weight loss for a majority of the participants" (p. 212). These consistent, lackluster results have fueled the development of nondicting alternatives.

Dieting Is Harmful

A second tenet of the nondieting movement is that dieting confers significant untoward consequences across several domains. Dieting is seen as a behavioral endorsement of the cultural norms that overvalue thinness and scorn obesity (Rothblum, 1994). Psychological consequences of dieting reportedly include depression, anxiety, anger, irritability, food and weight preoccupation, social isolation, and diminished body image and self-esteem (Carrier, Steinhardt, & Bowman, 1994; Garner & Wooley, 1991; McFarlane et al., 1999; Parham, 1996; Polivy & Herman, 1983). Cognitive impairments associated with dieting include diminished reaction time and increased distractibility (McFarlane et al., 1999). In addition, dieting is thought to lead to increases in disordered eating, particularly binge eating (Carrier et al., 1994; Ernsberger & Koletsky, 1999; McFarlane et al., 1999; Polivy & Herman, 1985).

Dieting is also believed to confer significant negative physical consequences, such as reduced metabolic rate, hypotension, dizziness, hair loss, and decreased bone mass (Berg, 1999; Garner & Wooley, 1991; Polivy & Herman, 1983). Berg (1999) noted the untoward consequences associated with various weight loss medications, such as increases in blood pressure and heart rate, as well as cardiac valvulopathy. In addition, she described the side effects associated with very-low-calorie diets, such as gallstone formation, anemia, constipation, headaches, dry skin, muscle cramps, bad breath, and even death. Based on data showing that weight loss has been associated with increased mortality, Gaesser (1999) has suggested that weight loss "may do more harm than good, particularly for persons with no pre-existing health conditions" (p. 1122).

"Weight cycling"—repeated cycles of weight loss and regain—is believed to magnify the ill effects of dieting and may even lead to the very conditions (e.g., heart disease, certain cancers) that dieting seeks to improve (Carrier et al., 1994; Gaesser, 1999). Ernsberger and Koletsky (1999) concluded that "during regain of lost weight, all of the short-term benefits of weight loss are undone, and in many cases risk factors become worse during weight regain than they were at the starting level" (p. 233). Many contend that dieting, rather than producing sustained weight loss, actually prevents weight loss (Ciliska, 1990) and promotes subsequent weight gain (Polivy & Herman, 1983). In other words, dieting can "make you fat" (Hirschmann & Munter, 1988, p. 82).

In summary, Polivy and Herman (1992) concluded that dieting can "create more problems than it solves" (p. 261). These negative consequences of dieting are even more disturbing given that dieters will not experience any sustained weight loss (as described above). Thus dieting is viewed as a treatment that is both harmful and ineffective (Wooley & Garner, 1991).

Long-Standing Beliefs Are Incorrect

A third guiding principle of the nondieting movement is that fundamental assumptions about the causes and consequences of overweight are incorrect (Garner & Wooley, 1991; Miller, 1999a; Parham, 1996). Nondieting proponents view the recent developments in the understanding of the genetics of body weight as evidence for a biological rather than a behavioral etiology of obesity. They argue that if excess weight were simply a matter of inappropriate eating habits, behavioral treatments that seek to modify those habits would work. The fact that they do not suggests a less behaviorally based etiology.

The nondieting movement also challenges the assumption that being overweight is unhealthy. Kano (1989) argued that "it is extremely misleading, if not plain wrong, to say that being fat is unhealthy" (p. 15). Many suggest that the association of overweight with certain medical conditions can be explained by a third factor, such as repeated dieting, inactivity, or smoking to suppress appetite (Ernsberger & Koletsky, 1999; Gaesser, 1999; Miller, 1999a). Based on the findings by Blair and colleagues (see Blair & Leermakers, Chapter 13, this volume) suggesting that fitness rather than fatness modifies risk, nondieting advocates suggest that increased fitness rather than decreased weight should be the principal means to improve health (Gaesser, 1999). Proponents further argue that moderate degrees of excess weight may actually diminish the risk of many conditions, such as osteoporosis and certain types of cancer (Ernsberger & Koletsky, 1999; Gaesser, 1999; Kano, 1989).

Independent of whether excess weight increases risk, many point to the lack of long-term data showing that weight loss improves health (Gaesser, 1999; Miller, 1999a). A *New England Journal of Medicine* editorial summarized the data linking weight loss to improved medical benefits as "limited, fragmentary, and often ambiguous" (Kassirer & Angell, 1998, p. 52). The belief that obesity is not harmful and weight loss is not beneficial makes dieting not only ineffective and harmful, but unnecessary as well.

NONDIETING PROGRAMS: GOALS AND METHODS

Goals

Although nondieting programs vary greatly in the methods they employ, they all generally seek to (1) increase awareness of dieting's ill effects; (2) educate patients about the biological basis of body weight; (3) use internal cues such as hunger and fullness, rather than external cues such as calories and fat grams, to guide eating behavior; (4) improve self-esteem and body image through self-acceptance rather than through weight loss; and (5) increase physical activity.

There is less consensus across programs about the goals for weight loss. Several programs recommend the attainment of an "optimal" or "natural" weight, defined loosely as the weight one's body is meant to maintain without dieting or restriction-induced overeating

(Hirschmann & Munter, 1988; Kano, 1989; Polivy & Herman, 1983). Some attempt to induce a slower weight loss than traditional approaches (Sbrocco, Nedegaard, Stone, & Lewis, 1999), while others seek to prevent weight gain (Rapoport, Clark, & Wardle, 2000). In general, most programs actively discourage weight loss for its own sake but acknowledge that a change in weight (either loss or gain) may occur when eating habits are normalized.

Methods

Although these general goals are consistent across nondieting programs the methods to achieve these outcomes vary considerably. This section reviews the various strategies advocated in nondieting programs relative to the goals described above.

Increasing Awareness of Dieting's Ill Effects

Most programs begin with participants' completing detailed dieting histories to underscore the central tenets that dieting is ineffective and harmful. Polivy (1991), for example, has participants complete detailed histories of all previous diets, including the amounts lost and regained, as well as the financial cost associated with each failed attempt. In group settings, members' experiences are summed to illustrate that thousands of dollars have been spent, only for the members to end up weighing more than they did before their first diet. Participants also complete symptom checklists concerning previous dieting attempts to underscore the deleterious physical and psychological consequences described above. Such histories are meant to personalize the concept that dieting has adverse consequences (e.g., lost money, food deprivation, physical symptoms) and does not produce long-term weight loss. In addition, nondieting interventions educate participants about the misguided motivations for dieting and/or weight loss, including social acceptance and unmet emotional needs (Kratina et al., 1996; Polivy, 1991; Roughan, Seddon, & Vernon-Roberts, 1990).

Education about the Biological Basis of Body Weight

Typically, participants are provided with written materials about the strong genetic influences on body weight. They are encouraged to use their own weight and dieting histories to find a "natural weight"—a stable weight that occurs when they are neither dieting nor overeating as a result of dieting (Polivy, 1991). Participants are also educated about the biological responses to energy restriction, such as decreases in resting energy expenditure and thyroid hormones. This information is used to emphasize that weight cannot be easily changed and to debunk the notion that everyone can or should be the same size or weight.

Guiding Eating Behavior

Instructions regarding dietary intake fall into two domains. The first concerns the process of eating (i.e., how to eat), while the second concerns the product (i.e., what to eat). Regarding the process of eating, a central recommendation in most programs is to "stop dieting" (Foreyt & Goodrick, 1992; Polivy & Herman, 1983). Participants are encouraged to abandon dieting behaviors, such as going long periods of time without eating, avoiding forbidden foods, and getting weighed frequently. The purpose of doing so is to shift from a dieting mentality, in which food is the enemy, to a state of mind in which food is enjoyed (Kano, 1989; Roughan et al., 1990). This shift is thought to normalize food consumption patterns, reduce disordered eating, and assist people in overcoming their preoccupation with food (Allen & Craighead, 1999; Carrier et al., 1994; Omichinski & Harrison, 1995;

TABLE 24.1. Studies of Nondieting Approaches

Study	Sample size[a]	Treatment duration and description	Baseline BMI and weight	Posttreatment outcomes			Follow-up		
				Medical	Behavioral/psychosocial	Weight	Length	% n[b]	Outcomes
			Descriptive studies						
Carrier (1994)	79/51[c] (23% M)	26 wk; designed to reduce restrained eating, improve self-acceptance, and increase self-esteem.[d]	F = 25 ± 5 kg/m², 69 ± 13 kg; M = 28 ± 4 kg/m², 86 ± 12 kg[e]	Not assessed	Improvements in mastery of internally directed eating style.[f]	Not assessed	36 mo	18%	3 groups.[g] All groups: Sig. ↑ in self-acceptance and physical activity; sig. ↓ in frequency of dieting behaviors. Groups 2 and 3: Sig. ↑ in self-esteem.
Lewis et al. (1992)	26/26	8 wk; encouraged modification of eating patterns rather than dieting; emphasized health risks of dieting.	31 kg/m², 79 kg	Not assessed	No sig. Δ in restraint; sig. ↑ in perceived body size, self-esteem, weight control self-efficacy, and food- and weight-related assertiveness.	−2 kg −1.5 kg	6 mo	92%	↑ in self-esteem, weight control self-efficacy, and food- and weight-related assertiveness maintained; −1 kg additional weight loss.
Mellin et al. (1997)[h]	29/22[i] (5% M)	12 wk; designed to train subjects in strong nurturing, effective limits, body pride, good health, balanced eating, mastery living.	33 ± 5 kg/m², 93 ± 19 kg	Sys. BP, −7; dia BP, −6 (both sig.)	↓ in depression; ↑ in physical activity.	−4 kg	24 mo	100%	Sys. BP, −15; dia. BP, −14; −8 kg in weight; no sig. changes in depression; sig. ↑ in physical activity.
Omichinski & Harrison (1995)	253/208 (6% M)	10 wk; promoted a nondieting lifestyle characterized by nourishing eating and activity patterns and self-acceptance.	Not reported	Not assessed	Sig. ↑ in self-acceptance, self-nourishment, and nondieting behaviors.[j]	Not assessed	None	None	None

Polivy & Herman (1992)	19/15	10 wk; designed to encourage subjects to stop dieting and adopt healthy eating practices.[k]	104 kg	Not assessed	Sig. ↓ in bulimia, depression, restraint, drive for thinness; sig. ↑ in self-esteem and interoceptive awareness. No sig. Δ in body dissatisfaction.	+6 kg[l]	6 mo	53%	+8 kg in weight; sig. ↓ in drive for thinness, restraint, depression, and ineffectiveness; sig. ↑ in interoceptive awareness and self-esteem.
Robinson & Bacon (1996)	58/47	11 tx. sessions[m]; designed to increase daily activity and self-esteem, and to decrease depression and fat-phobic attitudes.	34 kg/m², 94 kg	Not assessed	Sig. ↓ in fat phobia and depression; sig. ↑ in self-esteem	Not assessed	None	None	None
Roughan et al. (1990)	87/80[n]	10 wk; designed to increase eating in response to internal hunger cues and to develop body acceptance.	32 ± 8 kg/m², 87 ± 2 kg[o]	Not assessed	Sig. improvements in body image, depression, eating attitude, self-esteem, and self-image.	−2 kg	24 mo	70%	−3 kg[o] in weight; sig. improvements in psychological functioning maintained.
					Randomized controlled trials				
Allen & Craighead (1999)	29/20	8 wk; 2 groups: 1. Appetite awareness training (eat in response to internal hunger). 2. Wait-list control.	Not reported	Not assessed	Group 1 showed significantly greater ↓ in binge eating; depression; social anxiety; and urge to eat when food present, when experiencing negative emotions, or using food as a reward. Group 1 also showed a trend for greater ↑ in self-esteem relative to Group 2.	No sig. Δ for either group[p]	None	None	None

(*continued*)

501

TABLE 24.1. *continued*

				Posttreatment outcomes			Follow-up		
Study	Sample size[a]	Treatment duration and description	Baseline BMI and weight	Medical	Behavioral/psychosocial	Weight	Length	% n[b]	Outcomes

Randomized controlled trials (cont.)

Tanco et al. (1998)	62/50	8 wk (optional 3 add'l wk); 3 groups: 1. Cognitive group treatment (nondieting): Healthy eating w/out weight loss attempt; regular exercise (3×/wk). 2. Behavior therapy weight loss (dieting): 1,200–1,500 kcal/day; regular exercise (3×/wk). 3. Wait-list control.	Group 1: 39 ± 5 kg/m², 113 ± 19 kg; Group 2: 39 ± 6 kg/m², 104 ± 16 kg; Group 3: 41 ± 6 kg/m², 112 ± 20 kg	Not assessed	Group 1: Sig. ↓ in depression, anxiety, and eating-related psychopathology. Groups 2 and 3: No sig. Δ in above variables. Groups 1 and 2: Similar and sig. ↑ in proportion of regular exercisers. Group 3: Nonsig. ↓ in proportion of regular exercisers.	Group 1: –2 kg; Group 2: –3 kg; Group 3: ± 1 kg	6 mo	57%[v]	Group 1: –5 kg; Group 2: –9 kg; no sig. differences in proportion of regular exercisers.

Note. Only studies that were traditionally nondieting in nature were included (see "Nondieting Programs: Goals and Methods" section). Studies that shared some nondieting goals (e.g., Rosen's studies on improving body image) were not included if they did not also specifically address the need to stop dieting. All subjects were female except as noted; males expressed as % of completers. Data are presented as mean ± SD where SD was reported.

[a]Number of subjects who started study/number of subjects who completed study. [b]% of those who completed study. [c]Original number enrolled not defined; 79 completed pretreatment and 3-year follow-up questionnaires; 28 of 79 did not complete 26-week treatment program; 14 of 79 attended at least one follow-up meeting. [d]Based on Hirschmann and Munter's (1989) *Overcoming Overeating* approach. [e]Weights for both groups based on self-reports. [f]Measured ability to identify physiological vs. emotional hunger, ability to match hunger to a specific food, ability to identify an emotion associated with eating, and extent to which one kept food accessible throughout the day. [g](1) Dropouts: Didn't complete 26-week program. (2) Participants: Completed 26-week program. (3) Participants and follow-up: Completed 26-week program and at least 2 follow-up activities. [h]n = 13 for depression and BP data. [i]4 dropouts; 3 completed treatment but did not complete follow-up—no data included. [j]A 6-point Likert-type scale was developed for this program assessing prevalence of chronic dieting (higher score indicated a "more independent, nondieting lifestyle"). [k]Based on Polivy and Herman (1983) book *Breaking the Diet Habit.* [l]n = 13. [m]Length of treatment not reported. [n]Data collected on only 38 subjects at all five data points. [o]n = 72 for BMI/weight data. [p]No data given. [q]Mean ranges for three groups. [r]Brownell (1989) *LEARN Program for Weight Control.* [s]Group 3 not included in 18-month follow-up; given treatment after 6 months. [t]No comparisons of control and experimental groups were directly reported. [u]Values for Miller et al. (1993) are means ± SEM. [v]Group 3 not included in 6-month follow-up.

504

Controlled Comparisons

More recently, second-generation studies have employed randomized controlled trials to compare a variety of nondieting approaches to traditional dieting programs and/or no-treatment controls. Tanco and colleagues (1998) showed that an 8-week nondieting approach, compared to standard weight loss treatment and a wait-list control, produced greater improvements in mood and in some measures of eating-related psychopathology after treatment. Both the dieting and nondieting groups lost small amounts of weight (2.6 and 1.8 kg, respectively). Follow-up data at 6 months, available on only 57% of subjects, showed weight losses of 8.9 and 4.9 kg, respectively. Significant increases in the proportion of regular exercisers in both treatment groups at the end of treatment did not persist at follow-up.

Sbrocco and colleagues (1999) compared a traditional behavioral treatment program using a 1,200-kcal/day diet to a behavioral choice program that coupled elements of nondieting with a moderately restricted diet of 1,800 kcal/day. After the 13-week treatment, both groups experienced significant increases in self-esteem, but no changes in level of depression. The behavioral choice group showed a significantly greater decrease in restraint. The traditional group experienced greater weight loss (5.6 vs. 2.5 kg). At the 1-year follow-up, there were no significant differences between the groups in exercise frequency, restraint, eating disorder constructs, self-esteem, or depression. Interestingly, during the follow-up period the traditional group gained weight, while the behavioral choice group lost weight. Thus, at the 1-year follow-up, the behavioral choice group had a mean weight loss of 10.1 kg, compared to 4.3 kg for the traditional group.

In a recent study, Rapoport and colleagues (2000) compared a standard behavioral treatment to a nondieting approach that was focused on preventing weight gain and avoiding severe restriction. The study was noteworthy for its assessment of lipids, glucose, and blood pressure. After the 10-week treatment, the standard treatment produced a 3.8-kg weight loss, compared to 1.3 kg for the nondieting group. Both groups experienced significant improvements in measures of depression, self-esteem, and body image at 10 weeks. At 12 months, both groups showed small weight losses (2–4 kg), small but significant improvements in blood pressure and total and low-density lipoprotein cholesterol, and significant changes in self-esteem, depression, and body image. However, there were no differences between the groups at 12 months on any of these variables.

Two controlled trials have evaluated the efficacy of nondieting approaches in the treatment of binge-eating disorder (Allen & Craighead, 1999; Goodrick et al., 1998). Goodrick and colleagues (1998) compared a nondieting approach, a dieting approach, and a wait-list control. After 6 months of treatment, both the dieting and nondieting groups showed significant and similar improvements in binge eating. Both treatment groups, as well as the wait-list control, were within 1.4 kg of their baseline weight. Similar findings were observed at 18 months. These small weight losses in the dieting group may be attributable to the fact that subjects were not weighed at weekly sessions. Allen and Craighead (1999) compared an 8-week appetite awareness treatment, focused on responding to moderate signals of hunger and satiety, to a wait-list control. At the end of treatment, the appetite awareness group showed significant improvements in binge eating, self-esteem, and depression. Neither group showed any significant change in weight. These two studies suggest that nondieting programs appear to have favorable effects upon binge eating, but not greater than those of traditional dieting treatments.

Although these recent controlled trials have increased the fund of knowledge about nondieting approaches, they are limited by short interventions, incomplete follow-ups, small samples and high attrition. For example, most (five of seven) of the randomized studies in Table 24.1 employed interventions ranging from 8 to 13 weeks. Three studies reported no follow-up data (Allen & Craighead, 1999; Ciliska, 1998; Miller et al., 1993), and another included only 57% of subjects at follow-up (Tanco et al., 1998). Furthermore, three studies had fewer than 25 subjects (Allen & Craighead, 1999; Miller et al., 1993; Sbrocco et al., 1999), and three had attrition greater than 30% during treatment (Allen & Craighead, 1999; Ciliska, 1998; Miller et al., 1993).

Findings of the Research

Based on the available data, what can be concluded about the utility of nondieting approaches? One consistent finding is that nondieting approaches appear to have favorable effects on self-esteem. Faith, Fontaine, Cheskin, and Allison (2000) performed a meta-analysis on six (mostly uncontrolled) studies and found effect sizes for self-esteem ranging from 0.67 to 3.79, which yielded a weighted mean d value of 1.57 ($SE = 0.11$). In other words, self-esteem was increased by approximately 1.5 standard deviation units—an extremely strong effect. There are consistent but not universal findings for improvements in mood and body image. Some studies found that psychosocial changes in nondieting groups were similar to those in dieting groups (Rapoport et al., 2000; Sbrocco et al., 1999), while others found greater improvements in nondieting groups (Tanco et al., 1998).

Among the few studies that assessed physiological variables (Ciliska, 1998; Mellin et al., 1997; Miller et al., 1993; Rapoport et al., 2000), there were small but significant changes in blood pressure and lipids, although Rapoport and colleagues (2000) found no difference between dieting and nondieting groups. Interestingly, Ciliska (1998) reported a decrease in diastolic blood pressure in the absence of weight loss.

Most nondieting programs produce little or no change in body weight. The programs producing the larger weight losses are typically those that have incorporated some elements of traditional dieting (Miller et al., 1993; Sbrocco et al., 1999), with the exception of Mellin and colleagues (1997). It is interesting to note that in some studies, weight loss continued in the nondieting group during follow-up (Mellin et al., 1997; Sbrocco et al., 1999)—a pattern quite different from that of traditional dieting programs. In summary, it seems reasonable to conclude that nondieting programs favorably affect self-esteem, mood, and body image, but result in little change in body weight. The effects on medical outcomes are understudied, especially in controlled trials.

A CRITICAL VIEW

This section assesses the relative strengths and weaknesses of nondieting approaches, and suggests directions for future research and practice.

Strengths

A major strength of the nondieting movement is its continued emphasis on the long-term ineffectiveness of conventional, dieting-based treatments. Although increased physical activity and continued patient–practitioner contact following treatment significantly improve the maintenance of weight loss in the year following treatment, weight regain is the most frequent long-term outcome of dieting (NHLBI, 1998). This lack of long-term success for most persons should lead overweight persons to consider carefully the long-term benefits and risks of dieting before embarking on "another diet." In addition, the lack of long-term efficacy should prompt health care professionals to develop alternative treatment approaches aimed at improving the health of overweight persons. Unfortunately, multiple efforts to modify the dieting paradigm in some way have resulted in the same long-term result—weight regain. Clearly, there is a need for new approaches that are not based on the current dieting paradigm, and the nondieting movement has provided one such alternative.

Perhaps the greatest strength of the nondieting movement is the affirmation of a person's worth, no matter what he or she weighs. This message is so countercultural that it can seem ridiculous to suggest that obese persons should accept themselves or that overweight does not result from a lack of character or willpower. However, there are indeed many factors that influence body weight, some of which are not under one's control (see Price, Chapter 4, this volume). Overweight persons are not weak-willed, lazy, and undisciplined; nor are they morally inferior or deficient in character. Such stereotypes are not only inaccurate but cruel, and like other forms of discrimination and prejudice, they should not be tolerated. The nondieting movement has provided a great service by promoting these messages, which encourage overweight persons to live life now, rather than waiting until they lose weight (Johnson, 1995). In addition, these messages can prompt professionals to remember that as members of our society, they are likely to have antifat attitudes that need to be identified and modified (Price, Desmond, Krol, Snyder, & O'Connell, 1987; Yalom, 1993).

Weaknesses

The most significant weakness of the nondieting approaches is the lack of scientific support. It is troubling that nondieting books and programs have increased significantly, despite a dearth of studies demonstrating their effectiveness. No approach, no matter how well intentioned or sensible, should be marketed as effective when it has not been adequately studied. As for any other treatment, efficacy claims about nondieting programs should be supported by well-conducted studies. Unfortunately, the proliferation of nondieting books, videos, and clinic-based programs makes it difficult to distinguish these approaches from the multitude of new diet books and diet clinics that are also promoted without scientific evaluation. Overweight persons deserve better. They are entitled to know the short- and long-term results of alternative treatments, so they can make informed decisions about their health and weight.

The nondieting movement also suffers from a lack of empirical support for some of its basic beliefs. For example, it has been well known for over a decade that the psychosocial effects of dieting and weight loss are typically, although not universally, quite positive among obese persons receiving standard cognitive-behavioral treatment, despite reports in the 1950s of adverse effects in normal-weight men and obese psychiatric patients (Foster & Wadden, 2001). Yet nondieting programs continue to conclude that dieting is universally harmful, based largely on laboratory assessments of normal-weight, college-age women classified as "restrained eaters." Similarly, recent comprehensive reviews do not support claims that dieting leads to binge eating or other eating disorders among obese individuals (National Task Force on the Prevention and Treatment of Obesity, 2000).

Nondieting books often describe the harmful effects of weight cycling in unequivocal terms. The scientific literature reveals that some of the effects of weight cycling (i.e., decreased metabolic rate, increased body fat, depression) do not occur, while others (i.e., increased morbidity and mortality, psychological effects) are far from being clearly resolved (Brownell & Rodin, 1994; Foster, Sarwer, & Wadden, 1997; Gregg & Williamson, Chapter 7, this volume).

Finally, the belief that weight is not a risk factor for disease is contrary to a large body of literature that has controlled for multiple mediating factors (NHLBI, 1998). Some data do suggest that health may be more influenced by fitness than by fatness (Blair & Leermakers, Chapter 13, this volume); therefore, it may be possible to be fit and fat. However, many Americans, both overweight and lean, are not fit. Thus many overweight persons—the targets of most nondieting programs—are at higher risk. It remains to be seen whether changes in weight or fitness will be more effective in terms of health outcomes. In the absence of definitive data and the presence of substantial contradictory data, it seems misleading or even irresponsible to suggest that excess weight is unrelated to health. Whether increased risk is mediated by fat or fitness, obese, unfit people are at increased medical risk. Although psychosocial improvements are important in their own right, the lack of attention to reducing medical risk is troubling.

In addition, there is considerable evidence that weight loss among obese persons improves diabetes, hypertension, and dyslipidemia over 6–12 months (NHLBI, 1998; Pi-Sunyer, 1996). Although it is true that no studies have shown definitively that weight loss has long-term benefits on health, no such studies have been conducted. Most studies that have been reported about the effects of intentional weight loss were not designed to answer that question, and most rely on self-reports and/or retrospective recalls of weight, weight loss, and number of dieting attempts (Gregg & Williamson, Chapter 7, this volume). Among this flawed literature, some studies indicate that intentional weight loss has positive long-term effects, while others show no or adverse effects (Gregg & Williamson, Chapter 7). Fortunately, a 12-year prospective randomized controlled trial is being conducted in 5,000 obese individuals with Type 2 diabetes to address this critical question (see www.lookaheadstudy.org).

Similarly, although a large body of research suggests the importance of biological factors in the control of body weight, it is a mistake to minimize the role of environmental factors. The increase in the prevalence of obesity during the last decade cannot be explained by genetic factors. Clearly, biological and behavioral factors interact to influence body weight (Wadden, Brownell, & Foster, in press). Both should be considered when a person is attempting modest weight loss as a means to improve health.

Challenges

Given these strengths and weakness, the nondieting movement, as well as the entire scientific community with an interest in the health of overweight persons, is faced with a series of challenges. We believe that nondieting approaches merit further investigation in randomized controlled trials. In order to facilitate assessments of clinical utility, we make the following recommendations for future research.

The first is to define clearly what is meant by "dieting" and "nondieting" treatments, since standard cognitive-behavioral approaches and nondieting approaches for weight loss have more in common than might be thought (e.g., eating a variety of foods in moderation, consuming forbidden foods, increasing physical activity, limiting external cues to eating, self-acceptance). Such comparisons will be facilitated by the use of standardized treatment protocols for both nondieting and dieting treatments. Critical issues will include the goals and methods of dieting and nondieting approaches, as well as measurable outcomes to assess whether goals have been achieved. We agree with Parham (1996) that each program should be assessed relative to its unique goals, but we add that such goals need to be made explicit and measurable.

Since a common goal of nondieting programs is to stop dieting, it will be important to clearly define what is meant by "dieting." This may mean going long periods of time without eating, avoiding "fattening" or "forbidden" foods, or following a specific eating regimen. A recent recommendation is that dieting "refers to the intentional and sustained restriction of caloric intake for the purpose of reducing body weight or changing body shape"

(National Task Force, 2000, p. 2582). It is interesting to note that the word "diet" is derived from the Greek *diaita*, meaning "way of life." The treatment of many other medical conditions (e.g., hypertension, diabetes, lactose intolerance, celiac disease, dyslipidemia) consists of dietary management that requires limiting or even eliminating certain types of foods to improve health. Overweight persons will need guidance about how to distinguish "dieting" from other methods of healthy eating/living.

Optimal interventions are likely to be at least 6 months in duration, especially for nondieting programs that seek to challenge long-standing beliefs and behaviors about weight, eating, physical activity, self-esteem, and body image. Mastering the dialectic of acceptance and change can be quite challenging (Dougher, 1994; Wilson, 1996), and it is unlikely that sustained attitudinal and/or behavioral changes can be achieved after a few months of weekly meetings.

It would also be useful to include interventions that are variants on the dieting and nondieting paradigms. It may be that some blending of approaches, as reported by Sbrocco and colleagues (1999), will be helpful. Similarly, it may be useful to evaluate interventions that focus solely on improving fitness, with less concern about dieting or nondieting.

A critical issue in such research will be the measurement of both physical and psychological indices of health. If health at any weight is the desired paradigm shift, both dieting and nondieting programs must be compared on such risk factors as lipids, glucose tolerance, blood pressure, and fitness. Although changes in diet and physical activity may be interesting, the lack of valid assessment (without considerable expense) makes them less useful.

When investigators are reporting mean changes in physical and psychological variables, it is important to assess clinical significance. Reporting only mean values can obscure important information, such as changes in clinical status. For example, statistically significant changes in Beck Depression Inventory scores for a nondepressed sample (e.g., from 7 to 3) are much less meaningful than the percentage of patients who progressed from depressed to nondepressed categories. Assessing clinical significance will be enhanced by using reliable and valid psychosocial measures that have normative scores for clinical and nonclinical samples. This will allow readers to assess whether pre- and posttreatment values were in clinically significant ranges. Similarly, for physiological variables, it will be important to report subanalyses for patients who already have diabetes, dyslipidemia, or hypertension than for those who do not have such comorbidities.

In addition to the larger issue of relative efficacy, many other questions deserve research attention. For example, it is unclear whether nondieting approaches are best suited for overweight persons who have never dieted, for those who have dieted and given up, for average-weight persons who have neither dieted nor become overweight, or for those at risk for eating disorders. It is possible that nondieting approaches may be a useful tool in the prevention of eating disorders and obesity. Thus it may be best to teach people never to begin dieting than to teach them to stop dieting once they have begun.

A final challenge is to decrease the distance between dieting approaches typically used by professionals in the obesity field and nondieting approaches typically used by those in the eating disorders field. This division has sometimes resulted in misunderstandings that can lead to hostility and hyperbole. Overweight persons would be better served by active collaboration between the two fields. It is likely that the two fields may disagree about several issues, such as the effects of dieting and the ill effects of obesity. However, they are likely to agree about the long-term ineffectiveness of most dieting attempts, the value of enhancing body image and self-esteem without weight loss, the need to fight discrimination against obese persons, and the need to provide effective health care for overweight patients beyond weight loss.

CONCLUSION

The development of nondieting approaches represents an exciting advance in the care of overweight persons. However, these approaches should be carefully evaluated before being widely disseminated. Such information will help overweight persons make informed decisions about managing their health and weight. Ultimately, whether the decision is to diet or not to diet, we hope that professionals can help overweight persons realize that weight is just one factor that describes them; it doesn't define them.

REFERENCES

Allen, H. N., & Craighead, L. W. (1999). Appetite monitoring in the treatment of binge eating disorder. *Behavior Therapy, 30,* 253–272.

Berg, F. M. (1999). Health risks associated with weight loss and obesity treatment programs. *Journal of Social Issues, 55,* 277–297.

Blair, S. N. (1991). *Living with exercise: Improving your health through moderate physical activity.* Dallas, TX: American Health.

Brownell, K. D. (1989). *The LEARN program for weight control.* Dallas, TX: Brownell and Hager.

Brownell, K. D., & Rodin, J. (1994). Medical, metabolic, and psychological effects of weight cycling. *Archives of Internal Medicine, 154,* 1325–1330.

Burgard, D., & Lyons, P. (1994). Alternatives in obesity treatment: Focusing on health for fat women. In P. Fallon, M. A. Katzman, & S. C. Wooley (Eds.), *Feminist perspectives on eating disorders* (pp. 212–230). New York: Guilford Press.

Carrier, K. M., Steinhardt, M. A., & Bowman, S. (1994). Rethinking traditional weight management programs: A 3-year follow-up evaluation of a new approach. *The Journal of Psychology, 128,* 517–535.

Cash, T. F. (1997). *The body image workbook: An 8-step program for learning to like your looks.* Oakland, CA: New Harbinger.

Ciliska, D. (1990). *Beyond dieting.* New York: Brunner/Mazel.

Ciliska, D. (1998). Evaluation of two nondieting interventions for obese women. *Western Journal of Nursing Research, 20,* 119–135.

Dougher, M. J. (1994). The act of acceptance. In S. C. Hayes, N. S. Jacobson, V. M. Follette, & M. J. Dougher (Eds.), *Acceptance and change: Content and context in psychotherapy* (pp. 37–45). Reno, NV: Context Press.

Ernsberger, P., & Koletsky, R. J. (1999). Biomedical rationale for a wellness approach to obesity: An alternative to a focus on weight loss. *Journal of Social Issues, 55,* 221–260.

Faith, M. S., Fontaine, K. R., Cheskin, L. J., & Allison, D. B. (2000). Behavioral approaches to the problems of obesity. *Behavior Modification, 24,* 459–493.

Foreyt, J. P., & Goodrick, G. K. (1992). *Living without dieting.* Houston, TX: Harrison.

Foster, G. D. (2001). Non-dieting approaches. In C. G. Fairburn & K. D. Brownell (Eds.), *Eating disorders and obesity* (2nd ed., pp. 604–608). New York: Guilford Press.

Foster, G. D., Sarwer, D. B., & Wadden, T. A. (1997). Psychological effects of weight cycling in obese persons: A review and research agenda. *Obesity Research, 5,* 474–488.

Foster, G. D., & Wadden, T. A. (2001). Social and psychological effects of weight loss. In C. G. Fairburn & K. D. Brownell (Eds.), *Eating disorders and obesity* (2nd ed., pp. 500–504). New York: Guilford Press.

Gaesser, G. A. (1999). Thinness and weight loss: Beneficial or detrimental to longevity? *Medicine and Science in Sports and Exercise, 31,* 1118–1128.

Garner, D. M., & Wooley, S. C. (1991). Confronting the failure of behavioral and dietary treatments for obesity. *Clinical Psychology Review, 11,* 729–780.

Gast, J., & Hawks, S. R. (1998). Weight loss education: The challenge of a new paradigm. *Health Education and Behavior, 25,* 464–473.

Goodrick, G. K., & Foreyt, J. P. (1991). Why treatments for obesity don't last. *Journal of the American Dietetic Association, 91,* 1243–1247.

Goodrick, G. K., Poston, W. S. C., II, Kimball, K. T., Reeves, R. S., & Foreyt, J. P. (1998). Nondieting versus dieting treatment for overweight binge-eating women. *Journal of Consulting and Clinical Psychology, 66,* 363–368.

Hirschmann, J. R., & Munter, C. H. (1988). *Overcoming overeating: Living free in the world of food.* Reading, MA: Addison-Wesley.

Johnson, C. A. (1995). *Self-esteem comes in all sizes: How to be happy and healthy at your natural weight.* New York: Doubleday.

Kano, S. (1989). *Making peace with food: Freeing yourself from the diet/weight obsession.* New York: Harper & Row.

Kassirer, J. P., & Angell, M. (1998). Losing weight—an ill-fated New Year's resolution [Editorial]. *New England Journal of Medicine, 338,* 52–53.

Kratina, K., King, N. L., & Hayes, D. (1996). *Moving away from diets: New ways to heal eating problems and exercise resistance.* Lake Dallas, TX: Helm Seminars.

Lewis, V. J., Blair, A. J., & Booth, D. A. (1992). Outcome of group therapy for body-image emotionality and weight-control self-efficacy. *Behavioural Psychotherapy, 20,* 155–165.

Lyons, P., & Burgard, D. (1990). *Great shape: The first fitness guide for large women.* Palo Alto, CA: Bull.

Lyons, P., & Miller, W. C. (1999). Effective health promotion and clinical care for large people. *Medicine and Science in Sports and Exercise, 31,* 1141–1146.

McFarlane, T., Polivy, J., & McCabe, R. E. (1999). Help, not harm: Psychological foundation for a nondieting approach toward health. *Journal of Social Issues, 55,* 261–276.

Mellin, L., Croughan-Minihane, M., & Dickey, L. (1997). The solution method: 2-year trends in weight, blood pressure, exercise, depression, and functioning of adults trained in development skills. *Journal of the American Dietetic Association, 97,* 1133–1138.

Miller, W. C. (1999a). Fitness and fatness in relation to health: Implications for a paradigm shift. *Journal of Social Issues, 55,* 207–219.

Miller, W. C. (1999b). How effective are traditional dietary and exercise interventions for weight loss? *Medicine and Science in Sports and Exercise, 31,* 1129–1134.

Miller, W. C., Wallace, J. P., Eggert, K. E., & Lindeman, A. K. (1993). Cardiovascular risk reduction in a self-taught, self-administered weight-loss program called the nondiet diet. *Medicine and Exercise for Nutrition and Health, 2,* 218–223.

National Heart, Lung, and Blood Institute (NHLBI). (1998). Clinical guidelines on the identification, evaluation, and treatment of overweight and obesity in adults: The evidence report. *Obesity Research, 6*(Suppl.), 51S–220S.

National Task Force on the Prevention and Treatment of Obesity. (2000). Dieting and the development of eating disorders in overweight and obese adults. *Archives of Internal Medicine, 160,* 2581–2589.

Omichinski, L. (1999). *You count, calories don't.* Portage la Prairie, Manitoba, Canada: HUGS International.

Omichinski, L., & Harrison, K. R. (1995). Reduction of dieting attitudes and practises after participation in a non-diet lifestyle program. *Journal of the Canadian Diabetic Association, 56,* 81–85.

Parham, E. S. (1996). Is there a new weight paradigm? *Nutrition Today, 31,* 155–161.

Parham, E. S. (1999). Promoting body size acceptance in weight management counseling. *Journal of the American Dietetic Association, 99,* 920–925.

Pi-Sunyer, F. X. (1996). A review of long-term studies evaluating the efficacy of weight loss in ameliorating disorders associated with obesity. *Clinical Therapeutics, 18,* 1006–1035.

Polivy, J. (1991). *Stop dieting: A program to enhance self-acceptance.* Toronto: Author.

Polivy, J., & Herman, C. P. (1983). *Breaking the diet habit: The natural weight alternative.* New York: Basic Books.

Polivy, J., & Herman, C. P. (1985). Dieting and bingeing: A causal analysis. *American Psychologist, 40,* 193–201.

Polivy, J., & Herman, C. P. (1992). Undieting: A program to help people stop dieting. *International Journal of Eating Disorders, 11,* 261–268.

Price, J. H., Desmond, S. M., Krol, R. A., Snyder, F. F., & O'Connell, J. K. (1987). Family practice physicians' beliefs, attitudes and practices regarding obesity. *American Journal of Preventive Medicine, 3,* 215–220.

Rapoport, L., Clark, M., & Wardle, J. (2000). Evaluation of a modified cognitive-behavioural programme for weight management. *International Journal of Obesity, 24,* 1726–1737.

Robinson, B. E., & Bacon, J. G. (1996). The "If Only I Were Thin . . ." treatment program: Decreasing the stigmatizing effects of fatness. *Professional Psychology Research and Practice, 27*(2), 175–183.

Robison, J. I. (1997). Weight management: Shifting the paradigm. *Journal of Health Education, 28,* 28–34.

Robison, J. I., Hoerr, S. L., Petersmarck, K. A., & Anderson, J. V. (1995). Redefining success in obesity intervention: The new paradigm. *Journal of the American Dietetic Association, 95,* 422–423.

Rosen, J. C., Orosan, P., & Reiter, J. (1995). Cognitive behavior therapy for negative body image in obese women. *Behavior Therapy, 26,* 25–42.

Ross, J. (1999). *The diet cure.* New York: Penguin.

Rothblum, E. D. (1994). I'll die for the revolution but don't ask me not to diet: Feminism and the continuing stigmatization of obesity. In P. Fallon, M. A. Katzman, & S. C. Wooley (Eds.), *Feminist perspectives on eating disorders* (pp. 53–76). New York: Guilford Press.

Roughan, P., Seddon, E., & Vernon-Roberts, J. (1990). Long-term effects of a psychologically based group programme for women preoccupied with body weight and eating behavior. *International Journal of Obesity, 14,* 135–147.

Sbrocco, T., Nedegaard, R., Stone, J. M., & Lewis, E. L. (1999). Behavioral choice treatment promotes continuing weight loss: Preliminary results of a cognitive-behavioral decision-based treatment for obesity. *Journal of Consulting and Clinical Psychology, 67,* 260–266.

Tanco, S., Linden, W., & Earle, T. (1998). Well-being and morbid obesity in women: A controlled therapy evaluation. *International Journal of Eating Disorders, 23,* 325–339.

Tribole, E., & Resch, E. (1995). *Intuitive eating.* New York: St. Martin's Press.

Wadden, T. A. (1993). Treatment of obesity by moderate and severe caloric restriction: Results of clinical research trials. *Annals of Internal Medicine, 119,* 688–693.

Wadden, T. A., Brownell, K. D., & Foster, G. D. (in press). Obesity: Responding to the global epidemic. *Journal of Consulting and Clinical Psychology.*

Wilson, G. T. (1996). Acceptance and change in the treatment of eating disorders and obesity. *Behavior Therapy, 27,* 417–439.

Wooley, S. C., & Garner, D. M. (1991). Obesity treatment: The high cost of false hope. *Journal of the American Dietetic Association, 91,* 1248–1251.

Yalom, I. (1993). *Love's executioner and other tales of psychotherapy.* New York: Basic Books.

Young, M. E. (1995). *Diet breaking: Having it all without having to diet.* London: Hodder & Stoughton.

PART VI

CHILDHOOD OBESITY AND OBESITY PREVENTION

25

Development of Childhood Obesity

ROBERT I. BERKOWITZ
ALBERT J. STUNKARD

This chapter provides a brief overview of risk factors for the development of obesity early in life. Such knowledge is needed for prevention and treatment of the current epidemic of childhood and adolescent obesity.

"Obesity" has been defined as excess body fat and is often estimated by measures of weight (in kilograms) normalized by height (in meters) squared (body mass index, or BMI). Adult obesity, defined as a BMI $\geq$ 30 kg/m^2, is associated with increased morbidity or mortality (Pi-Sunyer, 1991). No specific level of excess body fat is associated with morbidity or mortality for children and adolescents. Thus, for children and adolescents, "overweight" (i.e., risk for obesity) has been estimated by a statistical approach; this consists of the age- and sex-specific 95th percentile of BMI of the population measured in the National Health Examination Surveys (NHES) II and III, conducted from 1963 to 1970 (Himes & Dietz, 1994; Troiano & Flegal, 1998; Troiano, Flegal, Kuczmarski, Campbell, & Johnson, 1995). Children and adolescents between the 85th and 95th percentiles of BMI have been described as being at "risk for overweight."

INCREASE IN PREVALENCE OF OBESITY IN CHILDHOOD AND ADOLESCENCE

A more recent survey, the National Health and Nutrition Examination Survey III (NHANES III), assessed weight and height for U.S. adults and children from 1988 to 1994 (Troiano et al., 1995). NHANES III allowed comparisons with earlier data from the NHES II and III (1963–1970), NHANES I (1971–1974), and NHANES II (1976–1980). Major increases in the prevalence of overweight and risk for overweight for children and adolescents occurred between the earlier (1963–1980) and later (1988–1994) surveys.

For children and adolescents, the prevalence of overweight (i.e., BMI at or above the 95th percentile, from the 1963–1970 surveys) in NHANES III (1988–1994) was 10.9%, and the risk for overweight (i.e., the 85th percentile of BMI) was 22% (Troiano et al.,

1995). For 6- to 11-year-old white girls, the increase from 5.1% prevalence of overweight in NHES II to 10.2% in NHANES III represents a 100% increase. The increase in prevalence from 15.7% to 22.0% for the 85th percentile is a 40% relative increase in risk for overweight (Troiano et al., 1995). Similar clinically significant increases for both percentiles were described for all gender, age, and racial groups. This increase in prevalence is in stark contrast to the period between NHES II and III (1963–1970) and NHANES II (1976–1980), when the prevalence increased only slightly for adolescents and somewhat more for children.

Using the definition of the 95th percentile for BMI from the 1963–1970 surveys, Troiano and colleagues (1995) have estimated that about 4.7 million children aged 6–17 years in the United States would have been classified as overweight during the period of NHANES III. An increase in positive energy balance accompanying modernization has been suggested as the most likely factor responsible for this increase in prevalence. Factors such as environmental shift, caloric consumption, and physical activity are discussed later in this chapter.

Is the entire population of children heavier, or are those who are overweight becoming heavier? In an innovative analysis, Troiano and Flegal (1998) described mean–difference plots (Cleveland, 1993) to see how the distributions of BMIs differed between NHES II–III and NHANES III. They found that the children who were overweight were much more so in NHANES III than in the earlier surveys. Children in the lighter distributions of BMI in NHES II–III remained lighter in NHANES III. This may suggest a gene–environment interaction, wherein only those children genetically susceptible to environmental change are becoming more overweight.

PREDICTION OF OBESITY IN ADULTHOOD FROM CHILDHOOD

It was once believed that infants would grow out of their "baby fat" and not become obese adults. Significant associations between measures of adiposity in childhood and adulthood have been found, but some overweight children do not become obese as adults. Rolland-Cachera and colleagues (1987) found that infants with a BMI over the 75th percentile had twice the risk of being overweight as adults as infants under the 25th percentile had. Another study reported that 55% of children who had a high BMI at 7 years of age developed adult obesity (Stark, Atkins, Wolff, & Douglas, 1981). Although BMI may not be an ideal way to measure adiposity in infants and children because it does not describe lean mass or fat mass, it does appear to predict BMI in adulthood.

Whitaker, Wright, Pepe, Seidel, and Deitz (1997) assessed the additive contributions of both parental and child weight status to the prediction of obesity in adulthood. Increased body fat early in childhood was a greater risk factor for children whose parents were overweight than for those with lean parents (Whitaker et al., 1997). A 1- to 2-year-old child who was at the 85th percentile or higher for weight, and who had an overweight parent, had a fourfold risk for adult obesity (40% became obese adults), compared with a child who was overweight at that age and had lean parents (8% became obese adults). As the age of the child increased, overweight increased the risk for adult obesity (see Figure 25.1). Thus a 3- to 5-year-old overweight child of overweight parents had a 60% chance of becoming an obese adult, while a lean child of overweight parents had a 20% chance. By age 10, however, the effect of parental overweight declined. Adolescents who were overweight remained at very high risk of adult obesity, regardless of parental weight status. Of note, a lean child of lean parents had the lowest risk of developing adult obesity.

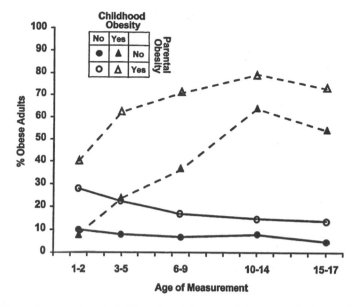

FIGURE 25.1. Effect of parental and childhood weight on weight status during early adulthood. Percentages of overweight adults are plotted in relation to whether the children were overweight at each age and whether the children had one or both parents overweight at the same time. When one parent was overweight, nonoverweight 1- to 2-year-old children had a much greater risk of becoming overweight as adults, compared to children with no overweight parents. This effect of parental weight status was no longer evident by ages 7–9. The effect of parental overweight declined as children entered adolescence, and the tracking of adolescent overweight into early adulthood became much stronger. Adapted from Whitaker, Wright, Pepe, Seidel, and Dietz (1997; copyright 1997 by the Massachusetts Medical Society; adapted by permission) by Bray (1998). Copyright 1998 by Handbooks in Health Care Co. Reprinted by permission.

ENERGY INTAKE

Breast and Bottle Feeding

The role of early feeding practices—such as breast or bottle feeding, or the timing of the introduction of solid foods—has been evaluated in relation to the development of obesity. Longitudinal studies found that although formula-fed infants had greater weight and length during infancy than did breast-fed infants, no differences in adiposity were observed later in childhood (Butte, Wong, Hopkinson, Smith, & Ellis, 2000; Fomon, Rogers, Ziegler, Nelson, & Thomas, 1984; Fomon, Thomas, Filer, Ziegler, & Leonard, 1971; Parsons, Power, Logan, & Summerbell, 1999). NHANES III found small differences between breast- and bottle-fed infants at 8–11 months that were reduced by 2 years of age, and no longer present by 5 years (Hediger, Overpeck, Ruan, & Troendle, 2000). Several other longitudinal studies similarly found no differences in adiposity later in childhood (Fomon et al., 1971, 1984; Parsons et al., 1999). Furthermore, neither the age of introduction of solid foods nor the macronutrient composition of the diet (i.e., percentages of carbohydrate, fat, and protein) in infancy appeared to be associated with the development of obesity (Parsons et al., 1999; Rosenbaum & Leibel, 1998). Thus mode of feeding early in infancy has no apparent effect on the development of obesity during childhood.

Caloric Consumption and Dietary Composition

It is difficult to obtain accurate measurement of dietary intake in infants and children, as it is in adults. Underreporting of food intake is common. The use of dietary history methods is inadequate for estimating caloric consumption, but such methods have been used to estimate macronutrient composition of the diet.

Three studies have reported that energy intake in infancy predicted later measures of body fatness; one study has not. In a study of children at high risk for obesity, infants who became overweight at 1 year consumed 42% more energy at 6 months of age than did 12 infants who remained lean (Roberts, 1991; Roberts, Savage, Coward, Chew, & Lucas, 1988). In a breast-feeding study, energy intake at 6 months predicted body fatness at 1 year (Dewey, Heinig, Nommsen, Peerson, & Lonnerdal, 1993). In a second study of high-risk children, caloric consumption at 3 months predicted weight and adiposity at 1 year (Stunkard, Berkowitz, Stallings, & Schoeller, 1999). In this latter study, food intake was estimated by weighing the baby bottle or the infant before and after each feeding over a 3-day period—a method presumably more valid than dietary recalls or histories. Only one study found that food intake or caloric consumption did not predict body fatness in early childhood (Wells, Stanley, Laidlaw, Day, & Davies, 1998).

Common sense suggests that children at risk for obesity consume greater amounts of calories and fat. Few studies have examined caloric consumption and macronutrient intake during childhood as predictors of obesity in adolescence or adulthood. In a thorough review, Parsons and colleagues (1999) reported that most studies found that neither caloric intake nor macronutrient intake (including fat consumption) was associated with the development of greater adiposity later in childhood or during adulthood. One major longitudinal study of children, the Bogalusa Heart Study (Shear et al., 1988), reported an increase in the prevalence of obesity over time, but did not find a relation between caloric consumption and adiposity. No increase in caloric consumption over time was reported. However, a more recent prospective study (Berkey et al., 2000) evaluated food intake in more than 10,000 children 9–14 years of age by using a food frequency questionnaire; for both boys and girls, a greater reported caloric intake predicted a greater increase in BMI a year later.

Four studies have found an association between dietary fat intake and body fat in children (Gazzaniga & Burns, 1993; Maffeis, Pinelli, & Schutz, 1996; Obarzanek et al., 1994; Tucker, Seljaas, & Hager, 1997). Four others, however, did not (Davies, 1997; Parsons et al., 1999; Ricketts, 1997). A recent study using the 4-day weighed food record method reported that body fat in children from 1.5 to 4.5 years of age was not associated with total energy intake or macronutrient intake (Atkin & Davies, 2000).

As with studies of the role of dietary fat, studies of dietary protein are in conflict. The age at which BMI rises after its trough in early childhood has been termed "adiposity rebound," and it may be a critical period for the development of obesity (Rolland-Cachera et al., 1987). Parizkova and Rolland-Cachera (1997) found that higher protein intake at 2 years of age predicted early adiposity rebound and increased body fatness at 8 years. However, another study of the dietary intake of 889 children from the United Kingdom reported no association between protein intake (or any other component of the diet) and adiposity rebound up to 5 years of age (Dorosty, Emmett, Cowin, & Reilly, 2000).

Rolls and colleagues (Bell, Castellanos, Pelkman, Thorwart, & Rolls, 1998) have proposed that energy density is the primary determinant of overconsumption, and that increased intake of high-fat diets may be due to their energy density rather than their fat content. This intriguing proposal has yet to be tested in children.

As noted earlier, a major limitation in the assessment of food intake is underreporting on food records (Stunkard & Waxman, 1981). Bandini, Schoeller, Cyr, and Dietz (1990), monitoring total energy expenditure with the doubly labeled water technique, found that both obese and nonobese adolescents underreported their food intake, but that underreporting was greater in the former group. The authors concluded that imprecision in adolescents' reports of food intake precludes the use of this method to assess the role of energy intake in the development of obesity.

In summary, the literature suggests that dietary intake during infancy, when it may be easier to assess, predicts early childhood adiposity. By contrast, dietary intake during childhood, which is more difficult to measure, may not predict later adiposity. The predictive value for adiposity in childhood of dietary composition (in particular, fat or protein intake) is unclear.

Feeding Style

In contrast to the equivocal predictive power of food intake, a vigorous feeding style is a strong predictor of later adiposity. In infants, this style is characterized by rapid, high-pressure nutritive sucking, with longer sucks and sucking burst durations, and with shorter intervals between bursts. Agras, Kraemer, Berkowitz, and Hammer (1990) found that this style, measured in the laboratory at 2 and 4 weeks of age, predicted adiposity at 1, 2, and 3 years of age in a representative cohort. We (Stunkard, Berkowitz, Stallings, & Schoeller, 1999) reported not only that infants of overweight mothers manifested a more vigorous feeding style than did infants of lean mothers, but that this style predicted adiposity at 12 months of age.

Studies of eating style in infancy are complemented by those in childhood. Drabman and colleagues reported that a rapid feeding style was associated with adiposity in children (Drabman, Cordua, Hammer, Jarvie, & Horton, 1979; Drabman, Hammer, & Jarvie, 1977). Obese boys (Waxman & Stunkard, 1980) and girls (Waxman, 1988) ate twice as rapidly as nonobese control subjects. Barkeling, Ikman, and Rossner (1992) found that 11-year-old obese children ate much more rapidly than nonobese children. Furthermore, the eating rate of obese children did not decelerate during the course of a meal, while that of the nonobese children did. The investigators suggested that this lack of deceleration of eating rate represented a problem with a satiety signal or with the response to that signal.

The vigorous or rapid eating style described in infancy and childhood may be a behavioral marker for a genetic propensity for increased food intake and for increased weight gain. Long-term studies of infants and children with this feeding style are required to assess the predictive power for adiposity of this promising measure.

The Modern Food Environment

The increase in the prevalence of obesity suggests that there has been a change toward a positive energy balance, either as a result of increased food consumption, less physical activity, or a combination of the two. Energy-dense foods are plentiful and relatively inexpensive in the United States. As compared to 1970, Americans now consume more meals outside the home; these meals tend to be more calorically dense and higher in fat (Life Science Research Office, 1989; Troiano et al., 1995). Adolescents, in particular, frequently consume high-fat and fried foods when eating out (McGinnis, 1992). Adolescents in southern European countries snack less often between meals and eat less often in fast-food restaurants than do adolescents in the United States (Cruz, 2000). The prevalence of overweight in southern Europe is less than that in the United States (i.e., 15% vs. 22%).

ENERGY EXPENDITURE

Physical Activity

Physical activity is a component of energy expenditure that may be a strong predictor of childhood obesity. The amount of energy expended during physical activity can vary, depending on the level of activity—from sleeping to running. Investigators have used a variety of methods to estimate the effects of physical activity on body fat development in childhood, including self-report instruments, computerized accelerometers, and the doubly labeled water technique.

As long ago as 1953, Mayer proposed that physical inactivity was clearly an important factor in the development of obesity. Most studies of physical activity in children and adolescents have been cross-sectional. Most found that obese subjects were less active than their lean peers (Berkowitz, Agras, Korner, Kraemer, & Zeanah, 1985; Bullen, Reed, & Mayer, 1964; Davies, Gregory, & White, 1995; Sallis, Patterson, Buono, & Nadar, 1988; Waxman, 1988; Waxman & Stunkard, 1980), although some did not (Parsons et al., 1999).

Two prospective studies failed to find a relationship between physical activity in infancy and the development of body fat in early childhood (Berkowitz et al., 1985; Parsons et al., 1999), although two studies of children did. The Framingham Children's Study prospectively evaluated 97 children aged 3–5 years, assessing physical activity with an electronic motion sensor twice yearly (Moore, Nguyen, Rothman, Cupples, & Ellison, 1995). When age, television viewing, energy intake, and baseline weight status (of the child and parents) were controlled for, inactive preschoolers were 3.8 times more likely than active children to have greater skinfold thicknesses over time. Berkey and colleagues (2000) evaluated physical activity patterns by questionnaire in over 10,000 children aged 9–14 years and found greater increases in BMI in those who reported lower levels of physical activity and higher levels of television viewing.

Television Viewing

Television viewing is an important aspect of modern life that may contribute to childhood obesity in children as a result of reducing energy expenditure (Dietz & Gortmaker, 1985; Robinson et al., 1993). American children spend more time watching television than they spend in school; they spend more time watching TV and videotapes and playing video games than engaging in any other activity except for sleeping (Annenberg Public Policy Center, 1997). In a nationally representative cohort of 746 children aged 10–15 years, Gortmaker and colleagues (1996) reported an association between the prevalence of overweight and television viewing. In this study, the odds of becoming overweight were 4.6 times greater for those children watching over 5 hours of TV a day than for those watching 0–2 hours a day. This finding held even when the investigators controlled for baseline weight, parental weight, and socioeconomic status (SES). Television viewing may contribute to the development of obesity both by reducing energy expenditure and by increasing food intake, either while watching TV or at a later time (as a result of food advertisements) (Birch & Fisher, 1998).

In the United States, most advertising during children's TV programming is for food (Birch & Fisher, 1998); furthermore, these foods are not of high nutritional value. Advertised foods are usually sugary breakfast cereals and snack foods with high levels of fat, sugar, and salt. Similar findings have been reported for British children (Lewis & Hill, 1998; Parsons et al., 1999).

An intervention study has yielded powerful evidence of the contribution of television watching to childhood obesity. Robinson (1999) showed that reduction of TV watching and video game usage resulted in significantly reduced BMI levels in third- and fourth-graders, compared to those students in control schools. Decreasing inactivity by reducing television viewing and video game playing may be an important new measure to prevent the development of obesity.

Metabolic Rate

There has been considerable interest in whether metabolic rate predicts the development of body fat in infancy and childhood. One hypothesis was that a low metabolic rate in infants and children, perhaps because of more efficient energy utilization, might lead to obesity.

Roberts and colleagues (1988) reported that six infants with a low total energy expenditure (TEE), who were born to obese mothers, became overweight at 1 year. Twelve children with a higher TEE (and either obese or nonobese mothers) did not. No association between resting energy expenditure (REE) and obesity was reported in this study.

Two subsequent studies of representative samples found no relationship between low TEE and the development of adiposity (Davies, 1997; Wells et al., 1998). A third study of 38 infants of lean mothers and 40 infants of obese mothers also found no relationship between TEE (as well as REE) and body weight (or weight gain) at 1 year of age (Stunkard, Berkowitz, Stallings, & Schoeller, 1999).

Griffiths and Payne (1976) reported that 4-year-old children of obese mothers had a lower REE than those of normal-weight mothers, and Griffiths, Payne, Stunkard, Rivers, and Cox (1990) found that low REE predicted adiposity in girls but not boys at age 15. Two other studies of children failed to find a relationship between low energy expenditure and adiposity. TEE and postprandial REE were not related to body fat in 73 children 5 years of age with either obese or lean parents (Goran et al., 1995). In a prospective study of preadolescents, Goran and colleagues (1998) found that neither REE nor TEE was inversely related to change in fat mass. In this same study, initial fatness, parental fatness, and female gender were predictive of greater increase in fat mass.

Thus the majority of studies suggest that low energy expenditure is not a risk factor for obesity in infancy or childhood (Goran et al., 1995). As noted earlier, parental obesity influences childhood adiposity (Whitaker et al., 1997), though it is not clear whether this effect is mediated via energy expenditure. Goran and colleagues (1995) and Salbe, Tataranni, Fontvieille, and Ravussin (1996) did not find an association between parental BMI and childhood TEE.

HEREDITY

A review of the relationship between measures of body weight of parents and their adult offspring revealed correlations between .20 and .30 (Meyer & Stunkard, 1993). What is the relation between parental adiposity and that of offspring in infancy and childhood?

One study examined the relationship between parental BMI and measures of body weight in children at 3, 12, and 24 months of age (Stunkard, Berkowitz, Stallings, & Cater, 1999). Neither paternal nor maternal BMI was related to weight or weight for length in these children through age 24 months. The relation between maternal and offspring weights has been evaluated more often at birth than during the first 2 years of life. Three large studies found significant correlations between mothers' weights and the birthweights of their infants (.21–.32) (Garn & Pesick, 1982; Love & Kinch, 1965; Weiss & Jackson, 1969). Oth-

girls. Surveys of 5,518 Australian children (7–11 years old) and Belgian youth (12–15 years old) found this inverse relationship for girls but not for boys (Booth, Macaskill, Lazarus, & Baur, 1999; DeSpiegelaere, Dramaix, & Hennart, 1998). Kinra, Nelder, and Lewendon (2000) reported on 20,793 children in the British city of Plymouth, where childhood obesity was twice that in Britain as a whole. The odds ratio for a girl of lower SES to be obese was 1.39; that for boys did not reach statistical significance.

As with studies of adults, investigators have suggested that the stresses of low SES may lead to the development of greater rates of obesity, though there are few reports about the eating behavior of children of low SES. Lower levels of physical activity as measured with an accelerometer, however, were associated with lower SES among obese children (Epstein, Paluch, Coleman, Vito, & Anderson, 1996).

Self-Regulation versus Parental Regulation of Food Intake

Birch and Fisher (1998) found that infants and children were able to regulate their own energy intake, and that day-to-day energy intake was stable. Fomon (1993) reported that infants given different densities of formula adjusted their intake, maintaining the same total energy intake. In a series of studies, Birch and Fisher varied the caloric density of a first meal and found that children would eat fewer calories in a second meal if the first meal was higher in calories. They caution, however, that further research is needed to determine whether children remain able to self-regulate food intake in the presence of a high-fat diet.

A desirable goal is the promotion of dietary habits in childhood that include moderation, nutritional balance, and low levels of consumption of fat and sugars (Birch & Fisher, 1998). This goal may not be easy to attain in modern cultures that encourage food intake. Birch, Zimmerman, and Hind (1980) found that using foods as rewards, or restricting preferred foods, increased children's preferences for these foods. Fisher and Birch (1995) found in girls, but not boys, that prior maternal restriction of snack foods was associated with their increased consumption.

Can child feeding practice reduce self-regulation of food intake in children? When children were rewarded for "cleaning their plates," their food intake was increased, compared with that of children not rewarded in the laboratory setting (Birch, McPhee, Shoba, Steinberg, & Krehbiel, 1987). Klesges, Malott, Boschee, and Weber (1986) reported that parental prompting to eat was associated with increased meal duration (measured in the home setting) and overweight in children. Furthermore, when a child's refusal to eat was met with a parental prompt, the child then ate more (Klesges et al., 1983). Prompting and rewarding eating behavior may override a child's self-regulation of food intake and foster overfeeding. Reduction of food prompts and rewards at mealtime may help to lower the risk of childhood obesity. This issue requires further study.

Johnson and Birch (1994) found that girls, but not boys, whose parents exerted more control over eating had greater body fatness. Mothers who exerted more control had greater dietary restraint and had more weight and dieting difficulties themselves. Parents reporting greater dietary disinhibition had children who failed to compensate in their eating when presented with increases in the caloric density of meals. It is not clear whether the parental control that is associated with childhood obesity is causative, disrupting a child's self-regulation of eating, or whether it represents an attempt to minimize weight gain in an already overweight child. On the other hand, this familial association may be inherited and may be a behavioral marker for a genetically mediated process of weight gain. Prospective studies are needed to understand the predictivenss of this parental style.

Psychological Factors

Three studies have obtained mixed results concerning the predictive power of temperament on later fatness in children. Carey, Hegvik, and McDevitt (1988) reported that decreased adaptability, increased intensity, and increased withdrawal predicted increased weight for height at the ages of 3–7 years. Examining infants earlier in life, Wells and colleagues (1997) found that an infant's "distress to limitations" (e.g., fussing or crying while waiting for food, being dressed/undressed, or being prevented from obtaining a desired object) was associated with body fatness at 2–3 years of age. Interestingly, those infants who were "soothable" (i.e., reduced their distress in response to parental soothing efforts) gained less body fat. A third study reported no association between infant temperament and later adiposity (Kramer et al., 1986). These findings need further investigation.

Gortmaker, Must, Perrin, Sobol, and Dietz (1993) found no differences between obese and nonobese adolescents in self-esteem, and other studies have found little or no relationship between obesity and depression or anxiety (Friedman & Brownell, 1995; Wadden, Foster, Stunkard, & Linowitz, 1989). However, obese children and adolescents have been found to have greater body image dissatisfaction than their average-weight peers (Wadden et al., 1989).

We (Berkowitz, Stunkard, & Stallings, 1993) observed symptoms of binge eating in about 30% of adolescent obese girls who sought weight reduction—a rate similar to that described in studies of adults. The histories of dieting in adolescents with and without binge eating were similar, suggesting that dieting is not a sufficient cause of this disorder. The percentage of adolescents who report binge eating increases with greater BMI (Moyer, De-Pietro, Berkowitz, & Stunkard, 1997), suggesting that disinhibited overeating contributes to weight gain. Obese adolescents who report binge eating also have higher levels of depression than do obese adolescents who do not binge (Berkowitz et al., 1993). Prospective studies are needed to assess whether children with a vigorous feeding style are more likely to develop binge eating in adolescence.

RARE CAUSES OF CHILDHOOD OBESITY

This chapter has not been able to review all aspects of the development of childhood obesity. Relatively uncommon syndromes may present as childhood obesity. Hypothalamic obesity, for example, may develop secondary to tumors, trauma, surgery, and inflammation of the ventral medial hypothalamus, resulting in hyperphagia (Bray, 1992). Endocrine disorders such as hypothyroidism and Cushing syndrome may also present with obesity, as may genetic disorders such as Prader–Willi syndrome. In addition, medications associated with weight gain include glucocorticoids (for immunological disease), lithium carbonate (for bipolar disorder), anticonvusants (such as divalproex sodium), and atypical antipsychotic medications. Putative genes and the biological development of adipose tissue in children are discussed elsewhere (Rosenbaum & Leibel, 1998).

SUMMARY

A significant increase in the prevalence of overweight children and adolescents has occurred in the United States, as reported in NHANES III (1988–1994). Susceptible children are significantly more overweight than in earlier surveys. There is evidence of an additive contribution of both parental and child weight status in the prediction of obesity from childhood into

Dorosty, A. R., Emmett, P. M., Cowin, S. D., & Reilly, J. J. (2000). Factors associated with early adiposity rebound: ALSPAC Study Team. *Pediatrics, 105,* 1115–1118.

Drabman, R. S., Hammer, D., & Jarvie, G. J. (1977). Eating styles of obese and non-obese black and white children in a naturalistic setting. *Addictive Behavior, 2,* 83–86.

Drabman, R. S., Cordua, G. O, Hammer, L. D., Jarvie, G. J., & Horton, W. (1979). Developmental trends in eating rates of normal and overweight preschool children. *Child Development, 50,* 211–216.

Epstein, L. H., Paluch, R. E., Coleman, K. J., Vito, D., & Anderson, K. (1996). Determinants of physical activity in obese children assessed by accelerometer and self-report. *Medicine and Science in Sports and Exercise, 28,* 1157–1164.

Esparza, J., Fox, C., Harper, I. T., Bennett, P. H., Schulz, L. O., Valencia, M. E., & Ravussin, E. (2000). Daily energy expenditure in Mexican and USA Pima Indians: Low physical activity as a possible cause of obesity. *International Journal of Obesity, 24,* 55–59.

Fisher, J. O., & Birch, L. L. (1995). Fat preferences and fat consumption of 3- to 5-year-old children are related to parental adiposity. *Journal of the American Dietetic Association, 95,* 759–765.

Fomon, S. J. (1993). *Nutrition of normal infants.* St. Louis, MO: Mosby–Year Book.

Fomon, S. J., Rogers, R., Ziegler, E., Nelson, S. E., & Thomas, L. N. (1984). Indices of fatness and serum cholesterol at age eight years in relation to feeding and growth during early infancy. *Pediatrics Research, 18,* 1233–1238.

Fomon, S. J., Thomas, L., Filer, L., Ziegler, E. E., & Leonard, M. T. (1971). Food consumption and growth of normal infants fed milk-based formulas. *Acta Paediatrica Scandinavica,* (Suppl. 223), 1–36.

Friedman, M. A., & Brownell, K. D. (1995). Psychological correlates of obesity: Moving to the next generation. *Psychological Bulletin, 117,* 3–20.

Frisancho, A. R., Klayman, J. E., & Matos, J. (1977). Newborn body composition and its relationship to linear growth. *American Journal of Clinical Nutrition, 30,* 704–711.

Gampel, B. (1965). The relationship of skeletal thickness in the neonates to sex, length of gestation, size at birth and maternal skinfold. *Human Biology, 37,* 29–35.

Garn, S. M., & Pesick, R. D. (1982). Relationship between various maternal body mass measures and size of the newborn. *American Journal of Clinical Nutrition, 36,* 664–668.

Gazzaniga, J. M., & Burns, T. L. (1993). Relationship between diet composition and body fatness, with adjustment for resting energy expenditure and physical activity, in preadolescent children. *American Journal of Clinical Nutrition, 58,* 21–28.

Goran, M. I., Carpenter, W. H., McGloin, A., Johnson, R., Hardin, J. M., & Weinsier, R. L. (1995). Energy expenditure in children of lean and obese parents. *American Journal of Physiology, 268,* E9170–E9240.

Goran, M. I., Shewchuk, R., Gower, B. A., Nagy, T. R., Carpenter, W. H., & Johnson, R. K. (1998). Longitudinal changes in fatness in white children: No effect of childhood energy expenditure. *American Journal of Clinical Nutrition, 67,* 309–316.

Gortmaker, S. L., Must, A., Perrin, J. M., Sobol, A. M., & Dietz, W. H. (1993). Social and economic consequences of overweight in adolescence and young adulthood. *New England Journal of Medicine, 329,* 1008–1012.

Gortmaker, S. L., Must, A., Sobol, A. M., Peterson, K., Colditz, G. A., & Dietz, W. H. (1996). Television viewing as a cause of increasing obesity among children in the United States, 1986–1990. *Archives of Pediatrics and Adolescent Medicine, 150,* 356–362.

Griffiths, M., & Payne, P. R. (1976). Energy expenditure in small children of obese and non-obese parents. *Nature, 260,* 698–700.

Griffiths, M., Payne, P. R., Stunkard, A. J., Rivers, J. P. W., & Cox, M. (1990). Metabolic rate and physical development in children at risk of obesity. *Lancet, 336,* 76–78.

Gross, T., Sokol, R. J., & King, K. C. (1980). Obesity in pregnancy: Risks and outcome. *Obstetrics and Gynecology, 56,* 446–450.

Harrison, G. G., Udall, J. N., & Morrow, G. (1980). Maternal obesity, weight gain in pregnancy and infant birthweight. *American Journal of Obstetrics and Gynecology, 136,* 411–412.

Hashimoto, N., Kawasaki, T., Kikuchi, T., Takahashi, H., & Uchiyama, M. (1995). Influence of parental obesity on the physical constitution of preschool children in Japan. *Acta Paediatrica Japonica, 37,* 150–153.

Heath, G. W., Pratt, M., Warren, C. W., & Kann, L. (1994). Physical activity patterns in American high school students. *Archives of Pediatrics and Adolescent Medicine, 148,* 1131–1136.

Hediger, M. L., Overpeck, M. D., Ruan, W. J., & Troendle, J. F. (2000). Early infant feeding and growth status of US-born infants and children aged 4–71 mo: Analyses from the third National Health and Nutrition Examination Survey, 1988–1994. *American Journal of Clinical Nutrition, 72,* 159–167.

Himes, J. H., & Dietz, W. H. (1994). Guidelines for overweight in adolescent preventive services: recommendations from an expert committee: The Expert Committee on Clinical Guidelines for Overweight in Adolescent Preventive Services. *American Journal of Clinical Nutrition, 59,* 307–316.

Johnson, S. L., & Birch, L. L. (1994). Parents' and children's adiposity and eating style. *Pediatrics, 94,* 653–661.

Kinra, S., Nelder, R. P., & Lewendon, G. J. (2000). Deprivation and childhood obesity: A cross sectional study of 20,973 children in Plymouth, United Kingdom. *Journal of Epidemiology and Community Health, 54,* 456–460.

Klesges, R. C., Coates, T. J., Brown, G., Sturgeon-Tillisch, J., Moldenhauer-Klesges, L. M., Holzer, B., Woolfrey, J., & Vollmer, J. (1983). Parental influences on children's eating behavior and relative weight. *Journal of Applied Behavior Analysis, 16,* 371–378.

Klesges, R. C., Malott, J. M., Boschee, P. F., & Weber, J. M. (1986). The effects of parental influences on children's food intake, physical activity, and relative weight. *International Journal of Eating Disorders, 5,* 335–346.

Kopelman, P. G. (2000) Obesity as a medical problem. *Nature, 404,* 635–643.

Kramer, M. S., Barr, R. G., Leduc, D. G., Boisjoly, C., McVey-White, L., & Pless, I. B. (1985). Determinants of body weight and adiposity in the first year of life. *Journal of Pediatrics, 106,* 10–14.

Kramer, M. S., Barr, R. G., Pless, I. B., Bolisjoyly, C., McVey-White, L., & Leduc, D. G. (1986). Determinants of weight and adiposity in early childhood. *Canadian Journal of Public Health/Revue Canadienne de Santé Publique, 77*(Suppl.), 98–103.

Lewis, M. K., & Hill, A. J. (1998). Food advertising on British children's television: A content and experimental study with nine-year olds. *International Journal of Obesity, 22,* 206–214.

Life Science Research Office, Federation of Associated Societies for Experimental Biology. (1989). *Nutrition monitoring in the United States: An update report on nutrition monitoring* (Publication No. PHS 89–255). Washington, DC: U.S. Department of Health and Human Services.

Love, E. J., & Kinch, R. A. H. (1965). Factors influencing birth weight in normal pregnancy. *American Journal of Obstetrics and Gynecology, 91,* 342–347.

Luepker, R. V. (1999). How physically active are American children and what can we do about it? *International Journal of Obesity, 23*(Suppl. 2), S12–S17.

Maffeis, C., Pinelli, L., & Schutz, Y. (1996). Fat intake and adiposity in 8 to 11-y-old obese children. *International Journal of Obesity, 20,* 170–174.

Mayer, J. (1953). Genetic, traumatic and environmental factors in the etiology of obesity. *Physiological Reviews, 33,* 472–508.

McGinnis, J. M. (1992). The public health burden of a sedentary lifestyle. *Medicine and Science in Sports and Exercise, 24*(Suppl.), S196–S200.

Meyer, J. M., & Stunkard, A. J. (1993). Genetics and human obesity. In A. J. Stunkard & T. A. Wadden (Eds.), *Obesity: Theory and therapy* (2nd ed., pp. 137–149). New York: Raven Press.

Moore, L. L., Nguyen, U. S., Rothman, K. J., Cupples, L. A., & Ellison, R. C. (1995). Preschool physical activity level and change in body fatness in young children: The Framingham Children's Study. *American Journal of Epidemiology, 142,* 982–988.

Morgan, J. (1986). Parental weight and its relation to infant feeding patterns and infant obesity. *International Journal of Nursing Studies, 23,* 255–264.

Moyer, D., DePietro, L., Berkowitz, R. I., & Stunkard, A. J. (1997). Childhood sexual abuse and precursors of binge eating in an adolescent female population. *International Journal of Eating Disorders, 21,* 23–30.

Obarzanek, E., Schreiber, G. B., Crawford, P. B., Goldman, S. R., Barrier, P. M., Frederick, M. M., & Lakatos, E. (1994). Energy intake and physical activity in relation to indexes of body fat: The National Heart, Lung, and Blood Institute Growth and Health Study. *American Journal of Clinical Nutrition, 60,* 15–22.

Parizkova, J., & Rolland-Cachera, M. F. (1997). High proteins early in life as a predisposition for later obesity and further health risks. *Nutrition, 13,* 818–819.

Parsons, T. J., Power, C., Logan, S., & Summerbell, C. D. (1999). Childhood predictors of adult obesity: A systematic review. *International Journal of Obesity, 23*(Suppl. 8), S1–S107.

Pi-Sunyer, F. X. (1991). Health implications of obesity. *American Journal of Clinical Nutrition, 53,* 1595S–1603S.

Prentice, A. M., & Jebb, S. A. (1995). Obesity in Britain: Gluttony or sloth? *British Medical Journal, 311,* 437–439.

Ravelli, G. P., Stein, Z. A., & Susser, M. W. (1976). Obesity in young men after famine exposure in utero and early infancy. *New England Journal of Medicine, 295,* 349–353.

Ravelli, A. C., van der Meulen, J. H., Osmond, C., Barker, D. J., & Bleker, O. P. (1999). Obesity at the age of 50 in men and women exposed to famine prenatally. *American Journal of Clinical Nutrition, 70,* 811–816.

Ricketts, C. D. (1997). Fat preferences, dietary fat intake and body composition. *European Journal of Clinical Nutrition, 51,* 778–781.

Roberts, S. B. (1991). Early diet and obesity. In W. Heird (Ed.), *Nutritional needs of the six to twelve month old infant* (Vol. 2, pp. 303–306). New York: Raven Press.

Roberts, S. B., Savage, J., Coward, W. A., Chew, B., & Lucas, A. (1988). Energy expenditure and intake in infants born to lean and overweight mothers. *New England Journal of Medicine, 318,* 461–466.

Robinson, T. N. (1999). Reducing children's television viewing to prevent obesity. *Journal of the American Medical Association, 282,* 1561–1567.

Robinson, T. N., Hammer, L. D., Killen, J. D., Kraemer, H. C., Wilson, D. M., Hayward, C., & Taylor, C. B. (1993). Does television viewing increase obesity and reduce physical activity?: Cross-sectional and longitudinal analyses among adolescent girls. *Pediatrics, 91,* 273–280.

Rolland-Cachera, M., Deheeger, M., Guilloud-Bataille, M., Avons, P., Patois, E., & Sempé, M. (1987). Tracking the development of adiposity from one month of age to adulthood. *Annals of Human Biology, 14,* 219–229.

Rosenbaum, M., & Leibel, R. L. (1998). The physiology of body weight regulation: Relevance to the etiology of obesity in children. *Pediatrics, 101,* 525–539.

Rush, D., Davis, H., & Susser, M. (1972). Antecedents of low birth weight in Harlem, New York City. *International Journal of Epidemiology, 1,* 375–387.

Salbe, A., Tataranni, P., Fontvieille, A., & Ravussin, E. (1996). Parental body size does not influence energy expenditure in 5-y old Pima Indian children. *Obesity Research, 4*(Suppl.), 17S.

Sallis, J. F., Patterson, T. L., Buono, M. J., & Nadar, P. R. (1988). Relation of cardiovascular fitness and physical activity to cardiovascular disease risk factors in children and adults. *American Journal of Epidemiology, 127,* 933–941.

Shear, C. L., Freedman, D. S., Burke, G. L., Harsha, D. W., Webber, L. S., & Berenson, G. S. (1988). Secular trends of obesity in early life: The Bogalusa Heart Study. *American Journal of Public Health, 78,* 75–77.

Sobal, J., & Stunkard, A. J. (1989). Socioeconomic status and obesity: A review of the literature. *Psychological Bulletin, 105,* 260–275.

Stark, O., Atkins, E., Wolff, O. H., & Douglas, J. W. (1981). Longitudinal study of obesity in the National Survey of Health and Development. *British Medical Journal, 283,* 13–17.

Stunkard, A. J., Berkowitz, R. I., Stallings, V. A., & Cater, J. R. (1999). Weights of parents and infants: Is there a relationship? *International Journal of Obesity, 23,* 159–162.

Stunkard, A. J., Berkowitz, R. I., Stallings, V. A., & Schoeller, D. A. (1999). Energy intake, not energy output, is a determinant of body size in infants. *American Journal of Clinical Nutrition, 69,* 524–530.

Stunkard, A. J., & Waxman, M. (1981). Accuracy of self-reports of food intake: A review of the literature and a report of a small series. *Journal of the American Dietetic Association, 79,* 547–551.

Troiano, R. P., & Flegal, K. M. (1998). Overweight children and adolescents: Description, epidemiology, and demographics. *Pediatrics, 101,* 497–504.

Troiano, R. P., Flegal, K. M., Kuczmarski, R. J., Campbell, S. M., & Johnson, C. L. (1995). Overweight prevalence and trends for children and adolescents. *Archives of Pediatrics and Adolescent Medicine, 149,* 1085–1091.

Tucker, L. A., Seljaas, G. T., & Hager, R. L. (1997). Body fat percentage of children varies according to their diet composition. *Journal of the American Dietetic Association, 97,* 981–986.

Wadden, T. A., Foster, G. D., Stunkard, A. J., & Linowitz, J. R. (1989). Dissatisfaction with weight and figure in obese girls: Discontent but not depression. *International Journal of Obesity, 13,* 89–97.

Waxman, M. (1988). *Fat families and thick description: A naturalistic study of obese girls and their nonobese sisters.* Unpublished doctoral dissertation, University of Pennsylvania.

Waxman, M., & Stunkard, A. J. (1980). Caloric intake and expenditure of obese boys. *Journal of Pediatrics, 96,* 187–193.

Weiss W., & Jackson, E. C. (1969). Maternal factors affecting birth weight. In *Perinatal factors affecting human development* (PAHO Pan American Health Organization Publication No. 185). Washington DC: Pan American Health Organization.

Wells, J. C. K., Stanley, M., Laidlaw, A. S., Day, J. M., & Davies, P. S. W. (1998). Energy intake in early infancy and childhood fatness. *International Journal of Obesity, 35,* 347–54.

Wells, J. C., Stanley, M., Laidlaw, A. S., Day, J. M., Stafford, M., & Davies, P. S. (1997). Investigation of the relationship between infant temperament and later body composition. *International Journal of Obesity, 21,* 400–406.

Whitaker, R. C., Wright, J. A., Pepe, M. S., Seidel, K. D., & Dietz, W. H. (1997). Predicting obesity in young adulthood from childhood and parental obesity. *New England Journal of Medicine, 337,* 869–873.

26

Treatment of Pediatric Obesity

GARY S. GOLDFIELD
HOLLIE A. RAYNOR
LEONARD H. EPSTEIN

The increasing prevalence of pediatric obesity represents a serious public health concern (see Berkowitz & Stunkard, Chapter 25, this volume; Gortmaker, Dietz, Sobol, & Wehler, 1987). In our previous review of the literature on treatment of pediatric obesity (Epstein, Myers, Raynor, & Saelens, 1998), we examined 32 clinic-based and 6 school-based outcome studies, as well as surgical and pharmacological interventions. The primary goal of this chapter is to update our previous review (Epstein et al., 1998) by adding seven new clinic-based obesity treatment studies. Since our previous review, there have been few published studies examining surgical, pharmacological, or school-based interventions for pediatric obesity that meet our inclusion criteria; thus these areas are not reviewed again in this chapter. In addition to including new clinic-based studies, we examine how duration of treatment influences patterns of weight change in obese children. Data from the treatment of obese adults suggest that longer therapy is associated with greater weight loss (Perri, Nezu, Patti, & McCann, 1989), but this relationship has not been investigated with the management of childhood obesity. In addition, we outline areas for future research, discuss several challenging issues that therapists encounter when providing treatment of childhood obesity, and provide suggestions for dealing with these clinical issues.

STUDIES OF THE TREATMENT OF CHILDHOOD OBESITY: ORGANIZATION OF OUR REVIEW

The goals for treating childhood obesity are regulating body weight through adequate nutrition for growth and development, and thereby allowing natural growth, minimizing loss of lean body mass, and preventing endocrine disturbances (Rees, 1990). In addition, treatments should be associated with positive changes in physiological and psychological sequelae of obesity. Treatments should modify eating and exercise behaviors, along with the factors that regulate these behaviors, so that new, healthier behaviors persist throughout development.

Our review in this chapter is organized according to major components of treating pediatric obesity, including dietary, activity, and behavior change components. In selecting the studies included in this review, we considered the quality of the study design, with a focus on randomized controlled studies. When studies did not provide sufficient detail to determine whether subjects were allowed to choose their preferred treatment, or whether they could have been placed in groups on the basis of factors that could bias interpretation of results, we erred on the conservative side and considered them not to be randomized studies. The seven studies that were added for this review were identified via computerized literature searches in several databases, including MEDLINE and PsycINFO, from January 1966 to February 2000.

The details of the randomized studies that were reviewed are presented in Tables 26.1 and 26.2. These tables include participant age, group assignment, sample size, sex distribution, dietary components, exercise intervention, and results. Several dependent measures were used across studies. The most common were changes in percentage of overweight, body mass index (BMI), body weight, and percentage of body fat. Where available, we have provided the baseline values, end-of-treatment changes, and end-of-follow-up changes. To provide a common definition of when treatment ends and follow-up begins, we considered treatment to be continuing as long as subjects were seen at least once every 6 weeks. The most relevant information is significance in the differential rate of change between groups over time, but if this information was not available, within-group differences are presented.

FINDINGS OF THE LITERATURE REVIEW

Dietary Interventions

Diet therapy for obesity is based on the hypothesis that obesity results when energy intake exceeds energy expenditure, and that negative energy balance needed for weight loss can be achieved more rapidly through caloric reduction than through increased energy expenditure. The general goals of most dietary interventions involve reducing and stabilizing caloric intake, decreasing fat intake, and restructuring dietary consumption to conform more closely to current dietary recommendations.

Amador, Ramos, Morono, and Hermelo (1990) demonstrated that the degree of caloric restriction is important by showing significantly larger weight loss with a more restricted diet (0.17 MJ/kg of expected body weight for height) than with a less restricted diet (0.25 MJ/kg of expected body weight for height), with treatment effects maintained at 12-month follow-up. Gropper and Acosta (1987) investigated the effects of dietary fiber in a sample of obese children and found that 15 g of fiber supplementation combined with a reduced-energy diet for 4 weeks did not significantly decrease energy intake or increase weight loss, compared with 4 weeks of the reduced-energy diet alone.

Several different dietary approaches designed to reduce caloric intake and/or develop healthier eating habits have been studied. One approach is to provide individualized dietary interventions. Hills and Parker (1988) found that preadolescents who were provided with individualized dietary recommendations for 16 weeks without caloric restriction showed no weight loss. Another approach is the diabetic exchange system, with a caloric level calculated to produce a weight loss of 1 pound (0.45 kg) per week. In two studies, diet-plus-exercise programs were associated with significantly better weight changes than those in the no-treatment control groups (Becque, Katch, Rocchini, Marks, & Moorehead, 1988; Rocchini et al., 1988).

TABLE 26.1. Characteristics of Child Obesity Treatment Studies

Authors	Age	Assign	Between-group variable	n	% girls	Diet	Exercise
Amador et al. (1990)	10–13	R	1. Restrictive diet 2. Nonrestrictive diet	47 47	47.9	Restricted to 30% of energy requirement (1), nutritional information (1, 2)	Exercise information (1, 2)
Aragona et al. (1975)	5–11	R	1. Response cost + reinforcement 2. Response cost 3. Control	5 3 5	100.0	Nutrition information (1, 2)	Daily exercise instructions and program for parents (1, 2)
Bacon & Lowrey (1967)	5–17	R	1. Fenfluramine 2. Placebo (Within-subject design, order randomized)	20 (total)	~71.4	1,000–1,200 kcal/day (1, 2)	None
Becque et al. (1988)	12–13	R	1. Exercise + diet 2. Diet 3. Control	11 11 14	58.3	ADA exchange for ↓ 1–2 lb/wk (1, 2)	Supervised aerobic activity @ 60%–80% maximal heart rate, 50 min, 3×/wk (1)
Brownell et al. (1983)	12–16	RS	1. Mother and child seen separately 2. Mother and child seen together 3. Child seen alone	14 15 13	78.6	Nutrition information (1, 2, 3)	Exercise information (1, 2, 3)
Coates, Jeffery, et al. (1982)	13–17	RS	1. Daily contact, reinforced for weight 2. Weekly contact, reinforced for weight 3. Daily contact, reinforced for calories 4. Weekly contact, reinforced for calories	8 8 11 11	68.4	Caloric goals estimated for ↓ 1–2 lb/wk (1, 2, 3, 4)	Minimal exercise information (1, 2, 3, 4)
Coates, Killen, & Slinkard (1982)	13–17	RS	1. Mother and child seen separately 2. Child seen alone	31 (total)	64.5	Nutrition information (1, 2)	Exercise information (1, 2)
Duffy & Spence (1993)	7–13	R	1. Cognitive treatment 2. Progressive relaxation	14 13	~78.6	Traffic-light diet (1, 2)	Lifestyle, aerobic, and calisthenic activity (1, 2)
Epstein et al. (1980)	6–12	RS	1. Behavior modification 2. Nutrition education	14 (total)	~38.5	Traffic-light diet, 900–1,200 or 1,500 kcal/day (1, 2)	Exercise information (1, 2)
Epstein et al. (1981); Epstein, Valoski, Wing, & McCurley (1994)	6–12	RS	1. Mother and child targeted 2. Child targeted 3. Nonspecific target	76 (total)	69.6	Traffic-light diet, limit 1,200–1,500 kcal/day (1, 2, 3)	Exercise information

534

Study	Ages	Design	Treatment groups	N	%	Diet	Activity
Epstein et al. (1982)	8–12	R	1. Aerobic activity + diet 2. Lifestyle activity + diet 3. Aerobic activity alone 4. Lifestyle activity alone	51 (total)	~78.4	Traffic-light diet, 900–1,200 or 1,500 kcal/day (1, 2)	Aerobic (1, 3) or lifestyle (2, 4) activity; isocaloric across groups
Epstein et al. (1984); Epstein, Valoski, et al. (1994)	8–12	R	1. Exercise + diet 2. Diet 3. Control	18 18 17	NR	Traffic-light diet (1, 2)	Lifestyle activity (200–400 kcal/day) (1)
Epstein, Wing, Koeske, & Valoski (1985); Epstein, Valoski, Wing, & McCurley (1994)	8–12	R	1. Programmed aerobic activity 2. Lifestyle activity 3. Calisthenics	41 (total)	~60.0	Traffic-light diet, 1,200 kcal/day (1, 2, 3)	Aerobic (1), lifestyle (2), or calisthenic (3) activity; isocaloric across groups
Epstein, Wing, Penner, & Kress (1985)	8–12	RS	1. Exercise + diet 2. Diet	23 (total)	100.0	Traffic-light diet, 900–1,200 kcal/day (1, 2)	Supervised exercise, 3-mile walk, 3×/wk (1)
Epstein, Wing, Woodall, et al. (1985)	5–8	R	1. Behavior modification 2. Education	8 11	100.0	Traffic-light diet, 900–1,000 or 1,200 kcal/day (1, 2)	Lifestyle activity (1, 2)
Epstein, Wing, et al. (1986); Epstein, Valoski, et al. (1994)	8–12	R, IV	1. Parent overweight 2. Parent normal-weight	41 (total)	NR	Traffic-light diet, 1,200 kcal/day (1, 2)	Lifestyle activity (1, 2)
Epstein, McKenzie, et al. (1994)	8–12	R	1. Mastery criteria 2. No mastery criteria (yoked)	44 (total)	~74.4	Traffic-light diet, from 900–1,800 to 900–1,200 kcal/day (1, 2)	Lifestyle activity (1, 2)
Epstein, Valoski, Vara, et al. (1995)	8–12	R	1. Reinforced for ↑ activity 2. Reinforced for ↓ sedentary behavior 3. Reinforced for both ↑ activity + ↓ sedentary	61 (total)	73.0	Traffic-light diet, 1,000–1,200 kcal/day (1, 2, 3)	↑ Activity (1), ↓ sedentary (2), or both ↑ activity and ↓ sedentary (3)
Epstein, Paluch, Gordy, Saelens, & Ernst (2000)	8–12	RS	1. Standard treatment + parent–child problem solving 2. Standard treatment + child problem solving 3. Standard treatment	17 18 17	51.9	Traffic-light diet, 1,200 kcal/day (1, 2, 3)	Lifestyle activity (1, 2, 3)

(*continued*)

TABLE 26.2. Outcomes of Child Obesity Treatment Studies on Clinical Samples

Authors	OW* (%)	BMI*	BW* (lb)	BF* (%)	Rx (mo)	OW† (%)	BMI†	BW† (lb)	BF† (%)	FU (mo)	OW† (%)	BMI†	BW† (lb)	BF† (%)	Results
Amador et al. (1990)	>97th %ile				0–6 1 2					0–12 1 2			↓14.9ᵃ ↓4.8ᵇ		BW, Rx, FU: 1 > 2 (analyzed by gender)
Aragona et al. (1975)	(29.6) (34.1) (41.7)	(21.7) (22.8) (23.1)	105.6 104.6 9.3		0–3 1 2 3	↓15.7ᵃ ↓14.2ᵇ ↓1.8ᵇ	↓2.4ᵃ ↓2.2ᵃ ↓0.2ᵇ	↓11.3ᵃ ↓9.6ᵃ ↑0.9ᵇ		0–11 1 2 3	(↓11.8) (↓7.1) (↓2.5)	(↓1.2) (↓0.3) (↓0.6)	↓0.7 ↑7.3 ↑5.3		BW, Rx: 1, 2 > 3 BW, FU: 1 = 2 = 3
Bacon & Lowrey (1967)	>97th %ile				0–2 1 2			(lb/mo) ↓4.3 ↓1.9		None					BW, Rx: 1 = 2
Becque et al. (1988)			149.4 169.8 151.1	38.3 44.0 39.8	0–5 1 2 3			↓3.5 ↓0.9 ↑7.0	↓3.0 ↓3.5 ↑0.7	None					BW, BF, Rx: 1 = 2 = 3
Brownell et al. (1983)	59.9 50.4 57.4	45.4 42.4 42.0	183.9 177.1 178.4		0–4 1 2 3	↓17.1ᵃ ↓7.0ᵇ ↓6.8ᵇ	↓4.7ᵃ ↓3.0 ↓2.0ᵇ	↓18.5ᵃ ↓11.7 ↓7.3ᵇ		0–12 1 2 3	↓20.5ᵃ ↓5.5ᵇ ↓6.0ᵇ	↓4.6ᵃ ↓0.1ᵇ ↓0.1ᵇ	↓16.9ᵃ ↑6.4ᵇ ↑7.0ᵇ		OW, Rx, FU: 1 > 2, 3 BMI, BW, Rx: 1 > 3 BMI, BW, FU: 1 > 2, 3
Coates, Jeffery, et al. (1982)	37.3 39.4 37.3 46.1				0–4 1 2 3 4	↓12.0‡ ↓5.2 ↓6.2 ↓5.0				0–10 1 2 3 4	↓8.0‡ ↑10.4 ↓2.4 ↑5.8				OW, Rx, FU: 1 > 2, 3, 4
Coates, Killen, & Slinkard (1982)	32.5 30.9				0–5 1 2	↓8.6 ↓5.1				0–18 1 2	↓8.4‡ ↓8.2‡				OW, Rx, FU: 1 = 2
Duffy & Spence (1993)	45.5 51.5		125.7 122.2		0–2 1 2	↓7.8‡ ↓9.1‡		↓3.1 ↓3.1		0–8 1 2	↓8.9‡ ↓9.2‡		↑7.1 ↑3.6		OW, BW, Rx, FU: 1 = 2

Reference	%OW	BMI	Wt	T1	#	Δ1a	Δ1b	T2	#	Δ2a	Δ2b	Results
Epstein et al. (1980)	68.4		129.1	0–5	1	↓17.5a	↓8.6	None				OW, Rx: 1 > 2
	60.9		135.4		2	↓6.4b	↓3.4					BW, Rx: 1 = 2
Epstein et al. (1981); Epstein, Valoski, Wing, & McCurley (1994)	39.0	24.1	106.4	0–8	1	↓16.0‡		0–120	1	↓15.3a		OW, Rx: 1 = 2 = 3
	41.2	25.0	117.9		2	↓17.0‡			2	↓3.0		OW, FU: 1 > 3
	45.4	25.1	119.8		3	↓19.0‡			3	↑7.6b		
Epstein et al. (1982)	37.2	24.1	110.1	0–6	1	↓10.3‡	↓1.3‡	0–17	1	↑0.1a	↑1.2a	OW, BMI, Rx: 1 = 2 = 3 = 4
	40.5	24.9	116.6		2	↓19.0‡	↓3.0‡		2	↓13.8b	↑1.5b	OW, BMI, FU: 2, 4 > 1, 3
	38.7	25.3	126.4		3	↓13.9‡	↓2.1‡		3	↓9.7a	↓0.7a	
	34.0	24.0	115.1		4	↓13.2‡	↓2.0‡		4	↓11.2b	↓1.0b	
Epstein et al. (1984); Epstein, Valoski, et al. (1994)	44.0			0–6	1	↓16.0a		0–120	1	↓8.4		OW, Rx: 1, 2 > 2
	44.0				2	↓21.0a			2	↓10.0		OW, FU: 1 = 2
	44.0				3	↑3.0b						
Epstein, Wing, Koeske, & Valoski (1985); Epstein, Valoski, et al. (1994)	47.8		123.9	0–12	1	↓16.3‡	↑2.4	0–120	1	↓10.9a		OW, BW: Rx: 1 = 2 = 3
	48.3		124.0		2	↓16.1‡	↓2.3		2	↓19.7a		OW, FU: 1, 2 > 3
	48.0		123.9		3	↓17.5‡	↓2.3		3	↑12.2a		
Epstein, Wing, Penner, & Kress (1985)	48.0		118.3	0–12	1	↓25.4‡	↓8.5‡	None				OW, Rx: 1 = 2
	48.1		118.7		2	↓18.7‡	↓3.0					BW, Rx: 1 > 2
Epstein, Wing, Woodall, et al. (1985)	41.9	22.8		0–12	1	↓26.3a	↓3.7a	None				OW, BMI, Rx: 1 > 2
	39.2	22.7			2	↓11.2b	↓1.3b					
Epstein, Wing, et al. (1986); Epstein, Valoski, et al. (1994)	20–80			0–12	1	↓7.7a		0–120	1	↑3.1		OW, Rx: 2 > 1
					2	↓16.3b			2	↓11.1		OW, FU: 1 = 2
Epstein, McKenzie, et al. (1994)	60.6		127.4	0–12	1	↓26.5a		0–24	1	↓15.4		OW, Rx: 1 > 2
	58.8		121.5		2	↓16.7b			2	↓10.6		OW, FU: 1 = 2

(continued)

TABLE 26.2. *continued*

Authors	OW* (%)	BMI*	BW* (lb)	BF* (%)	Rx (mo)	OW† (%)	BMI†	BW† (lb)	BF† (%)	FU (mo)	OW† (%)	BMI†	BW† (lb)	BF† (%)	Results
Senediak & Spence (1985)					1					0–7					OW, BW, Rx: 2 > 1 > 3, 4
	34.6		114.2		0–12	↓5.3^a		↓3.7^a		1	↓13.0^a		↓2.4^a		OW, BW, FU: 1, 2 > 3
	34.9		110.1		0–43	↓13.6^b		↓7.9^b		2	↓19.2^a		↓6.1^a		
	41.7		105.2		0–14	↓1.4^c		↓0.7^c		3	↓5.9^b		↑0.6^b		
	37.6		103.6		0–1	↑2.3^c		↑1.7^c							
Wadden et al. (1990)					0–10					None					BW, Rx: 1 = 2 = 3
		36.7	223.1	40.4	1			↑7.7							
		32.8	191.6	39.5	2			↑3.7							
		35.1	211.0	41.6	3			↑6.6							
Wheeler & Hess (1976)					0–7					None					OW, Rx: 1 > 2
	40.4				1	↓4.1^a									
	38.9				2	↑6.3^b									

Note. The following abbreviations are used: *, baseline; †, change from baseline; ‡, value significantly different from baseline value (not reported when group differences are reported); OW, over-weight; BMI, body mass index; BW, body weight; BF, body fat; Rx, treatment period; FU, follow-up period; NR, not reported. Values with different superscript letters differ significantly from each other. Values in parentheses were derived for this table from data provided by the authors.

A third dietary approach is the "traffic-light diet," which has been used for preschool children (Epstein, Valoski, Koeske, & Wing, 1986) and preadolescent children (Duffy & Spence, 1993; Epstein, Paluch, Gordy, & Dorn, 2000; Epstein, Paluch, Gordy, Saelens, & Ernst, 2000; Epstein, Valoski, Vara, et al., 1995; Epstein, Wing, Koeske, Andrasik, & Ossip, 1981; Epstein, Wing, Koeske, Ossip, & Beck, 1982; Epstein, Wing, Koeske, & Valoski, 1984, 1985; Epstein, Wing, Penner, & Kress,1985; Epstein, Wing, Steranchak, Dickson, & Michelson, 1980; Epstein, Wing, Woodall, et al., 1985; Flodmark, Ohlsson, Ryden, & Sveger, 1993; Graves, Meyers, & Clark, 1988; Hills & Parker, 1988; Senediak & Spence, 1985; Valoski & Epstein, 1990). The traffic-light diet is a structured eating plan (900–1,300 kilocalories [kcal]/day) designed to guide participants' eating patterns to meet age recommendations for the basic four food groups, and now the Food Guide Pyramid. The traffic-light diet groups foods into categories based on nutrient density. The current version classifies groups based on dietary fat: Green foods ("go") provide 0–1 g of fat per serving; yellow foods ("caution") contain 2–5 g per serving; and red foods ("stop") have more than 5 g of fat per serving or a high simple-carbohydrate content (e.g., candy).

Interventions using the traffic-light diet as part of a comprehensive pediatric treatment have produced a significant decrease in obesity (Epstein, Paluch, Gordy, & Dorn, 2000; Epstein, Paluch, Gordy, Saelens, & Ernst, 2000; Epstein, Valoski, Vara, et al., 1995; Valoski & Epstein, 1990), improvement in nutrient density (Valoski & Epstein. 1990), and improvement in eating patterns (Duffy & Spence, 1993; Epstein et al., 1981) in preadolescent children. Reductions in high-energy-density "red foods" have also been observed after treatment (Duffy & Spence, 1993; Epstein et al., 1981), with significant associations between changes in intake of "red foods" and weight loss (Epstein et al., 1981) or decrease in percentage of overweight (Duffy & Spence, 1993). Finally, obese children of elementary school age who were treated with the traffic-light diet showed healthier changes in food preferences than comparable lean children who were not treated, evidenced by decreased liking for high-fat/low-sugar, high-sugar/low-fat, and high-fat/high-sugar foods, as well as a greater increase in rated palatability for low-fat/low-sugar foods (Epstein et al., 1989). In addition to short-term effects, long-term reductions in obesity, extending from 5 to 10 years after initiation of treatment, have been observed with the traffic-light diet in combination with behavioral, exercise, and familial treatment components (Epstein, McCurley, Wing, & Valoski, 1990; Epstein, Valoski, Kalarchian, & McCurley, 1995; Epstein, Valoski, Wing, & McCurley, 1990, 1994).

A more restrictive diet that has been used to treat pediatric obesity is the protein-sparing modified fast (PSMF) (Figueroa-Colon, von Almen, Franklin, Schuftan, & Suskind, 1993). It typically provides (1) 600–900 kcal/day; (2) 1.5–2.5 g of protein per kilogram of ideal body weight, usually lean meat; and (3) vitamin and mineral supplementation. Consumption of at least 1.5 liters of water per day is recommended. The PSMF is designed to maximize weight loss, preserve mineral balance, and achieve positive nitrogen balance, thereby conserving lean muscle mass in growing individuals. PSMF diets are usually of short duration (4–12 weeks), conducted under close medical supervision, and not commonly used with prepubertal children. A PSMF diet consisting of 600–800 kcal/day has been shown to produce larger reductions in percentage of overweight than a less restrictive diet (800–1,000 kcal) at 10 weeks and 6 months; however, no group differences emerged at 15 months (Figueroa-Colon et al., 1993).

Exercise Interventions

In most obesity treatments, reduction of caloric intake is the most significant contribution to negative energy balance (Wing & Jeffery, 1979). Increased physical activity, however,

dren in the child-and-mother-separately group decreased their percentage of overweight significantly more than did children in either the child-and-mother-together or the child-alone groups, which did not differ (reductions of 20.5% vs. 5.5% and 6.0%, respectively). However, treating the child and mother separately did not improve outcome after 10 months in a sample of black adolescents who received the same intervention (Wadden et al., 1990).

Treatment Frequency

Behavioral treatments are designed to teach parents and children new habits that facilitate weight loss and maintenance of weight loss. The scheduling of sessions may influence the process of learning these new skills. Senediak and Spence (1985) assessed the effects of rapid (eight sessions in 4 weeks) or gradual (eight sessions over 15 weeks) behavioral treatment versus a nonspecific control condition and a wait-list control group. At a 26-week follow-up, the gradual behavioral group had more significant weight change than did the rapid group, which had more weight change than did the nonspecific control group. Mastery of sequential components of behavior change is another variable that could influence habit change. Epstein, McKenzie, Valoski, Klein, and Wing (1994) tested the hypothesis that families required to master behavior changes before they progressed in the program would achieve better outcomes than those who received the same intervention without mastery. As predicted, results indicated that children in the mastery group had a significantly better treatment outcome than did children in the nonmastery group at 12 months. These differences, however, were not significant at 24 months.

Among the most important components of behavior change are the specification of goals and the frequency of reinforcement for meeting goals. Coates, Jeffery, Slinkard, Killen, and Danaher (1982) contrasted groups in which changes in caloric intake or weight were targeted and reinforced according to meeting daily or weekly goals. At 10 months, the best results were obtained by adolescents who were reinforced for weight change on a daily basis. Research has also evaluated the role of perception of choice in therapeutic outcome of behavioral obesity treatment (Mendonca & Brehm, 1983). Children who perceived that they chose the type of treatment achieved a greater reduction in percentage of overweight than did children in the no-choice control condition at 12 weeks. No treatment effect was found at 9 months, but the small sample size and attrition precluded meaningful interpretation at this time point.

Problem Solving

Two studies have investigated the effects of problem solving on weight changes, based on the hypothesis that weight loss could be enhanced by providing instruction on identifying and solving potential situations that threaten adherence to diet and exercise protocols. Graves and colleagues (1988) found that families in which parents receiving a behavioral program plus problem-solving training, a component of many behavioral treatments, had significantly better outcomes at an 8-month follow-up than families who received the behavioral program without training in problem solving. However, Epstein, Paluch, Gordy, Saelens, and Ernst (2000) found that children who received standard behavior therapy showed larger weight losses at posttreatment and exhibited significantly less weight gain at 24 months, compared to children receiving a behavior therapy intervention that provided enhanced problem solving for parents and children. The standard behavior therapy group that targeted problem solving in children did not exhibit significantly different weight changes from the standard treatment group or the group that targeted problem solving in children and parents.

Aragona, Cassady, and Drabman (1975) have compared different ways to motivate children to change eating and activity behaviors. They compared the effects of response cost (loss of monetary deposit for failure to meet attendance, self-monitoring, and child weight loss criteria) with or without reinforcement for behavior change versus a no-treatment control group in a small sample of 5- to 11-year-old children. Both response cost groups (response cost alone and response cost plus reinforcement) showed greater weight loss than controls at 12 weeks posttreatment. However, no treatment effects were found at follow-up, although reinforcement appeared to reduce weight regain.

Since obesity has been conceptualized as a disorder of self-control, one would expect that self-management treatment would enhance weight loss. However, children who received comprehensive behavioral family-based programs with child self-control training did not show greater weight changes than those who received the comprehensive program alone (Epstein, Valoski, et al., 1994; Epstein, Wing, Koeske, & Valoski, 1986; Israel, Guile, Baker, & Silverman, 1994). Although cognitive-behavioral therapy has been found to enhance the treatment of eating disorders beyond behavior therapy alone (Fairburn, Jones, Peveler, Hope, & O'Connor, 1993), Duffy and Spence (1993) found no additional effects on weight change of cognitive therapy techniques, such as monitoring negative thoughts or restructuring maladaptive cognitions. Their obese children were assessed at 8 weeks posttreatment and an 8-month follow-up.

Length of Treatment and Weight Change

Although research has shown that longer obesity treatment is associated with larger weight losses in adults (Jeffery et al., 2000; Perri et al., 1989), no research has examined how the length of treatment influences outcome in obese children. We examined the effects of treatment duration on change in percentage of overweight across 55 treatment groups from 25 studies that employed percentage of overweight as an outcome measure. Percentage of overweight was selected because it was the most widely used outcome (in 64% of studies) and is well suited for pediatric samples. It accounts for changes in height as well as weight. The majority of treatment groups involved behavior therapy components and/or education concerning diet and exercise. Groups that were not given instruction on diet or exercise, such as no-treatment control groups and attention placebo groups, were excluded. Linear regression was used to test the association between treatment length (in months) and change in percentage of overweight, with the baseline percentage of overweight included in the model, in addition to length of treatment.

Results of the regression analysis indicate that the number of months of treatment was related to change in percentage of overweight at the end of treatment ($r = .45$, $p < .001$), with a β coefficient of $-.79$, suggesting that bigger decreases were observed with longer treatments. The reduction in percentage of overweight approached 0.80% for each month of treatment. When baseline percentage of overweight was included in the regression model, the multiple r increased to $r = .63$, $p < .001$. This relationship is displayed graphically in Figure 26.1. These results indicate that longer treatments were associated with greater reductions in percentage of overweight. Baseline percentage of overweight and length of treatment accounted for 40% of the variance in the change in percentage of overweight.

It is interesting that the pattern of change during treatment of childhood obesity is similar to the pattern of change reported in treatment of adult obesity (Jeffery et al., 2000; Per-

community health interventions are weak. The same could be said for obesity treatment. One solution may be studies that focus more on documentation of behavior change and less on weight change.

COMMON CLINICAL PROBLEMS IN THE CHILDHOOD WEIGHT CONTROL PROGRAM

We have been implementing controlled clinical trials in pediatric obesity for over 20 years, with our first study published in 1980 (Epstein et al., 1980). During that time we have seen over 500 families and have learned a lot about clinical issues that influence short- and long-term weight control. The problems in treatment that we have seen are similar across studies, and are addressed in this section. These clinical issues are probably similar to those experienced by other research groups and by other clinicians who treat pediatric obesity. However, there are several important ways in which we conduct clinical research that may influence the development and resolution of these clinical issues.

First, we provide both individual and group experiences during treatment. At each treatment meeting, families are seen by an individual counselor, and family members then participate in separate parent and child groups. Other programs may offer either individualized or group treatment. In addition, during the course of weekly treatment, the staff members meet weekly to discuss the progress of each family. The purposes of these meetings are to address clinical issues early (allowing time for the counselors to address the issues) and to maximize counselors' adherence to treatment protocol. The structure of treatment delivery and case review may be different in other programs. Finally, no family with current psychopathology or a history of eating disorders in the immediate family is included in our clinical trials. With such a family, an intensive individualized intervention may reduce some problems associated with pediatric obesity treatment and familial comorbid psychopathology.

Self-Monitoring

The most common problem concerning treatment adherence is failure to self-monitor accurately. This problem is complicated by the coordination needed between parent and child, as both are attempting to self-monitor behaviors they are changing, along with the parent's additional responsibility of providing structured support for the child. There is extensive research on the importance of self-monitoring in obesity treatment, but self-monitoring can be a burden to obese children, and their recording can be very inaccurate (Bandini et al., 1990). This inaccuracy can create problems in understanding how well participants are implementing treatment. It can be frustrating to both the counselor and the family when an intake of 800 kcal/day is reported, but the child is gaining weight. When this situation arises, it is important for the counselor to determine the reason for the inaccuracies, so that appropriate solutions can be provided. If the cause of the inaccuracies, for example, is waiting until the end of the day (or waiting for a couple of days!) to record eating behaviors, the family and counselor can develop feasible solutions to help the child record shortly after eating (e.g., the family keeps the monitoring book near eating areas, the parent and child meet consistently to discuss eating behaviors, the parent models appropriate self-monitoring behaviors). In addition, a reward system can be established that encourages the child to record all foods that are consumed, thereby improving the accuracy of the self-monitoring. If foods are recorded but measured inaccurately (or not measured at all), then recorded caloric intake may be underestimated because of mismeasured portion size, and this problem will need to be addressed.

Keeping measuring utensils in visible locations in the kitchen and/or using a reinforcement system may increase the frequency and accuracy of food measurement.

Motivation

Another difficult clinical issue is a reduction in a child's motivation to develop and maintain eating and activity changes. This decrement in motivation may come from several sources: (1) losing less weight than expected; (2) failure to see changes in areas that are influenced by obesity, such as social interactions with other children (e.g., teasing) and sports ability; (3) not being able to eat whatever a friend is eating; and (4) having less self-control over eating unhealthy foods than an adult might have (Green, Fry, & Myerson, 1994). One way to improve motivation is to set behavioral goals that the child feels are attainable. This may mean that larger program goals may need to be restructured into smaller goals that the child can achieve fairly rapidly. This would allow the development of behavioral goals that are still challenging to the child, but within his or her perceived ability. Furthermore, as the behavioral goals are achieved more rapidly, the child can be reinforced for the changes, which should provide increased motivation for additional behavior changes.

Family Treatment

A family-based program may be most effective when all family members are willing to make changes within the home. Unfortunately, this is not the case in all families. A spouse, other siblings, grandparents, or other relatives may keep unhealthy foods in the home, use food as a reward, or tease children about their weight, thereby providing different messages regarding the importance or methods of weight control than the child receives from program staff. In this situation, the counselor needs to identify the source of nonsupport and implement an appropriate intervention. This may require the staff member to meet with the entire family to discuss ways of fostering a healthy eating environment, provide education about factors relating to the etiology and maintenance of obesity, and/or delineate ways in which family members can provide support for behavior change.

Pediatric Reinforcement

Our pediatric obesity treatment program is based on using positive reinforcement to shape (and maintain) new behaviors that are targeted in the program. Families are given extensive training in the use of a point- or contract-based reinforcement system. One of the main challenges in implementing the program is having parents use positive reinforcement, perhaps because they are more aware of their children's misbehavior than of their good behavior. Some parents start the program using positive reinforcement, but over time they may fail to observe positive behavior change or to implement the point economy. Other parents may fail to recognize the importance of positive reinforcement in helping their child make behavior changes. They feel that their child should be intrinsically motivated to change his or her behavior, because weight loss will improve weight and health.

When parents do not use positive reinforcement to help with behavior change, they still use other techniques; however, some of these may involve aversive parent–child interactions, such as parents' using punishment to stop child behaviors they don't like (e.g., eating candy). It is easy for parents to revert to these disciplinary strategies, because they may produce behavior change more rapidly than positive reinforcement. For example, if parents want their child to clean his or her room, it may be easier to nag or yell until it is done than to provide praise for a clean room. However, the long-term danger of relying on aversive in-

Epstein, L. H., Valoski, A., Wing, R. R., Perkins, K. A., Fernstrom, M., Marks, B., & McCurley, J. (1989). Perception of eating and exercise in children as a function of child and parent weight. *Appetite, 12,* 105–118.

Epstein, L. H., Wing, R. R., Koeske, R., Andrasik, F., & Ossip, D. J. (1981). Child and parent weight loss in family-based behavior modification programs. *Journal of Consulting and Clinical Psychology, 49,* 674–685.

Epstein, L. H., Wing, R. R., Koeske, R., Ossip, D. J., & Beck, S. (1982). A comparison of lifestyle change and programmed aerobic exercise on weight and fitness changes in obese children. *Behavior Therapy, 13,* 651–665.

Epstein, L. H., Wing, R. R., Koeske, R., & Valoski, A. (1984). Effects of diet plus exercise on weight change in parents and children. *Journal of Consulting and Clinical Psychology, 52,* 429–437.

Epstein, L. H., Wing, R. R., Koeske, R., & Valoski, A. (1985). A comparison of lifestyle exercise, aerobic exercise and calisthenics on weight loss in obese children. *Behavior Therapy, 16,* 345–356.

Epstein, L. H., Wing, R. R., Koeske, R., & Valoski, A. (1986). Effect of parent weight on weight loss in obese children. *Journal of Consulting and Clinical Psychology, 54,* 400–401.

Epstein, L. H., Wing, R. R., Penner, B. C., & Kress, M. J. (1985). Effect of diet and controlled exercise on weight loss in obese children. *Journal of Pediatrics, 107,* 358–361.

Epstein, L. H., Wing, R. R., Steranchak, L., Dickson, B., & Michelson, J. (1980). Comparison of family based behavior modification and nutrition education for childhood obesity. *Journal of Pediatric Psychology, 5,* 25–36.

Epstein, L. H., Wing, R. R., Valoski, A., & Penner, B. (1987). Stability of food preferences in 8–12 year old children and their parents during weight control. *Behavior Modification, 11,* 87–101.

Epstein, L. H., Wing, R. R., Woodall, K., Penner, B. C., Kress, M. J., & Koeske, R. (1985). Effects of family-based behavioral treatment on obese 5–8 year old children. *Behavior Therapy, 16,* 205–212.

Fairburn, C. G., Jones, R., Peveler, R. C., Hope, R. A., & O'Connor, M. (1993). Psychotherapy and bulimia nervosa: Longer-term effects of interpersonal psychotherapy, behavior therapy, and cognitive behavior therapy. *Archives of General Psychiatry, 50,* 419–428.

Figueroa-Colon, R., von Almen, T. K., Franklin, F. A., Schuftan, C., & Suskind, R. M. (1993). Comparison of two hypocaloric diets in obese children. *American Journal of Diseases of Children, 147,* 160–166.

Flodmark, C. -E., Ohlsson, T., Ryden, O., & Sveger, T. (1993). Prevention of progression to severe obesity in a group of obese schoolchildren treated with family therapy. *Pediatrics, 91,* 880–884.

Garn, S. M., & Clark, D. C. (1976). Trends in fatness and the origins of obesity. *Pediatrics, 57,* 443–456.

Golan, M., Weizman, A., Apter, A., & Fainaru, M. (1998). Parents as exclusive agents of change in the treatment of childhood obesity. *American Journal of Clinical Nutrition, 67,* 1130–1135.

Gortmaker, S. L., Dietz, W. H., Sobol, A. M., & Wehler, C. A. (1987). Increasing pediatric obesity in the United States. *American Journal of Diseases of Children, 141,* 535–540.

Graves, T., Meyers, A. W., & Clark, L. (1988). An evaluation of problem-solving training in the behavioral treatment of childhood obesity. *Journal of Consulting and Clinical Psychology, 56,* 246–250.

Green, L., Fry, A. F., & Myerson, J. (1994). Discounting of delayed rewards: A life-span comparison. *Psychological Science, 5,* 33–36.

Gropper, S. S., & Acosta, P. B. (1987). The therapeutic effect of fiber in treating obesity. *Journal of the American College of Nutrition, 6,* 533–535.

Gutin, B., Owens, S., Slavens, G., Riggs, S., & Treiber, F. (1997). Effect of physical training on heart-period variability in obese children. *Journal of Pediatrics, 130,* 938–943.

Hills, A. P., & Parker, A. W. (1988). Obesity management via diet and exercise intervention. *Child: Care, Health and Development, 14,* 409–416.

Israel, A. C., Guile, C. A., Baker, J. E., & Silverman, W. K. (1994). An evaluation of enhanced self-regulation training in the treatment of childhood obesity. *Journal of Pediatric Psychology, 19,* 737–749.

Israel, A. C., Stolmaker, L., & Andrian, C. A. (1985). The effects of training parents in general child management skills on a behavioral weight loss program for children. *Behavior Therapy, 16,* 169–180.

Jeffery, R. W., Drewnowski, A., Epstein, L. H., Stunkard, A. J., Wilson, G. T., Wing, R. R., & Hill, D. R. (2000). Long-term maintenance of weight loss: Current status. *Health Psychology, 19,* 5–16.

Johnson, W. G., Hinkle, L. K., Carr, R. E., Anderson, D. A., Lemmon, C. R., Engler, L. B., & Bergeron, K. C. (1997). Dietary and exercise interventions for juvenile obesity: Long-term effect of behavioral and public health models. *Obesity Research, 5,* 257–261.

Kirschenbaum, D. S., Harris, E. S., & Tomarken, A. J. (1984). Effects of parental involvement in behavioral weight loss therapy for preadolescents. *Behavior Therapy, 15,* 485–500.

Kohl, H. W., & Hobbs, K. E. (1998). Development of physical activity behaviors among children and adolescents. *Pediatrics, 101,* 549–554.

Lichtman, S. W., Pisarska, K., Berman, E. R., Pestone, M., Dowling, H., Offenbacher, E., Weisel, H., Heshka, S., Matthews, D. W., & Heymsfield, S. B. (1992). Discrepancy between self-reported and actual caloric intake in obese subjects. *New England Journal of Medicine, 327,* 1893–1898.

McCrory, M. A., Fuss, P. J., McCallum, J. E., Yao, M., Vinken, A. G., Hays, N. P., & Roberts, S. B. (1999). Dietary variety within food groups: Association with energy intake and body fatness in men and women. *American Journal of Clinical Nutrition, 69,* 440–447.

Mellin, L. M., Slunkard, L. A., & Irwin, C. E. (1987). Adolescent obesity intervention: Validation of the SHAPEDOWN program. *Journal of the American Dietetic Association, 87,* 333–338.

Mendonca, P. J., & Brehm, S. S. (1983). Effects of choice on behavioral treatment of overweight children. *Journal of Social and Clinical Psychology, 1,* 343–353.

Owens, S., Gutin, B., Allison, J., Riggs, S., Ferguson, M., Litaker, M., & Thompson, W. (1999). Effect of physical training on total and visceral fat in obese children. *Medicine and Science in Sports and Exercise, 31,* 143–148.

Perri, M. G., Nezu, A. M., Patti, E. T., & McCann, K. L. (1989). Effect of length of treatment on weight loss. *Journal of Consulting and Clinical Psychology, 57,* 450–452.

Rees, J. M. (1990). Management of obesity in adolescence. *Medical Clinics of North America, 74,* 1275–1292.

Reybrouck, T., Vinckx, J., Van Den Berghe, G., & Vanderschueren-Lodeweyckx, M. (1990). Exercise therapy and hypocaloric diet in the treatment of obese children and adolescents. *Acta Paediatrica Scandinavica, 79,* 84–89.

Rocchini, A. P., Katch, V., Anderson, J., Hinderliter, J., Becque, D., Martin, M., & Marks, C. (1988). Blood pressure in obese adolescents: Effect of weight loss. *Pediatrics, 82,* 16–23.

Sallis, J. F., Simons-Morton, B. G., Stone, E. J., Corbin, C. B., Epstein, L. H., Faucette, N., Iannotti, R. J., Killen, J. D., Klesges, R. C., Petray, C. K., Rowland, T. W., & Taylor, W. C. (1992). Determinants of physical activity and interventions in youth. *Medicine and Science in Sports and Exercise, 24,* S248–S257

Sallo, M., & Silla, R. (1997). Physical activity with moderate to vigorous intensity in preschool and first-grade schoolchildren. *Pediatric Exercise Science, 4,* 44–54.

Senediak, C., & Spence, S. H. (1985). Rapid versus gradual scheduling of therapeutic contact in a family based behavioural weight control programme for children. *Behavioural Psychotherapy, 13,* 265–287.

Sidman, M. (1989). *Coercion and its fallout.* Boston: Authors Cooperative.

Valoski, A., & Epstein, L. H. (1990). Nutrient intake of obese children in a family-based behavioral weight control program. *International Journal of Obesity, 14,* 667–677.

Wadden, T. A., Stunkard, A. J., Rich, L., Rubin, C. J., Sweidel, G., & McKinney, S. (1990). Obesity in black adolescent girls: A controlled clinical trial of treatment by diet, behavior modification, and parental support. *Pediatrics, 85,* 345–352.

Wheeler, M. E., & Hess, K. W. (1976). Treatment of juvenile obesity by successive approximate control of eating. *Journal of Behavioral Therapy and Experimental Psychiatry, 7,* 235–241.

Wing, R. R., & Jeffery, R. W. (1979). Outpatient treatments of obesity: A comparison of methodology and results. *International Journal of Obesity, 3,* 261–279.

27

Prevention of Obesity

KATHRYN H. SCHMITZ
ROBERT W. JEFFERY

Among the *Healthy People 2010* top 10 "leading health indicators" is a goal to reduce the proportion of the U.S. population that is overweight or obese (U.S. Department of Health and Human Services, 2000). "Overweight" is defined as a body mass index (BMI) of 25.0–29.9 kg/m^2, and obesity as a BMI $\geq$ 30 kg/m^2. Because recent trends show a rise in obesity prevalence (Flegal, Carroll, Kuczmarski, & Johnson, 1998), this can be seen as a mandate to increase efforts to prevent obesity. Data from the third National Health and Nutrition Examination Survey (NHANES III) show that 54.9% of the general population over age 20 in the United States is overweight and 22.5% is obese (Flegal et al., 1998). Comparative data from Europe show prevalence rates ranging from lows of 7% and 9% in men and women, respectively, in Sweden to highs of 22% and 45% in men and women, respectively, in Lithuania. The averages across Europe are about 15% and 20% in men and women, respectively (Seidell, 1997). These figures suggest that the current obesity epidemic is not confined to the United States. The prevalence of U.S. adults with a BMI $\geq$ 30 has increased from 12.8% in the 1960s to 22.5% in the 1990s (Flegal et al., 1998). The costs associated with obesity treatment and comorbidities of obesity are high and predicted to grow (McIntyre, 1998). It has been estimated that the indirect and direct costs of obesity in the United States reached $100 billion per year by 1995 (Wolf, 1998).

In this chapter we briefly outline the known or suspected risk factors for (and correlates of) obesity, summarize a recently proposed three-tiered obesity prevention approach (Gill, 1997; World Health Organization, 1998), review prior studies that have focused on obesity prevention in the general population, and outline future research efforts toward obesity prevention. Because of the acknowledgment that there is an obesity epidemic in the United States and other developed nations, the focus of this chapter is on a public health approach to prevention of obesity (populations as units of analysis or treatment) rather than a clinical approach (individuals as units of treatment).

WHAT PREDICTS THE DEVELOPMENT OF OBESITY?

It is widely agreed that although there is certainly individual (genetic) variability in the susceptibility to obesity, the rapid increase in obesity prevalence over the past two decades cannot be primarily due to biology. There must be behavioral and environmental causes. Reviewers have used existing evidence to speculate on whether factors associated with increases in energy intake (eating) or decreases in energy expenditure (exercise) have caused a greater percentage of the rise in obesity prevalence (Dietz & Gortmaker, 1984; Gill, 1997; Harnack, Jeffery, & Boutelle, 2000; Popkin, Paeratakul, Zhai, & Ge, 1995a, 1995b; Prentice & Jebb, 1995; World Health Organization, 1998). Current data do not allow for a resolution of this debate. However, at the root of both conclusions is the concept that individual behaviors leading to energy imbalance (excess energy intake relative to expenditure) are mostly to blame for the increased prevalence of obesity. Furthermore, most authors conclude that although eating behavior and energy expenditure are the proximal causes, the more distal causes of the current obesity epidemic are obesogenic factors in our social, physical, and cultural environments (Gill, 1997; Grundy, 1998; Harnack et al., 2000; Hill, 2000; Hill & Peter, 1998; Nestle & Jacobson, 2000; Popkin et al., 1995a, 1995b; Poston & Foreyt, 1999, Prentice & Jebb, 1995; World Health Organization, 1998).

Risk Factors for Obesity

Prevention of a noncommunicable disease, such as obesity, requires an understanding of factors that predict the development of the disease. A "risk factor" for disease can be defined as "a measurable element in the chain of disease causation and a strong predictor of future risk" (Blackburn, 1994, p. 25). Classic risk factors have important statistical associations with future development of disease, but also have direct causal linkages with disease (Blackburn, 1994). "Risk indicators," by contrast, have statistical associations with future disease risk but no established causal pathway (Blackburn, 1994). "Correlates" of chronic disease may be physiological or behavioral characteristics that have been found to be associated with prevalent disease in cross-sectional analyses, but lack either the temporal association or plausible mechanism needed to support a causal interpretation. Risk factors, risk indicators, and correlates can be behavioral, physiological, demographic, or environmental. Extensive research on cardiovascular disease (CVD) has made it possible to broadly delineate the relative importance of risk factors, risk indicators, and correlates for CVD.

Unfortunately, the current state of obesity research does not allow for the same level of clarity regarding the proximal causes of obesity. Greater clarity about the relative importance of individual proximal as well as distal environmental factors for the development of obesity would assist in the development of cost-effective prevention efforts. Modifiable behavioral and physiological risk factors, indicators, and correlates of weight gain and obesity may include physical inactivity (low energy expenditure), high total caloric intake, high fat intake, high-glycemic-index diets, prenatal environment, birthweight, and childhood obesity (Abraham, Collins, & Nordsieck, 1971; Abraham & Nordsieck, 1960; Danforth, 1985; DiPietro, 1995; Gortmaker, Dietz, & Cheung, 1990; Grundy, 1998; Mathers & Daly, 1998; Morris & Zemel, 1999; Saltzman, 1999; Saris, 1998; Stephen & Wald, 1990). Childhood obesity is included as a modifiable risk factor because (at least in theory) it might be treated to prevent adulthood obesity (Epstein, Valoski, Kalarchian, & McCurley, 1995; Epstein, Valoski, Wing, & McCurley, 1994).

There are also a number of nonmodifiable factors that promote or predict the development of obesity. Although by definition these cannot be altered, they may be useful in discussing the groups for whom obesity prevention efforts will be most needed. Nonmodifiable risk factors, risk indicators, and correlates of weight gain and obesity may include weight gain during critical life periods, individual genetically determined physiological factors, physical environment (e.g., region of country, season, population density, area of residence), ethnicity, socioeconomic status (SES), and age (Abraham et al., 1971; Abraham & Nordsieck, 1960; Cairney & Wade, 1998; Curhan et al., 1996; De Spiegelaere, Dramaix, & Hennart, 1998; Dietz, 1994; Dietz & Gortmaker, 1984; Ellaway, Anderson, & Macintyre, 1997; Fisch, Bilek, & Ulstrom, 1975; Gross, Sokol, & King, 1980; Grundy, 1998; Jeffery, 1991; Kuczmarski, Flegal, Campbell, & Johnson, 1994; Lissau-Lund-Sørensen & Sørensen, 1992; Martikainen & Marmot, 1999; Pomerance & Krall, 1984; Power & Moynihan, 1988; Ravelli, Stein, & Susser, 1976; Rolland-Cachera et al., 1987; Sobal & Stunkard, 1989; Udall, Harrison, Vaucher, Walson, & Morrow, 1978; Vobecky, Vobecky, Shapcott, & Demers, 1983; Whitikar & Dietz, 1998; Williamson, Kahn, & Byers, 1991).

One perspective is that the observed differences in obesity prevalence according to ethnicity and SES may simply point to differential exposure to the obesogenic factors in our social, cultural, and physical environments (Jeffery, 1991). Support for this perspective comes from a Venezuelan study that found exposure to television food advertising to have a greater impact on family food purchases in low-SES families than in higher-SES families (Moya de Sifontes & Dehollain, 1986).

A number of specific environmental and secular changes have accompanied the recent increase in prevalence of obesity. For example, food portion sizes have increased (Harnack et al., 2000; Hill, 2000; Hill & Peter, 1998; Howard, 1997; Liebman & Hurley, 1996; Martson, 1996; Young & Nestle, 1995). Americans eat out with greater frequency now than ever before (Harnack et al., 2000). Public schools have allowed increasing student access to vending machine foods and fast foods, both of which are likely to be energy-dense (French, Jeffery, et al., 1997). There was a 147% increase in fast-food restaurants from 1972 to 1995 in the United States, with fast-food establishments totaling more than 180,000 nationwide by 1995 (French, Story, & Jeffery, 2001). Furthermore, there is observational evidence that increasing the frequency of visits to fast-food restaurants over a 3-year period is associated with significant increases in body mass in adult women (French, Harnack, & Jeffery, 2000). Television viewing time has also increased since the mid-20th century. Nielsen data estimated an average of 28 hours per week of television viewing by persons over 12 years old, compared to an estimate of 10.4 hours per week from a time use study of Americans conducted in 1965 (French et al., 2001). There is also ecological evidence that energy expended in non-leisure-time activities has decreased: increased use of automobiles for transportation, decreased use of public transportation, fewer children walking to school, and decreasing distances walked to school.

Primary, Secondary, and Tertiary Obesity Prevention

Recently, a three-tiered "bull's-eye" obesity prevention approach has been proposed (Gill, 1997; World Health Organization, 1998). The innermost, first tier is called "targeted prevention" and focused on weight gain prevention in obese patients and prevention/management of the comorbidities of obesity. The middle, second tier, called "selective prevention," focuses on individuals at high risk of developing obesity. The outermost, third tier is called "universal prevention" and focuses on prevention of obesity in the total population, regardless of risk factor status. In the subsequent sections, we review the literature relevant to the third-tier, "universal prevention" approach.

STUDIES OF OBESITY PREVENTION IN YOUTH

Outcomes in any obesity prevention or treatment studies in children must be placed in the context of nutritional adequacy to protect proper growth and development over time. Therefore, body weight or other obesity-related outcomes from interventions in children are not weight losses, but differences in the rate of weight increase in intervention versus control groups. Furthermore, obesity prevention and treatment efforts in children must acknowledge and address the potential risk of increasing negative eating and exercise habits associated with the development of eating disorders.

This review focuses on intervention studies that sought to improve eating and energy expenditure behaviors of children in the general population (not overweight or obese children or children at high risk for obesity), and that included measurement of some physiological obesity-related outcome. To identify intervention studies that fit these inclusion criteria, we conducted a computerized search of English-language peer-reviewed literature (in MEDLINE), searched our own files, and searched the references of identified papers. Table 27.1 includes the 22 completed interventions that were identified (Alexandrov et al., 1988; Bush et al., 1989; Donnelly et al., 1996; Dwyer, Coonan, Leitch, Hetzel, & Baghurst, 1983; Fardy et al., 1996; Flores, 1995; Gortmaker et al., 1999; Harrell et al., 1996; Killen et al., 1988; Lionis et al., 1991; Luepker et al., 1996; Mo-Suwan, Pongprapai, Junjana, & Puetpaiboon, 1998; Resnicow et al., 1992; Robinson, 1999; Sallis et al., 1997; Simonetti D'Arca & Sanarelli, 1986; Tamir et al., 1990; Tell & Vellar, 1987; Vandongen et al., 1995; Vartiainen & Puska, 1987; Walter, Hofman, Connelly, Barrett, & Kost, 1985; Worsley, Coonan, & Worsley, 1987).

Planet Health Intervention

We identified four completed trials in children in which one of the primary outcome variables was obesity-related (Donnelly et al., 1996; Gortmaker et al., 1999; Mo-Suwan et al., 1998; Robinson, 1999). Three of these studies included intervention strategies to alter physical activity and/or nutrition services in schools (Donnelly et al., 1996; Gortmaker et al., 1999; Mo-Suwan et al., 1998). Planet Health, an interdisciplinary intervention in sixth- to eighth-graders in Boston, showed significant treatment effects in girls (Gortmaker et al., 1999). Planet Health was conducted in 10 multiethnic public middle schools in Massachusetts (matched for community or school size and for ethnic composition) and focused on reducing television viewing time to 2 hours or less per day, increasing moderate and vigorous activity, decreasing high-fat food consumption, and increasing intake of fruits and vegetables. The intervention included staff training, classroom-based lessons (within language arts, math, science, and social studies), physical education curriculum, and monetary incentives to teachers to create lesson plans consistent with the program themes. The primary endpoint was change in an index that incorporated BMI and triceps skinfold thickness to indicate relative obesity. After 2 years of the intervention, the girls in the intervention schools were significantly less likely to be classified as obese than the girls in the control schools (odds ratio [OR] = 0.47, p = .03). There were no significant between-group differences for boys (OR = 0.85, p = .48). Between-group differences for decreases in television viewing time were 0.58 hours (p = .001) and 0.40 hours (p = .0003) per day in girls and boys, respectively. However, girls in the intervention group also improved fruit and vegetable intake by 0.32 servings per day more than the control group (p = .003), decreased total daily caloric intake more than the control group by 575.4 kilocalories (kcal) (p = .05), and marginally decreased percentage of calories from fat more than the control group by 0.67% (p = .07). By contrast, comparisons of between-group changes in these dietary fac-

TABLE 27.1. Interventions to Prevent Obesity in Youth

Author (year)	Description of the participants/setting	Intervention components	Length of intervention/ follow-up	Primary outcome variable	Outcomes/findings (mean ± SD or proportions)	Statistical significance
		Focus on obesity				
Robinson (1999)	San Jose, CA 192 children in grades 3–4 (approximately 9 years old) Two elementary schools, randomized	Classroom curriculum (18 sessions, 30–50 min each) to teach students in intervention group to "budget" television viewing time to 7 hours weekly Challenge to watch no television for 10 days at the end of curriculum Electronic television time manager device placed in homes of intervention group students Control school—no intervention	2 months/ 8 months	BMI (kg/m^2) Pre:	I: 18.38 ± 3.67 C: 18.10 ± 3.77	$p = .002$
				Post follow-up:	I: 18.67 ± 3.77 C: 18.81 ± 3.76	
				Tricep SF (mm) Pre:	I: 14.55 ± 6.06 C: 13.97 ± 5.43	$p = .002$
				Post follow-up:	I: 15.47 ± 5.95 C: 16.46 ± 5.27	
				Waist circum. (cm) Pre:	I: 60.48 ± 9.91 C: 59.51 ± 8.91	$p < .001$
				Post follow-up:	I: 63.57 ± 8.96 C: 64.73 ± 8.91	
Gortmaker et al. (1999)	Boston, MA Children in grades 6–8 10 schools, randomized	Planet Health: Interdisciplinary classroom curriculum with 32 core lessons incorporated into lessons in four major subjects and PE Focus on decreasing sedentary behavior, decreasing high-fat foods, increasing fruit and vegetable intake, and increasing moderate to vigorous activity Self-assessment, goal setting, evaluations, and incentives to teachers Control schools—no intervention	1–2 years	% of students defined as obese	I: Pre, 23.6%; post, 20.3% C: Pre, 21.5%; post, 23.7%	$p = .03$
				Odds ratio comparing % obese in intervention and control	Female: 0.47 Male: 0.85	$p = .48$
Mo-Suwan et al. (1998)	Southern Thailand 292 kindergarten children Eight classes, randomized	Superkids/Superfit school-based aerobic exercise program: 1-hour weekly PE class, plus 15-min walk and 20-min aerobic dance 3× weekly Control classes—1-hour weekly PE class	29.6 weeks	% of students with triceps skinfold thicknesses > 95th percentile	I: Pre, 12.2%; post, 8.8% C: Pre, 11.7%; post, 9.7%	$p = .058$ $p = .179$

Study	Setting/Population	Intervention	Duration	Outcome measure	Results	Significance
Donnelly et al. (1996)	Rural Nebraska Children in grades 3–5 2 schools (intervention and control school)	School-based obesity prevention intervention: Nutrition education—grade-specific curriculum Physical Best activity program—three weekly sessions (30–40 min), focus on individual, noncompetitive activities "LUNCHPOWER!" program—reduce fat and sodium in school lunches Control group—existing lunch program, team sports activity program	2 years	BMI (kg/m²): Baseline: Follow-up:	I: 17.9 ± 3.8 C: 18.1 ± 2.6 I: 18.9 ± 4.3 C: 19.3 ± 3.2	NSS

Focus on change in energy expenditure (physical activity)

Study	Setting/Population	Intervention	Duration	Outcome measure	Results	Significance
Sallis et al. (1997)	Poway, CA 955 children in grades 4–5 Seven elementary schools, randomization stratified by % minority in schools	SPARK (Sport, Play, and Active, Recreation for Kids): Three weekly PE classes—15 min health–fitness, 15 min skill–fitness activities Behavior change skills education (self-monitoring, reinforcement, goal setting, stimulus control, problem solving) Homework and monthly newsletters to parents, incentives for goal achievement Two treatment arms—I(s): SPARK led by specialist; I(t): SPARK led by classroom teacher Control schools—existing physical education class led by untrained teacher	2 school years	Mean sum of skinfolds (mm) Boys, pre: Boys, post: Girls, pre: Girls, post:	I(s): 26.9 ± 3.72 I(t): 26.8 ± 1.33 C: 27.1 ± 0.87 I(s): 26.4 ± 1.38 I(t): 25.5 ± 2.40 C: 28.0 ± 0.90 I(s): 28.7 ± 2.14 I(t): 30.4 ± 1.53 C: 31.2 ± 1.28 I(s): 30.0 ± 0.61 I(t): 28.0 ± 1.22 C: 30.1 ± 0.56	$p = .55$ $p = .14$
Flores (1995)	Palo Alto, CA Four grade 7 PE classrooms were randomized 43% African American, 43% Hispanic	Dance for Health: 50-minute aerobic dance class three times weekly 30-min health education class two times weekly—nutrition, exercise, obesity, smoking prevention, substance abuse, stress management, peer pressure Control classes—usual PE class	12 weeks	BMI (kg/m²): Girls (n = 49), pre: Girls, post: Girls, difference: Boys (n = 32), pre: Boys, post: Boys, difference:	I: 22.9 ± 6.1 C: 22.2 ± 4.4 I: 22.1 ± 6.0 C: 22.5 ± 4.4 I: −0.8; C: 0.3 Not reported Not reported I: −0.20; C: −0.06	$p < .05$ NSS

(continued)

TABLE 27.1. *continued*

Author (year)	Description of the participants/setting	Intervention components	Length of intervention/follow-up	Primary outcome variable	Outcomes/findings (mean ± SD or proportions)	Statistical significance
		Focus on change in energy expenditure (physical activity) *(cont.)*				
Worsley et al. (1987)	Adelaide, Australia 420 students, 10 years old, grades 4–5 Eight schools: Six treatment, two control (convenience sample)	First Body Owner's Program: Intervention schools had daily PE for 50 min with balanced focus on skills and endurance training. Four treatment arms: I(sm)—self-monitoring of physical activity and diet I(he)—health education/nutrition curriculum, 30 min twice weekly I(sm + he)—combined self-monitoring and health education I—daily physical activity only Control schools—no daily physical activity, no other interventions	5 months	Sum four skinfolds postintervention (adjusting for preintervention levels)	I(sm): Boys: 25.5, girls: 28.9 I(he): Boys, 28.2; girls, 32.2 I(sm + he): Boys, 29.7; girls, 29.9 I: Boys, 31.8; girls, 36.9 C: Boys, 30.8; girls, 31.8	Sex-adjusted F test comparing post-intervention sum of skinfolds for all groups, $p = .03$
Dwyer et al. (1983)	Adelaide, Australia Phase 1: 7 schools, grade 5, 510 students (10 years old) Three classes in each school randomized to one of three treatment conditions Phase 2: 2 years later, 216 students in grade 5 assessed again in five schools	Phase 1: Daily physical activity in two treatment groups: I(F) classes—75-min daily endurance-focused PE I(S) classes—75-min daily skill-focused PE Control classes—30 min of traditional PE three times weekly Phase 2: repeated measurements 2 years later in schools that adopted a combination of I(F) and I(S)	14 weeks/2 years	Phase 1: Δ, sum of four skinfolds Phase 2: Sum of four skinfolds 1978: 1980:	C: 0.93 ± 0.46 I(S): 0.39 ± 0.33 I(F): −1.26 ± 0.40 Boys: 31.90 ± 15.0, Girls: 40.24 ± 15.4 Boys: 28.62 ± 11.88, Girls: 36.23 ± 14.0	$p < .05$ $p < .05$
		Focus on nutrition only				
Simonetti, D'Arca, & Sanarelli (1986)	Rome, Italy Children aged 3–9 years Three schools, one per treatment condition	Two treatment arms, both focused on nutrition education: Multimedia Action (MA) school—distribution of printed materials, audiovisuals, discussion meetings with families and teachers Written Action (WA) school—printed material only Control school—no intervention	1 year	Δ in % obese, overweight, or normal-weight, using BMI values	Change in: % obese: MA, −12.2%; WA, 5.3%; C, 5.9% % overweight: MA, −12.1%; WA, −2.3%; C, 0.8% % normal: MA, 7.2%; WA, −0.7%; C, −3.8%	Not reported

Multiple-risk-factor interventions

Study	Description	Duration	Measure	Values	Significance
Luepker et al. (1996)	96 elementary schools in CA, MN, LA, TX 5,106 students in grades 3–5 28 schools randomized to school-only intervention 28 schools randomized to school and family intervention 40 control schools	CATCH (Child and Adolescent Trial for Cardiovascular Health): School intervention—increase moderate to vigorous activity in PE; nutrition and health education (classroom curricula: "Adventures of Hearty Heart and Friends," "F.A.C.T.S. for Five," and "CATCH"); food service modification ("Eat Smart" program: decrease fat, sodium) Family involvement—19 activity packets, family fun nights Control schools—usual PE, school food service, and health education	3 years	BMI (kg/m²) Baseline: Postintervention: Δ in BMI from baseline to follow-up	I: 17.68 ± 3.23 C: 17.58 ± 2.90 I: 19.74 ± 4.03 C: 19.66 ± 4.35 I: 2.06 ± 2.02 C: 2.13 ± 1.93	$p < .32$
Harrell et al. (1996)	North Carolina 1,274 children in grades 3–4 12 schools—6 urban, 6 rural Randomization by school, stratified by urban–rural	CHIC (Cardiovascular Health In Children): Twice-weekly classroom curriculum on nutrition, exercise, smoking avoidance, peer pressure Three weekly activity sessions—warm-up, 20 min of noncompetitive aerobic activities, cool down Control schools—usual health instruction	8 weeks	Between-group difference in: Δ BMI (kg/m²) Δ sum of triceps and subscapular skinfolds (mm)	I vs. C: −0.04 ± 0.04 I vs. C: 0.05 ± 0.07	NSS NSS
Fardy et al. (1996)	New York City 346 students in grades 9–12 Randomization by classrooms Inner-city school	PATH (Physical Activity and Teenage Health) program: Five health promotion classes weekly—20–25 min of step aerobics, jump rope, cycling, and/or resistance training; 5-min "minilecture" on exercise, nutrition, smoking avoidance, stress management, heart disease, cancer, or motivation Control classes—usual PE class (usually volleyball)	11 weeks	Δ BMI (kg/m²), Δ body fat estimated by skinfolds	No specific values reported	NSS
Vandongen et al. (1995)	Western Australia 971 children aged 10–12 years 30 schools randomized to five treatment conditions	Five treatment conditions: Fitness (F)—Six 30-min classroom lessons on the importance of physical activity, 15 min of daily physical activity School nutrition (SN)—10 lessons (1 hour each) to improve knowledge, attitudes, and eating habits	1 school year	Pre–post change in % body fat, triceps skinfolds (mm), subscapular skinfolds (mm), and BMI (kg/m²)	(Specific values not available) Δ in: % body fat Subscapular skinfolds Tricep skinfolds BMI	NSS NSS $p < .05$ for F&SN vs. C in boys and girls NSS (continued)

TABLE 27.1. *continued*

Author (year)	Description of the participants/setting	Intervention components	Length of intervention/ follow-up	Primary outcome variable	Outcomes/findings (mean ± SD or proportions)	Statistical significance
		Multiple-risk-factor interventions (cont.)				
Vandongen et al. (1995) (*cont.*)		Home nutrition (HN)—Five nutrition messages via comic books delivered to students at school and including information for parents School and home nutrition (S&HN)—combination of above-described interventions Fitness and school nutrition (F&SN)—combination of above-described interventions Control schools—no treatment				
Resnicow et al. (1992)	Bronx, NY 1,209 children, grades 1–6 4 schools—three assigned to receive intervention, 1 assigned to control condition Houston, TX One control to condition school Inner-city, low-SES, predominantly African American	Know Your Body program for CVD risk factor reduction: Health education curriculum, 30–45 min weekly School cafeteria food modifications—increase fiber, decrease fat Peer leader training, student health committees, food-tasting parties, drug and nutrition education Poster and essay contests, student aerobics, special health lectures Control schools—existing health, science curricula	2.5 years	BMI (kg/m^2) Pre: Post:	C: 17.9; I(low): 17.2; I(med.): 17.3; I(high): 17.4 C: 19.1; I(low): 19.1; I(med):19.6; I(high): 19.2	NSS
Lionis et al. (1991)	Rural Crete 171 children aged 13–14 years Five schools—three assigned to treatment, two assigned to control condition	Greek modification of Know Your Body: Health education curriculum, 10 sessions, 2 hours each Parental involvement Control schools—no health education counseling	9 months (1 school year)	BMI (kg/m^2) Δ Triceps skinfold Δ (mm)	I: 0.21 ± 1.43 C: 0.72 ± 0.97 I: −0.40 ± 2.77 C: −1.02 ± 2.72	$p < .05$ NSS
Tamir et al. (1990)	Jerusalem, Israel 406 children, grade 1, 7–9 years old 16 schools (8 control, 8 intervention)	SEGEV program—Israeli version of Know Your Body: Health education curriculum, 10 sessions, 12–20 hours total instruction per school year Parental involvement and community health fairs Control group—no health education or counseling	2 years	Post BMI (kg/m^2) residual scores, controlling for pre-BMI values	Jewish: I (boys): 0.00 ± 1.10 I (girls): −0.20 ± 0.93 C (boys): 0.14 ± 0.91 C (girls): 0.11 ± 1.05	Three-way ANOVA comparing Jewish, Arab, and control

Study	Setting/Sample	Intervention	Duration	Outcome measure	Results	Significance
					Arab: I (boys): −0.11 ± 0.77 I (girls): −0.68 ± 0.21 C (boys): 0.27 ± 1.26 C (girls): 0.31 ± 0.91	students, $p < .01$
Bush et al. (1989)	Washington, DC Grades 4–6, nine schools Randomization stratified according to tertiles of % of students eligible for federal school lunch program Three schools randomized to control condition Three schools each randomized to two treatment conditions	Know Your Body: Health education curriculum, 45-min periods twice weekly throughout school year Parental involvement Two treatment arms: Full intervention—health education curriculum and health passport Partial intervention—health education curriculum and cholesterol screening results to parents Control schools—no health education, no health passport	2 years	Between-group difference for Δ in: Ponderosity index (kg/m$^{2.77}$) Triceps skinfold (mm)	0.23 ± 2.7 0.24 ± 10.6	$p = .07$ $p = .64$
Walter et al. (1988)	Bronx, NY (22 schools) Westchester County, NY (15 schools) Grade 4 students at baseline, 1,769 children at follow-up Schools randomized to treatment or control condition: 14 treatment, 8 control schools in Bronx 8 treatment, 7 control schools in Westchester	Know Your Body: Health education curriculum, 2 hours per week throughout school year	5 years	Between-group difference for yearly Δ in: Ponderosity index (kg/m$^{2.77}$)	Westchester: I: 0.00 ± 0.1 C: 0.1 ± 0.1 Bronx: I: 0.1 ± 0.1 C: 0.2 ± 0.1	NSS NSS
Killen et al. (1988)	Northern California 1,447 grade 10 students from four high schools Schools randomized within two school districts	Stanford Heart Health Program: Three sessions per week for 7 weeks, as part of regular PE class 20 classroom sessions (50 min each) focusing on physical activity, nutrition, cigarette smoking, stress, personal problem solving	7 weeks	BMI (kg/m^2) Pre: Post (2-month follow-up):	I (boys): 21.6 ± 3.5 I (girls): 22.1 ± 3.9 C (boys): 20.9 ± 2.7 C (girls): 21.4 ± 3.0 I (boys): 21.7 ± 3.6 I (girls): 21.9 ± 3.8 C (boys): 21.3 ± 2.7 C (girls): 21.4 ± 3.1	$p = .05$

(continued)

1992; Vartiainen & Puska, 1987); and one involved a community health fair (Tamir et al., 1990). The earlier studies were less methodologically stringent, including one with assigned treatment conditions (as opposed to randomization) (Alexandrov et al., 1988). The more recent studies have all been randomized controlled trials. The length of intervention has ranged from 8 weeks (Harrell et al., 1996) to 5 years (Walter et al., 1985). The obesity-related outcomes from these studies were between-group differences in BMI or skinfolds and were mostly small, inconsistent across specific outcome variables, and (with few exceptions) nonsignificant. On the other hand, many of them were successful in improving eating and/or exercise behaviors in the intervention schools.

The largest completed multiple-risk-factor intervention in children that included physical activity and nutrition intervention components was the Child and Adolescent Trial for Cardiovascular Health (CATCH; Luepker et al., 1996), which was conducted in 96 elementary schools in California, Minnesota, Louisiana, and Texas (56 intervention, 40 control schools). The CATCH intervention components included modifications to school food services, increases in moderate to vigorous activity in PE classes, and classroom-based nutrition and PE curricula. Family involvement was included in 28 schools. There were no between-group differences in BMI changes after 3 years of the intervention. However, like many of the other multiple-risk-factor intervention trials in school children, the CATCH showed the feasibility of delivering classroom-based and environmental changes to PE curriculum and cafeteria modifications within a school setting.

All of the studies in Table 27.1 included a strong school-based intervention component. Schools are an attractive setting for obesity prevention efforts in children, because of the large amount of time children spend in school; the ability to use existing organizational, communication, and social structures; and the ability to reach a large portion of children in the general population. In addition, one to two meals per day are eaten at school for 5 days of the week. On the other hand, as attractive as schools are for intervening in children's eating and physical activity behaviors, other social settings, such as the family and community, also have significant influences on youth behaviors. As noted above, six of the multiple-risk-factor interventions included home, family, or community intervention components (Bush et al., 1989; Lionis et al., 1991; Luepker et al., 1996; Tamir et al., 1990; Tell & Vellar, 1987; Vandongen et al., 1995). However, for the most part, the family, home, and community components of the reviewed youth interventions were minimal. Luepker and colleagues (1996) noted that if a family component of a school-based physical activity and nutrition intervention was to be successful, it would have to be more intensive than the minimal-contact intervention included in the CATCH.

Interventions in Diverse Settings

Recent Centers for Disease Control and Prevention (1996, 1997) guidelines for promoting physical activity and healthy eating note the importance of including community and family efforts, in addition to school-based programs. The National Heart, Lung, and Blood Institute (NHLBI) has funded several ongoing community-based interventions for youth in specific high-risk minority groups, including one in Native American children (Davis et al., 1999). Furthermore, a multicenter study funded by the NHLBI called the Trial of Activity in Adolescent Girls (TAAG) will test a school- and community-linked intervention to prevent the decline in physical activity in adolescent girls. Efforts such as these are needed to evaluate the usefulness of underutilized social settings for obesity prevention efforts in youth.

Of the studies included in Table 27.1, those conducted in less diverse settings were more likely to show significant obesity-related treatment effects (Alexandrov et al., 1988;

Dwyer et al., 1983; Flores, 1995; Killen et al., 1988; Lionis et al., 1991; Mo-Suwan et al., 1998; Robinson, 1999; Simonetti D'Arca & Sanarelli, 1986; Tamir et al., 1990; Worsley et al., 1987). This was particularly true for studies for which the outcomes included multiple chronic disease risk factors or multiple behaviors. Planet Health is the first successful school-wide intervention that has reported significant treatment effects for obesity-related outcomes and that took place in a diverse setting (30% of students were not European American) (Gortmaker et al., 1999). Despite the success of Planet Health in girls, the challenge of developing successful interventions for obesity prevention in multicultural settings should remain a high priority, given the general lack of prior success in studies conducted in diverse settings.

The absence of long-term treatment effects from the studies included in Table 27.1 makes it difficult to evaluate the efficacy of these interventions for population-wide effects on obesity prevalence. Most of the studies were able to show improvements in children's eating and/or exercise habits, and the large trials indicate the feasibility of implementing school-wide changes for the purpose of obesity prevention. Future studies will need to evaluate the cost-effectiveness of school- and/or community-based obesity prevention interventions in youth, including long-term follow-up of obesity prevalence and incidence. Despite the encouraging results of some school-based physical activity or nutrition programs, their political feasibility has not been clearly demonstrated. Furthermore, effects of these interventions on adult behaviors or adulthood obesity-related outcomes remain to be shown.

STUDIES OF OBESITY PREVENTION IN ADULTS

Community Trials Focused on Multiple Risk Factors

There have been a number of large community trials to influence multiple noncommunicable disease risk factors. These include the Minnesota Heart Health Program, the Pawtucket Heart Health Program, the North Karelia Project, a national program on the island of Mauritius, and the two community trials that originated out of Stanford University (Carleton, Lasater, Assaf, Feldman, & McKinlay, 1995; Dowse et al., 1995; Fortmann, Williams, Hulley, Haskell, & Farquhar, 1981; Jeffery et al., 1995; Stern, Farquhar, Maccoby, & Russell, 1976; Taylor, Fortmann, & Flora, 1991). Like the interventions in children, community-based interventions with significant nutrition and exercise education efforts aimed at adults make these trials potential population-based obesity prevention (or treatment) studies. However, like the studies in children, the multiple-risk-factor approach has not shown much promise in affecting obesity-related outcomes in adults.

The six studies cited above implemented community-wide intervention efforts to reduce CVD risk factors, including improving eating and physical activity. The interventions were delivered through mass media, as well as school, church, social organizations, and worksites. Some included a population-wide risk factor screening and environmental interventions to promote healthy eating choices in grocery stores and restaurants. Some studies promoted environmental changes to promote physical activity in the community, including building additional community exercise facilities. All of these studies included assessments of obesity-related outcomes, but none of them focused exclusively on obesity. Encouraging self-reported changes in exercise and eating behaviors have been reported from many of the large trials. Unfortunately, these did not translate into meaningful long-term changes in physiological endpoints related to obesity, despite scattered reports of small statistically significant obesity-related changes (Carleton et al., 1995; Fortmann et al., 1981).

By contrast, most of the large community trials showed significant intervention effects

The women in the weekly group meetings and correspondence course treatment groups lost 1.9 ± 1.18 and 1.1 ± 2.1 kg, respectively, compared with a loss of 0.2 ±1.3 kg in the lifestyle brochure group ($p < .03$). However, there was some weight regain in both the weekly meeting and correspondence course groups by the 6-month follow-up ($n = 50$), so that there were no longer any statistically significant treatment effects. This suggests a lack of long-term efficacy for these types of programs. Furthermore, with a 50% dropout rate at 6 months, the acceptability of any of the three treatment formats might be questioned.

Participants in the Pound of Prevention study were surveyed as to preferences for treatment approaches (Sherwood et al., 1998). Among suggestions made to improve community-based weight control interventions were the possibilities of more individualized diet and physical activity programming and a more specific and demanding intervention message than typical public health messages emphasizing moderation. Participants also expressed a preference for minimal-contact education approaches over face-to-face class formats. Perhaps emerging electronic communication technologies could be used in future health education interventions to address the preference for both minimal contact and individualized programming in a cost-effective manner. Future studies on preventing weight gain in adults should focus on a programmatic approach to creating a balance between acceptability and efficacy that will translate into an effective, widely usable obesity prevention program.

ENVIRONMENTAL STUDIES RELATED TO OBESITY PREVENTION

Recent commentaries have consistently concluded that the current obesity epidemic has at its root widespread physical, social, and cultural factors (Gill, 1997; Grundy, 1998; Harnack et al., 2000; Hill, 2000; Hill & Peter, 1998; Nestle & Jacobson, 2000; Popkin et al., 1995a, 1995b; Poston & Foreyt, 1999; Prentice & Jebb, 1995; World Health Organization, 1998). This has led to a burgeoning list of suggested approaches to intervene on these environmental factors—including mass media campaigns, taxes on high-fat foods, price supports for fruits and vegetables, and federal funding for daily PE in public schools, just to name a few (Nestle & Jacobson, 2000). Mass media campaigns are the only "macroenvironmental" interventions that have been conducted thus far to influence eating and physical activity choices in the general population.

Mass Media Campaigns

To identify mass media campaigns to promote healthy eating or physical activity (which included some evaluation of the programs' efficacy), we conducted a computerized search of the English-language peer-reviewed literature (MEDLINE), a search of our own files, and review of the references in identified papers. Few such mass media programs have evaluated program efficacy. Those that have evaluated efficacy have done so by evaluating behavior change, not by assessing obesity-related physiological outcomes in the target population. Several of the multiple-risk-factor community trials reviewed earlier also included mass media campaigns to promote healthy eating and physical activity (Flora, Maccoby, & Farquhar, 1989; Puska et al., 1985, 1987). These have not been included here, because it is impossible to determine whether the impact of these programs was due to the mass media campaign or to some other part of the community intervention. The two nutrition education interventions and one physical activity promotion intervention that were identified in this search are included in Table 27.2 (Booth, Bauman, Oldenburg, Owen, & Magnus, 1992; Levy & Stoker, 1987; Owen, Bauman, Booth, Oldenburg, & Magnus, 1995; Reger, Wootan, & Booth-Butterfield, 1999).

TABLE 27.2. Mass Media Campaigns to Promote Healthy Eating and Physical Activity

Author (year)	Setting	Design or evaluation method	Duration	Goal	Strategy	Outcomes	Statistical significance
				Nutrition			
Reger et al. (1999)	Mass media	Controlled intervention	6-week intervention/ 6-month follow-up	Mass media promotion of low-fat milk purchases	Paid advertisements, public relations	Increased supermarket sales of low-fat milk at the end of the intervention and at 6-month follow-up, compared to control city	$p < .0003$
						Greater % of phone interviewees who reported switching to low-fat milk in intervention vs. control city	$p < .0001$
Levy & Stoker (1987)	Mass media	Uncontrolled intervention: Evaluation of sales prior to and during intervention	64 weeks—16-week baseline (preintervention)	Mass media promotion of high-fiber cereal consumption	Mass media	Increased sales of high-fiber cereals during 48-week evaluation period	Not reported
				Physical activity			
Owen et al. (1995), Booth et al. (1992)	National mass media campaign	Uncontrolled intervention: Phone surveys before and after campaign	1 month; intervention repeated a 2nd year	Promotion of walking as a form of exercise	Mass media, promotional items (stickers, T-shirts), promotional tours, and inclusion of the theme in scripts on two episodes of popular soap opera	Significant increase in self-report of walking over past 2 weeks for year 1 of campaign, but not for year 2	Year 1, $p < .01$; year 2, NSS

Note. NSS, not statistically significant.

573

TABLE 27.3. *continued*

Author/ (year)	Setting	Design or evaluation method	Duration	Goal	Strategy	Outcomes	Statistical significance
Buscher et al. (2001)	University dining hall cafeteria	Uncontrolled interventions Study—ABA Study 2—ABA	Study 1—A = 13 days; B = 28 days with 7 days each for promoting four separate foods Study 2—A = 14 days; B = 15 days	Study 1: Increase healthy snacking in four food groups: yogurt, pretzels, fruit shakes, vegetable baskets Study 2: Increase yogurt purchases	Study 1: Point of purchase messages that focused on "BEST" (Budget friendly, Energizing, Sensory satisfaction, Time efficiency) messages were specific for each of the four food groups Study 2: Same as study 1, but just for yogurt.	Study 1: Sales of the four food groups during intervention compared to baseline and follow-up Study 2: Yogurt sales during baseline compared to intervention and follow-up	Study 1: Higher yogurt and pretzel sales during intervention and follow-up weeks than during baseline ($p < 0.001$); however, no differences for fruits or vegetables. Study 2: Yogurt sales were greater during intervention and follow-up than during baseline ($p < 0.01$)
French, Story, et al. (1997)	Two high school cafeterias	Uncontrolled intervention: A_1BA_2, where $A_1 = 4$ weeks, B and $A_2 = 3$ weeks	10 weeks total	Increasing consumption of fruits and vegetables by lowering price, increasing availability, and promotional signs	50% price reduction on fruits and vegetables, signs	Significant increases in sales during intervention Return to baseline levels at follow-up	$p < .01$ $p = .85$
Perlmutter et al. (1997)	Worksite cafeteria	Uncontrolled intervention: ABCDA, testing of several types of interventions	9 months total	Acceptance of entrees modified to reduce fat and sodium	Modification of seven entrees, marketing of modified entrees	Greater acceptance of modified entrees after than before marketing, but no significant increase in sales of entrees	NSS

576

Study	Setting	Design	Intervention focus	Intervention materials	Results	Significance
Jeffery et al. (1994)	Worksite cafeteria	Uncontrolled intervention: ABA, where A and B were each 3 weeks long	9 weeks total	Price and availability changes to increase consumption of fruits and vegetables	50% increase in availability of fruits and vegetables, 50% reduction in price	Significant increases in fruit and salad purchases during intervention ($p = .0001$); Increases in salad sales were still higher than baseline during follow-up phase ($p = .01$)
Casarez et al. (1994)	University cafeteria	Uncontrolled intervention: ABA	10 weeks	Point-of-purchase information on low-fat menu items	Posters, menu marquees, flyers	Increased low-fat sales that were maintained in follow-up survey ($p < .001$)
Mayer et al. (1987)	Worksite cafeteria	Uncontrolled intervention: ABA	A = 4 weeks, B = 4 weeks	Point-of-purchase nutrition education	Caloric content labels, nutrition awareness game, incentive raffles	No significant decrease in calories per tray, but some increases in targeted foods (Not reported)
Mayer et al. (1986)	Public cafeteria	Uncontrolled intervention: ABAB	9 weeks total	Point-of-purchase nutrition education regarding "low-fat" entrees	Posters, menu of low-fat choices in entree section, table fliers	Significant increase in sales of low-fat entrees during intervention phases ($p < .005$)
Schmitz & Fielding (1986)	Worksite cafeteria	Uncontrolled intervention: Pre- and posttest	6 months	Nutrition education regarding calories, fat, sodium, and cholesterol	Food labels with calories, fat, sodium, and cholesterol information placed at 15 stations	Significant decreases in calories, fat, and sodium, but not cholesterol, values per tray ($p < .01$, $p < .01$, $p = .00$, and $p = .47$, respectively)
Davis-Chervin et al. (1985)	Two dormitory cafeterias	Uncontrolled intervention: ABABABA, where A = no intervention period and B = intervention period; both A and B were 5 weeks long	1 academic year total	Nutrition education: Total calories, cholesterol, and % fat for selected cafeteria items	Posters, nutrient display cards	Increases in selection of low-cholesterol and low-calorie entrees in one dorm, but not the other (Inconsistent statistical significance over multiple comparisons)

577

(continued)

TABLE 27.3. *continued*

Author/(year)	Setting	Design or evaluation method	Duration	Goal	Strategy	Outcomes	Statistical significance
French, Jeffery, et al. (1997)	Vending machines	Uncontrolled intervention: ABA	10 weeks total	Promotion of low-fat snacking choices	Bright orange signs on vending machines noting that low-fat items were labeled, and labels on specific low-fat items; 50% price reduction on low-fat items	Increase in sales of low-fat items during intervention, but not at follow-up	$p < .02$
Hoerr and Louden (1993)	Vending machines	Uncontrolled intervention: Vending sales prior to and after introduction of healthy snacks, and after addition of nutrition labels to new snacks	3 years total	Promotion of healthy snacks	Introduction of healthy snacks in year 2; addition of nutrition information posted above snacks	Decrease in vending sales in year 2 to 85.7% of year 1 sales; increased in year 3 to 92.5% of year 1 sales	$p < .01$ for year 1 to 2 difference
Wilbur et al. (1981)	Vending machines	Controlled intervention	6 months total	Point-of-purchase promotion of low-fat snacks	Nutrition information and introduction of new low-fat snack items	Increased vending sales at intervention sites compared to control sites	$p < .01$
Larson-Brown (1978)	Vending machines	Uncontrolled intervention: Pre–post testing	1 month of intervention, 1 month of follow-up	Point-of-purchase nutrition information to promote healthy snack choices	Nutritive value card graphs for all foods in vending machines posted on machine	More nutritious foods accounted for 49.8% vs. 53.7 of total sales pre- and postintervention, respectively	$p < .01$

Note. NSS, not statistically significant.

580

1987; Casarez, Lee, Jacob, Lee, & Medora, 1994; Cinciripini, 1984; Colby, Elder, Peterson, Kinsley, & Carleton, 1987; Davis & Rogers, 1982; De Spiegelaere et al., 1998; Dubbert, Johnson, Schlundt, & Ward Montague, 1984; Ernst et al., 1986; French et al., 2001; French, Jeffery, et al., 1997; Hoerr & Louden, 1993; Jeffery, French, Raether, & Baxter, 1994; Jeffery, Pirie, Rosenthal, Gerber, & Murray, 1982; Larson-Brown, 1978; Mayer et al., 1986; Mayer, Brown, Heins, & Bishop, 1987; Muller, 1984; Olson, Bisogni, & Thonney, 1982; Perlmutter, Canter, & Gregoire, 1997; Russo, Staelin, Nolan, Russell, & Metcalf, 1986; Schmitz & Fielding, 1986; Scott, Foreyt, Manis, O'Malley, & Gotto, 1979; Soriano & Dozier, 1978; Wagner & Winett, 1988; Wilbur, Zifferblatt, Pinski, & Zifferblatt, 1981; Zifferblatt, Wilbur, & Pinsky, 1980). Like the mass media campaigns, none of these microenvironmental interventions included physiological measurements of obesity-related endpoints. Participant behavior in these studies was observed in a manner that imposed no burden or only low burden, such as evaluating sales at a vending machine. In addition, many of these studies were short in duration; the interventions ranged in length from 6 days (Muller, 1984) to 3 years (Hoerr & Louden, 1993). Despite these limitations, there may be lessons from these microenvironmental interventions that could inform population-based obesity prevention efforts.

The nutritional microenvironmental interventions included in Table 27.3 promoted healthy eating with point-of-purchase educational campaigns, as well as changes in availability and cost of healthy foods. These interventions have taken place in a variety of settings, including supermarkets, vending machines, school and office cafeterias, and restaurants. The majority of these interventions focused on providing nutrient information to customers in each of these settings. Supermarkets were the sites of seven nutrition education interventions, ranging in length from 6 days to 1 year (Ernst et al., 1986; Jeffery et al., 1982; Muller, 1984; Mullis et al., 1987; Olson et al., 1982; Russo et al., 1986; Soriano & Dozier, 1978). The primary outcome for most of the nutrition education programs in supermarkets was sales of targeted items. A supermarket may not be a particularly promising environment for this style of intervention, since only a few studies reported small positive changes in sales of targeted items (Ernst et al., 1986; Muller, 1984; Olson et al., 1982). Given that marketing departments of for-profit food manufacturers are likely to have budgets that are much larger than the budgets of these intervention studies, it is possible that the intervention materials developed to promote low-calorie, low-fat, low-cholesterol, or some other healthful eating habit had difficulty competing for consumer attention.

Cafeteria-Based Interventions

We identified 13 point-of-choice nutrition intervention studies in cafeterias in a variety of settings: worksites (Jeffery et al., 1994; Mayer et al., 1987; Perlmutter et al., 1997; Schmitz & Fielding, 1986; Zifferblatt et al., 1980), high schools (French, Story, et al., 1997), dormitories (Buscher et al., 2001; Casarez et al., 1994; Cinciripini, 1984; Davis & Rogers, 1982; Davis-Chervin, Rogers, & Clark, 1985), and for-profit settings (Dubbert et al., 1984; Mayer et al., 1986). Most of these studies involved pre- and postintervention assessments of the eating behaviors of cafeteria patrons, sometimes before and after multiple versions of the intervention. The interventions were generally short, ranging in length from 3 weeks (French, Story, et al., 1997; Jeffery et al., 1994) to 18 weeks (Dubbert et al., 1984). The older studies focused on point-of-purchase nutrition education through labels on food choices, games, signs, and table placards promoting healthy eating choices. Three more recent studies focused on changing the price and availability of healthier food choices in school and worksite cafeterias. Entrees modified to reduce fat and sodium were found to be acceptable to worksite cafeteria patrons, according to sales data, especially after the changes were mar-

TABLE 27.4. Microenvironmental Interventions: Physical Activity

Author (year)	Setting	Design	Duration	Goal	Strategy	Outcomes	Statistical significance
Andersen et al. (1998)	Shopping mall	Uncontrolled intervention: ABB	1 month per phase, 3 months total	To increase stair usage	Sign at stairs/escalator focused on heart disease or weight control	Increase in proportion of people who used stairs vs. escalator	$p < .05$
Blamey et al. (1995)	Subway station	Uncontrolled intervention: ABA	3-week intervention	To increase stair usage	Sign at stairs/escalator to "stay healthy, save time, use the stairs"	Increase in proportion of people who used stairs vs. escalator during intervention and at follow-up	$p < .05$
Boutelle et al. (2001)	Office building	Uncontrolled intervention: A_1BCA_2; where A_1 = 3 weeks; B, C, and A_2 = 4 weeks	2 months total	To increase stair usage	Signs to promote stair usage; signs plus music and artwork to improve attractiveness of stairway	Increases in proportion of people using stairs vs. elevators	$p < 0.05$ comparing C to A_1 and A_2 to A_1
Brownell et al. (1980)	Shopping mall, train station, bus terminal	Uncontrolled intervention: Study 1: ABAB, where A = 2 weeks and B = 2 weeks Study 2: A_1BA_2, where A_1 = 5 days, B = 15 days, A_2 = 3 months	Study 1: 8 weeks total Study 2: 3.5 months total	To promote use of stairs vs. escalator	Signs to promote stair usage	Increase in stair usage during interventions (studies 1 and 2); increase maintained at 1-month but not 3-month follow-up	Increase during intervention: $p < .0001$; increase at 1-month follow-up, $p < .05$; increase at 3-month follow-up, NSS

Study	Setting	Design	Duration	Purpose	Intervention	Results	Significance
Vuori et al. (1994)	Industrial worksite	Uncontrolled intervention: Survey of workers before and after intervention	6 months	To increase physically active commuting to work	Information dissemination through bulletins, leaflets, and company newsletter; activity diaries, lotteries, and chances for fitness testing; improved facilities for showering and changing clothes	7% of surveyed employees reported increasing physically active commuting as a result of the intervention	Not reported
Mayer & Geller (1982)	Community bike path	ABA, quasi-experimental with convenience control setting	9 weeks total	To promote biking as a mode of commuting to a university	Contest to win prizes (eligibility depended on use of bike path); announcements of contest in media	Significant increase in use of bike path during intervention phase, which was not maintained at follow-up	$p < .01$ and NSS, respectively
Titze et al. (2001)	Four office buildings	Uncontrolled intervention: ABA	4 month intervention, 2–3 weeks of measurements pre- and post-intervention	To increase stair usage	Intervention varied by office according to the internal committee formed at each office site, but included games on stairwells, offerings of fresh fruit on stairwells, and at least 1 day on which the elevator was closed/unusable at each office site	Increases in the proportion of people using stairs vs. elevators	$p = .03$ using observations; $p = 0.27$ using automatic counter method

Note. NSS, not statistically significant.

Colby, J. J., Elder, J. P., Peterson, G., Kinsley, P. M., & Carleton, R. A. (1987). Prompting the selection of healthy food through menu item description in a family-style restaurant. *American Journal of Preventive Medicine, 3*(3), 171–177.

Curhan, G. C., Chertow, G. M., Willett, W. C., Spiegelman, D., Colditz, G. A., Manson, J. E., Speizer, F. E., & Stampfer, M. J. (1996). Birthweight and adult hypertension and obesity in women. *Circulation, 94,* 1310–1315.

Danforth, E. (1985). Diet and obesity. *American Journal of Clinical Nutrition, 41,* 1132–1145.

Davis, D. Z., & Rogers, T. (1982). Point-of-choice nutrition information for the modification of milk selection. *Journal of American College Health, 30,* 275–278.

Davis, S. M., Going, S. B., Helitzer, D. L., Teufel, N. I., Snyder, P., Gittelsohn, J., Metcalfe, L., Arviso, V., Evans, M., Smyth, M., Brice, R., & Altaha, J. (1999). Pathways: A culturally appropriate obesity-prevention program for American Indian schoolchildren. *American Journal of Clinical Nutrition, 69*(45), 7965–8025.

Davis-Chervin, D., Rogers, T., & Clark, M. (1985). Influencing food selection with point-of-choice nutrition information. *Journal of Nutrition Education, 17*(1), 18–22.

De Spiegelaere, M., Dramaix, M., & Hennart, P. (1998). The influence of socioeconomic status on the incidence and evolution of obesity during early adolescence. *International Journal of Obesity, 22,* 268–274.

Dietz, W. H. (1994). Critical periods in childhood for the development of obesity. *American Journal of Clinical Nutrition, 59,* 955–959.

Dietz, W. H., & Gortmaker, S. L. (1984). Factors within the physical environment associated with childhood obesity. *American Journal of Clinical Nutrition, 39,* 619–624.

DiPietro, L. (1995). Physical activity, body weight, and adiposity: An epidemiologic perspective. *Exercise and Sport Science Reviews, 23,* 275–304.

Donnelly, J. E., Jacobsen, D. J., Whatley, J. E., Hill, J. O., Swift, L. L., Cherrington, A., Polk, B., Tran, Z. V., & Reed, G. (1996). Nutrition and physical activity program to attenuate obesity and promote physical and metabolic fitness in elementary school children. *Obesity Research, 4*(3), 229–243.

Dowse, G. K., Gareeboo, H., Alberti, K. G., Zimmet, P., Tuomilehto, J., Purran, A., Fareed, D., Chitson, P., & Collins, V. R. (1995). Changes in population cholesterol concentrations and other cardiovascular risk factor levels after five years of the Noncommunicable Disease Intervention Programme in Mauritius. *British Medical Journal, 311*(7015), 1255–1259.

Dubbert, P. M., Johnson, W. G., Schlundt, D. G., & Ward Montague, N. (1984). The influence of caloric information on cafeteria food choices. *Journal of Applied Behavior Analysis, 17*(1), 85–92.

Dunn, A. L., Marcus, B. H., Kampert, J. B., Garcia M. E., Kohl, H. W., & Blair, S. N. (1997). Reduction in cardiovascular disease risk factors: 6-month result from Project Active. *Preventive Medicine, 26,* 883–892.

Dwyer, T., Coonan, W. E., Leitch, D. R., Hetzel, B. S., & Baghurst, R. A. (1983). An investigation of the effects of daily physical activity on the health of primary school students in South Australia. *International Journal of Epidemiology, 12*(3), 308–313.

Ellaway, A., Anderson, A., & Macintyre, S. (1997). Does area of residence affect body size and shape? *International Journal of Obesity, 21*(4), 304–308.

Epstein, L. H., Valoski, A. M., Kalarchian, M. A., & McCurley, J. (1995). Do children lose and maintain weight easier than adults?: A comparison of child and parent weight changes from six months to ten years. *Obesity Research, 3,* 411–417.

Epstein, L. H., Valoski, A. M., Vara, L. S., McCurley, J., Wisniewski, L., Kalarchian, M. A., Klein, K. R., & Shrager, L. R. (1995). Effects of decreasing sedentary behavior and increasing activity on weight change in obese children. *Health Psychology, 14*(2), 109–115.

Epstein, L. H., Valoski, A. M., Wing, R. R., & McCurley, J. (1994). Ten-year outcomes of behavioral family-based treatment for childhood obesity. *Health Psychology, 13*(5), 373–383.

Ernst, N., Wu, M., Frommer, P., Katz, E., Matthews, O., Moskowitz, J., Pinsky, J., Pohl, S., Schreiber, G., Sondik, E., Tenney, J., Wilbur, C., & Zifferblatt, S. (1986). Nutrition education at the point of purchase: The Foods for Health project evaluated. *Preventive Medicine, 15,* 60–73.

Fardy, P. S., White, R. E., Haltiwanger-Schmitz, K., Magel, J. R., McDermott, K. J., Clark, L. T., & Hurster, M. M. (1996). Coronary disease risk factor reduction and behavior modification in minority adolescents: The PATH program. *Journal of Adolescent Health, 18,* 247–253.

Fisch, R. O., Bilek, M. K., & Ulstrom, R. (1975). Obesity and leanness at birth and their relationship to body habits in later childhood. *Pediatrics, 45,* 521–528.

Flegal, K. M., Carroll, M. D., Kuczmarski, R. J., & Johnson, C. L. (1998). Overweight and obesity in the United States: Prevalence and trends, 1960–1994. *International Journal of Obesity, 22*(1), 39–47.

Flora, J. A., Maccoby, N., & Farquhar, J. W. (1989). Communication campaigns to prevent cardiovascular disease: The Stanford Three-Community study. In R. E. Rice & C. K. Atkin (Eds.), *Public communication campaigns* (pp. 233–252). Beverly Hills, CA: Sage.

Flores, R. E. (1995). Dance for Health: improving fitness in African American and Hispanic adolescents. *Public Health Reports, 110*(2), 189–193.

Forster, J. L., Jeffery, R. W., Schmid, T. L., & Kramer, F. M. (1988). Preventing weight gain in adults: A Pound of Prevention. *Health Psychology, 7*(6), 515–525.

Fortmann, S. P., Williams, P. T., Hulley, S. B., Haskell, W. L., & Farquhar, J. W. (1981). Effect of health education on dietary behavior: The Stanford Three-Community Study. *American Journal of Clinical Nutrition, 34*(10), 2030–2038.

French, S. A., Harnack L., Jeffery, R. W. (2000). Fast food restaurant use among women in the Pound of Prevention study: Dietary, behavioral and demographic correlates. *International Journal of Obesity, 24,* 1353–1359.

French, S. A., Jeffery, R. W., Story, M., Breitlow, K. K., Baxter, J. S., Hannan, P., & Snyder, M. P. (1997). A pricing strategy to promote low-fat snack choices through vending machines. *American Journal of Public Health, 87*(5), 849–851.

French, S. A., Jeffery, R. W., Story, M., Breitlow, K. K., Baxter, J. S., Hannan, P., & Snyder, M. P. (2001). Pricing and promotion effects on low fat vending snack purchases: The CHIPs study. *American Journal of Public Health, 91,* 112–117.

French, S. A., Story, M., & Jeffery, R. W. (2001). Environmental influences on eating and physical activity. *Annual Review of Public Health, 22,* 309–355.

French, S. A., Story, M., Jeffery, R. W., Snyder, P., Eisenberg, M., Sidebottom, A., & Murray, D. (1997). Pricing strategy to promote fruit and vegetable purchase in high school cafeterias. *Journal of the American Dietetic Association, 97*(9), 1008–1010.

Gill, T. P. (1997). Key issues in the prevention of obesity. *British Medical Bulletin, 53*(2), 359–388.

Glanz, K., & Mullis, R. M. (1988). Environmental interventions to promote healthy eating: A review of models, programs, and evidence. *Health Education Quarterly, 15*(4), 395–415.

Gortmaker, S. L., Dietz, W. H., & Cheung, L. W. Y. (1990). Inactivity, diet, and the fattening of America. *Journal of the American Dietetic Association, 90,* 1247–1252, 1255.

Gortmaker, S. L., Peterson, K., Wiecha, J., Sobol, A. M., Dixit, S., Fox, M. K., & Laird, N. (1999). Reducing obesity via a school-based interdisciplinary intervention among youth. *Archives of Pediatrics and Adolescent Medicine, 153,* 409–418.

Gross, T., Sokol, R. J., & King, K. C. (1980). Obesity in pregnancy: Risks and outcome. *Obstetrics and Gynecology, 56,* 446–450.

Grundy, S. M. (1998). Multifactoral causation of obesity: Implications for prevention. *American Journal of Clinical Nutrition, 67*(Suppl.), 563S–572S.

Harnack, L. J., Jeffery, R. W., & Boutelle, K. N. (2000). Temporal trends in energy intake in the United States: An ecological perspective. *American Journal of Clinical Nutrition, 71,* 1478–1484.

Harrell, J. S., McMurray, R. G., Bangdiwala, S. I., Frauman, A. C., Gansky, S. A., & Bradley, C. B. (1996). Effects of a school-based intervention to reduce cardiovascular disease risk factors in elementary school children: The Cardiovascular Health in Children Study (CHIC). *The Journal of Pediatrics, 128*(6), 797–805.

Hennrikus, D. J., & Jeffery, R. W. (1996). Worksite interventions for weight control: A review of the literature. *American Journal of Health Promotion, 10*(6), 471–498.

Hill, J. (2000). Environmental and genetic contributions to obesity. *Medical Clinics of North America, 84*(2), 333–346.

grante, J. P. (1992). A three-year evaluation of the Know Your Body program in inner-city schoolchildren. *Health Education Quarterly, 19*(4), 463–480.

Robinson, T. N. (1999). Reducing children's television viewing to prevent obesity: A randomized controlled trial. *Journal of the American Medical Association, 282*(16), 1561–1567.

Rolland-Cachera, M. F., Deheeger, M., Guilloud-Bataille, M., Avons, P., Patois, E., & Sempé, M. (1987). Tracking the development of adiposity from one month of age to adulthood. *Annals of Human Biology, 14*(3), 219–229.

Russo, J. E., Staelin, R., Nolan, C. A., Russell, G. J., & Metcalf, B. L. (1986). Nutrition information in the supermarket, *Journal of Consumer Research, 13,* 48–70.

Sallis, J. F., McKenzie, T. L., Alcaraz, J. E., Kolody, B., Faucette, N., & Hovell, M. F. (1997). The effects of a 2-year physical education program (SPARK) on physical activity and fitness in elementary school students. *American Journal of Public Health, 87*(8), 1328–1334.

Saltzman, E. (1999). The low glycemic index diet: Not yet ready for prime time. [Letter to the Editor]. *Nutrition Reviews, 57*(Pt. 1), 297.

Saris, W. H. M. (1998). In search of factors regulating body weight. *Current Opinion in Clinical Nutrition and Metabolic Care, 1,* 549–551.

Schmitz, M. F., & Fielding, J. E. (1986). Point-of-choice nutritional labeling: Evaluation in a worksite cafeteria. *Journal of Nutrition Education, 18*(1), S65-S68.

Scott, L. W., Foreyt, J. P., Manis, E., O'Malley, M. P., & Gotto, A. M. (1979). A low-cholesterol menu in a steak restaurant. *Journal of the American Dietetic Association, 74,* 54–56.

Seidell, J. C. (1997). Time trends in obesity: An epidemiological perspective. *Hormones and Metabolic Research, 29,* 155–158.

Sherwood, N. E., Morton, N., Jeffery, R. W., French, S. A., Neumark-Sztainer, D., & Falkner, N. H. (1998). Consumer preferences in format and type of community-based weight control programs. *American Journal of Health Promotion, 13*(1), 12–18.

Simkin-Silverman, L., Wing, R. R., Hansen, D. H., Klem, M. L., Pasagian-Macaulay, A., Meilahn, E. N., & Kuller, L. H. (1995). Prevention of cardiovascular risk factor elevations in health premenopausal women. *Preventive Medicine, 24,* 509–517.

Simkin-Silverman, L., Wing, R. R., Boraz, M. A., Meilahn, E. N., & Kuller, L. H. (1998). Maintenance of cardiovascular risk factor changes among middle-aged women in a lifestyle intervention trial. *Women's Health, 4*(3), 255–271.

Simonetti D'Arca, A., & Sanarelli, G. (1986). Prevention of obesity in elementary and nursery school children. *Public Health, 100,* 166–173.

Sobal, J., & Stunkard, A. J. (1989). Socioeconomic status and obesity: A review of the literature. *Psychological Bulletin, 105*(2), 260–275.

Soriano, E., & Dozier, D. M. (1978). Selling nutrition and heart healthy behavior at the point-of-purchase. *Journal of Applied Nutrition, 30,* 56–65.

Stephen, A. M., & Wald, N. J. (1990). Trends in individual consumption of dietary fat in the United States, 1920–1984. *American Journal of Clinical Nutrition, 52,* 457–469.

Stern, M. P., Farquhar, J. W., Maccoby, N., & Russell, S. H. (1976). Results of a two-year health education campaign on dietary behavior: The Stanford Three-Community study. *Circulation, 54*(5), 826–833.

Tamir, D., Feurstein, A., Brunner, S., Halfon, S., Reshef, A., & Palti, H. (1990). Primary prevention of cardiovascular diseases in childhood: Changes in serum total cholesterol, high density lipoprotein, and body mass index after 2 years of intervention in Jerusalem schoolchildren age 7–9 years. *Preventive Medicine, 19,* 22–30.

Taylor, C., B. Fortmann, S. P., & Flora, J. (1991). Effect of long-term community health education on body mass index: The Stanford Five-City Project. *American Journal of Epidemiology, 134,* 235–249.

Tell, G. S., & Vellar, O. D. (1987). Noncommunicable disease risk factor intervention in Norwegian adolescents: The Oslo Youth Study. In B. Hetzel & G. S. Berenson (Eds.), *Cardiovascular risk factors in childhood: Epidemiology and prevention* (pp. 203–217). New York: Elsevier.

Titze, S., Martin, B. W., Seller, R., & Marti, B. (2001). A worksite intervention module encouraging the use of stairs: Results and evaluation issues. *Sozial-und Praventivmedizin, 46,* 13–19.

U.S. Department of Health and Human Services. (2000). *Healthy people 2010: National health promotion and disease prevention objectives.* Atlanta, GA: Centers for Disease Control and Prevention.

Udall, J. N., Harrison, G. G., Vaucher, Y., Walson, P. D., & Morrow, G. (1978). Interaction of maternal and neonatal obesity. *Pediatrics, 62,* 17–21.

Vandongen, R., Jenner, D., Thompson, C., Taggart, A., Spickett, E. E., Burke, V., Beilin, L. J., Milligan, R. A., & Dunbar, D. L. (1995). A controlled evaluation of a fitness and nutrition intervention program on cardiovascular health in 10- to 12-year-old children. *Preventive Medicine, 24,* 9–22.

Vartiainen, E., & Puska, P. (1987). The North Karelia Youth Project 1978–80: Effects of two years of educational intervention on cardiovascular risk factors and health behavior in adolescence. In B. Hetzel & G. S. Berenson (Eds.), *Cardiovascular risk factors in childhood: Epidemiology and prevention* (pp. 203–217). New York: Elsevier.

Vobecky, J. S., Vobecky, J., Shapcott, D., & Demers, P. P. (1983). Nutrient intake patterns and nutritional status with regard to relative weight in early infancy. *American Journal of Clinical Nutrition, 38,* 730–738.

Vuori, I. M., Oja, P., & Paronen, O. (1994). Physically active commuting to work: Testing its potential for exercise promotion. *Medicine and Science in Sports and Exercise, 26*(7), 844–850.

Wagner, J. L., & Winett, R. A. (1988). Prompting one low-fat, high-fiber selection in a fast-food restaurant. *Journal of Applied Behavior Analysis, 21*(2), 179–185.

Walter, H. J., Hofman, A., Vaughn, B. A., & Wyader, E. L. (1988). Modification of risk factors for coronary heart disease: Five-year results of a school-based intervention trial. *New England Journal of Medicine, 318,* 1093–1100.

Whitikar, R. C., & Dietz, W. H. (1998). Role of the prenatal environment in the development of obesity. *Journal of Pediatrics, 132,* 768–776.

Wilbur, C. S., Zifferblatt, S. M., Pinsky, J. L., & Zifferblatt, S. (1981). Healthy vending: A cooperative pilot research program to stimulate good health in the marketplace. *Preventive Medicine, 10,* 85–93.

Williamson, D. F., Kahn, H. S., & Byers, T. (1991). The 10-y incidence of obesity and major weight gain in black and white US women aged 30–55 y. *American Journal of Clinical Nutrition, 53*(6, Suppl.), 1515S–1518S.

Wolf, A. M. (1998). What is the economic case for treating obesity? *Obesity Research, 6*(Suppl. 1), 2S–7S.

World Health Organization. (1998). *Obesity: Preventing and managing the global epidemic* (Publication No. WHO/NUT/NCD 98.1) Geneva: Author.

Worsley, A., Coonan, W., & Worsley, A. (1987). The First Body Owner's Programme: An integrated school-based physical and nutrition education programme. *Health Promotion, 2*(1), 39–49.

Young, L., & Nestle, M. (1995). Portion sizes in dietary assessment: Issues and policy implications. *Nutrition Reviews, 53,* 149–158.

Zifferblatt, S. M., Wilbur, C. S., & Pinsky, J. L. (1980). Changing cafeteria eating habits. *Journal of the American Dietetic Association, 76,* 15–20.

Auslander, W., 436
Avellone, M. E., 148
Averett, S., 146
Avila, P., 433, 437

Bachi, V., 341
Back, K., 145
Bacon, J. G., 501
Baez, M., 319
Baghurst, R. A., 559
Baik, J. H., 30
Bailey, B. A., 234, 399
Bailey, C., 262, 263
Bailey, R. C., 549
Bailey, S. M., 457
Bain, R. P., 129
Bajema, C. J., 8
Baker, J. E., 547
Baker, J. R., 11
Balkan, B., 20
Ballard-Barbasch, R., 7
Bandini, L. G., 48, 236, 549, 550
Bandura, A., 288
Banzet, M. N., 195
Barak, Y., 23
Baranowski, T., 437, 549
Barclay, D., 312
Baritussio, A., 322
Barker, D. J., 522
Barlascini, C. O., 330
Barlow, C. E., 286, 293, 294, 295, 297
Barnard, H. C., 258
Barnard, R. J., 404
Barnett, R. A., 263
Barofsky, I., 13, 149, 195
Baron, P. L., 350
Barr, V., 26
Barroso, I., 23
Barrows, K., 401
Barsh, G. S., 28
Bartlett, S. J., 126, 158, 161, 162, 187, 190, 197, 237, 255, 308, 401, 583
Barzilai, N., 25
Basdevant, A., 12, 111, 149, 195
Baskin, D. G., 27
Bass, J. J., 21
Bauer, B., 158
Baum, J. G., 364, 365
Bauman, A., 572
Baumann, H., 26
Baur, C. P., 22
Baur, L. A., 524
Baxter, J. S., 102, 581
Beck, A. T., 151, 153, 156, 186, 196, 450, 465
Beck, B., 28
Beck, S., 543
Becque, M. D., 533, 534, 538, 544
Beebe, C., 257
Begley, C. E., 395
Beirman, E. L., 4
Beliard, D., 372
Bell, E. A., 263, 389, 518
Bell, S. T., 360, 396
Benedict, F. G., 46
Bengtsson, C., 9
Bennett, G. A., 361

Bennett, P. H., 59, 97, 424
Bennett, S. M., 453
Bennett, W. M., 58, 333
Benson, K. F., 24
Benzinger, T. H., 43
Berg, F. M., 494, 495
Bergstrom, R., 10
Berkey, C. S., 518, 520
Berkowitz, R. I., 56, 57, 110, 111, 112, 113, 157, 202, 236, 239, 240, 242, 358, 460, 518, 519, 520, 521, 522, 525
Berkowitz, S., 242, 243
Berkson, J., 46
Bernlohr, D. A., 26
Berry, E. M., 116, 188, 189
Bessard, T., 50
Bessesen, D. H., 323
Betancourt, S., 154
Bhatnagar, D., 98
Bhopal, R., 417
Biddle, T. L., 252
Bienengraeber, M., 22
Bierman, E. L., 47
Bigaoutte, J. M., 112
Bilek, M. K., 558
Bindon, J. R., 523
Binyamini, J., 340
Birch, L. L., 520, 524, 549
Bird, A. P., 13
Birkenhauer, R. A., 342, 343, 344
Birketvedt, G., 114, 115, 116, 117
Bishop, D. B., 581
Bisogni, C. A., 581
Bissett, L., 427
Bistrian, B. R., 50
Bjorntorp, P., 95, 97, 188, 189, 340
Björvell, H., 358, 359, 370, 371, 373, 468
Black, A. E., 48, 236
Black, S., 151
Blackard, W. G., 330
Blackburn, G. A., 127
Blackburn, G. L., 50, 237, 256, 387, 466
Blackburn, H., 557
Blackman, L. R., 148
Blair, E. H., 155, 237, 305, 310, 361, 369, 401
Blair, S. N., 13, 125, 193, 194, 283, 286, 293, 294, 295, 296, 297, 372, 499
Blamey, A., 583, 584
Blaza, S., 47
Bleker, O. P., 522
Blier, P., 30
Blocher, C. R., 178
Block, G., 192
Blohme, G., 9
Blomquist, B., 544
Bloomfield, G. L., 178
Blumberg, M. S., 24
Blundell, J. E., 258, 323
Bø, O., 343
Bogardus, C., 43, 45, 46, 49, 56, 59, 61, 189, 425
Boman, L., 341
Bonaluni, U., 341
Bonnet, G., 345
Booth, M. L., 524, 572, 573, 574
Booth-Butterfield, S., 572
Boothby, W. M., 46

Boozer, C. N., 383
Boraz, M. A., 571
Borecki, I. B., 78
Borel, M. J., 44
Borjeson, M., 544
Borrud, L. G., 439
Boschee, P. F., 524
Bouchard, C., 46, 58, 61, 76, 77, 78, 81, 97, 173, 175, 189, 191, 283
Bougneres, P., 57
Boureau, F., 177
Boutelle, K. N., 557, 583, 584
Bouter, M., 340
Bouton, M. E., 439
Bowman, S., 495
Boyd, F., 159
Bradfield, R. B., 44
Bradley, L., 158
Bradylak, S. J., 46
Brand, J. C., 99, 258, 259, 267, 268
Brand-Miller, J. C., 257, 258
Brannick, M. T., 453
Braun, G. M., 116
Bray, G. A., 8, 25, 47, 50, 52, 75, 174, 175, 180, 237, 239, 317, 318, 320, 322, 323, 324, 325, 326, 327, 329, 330, 331, 333, 383, 389, 390, 517, 525
Brehm, S. S., 537, 541, 546
Breininger, J. F., 27
Brennan, M. B., 28
Breum, L., 332
Brewer, G., 201, 202, 240, 373, 387, 460
Brewerton, T. D., 154, 198
Briefel, R. R., 284
Brill, P. A., 424
Brinkman, V. L., 402
Brinkman-Kaplan, V., 402
Brittain, E., 126
Brobeck, J. R., 20
Broberger, C., 27, 28
Brodie, D., 453
Brodney, S., 13, 295
Brodoff, B. N., 255
Brody, J. E., 98
Brody, M. L., 111, 151
Brolin, R. E., 158, 343, 351
Brook, R. H., 147
Broomfield, P. H., 236, 401
Brouns, F., 258
Brown, A. M., 189
Brown, G. K., 186
Brown, I. R., 329
Brown, J. A., 27, 29
Brown, T. A., 149, 159, 450
Brown, T. P., 580, 581, 582
Brownell, K. D., 96, 99, 101, 102, 109, 110, 125, 146, 147, 150, 152, 153, 155, 157, 161, 162, 191, 192, 193, 195, 199, 230, 234, 235, 236, 240, 245, 305, 358, 360, 373, 386, 388, 392, 406, 407, 410, 428, 450, 456, 504, 507, 508, 525, 534, 538, 544, 545, 583, 584
Brozek, J., 57, 154
Bruce, A. C., 55
Bruce, B., 111
Brundin, T., 47
Brunner, R. L., 161
Brunzell, J. D., 44

Bruvold, W., 287, 367
Buemann, B., 55
Bullen, B. A., 520
Bultman, S. J., 28
Bunker, C., 8
Buono, M. J., 520
Burgard, D., 498
Burge, J. C., 161
Burke, L., 311, 313
Burland, T., 264
Burlet, C., 28
Burn, P., 27, 59, 374, 383
Burns, T. L., 518
Burt, P., 58
Burt, V., 482
Burton, L. C., 309
Burton, L. R., 155, 364, 368
Buscher, L. A., 576, 581
Bush, P. J., 559, 565, 567, 568
Butler, B. A., 162, 288, 309, 388
Butler, C., 438
Butte, N. F., 517
Butters, J. W., 455
Button, E. J., 448
Byers, T. E., 232
Byers, T., 129, 428, 558
Byrne, L., 323

Caballero, B., 116
Cachelin, F. M., 113, 428
Cairney, J., 558
Caldwell, M. B., 428
Callaway, C. W., 257
Calloway, D. H., 46, 251
Camoin, L., 59, 189
Campbell, I. T., 44
Campbell, I. W., 329
Campbell, L., 4
Campbell, R. G., 47
Campbell, S. M., 4, 76, 126, 416, 435, 515, 558
Campfield, L. A., 27, 59, 258, 374, 383
Camus, M. C., 27
Canning, H., 145
Canovatchel, W., 328, 329
Canter, D. D., 581
Cao, G., 420
Cao, H., 23
Cardon, L. R., 78
Carey, G., 80
Carey, V. J., 9
Carey, W. B., 525
Cargill, B. R., 152
Carleton, R. A., 569, 581
Carlton, E., 429
Carmack, C., 549
Carman, W. J., 4
Carmelli, D., 78
Carmillo, E., 50
Caro, J. F., 56
Caroll, M. D., 3
Carpenter, K. M., 147, 148, 149
Carrier, K. M., 495, 497, 498, 499, 500
Carroll, M. D., 95, 125, 418, 556
Carstensen, J. M., 3, 10
Carter, J. C., 111, 113
Carter, J. K., 173, 176

Carter, J. P., 430
Carter, P. L., 343
Carter, R., 12
Carty, J., 360
Casarez, A. J., 577, 581
Cash, T. F., 152, 158, 159, 195, 448, 449, 450, 453,
    454, 455, 456, 457, 458, 470, 484, 498
Castellani, J., 257
Castellanos, V. H., 518
Castro Cabezas, M., 327
Cater, J. R., 521, 522
Cattlett, H. N., 437
Cauley, J. A., 128
Cha, M. C., 383
Chada, K., 23, 24
Chagnon, Y. C., 61, 74, 78, 81, 85, 173, 175
Chaimoff, C., 340
Chalmers, J., 329
Chambers, J., 29
Chan, J. M., 9
Chappuis, P. H., 47
Chaput, Y., 30
Charbonnier, A., 43
Charles, M. A., 76
Charleston, J. B., 432, 437
Charnock, D. J. K., 110
Chascione, C., 50
Cheadle, A., 427
Chehab, F. F., 75
Chen, A. S., 76
Chen, G., 24, 26
Chen, H. C., 76
Chen, H., 23
Cherny, S., 404
Cheskin, L. J., 13, 149, 195, 200, 506
Cheung, L. W. Y., 557
Chew, B., 57, 518
Chew, I., 259
Chien, S., 284
Chipkin, S. R., 427
Cho, N. H., 173
Choate, M., 99
Choban, P. S., 161
Chomitz, V. R., 457
Chopra, I. J., 331
Christakis, G., 398, 399
Christensen, N. J., 55, 331
Christin, L., 43, 55, 56
Chua, S. C., 26, 27, 28, 29
Chumlea, W. C., 190
Chung, W. K., 22, 26
Cicuttini, F. M., 11
Ciliska, D., 484, 496, 498, 502, 506
Cinciripini, P. M., 578, 581
Civalleri, D., 341
Clark, A. G., 84, 87
Clark, D. C., 545
Clark, D. G., 203
Clark, D. M., 465
Clark, G. W., 346
Clark, H. B., 364
Clark, L. T., 581
Clark, L., 543
Clark, M. M., 152, 203, 497, 581
Clay-Williams, G., 425
Clement, K., 25, 27, 28, 59, 60, 83

Cleveland, W. S., 516
Clifford, C., 192
Clifton, P. G., 30
Clore, J. N., 330
Coakley, E. H., 12, 13, 177
Coates, T. J., 534, 538, 545, 546
Cockett, N. E., 22
Cody, R. P., 343
Coe, N. R., 26
Cohen, L. R., 111
Cohn, S. H., 46
Colagiuri, S., 257
Colby, J. J., 579, 581, 582
Colditz, G. A., 3, 4, 7, 9, 11, 12, 13, 42, 52, 96, 126,
    129, 177, 269
Cole, T. J., 43, 48, 190, 236
Coleman, D. L., 24, 25, 27, 59, 77, 84
Coleman, K. J., 524
Coleman, R. A., 24
Collins, A., 86
Collins, G., 125, 126, 127, 557
Collins, M. E., 232, 454
Collins, V. R., 557
Coltorti, A., 47
Comuzzie, A. G., 60, 61, 81, 82, 88
Cone, R. D., 28
Conill, A., 230
Connacher, A. A., 333
Connolly, H. M., 239, 318
Considine, R. V., 56, 59
Contaldo, F., 47
Conte, H. R., 150
Conway, J. M., 43
Cook, M. E., 173
Cook, S., 436
Coonan, W. E., 559
Cooper, C., 11
Cooper, K. H., 286, 290, 293, 294
Cooper, P. J., 449, 453, 454
Cooper, R. S., 420
Cooper, Z., 109, 113, 374, 449, 468, 472, 473
Cordua, G. O., 519
Cornwell, B., 487
Costa, D., 116
Couceyro, P., 60
Coulston, A. M., 258
Counts, B., 152
Cousins, J. H., 432, 436
Covi, L., 150
Coward, W. A., 45, 48, 57, 236, 518
Cowin, S. D., 518
Cox, M., 57, 521
Cox, N. J., 77
Craighead, L. W., 155, 239, 497, 498, 501, 505, 506
Crandall, C. S., 487
Crepaldi, G., 322
Crisp, A. H., 147
Crocker, J., 486, 487, 488
Crosby, L. A., 103
Croughan-Minihane, M., 498
Cruz, J. A., 519
Csikszentmihalyi, M., 161
Cummings, S. R., 128
Cunningham, J. J., 46
Cupples, L. A., 520
Curhan, G. C., 558

Curry, T. K., 343
Cusin, I., 28
Cutler, J. A., 126
Cutter, G., 161
Cyr, H. N., 48, 236, 549

D'Adamo, P., 264
Dai, H., 361
D'Alessio, D. A., 47
Daling, J. R., 10
Dallal, G. E., 8, 263
Daly, M. E., 557
Danaher, B. G., 546
Danforth, E., 47, 56, 331, 557
Dannhauser, A., 258
Dansky, B. S., 154, 198
Darga, L., 422, 424
Daria, H. L., 46
Darmaun, B., 50
Daston, S., 151
Dauncey, Y. M. J., 43
Davidson, M. H., 237, 243, 327, 390
Davies, J., 448
Davies, P. S. W., 518, 520, 521, 522
Davis, C. J., 448, 453, 457
Davis, D. Z., 578, 581
Davis, G. L., 341
Davis, J. R., 46
Davis, M. A., 4, 10
Davis, S. M., 568
Davis, S., 4, 10
Davis-Chervin, D., 577, 581
Day, J. M., 518
de Bruin, T. W., 327
de Courten, M., 57
de Jonge, L., 47
De Maria, E. J., 349
de Montigny, C., 30
De Spiegelaere, M., 558, 581
de Techtermann, F., 47
de Zwaan, M., 152
Deaver, K., 24
DeBacker, G., 147
Deeb, S. S., 23
Dehollain, P. L., 558
Delargy, H. J., 258
DeLeon, P. H., 103
DeLucia, J. L., 466
Demers, P. P., 558
Dengel, J. L., 126, 127
Dennis, S., 46
Derogatis, L. R., 150
Desgrey, J. M., 263
Desmond, S. M., 175, 483, 507
DeSpiegelaere, M., 524
Despres, J. P., 58, 76, 189
Devlin, M. J., 111, 151
Devos, R., 26, 27, 59, 374
Dewey, K. G., 518
Dewey, M. E., 453
DeWit, T. L., 345
Dhurandhar, N. V., 173, 176
Diamond, H., 264
Diamond, M., 264
Dibb, S., 99

Dickey, L., 498
Dickie, M. M., 27
Dickson, B., 543
DiClemente, C. C., 288
Didie, E. R., 449, 451, 460
Diehl, N., 28
Diehr, P., 130, 132
Dietz, W. H., 4, 7, 8, 12, 48, 56, 99, 102, 145, 190, 236, 269, 283, 416, 515, 517, 518, 520, 525, 532, 557, 558
Diez-Roux, A. V., 427
DiGuiseppi, C., 523
Dionne, M., 457
DiPietro, L., 286, 557
Ditschuneit, H. H., 236, 306, 408, 411, 412
Doak, C. C., 438
Doak, C. M., 97
Doak, L. G., 438
Dockray, G. J., 31
Doherty, J. U., 401
Dohm, G. L., 24
Dolivo, M., 43
Doll, H. A., 113, 149
Domel, S. B., 431, 437
Domelloff, L., 341
Donahoe, C. P., 46
Donaldson, L., 417
Donnelly, J. E., 559, 561
Doring, H., 24
Dorn, J., 536, 540, 543, 544
Dornbusch, S. M., 145
Dorner, G., 20
Dorosty, A. R., 518
Dougher, M. J., 509
Douglas, J. W., 516
Douglass, J., 60
Douketis, J. D., 96, 100
Dourish, C. T., 30
Dowling, M. T., 77
Dowse, G. K., 569
Dozier, D. M., 575, 581
Drabman, R. S., 519
Dramaix, M., 147, 524, 558
Drcnick, E., 96
Drent, M. L., 173
Drougas, H., 372
Drouin, P., 323
Drucker, E., 285
Dry, J., 177
Dubbert, B. K., 109, 152
Dubbert, P. M., 578, 581
Dublin, L. I., 127
Duffy, G., 534, 538, 543, 547
Duggirala, R., 83
Dugoni, B. L., 145
Dulloo, A. G., 43, 47, 360
Dunbar, J. M., 241
Duncan, L. J. P., 243, 322
Dunn, A. L., 288, 291, 292, 571
Dunn, H. L., 46
Dunn-Meynell, A. A., 20
Durnin, J. V. G. A., 44, 45, 58, 457
Durrington, P. N., 98
Dwyer, J. T., 256, 264
Dwyer, T., 559, 562, 567, 569
Dzumbira, T. M. O., 44

Eades, M. R., 259
Earle, T., 467, 498
Eaton, C. A., 203
Eberhardt, N. L., 48, 177
Echtay, K. S., 22
Eckel, R. H., 55
Edelsberg, J., 13
Edholm, O. G., 44, 45
Egger, G., 99, 101, 426
Eggers, H., 328
Eggert, K. E., 498
Ehm, M. G., 61
Eichwort, K., 12
Eipper, B. A., 28
Eisenstein, A. B., 27
Eisenthal, S., 405
Elashoff, R. M., 407
Elder, J. P., 581
Elder, K. A., 428
Eldredge, K. L., 152
Elias, C. F., 21, 27, 28
El-Kebbi, I. M., 427
Ellaway, A., 558
Elliot, D. L., 58
Ellis, K. J., 517
Ellison, R. C., 520
Ellsinger, B., 128
Elmer, P. J., 358, 359
Elmquist, J. K., 21, 24
Emerson, C. H., 27
Emmett, P. M., 518
Enerback, S., 22
Ensrud, K. E., 128, 131, 133
Enzi, G., 322
Epstein, L. H., 155, 194, 237, 245, 305, 361, 401,
    524, 532, 534, 535, 536, 539, 540, 543, 544,
    545, 546, 547, 549, 550, 557, 567
Erickson, J. C., 29
Erikson, H., 128
Eriksson, J. G., 139
Eriksson, K.-F., 126, 133, 134, 135
Erkelens, D. W., 327
Ernsberger, P., 494, 495, 496
Ernst, M. M., 535, 540, 543, 546
Ernst, N., 575, 581
Esparza, J., 97, 424, 523
Ettinger, W. H., 4
Evans, C. R., 350
Evans, R. M., 23, 30
Everhart, J. E., 125, 126, 129

Fabsitz, R. R., 78
Fainaru, M., 545
Fairburn, C. G., 109, 111, 112, 113, 114, 157, 374,
    449, 458, 459, 465, 467, 468, 469, 472, 473,
    477, 547
Fairman, R. P., 350
Faith, M. S., 86, 147, 149, 428, 506
Falkner, N. H., 12
Fan, H., 25
Fardy, P. S., 559, 563, 567
Farndsen, J., 341
Farooqi, I. S., 326
Farquhar, J. W., 100, 569, 572
Farrow, D. C., 10

Fathi, Z., 30
Favaro, A., 448
Favre, R., 43
Feightner, J. W., 96
Felber, J. P., 47
Feldman, H. A., 569
Feldman, J. J., 7
Feldman, W. F., 96
Felitti, V. J., 154, 156, 175, 198
Felson, D. T., 128
Felton, W. L., 178
Fenton, P. F., 77
Ferguson, C., 264
Ferguson, J. M., 155, 264
Ferrara, S., 448
Ferraro, R. T., 46, 55
Ferster, C. B., 301
Field, A. E., 8, 96
Field, C. R., 47, 192
Fielding, J. E., 577, 581
Figueroa-Colon, R., 536, 540, 543
Filer, L., 517
Fine, J. T., 4, 12, 128
Fine, M. A., 198
Finigan, K. M., 349
Finley, R. J., 255
First, M., 151
Fisch, R. O., 558
Fisher, E., 112, 157
Fisher, J. O., 520, 524, 549
Fishman, P., 340
Fitzgibbon, M. L., 148, 150, 372, 428
Flancbaum, L., 161
Flaten, H., 237, 238
Flatt, J. P., 50, 51, 52, 55
Flechtner-Mors, M., 236, 237, 306, 408, 410
Flegal, K. M., 3, 4, 42, 76, 95, 125, 126, 416, 418,
    515, 516, 556, 558
Fletcher, G. F., 288
Flier, J. S., 24, 27, 76
Flint, A., 326
Flodmark, C., 536, 540, 543, 545
Flora, J. A., 569, 572, 574
Flores, R. E., 559, 561, 567, 569
Flynn, K. J., 428
Folsom, A. R., 8, 129, 132, 374
Fomon, S. J., 517, 524
Fontaine, K. R., 13, 96, 149, 173, 195, 200, 308, 357,
    506, 583
Fontbonne, A., 329
Fontvieille, A. M., 57, 521
Ford, E. S., 10, 249
Foreyt, J. P., 96, 101, 112, 154, 161, 234, 360, 466,
    494, 497, 498, 499, 557, 572, 581
Forman, B. M., 23
Forse, R. A., 343
Forsen, T., 176
Forster, J. L., 358, 571
Fortmann, S. P., 100, 569, 574
Foster, G. D., 109, 112, 147, 151, 152, 154, 155, 158,
    159, 161, 162, 186, 193, 195, 201, 202, 230,
    231, 234, 236, 237, 238, 240, 245, 305, 306,
    358, 361, 372, 373, 387, 401, 425, 449, 450,
    451, 456, 459, 460, 482, 494, 507, 508, 525
Foster-Powell, K., 257
Fournier, G., 46, 58

Franckowiak, S. C., 583
Frank, A., 232, 383
Frank, R. G., 103
Franklin, F. A., 543
Frankowiak, S., 308
Franz, M. J., 257
Franzini, D. A., 341
Frayn, K. N., 52, 55
Frederich, R. C., 24
Freeman, V., 438
Freimuth, V. S., 426, 438
French, S. A., 77, 80, 81, 82, 83, 98, 100, 101, 102,
    129, 131, 132, 152, 153, 286, 287, 360, 367,
    558, 571, 576, 579, 580, 581, 582
Frey, D. L., 402
Friedman, M. A., 146, 147, 150, 152, 162, 195, 199,
    525
Frieze, I. H., 145
Frigeri, L. G., 28
Friis-Hansen, L., 31
Frisancho, A. R., 522
Fristal, A., 10
Froguel, P., 28, 60
Froidevaux, F., 55
Fry, A. F., 551
Frye, N., 398
Fujii, J., 22
Fujisawa, T., 86
Fuller, P. R., 358, 361
Funakoshi, A., 30

Gaesser, G. A., 495, 496
Gallagher, D., 19
Gallant, E. M., 22
Galuska, D. A., 249
Gampel, B., 522
Gandolfo, P., 158
Gantz, I., 60
Gardner, J. C., 190
Garfinkel, L., 128
Garfinkel, P. E., 116
Garn, S. M., 75, 521, 545
Garner, D. M., 110, 154, 448, 449, 450, 453, 454,
    494, 495, 496
Garrow, G., 177
Garrow, J. S., 44, 47
Garry, M., 102
Garthwaite, P. H., 133
Gasparello, L., 102
Gast, J., 498
Gautier, J. F., 61
Gavrilova, O., 26
Gazzaniga, J. M., 518
Ge, K., 557
Geissler, C. A., 44
Geller, E. S., 583, 585
Gench, B. E., 437
Gerard, R. J., 145
Gerber, W. M., 581
Ghilardi, N., 26, 27
Gianetta, E., 341, 346
Gibbon, M., 151
Gibbons, K., 448
Gibbons, L. W., 293, 294, 295, 297
Gill, A. M., 28
Gill, J. L., 77

Gill, T. P., 556, 557, 558, 572
Giovannucci, E. L., 10, 11
Gittleman, A. L., 263
Gladis, M. M., 112, 114, 155, 156, 193, 197
Glanz, K., 574
Gleaves, D. H., 453
Glynn, S. M., 203
Golan, M., 536, 540, 545
Golay, A., 47
Goldberg, A. N., 177
Goldberg, A. P., 126
Goldberg, J. P., 457
Goldberg, L., 58
Goldbourt, U., 130, 132
Golden, P. M., 420
Goldfield, G. S., 544
Goldfried, A. P., 474
Goldfried, M. R., 474
Goldstein, D. J., 178, 466
Goldstein, R. B., 127
Golik, A., 323
Golub, M. S., 9
Gonzalez, J. T., 438
Gonzalez, V. M., 438
Good, D. C., 145
Goodman, N., 145
Goodrick, G. K., 96, 101, 154, 161, 234, 360, 494,
    497, 498, 499, 502, 505
Goran, M. I., 57, 193, 425, 521
Gordy, C. C., 535, 536, 540, 543, 544, 546
Goreczny, A. J., 453
Gormally, J. F., 151, 157
Gorman, B. S., 110
Gorsky, R., 13
Gortmaker, S. L., 12, 99, 145, 416, 520, 525, 557,
    558, 559, 560, 567, 569
Gosztonyi, G., 173, 176
Gottesman, I. I., 75
Gotto, A. M., 581
Gotz, F., 20
Goudey-Lefevre, J., 77
Gouma, D. J., 345
Gower, B. A., 57
Grace, M., 198
Grace, W. J., 114, 193
Grady, K. E., 483
Graham, L. E., 358, 359
Grande, F., 46
Graves, T., 312, 536, 540, 543, 546
Gray, J. A., 323
Gray, J. J., 453, 454
Green, L., 543, 551
Green, R. D., 22
Green, S. M., 258
Greenberg, B., 99
Greene, H., 330
Greenstein, R. J., 345
Greenway, F. L., 239, 317, 318, 320, 322, 323, 325,
    326, 327, 329, 330, 331, 333, 383
Greenwood, M. R., 20
Gregoire, M. B., 581
Gregory, J., 520
Griffen, W. O., 351
Griffith, J., 428
Griffiths, M., 57, 521
Grilo, C. M., 110, 116, 153, 157, 195, 388, 450

Grobet, L., 21
Gropper, S. S., 533, 536, 540
Gross, T., 522, 558
Grossbart, S. L., 103
Grossbart, T. A., 451
Growdon, J. H., 116
Gruen, D., 154, 339, 451
Grundy, S. M., 557, 558, 572
Guenet, J. L., 27
Guerciolini, R., 326, 327
Guido, N. J., 73
Guile, C. A., 547
Guilford-Davenport, M., 448
Guilleminault, C., 177
Guisez, Y., 27, 59, 374
Guo, S. S., 190
Gustafsson, K., 258
Gutfeld, G., 481
Gutin, B., 47, 536, 540, 544
Gutzwiller, J. P., 326, 327
Guy-Grand, B., 28
Guzelhan, C., 326
Gwinup, G., 177
Gwirtsman, H. E., 157

Haas, M. H., 574, 578, 582
Hagander, B., 258
Hagen, R. L., 406
Hager, D. L., 99, 100
Hager, J., 61, 80, 81, 82, 83
Hager, R. L., 518
Hahn, T. M., 27
Haire-Joshu, D., 436
Hajak, G., 116
Halaas, J. L., 24, 27
Halford, J. C. G., 323
Hall, J. C., 343
Hallberg, D., 47
Hallstrom, T., 147
Halmi, K. A., 457
Halter, J. B., 47
Hamaday, V., 145
Hamilton, C. C., 402
Hamilton, E. J., 286
Hamilton, J. G., 329
Hamm, P. B., 125
Hamman, R. F., 55
Hammer, L. D., 519
Hammer, V. A., 263
Hammond, E. C., 128
Hampton, L. L., 31
Han, T. S., 149, 269
Hankin, J. H., 10
Hannan, P. J., 360
Hanotin, C., 323
Hansen, D. L., 192, 243, 323
Hansky, J., 258
Hanson, R. L., 61, 81, 85
Harbron, C. G., 263
Harnack, L. J., 557, 558, 572
Harper, I. T., 45
Harper, M. E., 22
Harrell, J. S., 559, 563, 567, 568
Harris, E. S., 545
Harris, J. A., 46
Harris, J. E., 145

Harris, J. K., 367
Harris, J. R., 43, 75, 189
Harris, T. B., 7, 12, 128, 340
Harrison, D. J., 102
Harrison, G. G., 522, 558
Harrison, K. R., 497, 498, 499, 500
Hart, D. J., 11
Hartmann, D., 326
Hartz, A. J., 9, 405
Harvey, J., 155, 237, 305, 361, 401
Hashimi, M. W., 8
Hashimoto, N., 190, 522
Hasin, D., 147, 149
Haskell, W. L., 100, 126, 569, 571
Hasstedt, S. J., 78
Hastorf, A. H., 145
Hasty, P., 22
Hathaway, S., 150
Hauck, W. W., 4
Hauptman, J. B., 326, 327
Hawkins, M., 25
Hawks, S. R., 498
Hawthorne, V. M., 4
Hayes, D., 494
Hayes, S. C., 407
He, W., 23
Heal, D. J., 323, 325
Heath, G. W., 430, 436, 523
Heatherton, T. F., 487
Heaton, A. W., 451
Heber, D., 407, 420
Hebert, P. R., 420
Hebl, M. R., 487
Heckemeyer, C. M., 201, 310, 371, 438
Heckerman, C. L., 407
Hediger, M. L., 517
Hegele, R. A., 23
Hegvik, R. L., 525
Hein, P., 332
Heinberg, L. J., 451, 452
Heini, A. F., 95, 193
Heinig, M. J., 518
Heins, J. M., 581
Heitmann, B. L., 128
Heldmaier, G., 22
Heliovaara, M., 11
Heller, P. A., 46
Heller, R. F., 259
Hellerstedt, W. L., 52, 312, 364
Helton, L. A., 319
Hendler, R., 255
Hennart, P., 524, 558
Hennrikus, D. J., 570
Henriksson, V., 340
Henry, P., 448
Henschel, A., 57, 154
Henson, M. C., 26
Heo, M., 86
Herman, C. P., 110, 147, 154, 157, 457, 494, 495, 496, 497, 498, 499, 501, 504
Hermansen, K., 259
Hermelo, M. P., 533
Hervey, G. R., 19
Herzog, D., 405
Herzog, J., 27
Heshka, S., 233, 398

Heska, S., 58
Heslin, J. A., 257
Hess, D. S., 347
Hess, D. W., 347
Hess, K. W., 537, 542
Hetherington, A. W., 20
Hetzel, B. S., 559
Hey, C., 345
Heyman, R. A., 23
Heymsfield, S. B., 24, 45, 59, 179, 326, 330, 374
Higgins, A. J., 102
Higgins, M., 126
Hill, A. J., 520
Hill, J. O., 46, 62, 129, 156, 177, 191, 193, 202, 244, 269, 287, 310, 323, 327, 330, 360, 367, 372, 475, 557, 558, 572
Hills, A. P., 533, 536, 541, 543, 544
Hilner, J. E., 456
Himes, J. H., 515
Himms-Hagen, J., 22
Hind, H., 524
Hindsberger, C., 55
Hinney, A., 24, 60, 81
Hirsch, J., 4, 19, 20, 29, 44, 188, 189, 360, 388
Hirschmann, J. R., 494, 496, 497, 498, 504
Hirvonen, M. D., 20
Hitman, G. A., 85
Hixson, J. E., 81
Ho, G., 28
Ho, K. S. I., 112
Hoag, S., 55
Hobbs, K. E., 549
Hochgeschwender, U., 28
Hocking, M., 341
Hodge, A. M., 77
Hoerr, S. L., 494
Hoerr, S. M., 580, 581, 582, 583
Hofman, A., 559
Hokfelt, T., 27
Holbrook, T. L., 9
Holden, J. H., 424
Hollander, P., 327, 328
Hollopeter, G., 29
Holly, R. G., 404
Holm, R. P., 429
Holst, J. J., 326
Holt, S. H., 258
Hope, R. A., 547
Hopkins, J., 109, 151, 193
Hopkinson, J. M., 517
Horgen, K. B., 96, 99, 101, 102
Horikawa, Y., 77
Horton, W., 519
Hotamisligil, G. S., 25
Houser, R. F., 457
Houston, C., 112, 157, 432, 436
Hovell, M. F., 358, 433, 437
Howard, B. V., 420
Howard, I. J., 112
Howard, T., 558
Howard-Pitney, B., 438
Hsu, L. K. G., 154, 158
Hsueh, W. C., 81
Huang, Z., 3, 8, 10
Hubbard, V. S., 239
Hudson, J. I., 112, 113

Huffine, C. E., 152
Hughes, P. C., 20, 75
Hulley, S. B., 100, 569
Hummel, K. P., 27, 77, 84
Hunter, G. R., 57, 193
Huntzicker, P. B., 44
Hurley, J., 558
Huszar, D., 28, 60
Hwang, C. S., 25
Hyde, R. T., 193, 293

Ikeda, Y., 237
Ikegami, H., 86
Ingram, D. D., 12
Inoue, S., 317, 323
Insull, W., 372
Israel, A. C., 536, 541, 545, 547
Israel, B. A., 173
Issad, T., 59, 189
Istvan, J., 147, 148
Ito, C. C., 341
Iverius, P. H., 44
Ives, D. G., 571

Jackson, A. S., 294, 296, 372
Jackson, E. C., 521
Jackson, S. P., 22
Jacob, M., 581
Jacobsen, D. J., 586
Jacobson, M. F., 102, 557, 570, 572
Jacques, P. F., 8
Jacquet, J., 47, 360
Jaeger, L. F., 46
Jaffin, B., 345
Jain, A., 427
Jakicic, J. M., 126, 162, 288, 291, 303, 307, 309, 310, 361, 363, 366, 369, 388, 407
James, W. P. T., 24, 55, 76, 77, 88, 237, 243, 324
Jarvie, G. J., 519
Jazwinski, C., 110
Jeanrenaud, B., 29
Jebb, S. A., 47, 193, 523, 557, 572
Jeffery, R. W., 8, 52, 77, 100, 101, 102, 103, 129, 132, 152, 157, 193, 200, 244, 245, 287, 301, 303, 309, 310, 311, 312, 314, 358, 360, 364, 366, 367, 368, 408, 466, 534, 538, 543, 546, 547, 557, 558, 569, 570, 571, 575, 577, 580, 581, 582, 583
Jenkins, A. L., 257
Jenkins, D. J. A., 257, 258
Jensen, D. R., 55
Jensen, M. D., 48, 177, 262
Jequier, E., 43, 46, 47, 50, 51, 55
Jerrett, I., 150
Jessop, D. S., 31
Jeunet, F. S., 326
Jhanwar-Uniyal, M., 29
Joanes, D., 258
Johansen, J., 27
Johansson, C., 27
Johansson, S.-E., 55
Johnson, C. A., 451, 488, 498, 507
Johnson, C. L., 3, 4, 76, 95, 126, 416, 418, 515, 556, 558
Johnson, D., 96
Johnson, K. C., 126

Johnson, M. S., 57
Johnson, P. R., 20
Johnson, R. K., 57
Johnson, S. L., 524
Johnson, T. D., 236, 306, 408
Johnson, W. G., 537, 541, 545, 581
Joly, R., 328
Jonderko, K., 331
Jones, P. J. H., 45
Jones, R. H., 55
Jones, R., 547
Jones, S. P., 323, 324
Jones, S. R., 30
Jonkmann, J. H., 326
Jonsson, E., 12
Jorde, L. B., 84
Josse, R. G., 257
Jozefowicz, R., 330
Jung, R. T., 333
Junjana, C., 559
Just, B., 50

Kafer, K. E., 29
Kahn, H. S., 558
Kaiser, P., 323
Kalarchian, M. A., 158, 543, 557
Kalkhoff, R. D., 9
Kalkwarf, H. J., 263
Kalodner, C. R., 466
Kalra, S. P., 326
Kambadur, R., 21
Kanatani, A., 29
Kandela, P., 98
Kanders, B. S., 237, 256, 432, 436, 437, 466
Kann, L., 523
Kano, S., 494, 496, 497, 498, 499
Karason, K., 135
Karaus, T. G., 150
Karlsson, J., 149, 160, 161
Karrison, T., 436
Kasser, T., 191
Kassirer, J. P., 494, 495, 496
Kastrup, J., 180
Katahn, M., 257, 262, 263, 264
Katch, F. I., 287
Katch, V. L., 533
Katona, G., 176
Katz, L. F., 30
Katz, S., 349
Katzel, L. I., 126
Katzman, M., 448
Kauer, J. A., 30
Kaul, L., 435
Kavanagh, K. H., 438
Kawachi, I., 177
Kawaguchi, Y., 86
Kawai, M., 26
Kawasaki, T., 190, 522
Kaye, S. A., 8
Kaye, W., 109, 111
Kayman, S., 287, 367
Keesey, R. E., 20, 46, 190
Keeton, W. P., 453, 455
Kehayias, J. J., 252
Kellum, J. M., 178, 347, 349, 350, 391
Kelly, D. L., 351

Kelly, F., 323
Kelly, J., 24
Kelman, S. H., 545
Kenardy, J., 111
Kendall, A., 263
Kendall, P. C., 161, 373
Kendrick, J. S., 436
Kenler, H. A., 343
Kennedy, P. H., 438
Kennedy, S. H., 116
Kern, P. A., 360
Kerver, J., 436
Kerzner, A. B., 358
Kessler, R. C., 148
Key, P., 400
Keyou, G., 98
Keys, A., 46, 51, 57, 58, 154, 157
Khoury, M. J., 86
Kideda, Y., 237
Kiemle, G., 453
Kikuchi, T., 190, 522
Killen, J. D., 534, 538, 545, 546, 559, 565, 569
Kilpatrick, D. G., 154, 198
Kimball, K. T., 234
Kinch, R. A. H., 521
King, A. C., 425, 426, 427, 571
King, K. C., 522, 558
King, N. L., 494
Kinra, S., 524
Kinsley, P. M., 581
Kirby, J., 264, 265
Kirby, R. F., 24
Kirkpatrick, J. R., 343
Kirkwood, S. P., 46
Kirsch, I., 466
Kirschenbaum, D. S., 46, 150, 372, 537, 541, 545
Kishimoto, T., 23
Kissebah, A. H., 81
Kittel, F., 147
Kittler, P. G., 417, 426, 427, 438
Kitzinger, G., 43
Kiwan, D., 487
Klaus, S., 22
Klayman, J. E., 522
Klein, E. R., 45
Klein, K. R., 546
Klein, P. D., 45
Kleiner, S. M., 252
Klem, M. L., 129, 156, 177, 202, 244, 269, 287, 310, 475, 571
Klem, M., 367
Klesges, R. C., 524
Kliewer, S. A., 23
Klingenberg, M., 22
Kneer, N., 330
Knowler, W. C., 53, 76, 81, 85
Kobes, S., 81
Koceja, D. M., 286
Koeske, R., 194, 535, 539, 543, 544, 547
Kohl, H. W., 286, 293, 294, 295, 297, 549
Kolaczynski, J. W., 56
Kolesar, J. M., 173
Koletsky, R. J., 494, 495, 496
Koletsky, S., 27
Kolonel, L. N., 10
Kopelman, P. G., 523

Kopin, A. S., 30
Koplan, J. P., 13, 269, 283
Korenman, S., 146
Korner, A. F., 520
Korner, J., 27, 28
Kornitzer, M., 147
Koss-Twardy, S. G., 326
Kovacs, E., 258
Kowalski, K., 156
Kowalski, T. J., 29
Kraemer, H. C., 416, 419, 426, 519, 520
Kral, J. G., 158, 391, 451
Krall, J. M., 558
Kramer, F. M., 358, 359, 360, 571
Kramer, M. S., 522, 525
Kratina, K., 494, 497
Kratt, P. P., 201, 310, 371, 438
Kravitz, M., 428
Krebill, H., 436
Krebs-Smith, S. M., 427
Krehbiel, R., 524
Kress, M. J., 535, 539, 543, 544
Krey, S., 367, 388
Kriketos, A. D., 330
Kristal, A. R., 439
Kristensen, P., 60
Krol, R. A., 175, 483, 507
Kromhout, D., 8
Krotkiewski, M., 188
Krude, H., 28, 60
Kruglyak, L., 84, 86, 87
Kruijer, H., 237
Krupka, L. R., 145
Krupp, J. R., 129
Kryscio, R. J., 236, 402
Kucio, C., 331
Kuczmarski, R. J., 3, 4, 76, 95, 126, 416, 418, 515, 556, 558
Kuehl, K. S., 58
Kuehnel, R. H., 109, 151, 161
Kuida, H., 78
Kulkarni, P. R., 173
Kuller, L. H., 8, 571
Kumanyika, S. K., 126, 175, 416, 417, 419, 420, 421, 423, 424, 426, 427, 432, 435, 436, 437, 438, 448, 487
Kupfer, D. J., 155
Kursar, J. D., 319
Kushi, A., 29
Kushner, R. F., 161, 177, 372
Kuyl, J. M., 258
Kuzmak, L. I., 343
Kyogoku, S., 10
Kyzer, S., 340

LaFleur, W. R., 144
Lagergren, J., 10
Lahlon, W., 111
Laidlaw, A. S., 518
Lake, J. K., 190
Lamoreux, M. L., 28
Lamporski, D. M., 109
Lander, E. S., 73, 86
Lane, M. D., 25
Lang, K., 176
Lang, W., 126, 291, 307, 361, 367, 407

Langlois, J. A., 128
Lapidus, L., 9
Laporte, D. J., 112
LaPorte, D., 158
Lardy, H. E., 330
Larkin, J., 12
Larsen, P. J., 31
Larson, D. E., 46, 55
Larson, K., 46
Larson-Brown, L. B., 581, 582
Larsson, B., 12, 128, 135, 147
Larsson, Y., 544
Lasater, T. M., 569
Lasco, R. A., 431, 436, 437
Latner, J. D., 233, 405, 406, 468
Lattimore, L., 404
Lauderdale, D. S., 419
Lauer, J. B., 368
Launer, L. J., 128
Lavin, P. T., 237
Lawren, B., 259
Lazarus, R., 524
Le Pen, C., 12
Le Stunff, C., 57
Lean, M. E. J., 131, 133, 149, 256, 266, 269, 323
Lec, E. S., 112
Lechan, R. M., 27
Lee, A., 329
Lee, C. D., 294, 296, 372
Lee, E. T., 420
Lee, G. H., 26, 61
Lee, H. C., 581
Lee, I. M., 372, 420
Lee, I., 125, 128, 129
Lee, I.-M., 293
Lee, J. H., 61, 73, 75, 81, 82, 83
Lee, J., 127, 581
Lee, S. J., 21
Leermakers, E. A., 308, 310, 361, 363, 366, 369
Lefebvre, P. J., 329
Legradi, G., 27
Lehmann, J. M., 23
Leibel, R. L., 19, 24, 26, 27, 28, 29, 44, 59, 74, 188, 189, 360, 383, 388, 517, 525
Leiderman, V. R., 175, 483
Leininger, M., 417, 438
Leitch, D. R., 559
Leiter, E. H., 27
Lembertas, A. V., 82
Lembo, P. M., 29
Lemonnier, D., 27
Lennon, D., 46
Lentz, L. R., 22
Leonard, B. E., 436
Leonard, M. T., 517
LePen, C., 149, 195
Lesser, M. S., 157
Letiexhe, M. R., 329
Letizia, K. A., 109, 112, 151, 155, 158, 161, 193, 200, 237, 305, 358, 361, 374, 401
Leutenegger, E., 323
Levelnson, S. M., 427
Levin, B. E., 20
Levine, J. A., 48, 54, 58, 177
Levitsky, D. A., 263
Levitt, E. B., 301

Levitz, L. S., 405
Levy, A. S., 285, 451, 572, 573, 574
Levy, A., 428
Levy, E., 12, 149, 195
Levy, P., 12
Lewendon, G. J., 524
Lewis, E. L., 467, 497
Lewis, M. K., 520
Lewis, R. J., 453, 455
Lewis, V. J., 500
Li, L., 523
Li, W., 83, 84, 87
Liao, Y., 420
Lichtman, S. W., 45, 48, 192, 330, 549
Licinio, J., 24
Liddle, R. A., 127
Liebman, B., 558
Liebschutz, J., 358
Liederman, V., 145
Lifson, N., 45
Lillioja, S., 43, 45, 46, 48, 50, 52, 53, 54, 55, 189
Lin, L., 60
Lindeman, A. K., 498
Linden, W., 477, 498
Lindgärde, F., 126, 133, 134, 135
Lindroos, A. K., 237
Linowitz, J. R., 147, 451, 525
Lionis, C., 559, 564, 567, 568, 569
Lipman, R. S., 150
Lipton, R. B., 420
Liska, T. G., 347
Lissau-Lund-Sørensen, I., 558
Lissner, L., 56, 96, 125, 135, 201, 237, 263, 351
Liss-Resnick, J., 457
Liu, R., 25
Liu, S. M., 26
Livingstone, M. B., 176
Loan, P., 448
Lockene, A., 326, 327
Lockwood, D. H., 252
Logan, S., 517
Logue, S. F., 30
Long, J. C., 85
Long, M., 457
Long, S. D., 133, 134
Lonnerdal, B., 518
Loos, F., 149, 195
Lord, G. M., 27
Louden, V. A., 580, 581, 582, 583
Love, E. J., 521
Love, R. J., 383
Lovejoy, J. C., 331
Lowe, M. R., 154, 398
Lowell, B. B., 22
Lozano, D. V., 102
Lu, D., 256, 264
Lucas, A., 45, 57, 518
Lucas, C. P., 424
Ludwig, D. S., 60, 257, 258, 388
Ludwig, H., 173, 176
Ludwig, W. W., 364
Luepker, R. V., 523, 559, 563, 567, 568
Lundgren, H., 9
Lundsgaard, C., 331
Lustig, R. H., 326
Lutjens, A., 329

Lyon, J. L., 10
Lyons, M. J., 173, 176
Lyons, P., 498
Lyu, L. C., 10

Macaskill, P., 524
Maccoby, N., 569, 572
MacCuish, A. C., 243, 322
Macdonald, I. A., 192, 194, 243, 323
MacDonald, K. G., 133, 134
Macgregor, A. M. C., 145, 450, 457, 483
Macgregor, M. D., 114
Macintyre, S., 558
MacKenzie, R. G., 28
MacLean, L. D., 343, 349
MacLennan, D. H., 22
Maclure, K. M., 4, 11
Madans, J., 7, 12, 128
Maddox, G. L., 145, 175, 483
Madsen, J., 331
Mafeis, C., 190
Maffei, M., 59
Maffeis, C., 518
Maggio, C. A., 125, 126
Magnus, P., 572
Mahler, R. J., 9
Mahowald, M. W., 116
Mains, R. E., 28
Major, B., 487
Makela, P., 11
Makue, D. M., 7
Maldonado, R., 30
Malenbaum, R., 405
Malone, K. E., 10
Maloney, S. K., 438
Malott, J. M., 524
Manibay, E., 428
Manis, E., 581
Manji, S., 50
Mann, G. V., 4
Manni, R., 116
Manninen, P., 11
Manson, J. E., 3, 4, 5, 6, 9, 11, 96, 129, 153, 173, 357
Mantazoros, C. S., 325
Marchiori, E., 322
Marckmann, P., 262
Marcus, M. D., 108, 109, 110, 111, 112, 151, 155, 157, 162, 193, 237, 305, 361, 401, 467
Marcus-Samuels, B., 26
Marin, P., 330, 331
Marks, B. L., 257
Marks, C. R., 533
Marks, H. H., 127
Marmarou, A., 178
Marmot, M. G., 558
Marsh, D. J., 29
Marshall, J. A., 55
Marti, B., 583
Martikainen, P. T., 558
Martin, A. D., 308, 361
Martin, B. W., 583
Martin, C. K., 152
Martin, L. F., 349
Martin, M., 99
Martinez, E. T., 448
Martinez, M. E., 10

Marton, K. I., 129
Martson, W., 558
Marwah, P., 330
Masheb, R. M., 110, 157
Mason, D. A., 201, 371, 438
Mason, D., 310
Mason, E. E., 341
Mason, E., 457
Mason, P., 438
Massari, M., 47
Matheny, M., 24
Mathers, J. C., 557
Mathus-Vliegen, L., 345
Matos, J., 522
Matsuda, M., 61
Maude, D., 448
Mauriege, P., 189
Mayer, J. A., 145, 520, 577, 581, 583, 585
Mayer, R. R., 200
Mayo, K., 428
Mazel, J., 264
Mazzuca, S. A., 429
McAdoo, W. G., 364, 365, 368
McAllister, D. A., 368
McArdle, W. D., 287
McBain, A. M., 329
McCabe, R. E., 494
McCance, D. R., 56
McCance, R. A., 20
McCann, K. L., 361, 532
McCann, U. D., 112
McClearn, G. E., 43, 75, 189
McCrory, M. A., 263, 549
McCurley, J., 534, 535, 539, 543, 557
McDevitt, S. C., 525
McDowell, M. A., 284
McElroy, S. L., 112, 113
McFarlane, T., 494, 495
McGee, D., 420
McGinnis, J. M., 519
McGovern, P. G., 367
McGuiness, B., 147
McGuire, M. T., 129, 156, 177, 202, 244, 269, 287, 310, 367, 475
McIntyre, A. M., 556
McKenzie, S. J., 535, 539, 546, 549
McKinlay, S. M., 569
McKinzie, A. A., 60
McKnight, S. L., 23
McLean, A. P., 349
McMahon, M., 50
McMahon, S., 126
McNabb, W. L., 429, 433, 434, 435, 436, 437
McNeely, M. J., 56
McNeil, G., 55
McPhee, L., 524
McPherron, A. C., 21
McQuillan, G. M., 340
McQuillan, S., 265
Medora, N., 581
Meilahn, E. N., 571
Meillin, L., 264
Melanson, E. L., 191, 192, 193
Melanson, K. J., 258
Melby, C. L., 46
Melia, A. T., 326, 328

Mellin, L. M., 498, 499, 500, 506, 537, 541
Melnyk, A., 22
Meltzer, A. A., 125, 126, 129
Melvin, K. E., 331
Mendelson, B. K., 454, 456
Mendelson, M. J., 152, 153, 159, 195, 447
Mendonca, P. J., 537, 541, 546
Menzies, D. G., 329
Merikangas, K., 86
Mertz, W., 48
Messick, S., 110, 192
Messing, B., 50
Metcalf, B. L., 581
Mettger, W., 426, 438
Metz, J. A., 408
Metzger, B. E., 173
Meyer, J. M., 521
Meyers, A. W., 543
Meyers, A., 312
Michalek, A. V., 112
Michaud, E. J., 28
Michel, Y., 428
Michelson, J., 543
Mickelsen, F., 57, 154
Mickelsen, O., 77
Mifflin, L., 99
Mikelsen, K. L., 128
Mikhail, N., 9
Mikulka, P. J., 159, 450
Miles, P. D., 23
Millen, B., 427
Miller, C. T., 487
Miller, D. S., 44, 45
Miller, M. F., 22
Miller, M. W., 59
Miller, O. N., 329
Miller, P., 264
Miller, W. C., 286, 494, 495, 496, 498, 499, 502, 504, 506
Miller, W. R., 371
Miller-Kovach, K., 398, 399
Miltenberger, R. J., 28
Mingheli, G., 43
Mitchell, B. D., 81
Mitchell, J. E., 109, 152
Miura, J., 237
Mochan, E., 145
Modalsli, Ø., 343
Moe, P. W., 43
Mokdad, A. H., 42, 56, 77, 269, 283, 285, 357
Monsen, E. R., 44
Montague, C. T., 24, 25, 59, 189, 325
Montgomery, G., 466
Monti, P. M., 407
Montignac, M., 258, 261
Moore, D. J., 426, 428
Moore, L. L., 520
Moore, M. E., 146, 147
Moorehead, C., 533
Moran, T. H., 30
Morgan, J., 522
Morino, M., 345
Morley, J. E., 329
Morono, M., 533
Morris, D. H., 257
Morris, K. L., 557

Morris, L. K., 129
Morris, R. D., 405
Morrow, G., 522, 558
Morssink, C. B., 416, 417, 426, 435, 438
Mortola, J. F., 330
Morton, N. E., 86
Mortrud, M. T., 28
Mo-Suwan, L., 559, 560, 569
Mount, M. A., 429
Mountjoy, K. G., 28
Moya de Sifontes, M. Z., 558
Moyer, D., 525
Moynihan, C., 558
Muller, D. C., 55, 125
Muller, T. E., 575, 581
Mullis, R. M., 574, 575, 581
Munro, J. F., 243, 322
Munter, C. H., 494, 496, 497, 498
Munzberg, H., 22
Muoio, D. M., 24, 25
Murgatroyd, P. R., 43, 263
Murray, D. M., 52, 581, 583
Mussell, M. P., 109, 110, 151, 152, 153
Must, A., 8, 10, 12, 42, 96, 145, 269, 420, 525
Mutrie, N., 583
Myers, M. D., 532
Myerson, J., 551
Mynatt, R. L., 28

Nabeshima, Y., 22
Nadar, P. R., 520
Nadeau, A., 46
Nader, P. R., 99
Nagle, F., 46
Nagy, L., 23
Nagy, T. R., 24, 57
Nahon, J. L., 29
Naimark, A., 128
Narayan, K. M., 434, 436
Narbro, K., 12
Naslun, I., 188
Naslund, I., 47
Natow, A., 257
Naveilhan, P., 29
Nedegaard, R. C., 467, 497
Needham, M. L., 428
Neel, J. V., 76, 88, 424
Nelder, R. P., 524
Nelson, D. L., 319
Nelson, J. A., 99
Nelson, J. E., 109, 152
Nelson, S. E., 517
Nestle, M., 557, 558, 570, 572, 586
Nestler, J. E., 330
Neuhaus, J. M., 4
Neumann, L., 484
Neumark-Sztainer, D., 145, 152
Newcomb, P. A., 3, 10
Newton, T., 453
Nezin, L. E., 425
Nezu, A. M., 357, 361, 532
Nguyen, U. S., 520
Niaura, R. S., 152, 203
Nichaman, M. Z., 112
Nicholas, G., 327
Nickerson, D. A., 87

Nicolas, J. P., 28
Nidiry, J. J., 435
Nielsen, B., 331
Niestijl Jansen-Zuidema, J. J., 326
Nigra, I., 345
Nir, Z., 484
Nissan, A., 345
Noble, R. E., 190
Nohr, C., 349
Nohria, V., 45
Nolan, C. A., 581
Nommsen, L. A., 518
Nonas, C. A., 109, 157
Noonan, D. J., 23
Noor, M. I., 44
Noppa, H., 147
Nordsieck, M., 557, 558
Norgan, N. G., 58
Norman, P. A., 113
Norman, R. A., 61, 82
Norris, A. H., 46
Notelovitz, M., 308, 361
Nuesslein-Hildesheim, B., 24
Nurnberger, J. I., 301
Nyman, A., 47
Nyman, M., 258
Nyomba, B. L., 46
Nyren, O., 10

Obarzanek, E., 420, 518
O'Brien, R. M., 155, 239
O'Connell, J. K., 175, 483, 507
O'Connell, M., 47, 56
O'Conner, M., 457
O'Connor, M. E., 113
O'Connor, M., 547
Odeleye, O. E., 57
Odink, J., 326
Ogihara, T., 86
O'Hare, W., 417, 418
Ohki-Hamazaki, H., 30, 31
Ohlson, L. O., 9
Ohlsson, T., 543
Ohman, M., 81, 83
Ohno, M., 237
Oja, P., 583
Oka, R. K., 571
Olbort, M., 24
Oldenburg, B., 572
Olefsky, J. M., 23
Olivecrona, G., 326
Ollmann, M. M., 28
Olmsted, M. P., 110, 453
Olson, C. L., 145
Olson, C. M., 575, 581
Olson, J. E., 145
O'Malley, M. P., 581
Omichinski, L., 497, 498, 499, 500
O'Neil, J. S., 26
O'Neil, P. M., 154, 198, 339, 451
O'Neill, M., 157
Ong, J. M., 360
Onyejekwe, J., 161
O'Rahilly, S., 25
Ornish, D., 137, 262
Orosan, P., 159, 201, 449, 499

Osborne, D., 150
Osmond, C., 522
Ossip, D. J., 543
Oster, G., 13
Osuga, J., 26
Overpeck, M. D., 517
Ow, C. L., 173
Owen, N., 572, 573, 574
Owens, S., 537, 541, 544
Ozata, M., 24, 25, 59, 189
Ozdemir, I. C., 24

Pace, P. W., 360
Pack, A. I., 177
Paeratakul, S., 98, 557
Paffenbarger, R. S., 125, 128, 129, 193, 293, 372
Palmiter, R. D., 29
Paluch, R. A., 535, 536, 540, 543, 544, 546
Paluch, R. E., 524
Pamuk, E. R., 13, 127, 128, 129, 232
Pamuk, E., 13, 127, 128, 129
Pan, X., 136, 137
Pargaman, D., 145
Parham, E. S., 494, 495, 496, 498, 508
Parienti, V., 116
Parizkova, J., 518
Parker, A. W., 533, 536, 541, 543, 544
Parker, S., 487
Paronen, O., 583
Parsons, T. J., 517, 518, 520, 523
Partridge, B., 330
Pasman, W. J., 249, 260
Passemore, R., 44
Pate, R. R., 288
Patel, D. J., 98
Patel, I. H., 328
Patterson, R. E., 439
Patterson, T. L., 99, 520
Patti, E. T., 371, 532
Patton, M. L., 252
Pavlou, K. N., 367, 388, 400
Paxton, S., 448
Payne, J. H., 340
Payne, P. R., 57, 521
Peacock, S. L., 10
Pearson, J. S., 150
Pedersen, N. L., 43
Pedersen, S. B., 341
Pederson, N. L., 75, 189
Peerson, J. M., 518
Pelkman, C. L., 518
Pelleymounter, M. A., 27
Peltonen, M., 135
Penner, B. C., 535, 539, 543, 544, 549
Pepe, M. S., 102, 190, 516, 517
Pera, V., 152
Perez, A., 159
Perlmutter, C. A., 576, 581, 582
Perola, M., 81
Perri, M. G., 237, 244, 303, 308, 309, 314, 357, 358, 361, 362, 364, 365, 367, 368, 369, 371, 372, 466, 467, 468, 532, 547
Perrin, J. M., 12, 145, 525
Persson, B., 544
Pertschuk, M. J., 449
Perusse, L., 61, 74, 78, 79, 81, 85, 88, 173

Pesick, R. D., 521
Peter, J., 557, 558, 572
Peters, J. C., 62, 360, 372
Petersen, P., 180
Petersen, S. E. K., 149
Petersmarck, K. A., 494
Peterson, A. C., 455
Peterson, C. B., 151, 152, 153
Peterson, G., 581
Petocz, P., 258
Pettitt, D. J., 57, 61, 76
Peveler, R. C., 547
Phelan, S. P., 398
Phillipson, E. A., 177
Pierce, J. W., 487
Pietrobelli, A., 86, 179, 181, 182
Pinelli, L., 518
Pines, H., 12
Pingitore, R., 145
Pinsky, J. L., 581
Pirie, P. L., 581
Pi-Sunyer, F. X., 47, 58, 96, 125, 126, 127, 173, 180, 358, 372, 508, 515
Pittet, P. H., 47
Plata-Salaman, C. R., 30
Pleas, J., 430, 437
Plutchik, R., 150
Poehlman, E. T., 46
Polivy, J., 110, 147, 154, 157, 453, 457, 494, 495, 496, 497, 498, 499, 501, 504
Pollard, K., 417, 418
Polley, B. A., 126, 307, 361, 407
Pollock, B. H., 24
Pollock, M. L., 293
Pomerance, H. H., 558
Pongprapai, S., 559
Pope, J., 262, 263
Pope-Cordle, J., 191
Popkin, B. M., 3, 97, 98, 557, 572
Pories, W. J., 133, 244, 343, 350
Porte, D., 383
Porter, C. L., 343
Porter, J. R., 330
Porzelius, L. K., 112, 157
Poston, W. S. C., 234, 466, 498, 557, 572
Potosky, A., 192
Potvin, J. H., 178
Pouillon, M., 111
Powell, K. E., 436
Power, C., 190, 517, 558
Powers, P. S., 159
Powrie, J. K., 133
Pradalier, A., 177
Pratt, M., 523
Prentice, A. M., 47, 48, 193, 236, 263, 523, 557, 572
Price, J. H., 173, 175, 483, 507
Price, J. M., 189
Price, R. A., 73, 74, 75, 76, 77, 78, 81, 189
Prineas, R. J., 8
Pritikin, N., 403, 404
Pritikin, R., 263
Prochaska, J. O., 288
Pronk, N. P., 193, 306
Prus-Wisniewski, R. P., 202, 239, 240, 242, 460
Pudel, V., 110

Puetpaiboon, A., 559
Puhn, A., 264
Puska, P., 559, 566, 568, 572

Qian, W., 236, 402
Qu, D., 29, 60
Quaade, F., 332
Quinn, D., 486, 487
Quinn, M. T., 429, 436

Raben, A., 262, 326
Raczynski, J. M., 456
Rademaker, B., 345
Radloff, S., 147, 148
Raether, C., 102, 581
Rajan, U., 567
Ralph, A., 55
Ramirez, E. M., 458, 459, 484
Ramirez, M. E., 78
Ramos, L. T., 533
Rand, C. S. W., 114, 145, 156, 450, 457, 483
Rankinen, T., 61, 173
Ranson, S. W., 20
Rao, D. C., 78, 173
Rapoport, L., 466, 497, 498, 503, 505, 506
Rardin, D., 151
Rasmussen, O., 259
Rathouz, P. J., 419
Ratti, M. T., 116
Rau, H., 25
Ravelli, A. C., 522
Ravelli, G. P., 522, 558
Ravussin, E., 42, 43, 45, 46, 47, 48, 49, 50, 51, 52,
    53, 54, 55, 56, 57, 59, 61, 74, 81, 97, 189, 193,
    194, 360, 424, 425, 521
Rawls, A., 22
Raymond, N., 152
Raynaud, A. S., 360
Raynor, H. A., 532
Reading, J. C., 155
Reaven, G. M., 259
Reaves, B. J., 25
Reed, D. L., 453, 455
Reed, D. R., 73, 75, 83
Reed, R. B., 520
Reed, T., 78
Rees, J. M., 532
Reeves, R. S., 234, 498
Reger, B., 572, 573, 574
Reich, D. E., 85, 86, 87
Reilly, J. J., 518
Reiss, E., 111, 113
Reiss, G. K., 22
Reiter, J., 152, 159, 195, 201, 449, 456, 499
Reitman, M., 26
Reitsma, J. B., 327, 328
Renjilian, D. A., 235
Resch, E., 264, 494
Resnicow, K., 559, 564, 567
Rexrode, K. M., 3, 8
Reybrouck, T., 537, 541, 544
Rhode, B. M., 343, 349
Rice, T., 74, 78, 81, 173
Richardson, S. A., 145
Rich-Edwards, J. W., 13
Richelsen, B., 341

Ricketts, C. D., 518
Ridings, P. C., 178
Riggs, S., 544
Riihimaki, H., 11
Riley, R. E., 44
Rimm, A. A., 9, 405
Rimm, E. B., 7, 9, 177
Rippe, J. M., 161, 202, 257, 398
Risch, N., 86
Rising, R., 45, 46, 49, 51, 52
Rissanen, A., 177
Ritenbaugh, C., 428, 441
Rivers, J. P. W., 57, 521
Rizzo, T. A., 173
Robbins, D. C., 47
Robbins, L. S., 28
Roberts, I., 523
Roberts, S. B., 45, 57, 263, 518, 521
Robertson, D. S., 55
Robertson, R. J., 288, 309, 388
Robinson, B. E., 501
Robinson, T. N., 57, 416, 520, 521, 522, 559, 560,
    567, 569
Robison, J. I., 494
Rocchini, A. P., 533, 537, 541, 544
Roche, A. F., 190
Rodefer, J. S., 544
Rodin, J., 152, 153, 195, 360, 448, 450, 507
Rodriguez, M. L., 437
Roe, D. A., 12, 145, 263
Roehling, M. V., 145, 146
Roger, P. J., 191
Rogers, R., 517
Rogers, T., 578, 581
Rohde, W., 20
Rohner-Jeanrenaud, F., 29
Rolland-Cachera, M. F., 516, 518, 558
Rollnick, S., 371, 438
Rolls, B. J., 263, 323, 389, 518
Romieu, I., 48
Romsos, D. R., 24, 30
Rongier, M., 50
Root, J. H., 438
Rosemurgy, A., 159
Rosen, J. C., 152, 158, 159, 195, 201, 449, 453, 455,
    456, 457, 458, 459, 467, 470, 484, 499
Rosen, R. C., 127
Rosenbaum, M., 19, 24, 360, 388, 517, 525
Rosenberg, M., 153, 450
Rosenblum, G. D., 109, 157
Rosenthal, B. S., 581
Rosing, L., 429
Ross, J., 494
Rossetti, L., 25
Rossi, J. S., 203
Rossiter, F. M., 108, 111
Rössner, S., 358, 359, 370, 372, 373, 468
Roth, H., 83
Rothblum, E. D., 495, 498
Rothman, K. J., 520
Rothman, R. A., 242, 243
Rotimi, C. N., 82
Rotnitsky, A., 9
Rotnitzky, A., 129
Roubenoff, R., 252
Roughan, P., 457, 497, 498, 499, 501

Roza, A. M., 46
Ruan, W. J., 517
Rubio, A., 323
Ruderman, A. J., 203
Rudnicki, M. A., 22
Rumpel, C., 12, 128
Rumpler, W. V., 43
Rupley, D. C., 9, 405
Rush, D., 522
Rush, J., 155
Russell, C. D., 25
Russell, G. J., 581
Russell, S. H., 569
Russo, J. E., 575, 581
Rustin, R. M., 147
Rutan, G., 8
Ryan, D. H., 318, 323
Ryden, O., 543
Ryttig, K. R., 237, 238

Saad, M. F., 46
Sacco, W. P., 453
Saelens, B. E., 532, 535, 540, 543, 544, 546
Saffari, B., 360
Saggi, B. W., 178
Saito, M., 25
Saito, Y., 29
Sakurai, T., 60
Sala, A., 448
Salamone, L. M., 127
Salbe, A. D., 57, 521
Sallis, J. F., 99, 520, 549, 559, 561, 567
Sallo, M., 549
Saltzberg, E., 453
Saltzman, E., 263, 557
Salvant, J. B., 178
Sampalis, J., 343
Sanarelli, G., 559, 562, 569
Sande, K. J., 44
Sandiford, I., 46
Sandler, J., 364
Sandstrom, B., 262
Sansone, L. A., 198
Sansone, R. A., 198
Santelli, R., 109
Santonastaso, P., 448
Saper, C. B., 21
Sapirstein, G., 466
Saris, W. H. M., 249, 258, 557
Sarlio-Lahteenkorva, S., 177
Sarwer, D. B., 152, 154, 161, 162, 195, 201, 202,
    230, 239, 240, 242, 243, 244, 339, 358, 449,
    450, 451, 456, 459, 460, 482, 507
Savage, J., 57, 518
Savard, R., 76
Saxton, J., 127
Sbrocco, T., 191, 467, 477, 497, 498, 499, 503, 505,
    506, 509
Scalfi, L., 47
Scarpace, P. J., 24
Schall, R., 258
Schalling, M., 27
Schank, D., 360
Scheen, A. J., 329
Scheinbaum, M. L., 323
Schemmel, R., 77

Schenk, C. H., 116
Schlingenseigpen, K. H., 45
Schlundt, D. G., 191, 192, 581
Schmid, T. L., 360, 571
Schmidt, I., 24
Schmidtke-Schrezenmeier, G., 326
Schmitz, K. H., 583
Schmitz, M. F., 577, 581
Schmitz, O., 259
Schoeller, D. A., 45, 47, 48, 56, 177, 192, 236, 287,
    518, 519, 521, 549
Schofield, W. N., 46
Schork, N. J., 86
Schrauwen, P., 46, 60
Schteingart, D. E., 323
Schuftan, C., 543
Schumaker, H. D., 145
Schulsinger, F., 453
Schulz, L. O., 46, 47, 97, 424
Schutz, Y., 43, 46, 47, 50, 51, 52, 55, 518
Schwab, R. J., 177
Schwalberg, M. D., 112
Schwartz, G. J., 27, 30
Schwartz, M. B., 162
Schwartz, M. H., 109
Schwartz, M. W., 27, 30
Schwartz, R. S., 46, 47, 56
Schwartz, R. W., 351
Schweizer, T., 258
Scopinaro, N., 158, 341, 346
Scott, L. W., 579, 581, 582
Scrocchi, L. A., 31
Seagle, H. M., 156, 177, 202, 244, 269, 287, 310, 323
Seale, J. L., 43
Sears, B., 259
Sears, S. F., 308, 361
Sebok, A., 176
Sebring, N. G., 110, 157, 162
Seddon, E., 457, 497
Seeley, R. J., 27
Segal, K. R., 47
Segal, L., 12
Seidel, K. D., 102, 190, 516, 517
Seidell, J. C., 8, 12, 55, 149, 269, 556, 583
Self, M. S., 440
Seligman, M. E. P., 161
Seljaas, G. T., 518
Sell, S., 193
Seller, R., 583
Sellers, T. A., 78
Sempos, C. T., 284
Senediak, C., 537, 542, 543, 546
Serdula, M. K., 56, 232, 249, 428
Shackleton, S., 23
Shaffer, P., 13
Shah, M., 360
Shapcott, D., 558
Shapiro, R. M., 364, 365, 367, 369
Sharma, M., 21
Shaten, J., 125
Shattuck, A. L., 439
Shay, K., 177
Shear, C. L., 518
Shekelle, R. B., 125
Shelmet, J. J., 52
Sherbourne, C. D., 149, 161, 195

Sherikar, A. A., 173
Sherwood, N. E., 152, 157, 193, 367, 572
Shide, D. J., 323
Shields, T. W., 46
Shigaki, C. L., 361
Shikora, S., 50
Shimomura, I., 23
Shimomura, Y., 29
Shizgal, H. M., 46
Shoba, B. C., 524
Shock, N. W., 46
Shoff, S. M., 3, 10
Shrago, E., 46
Shutter, J. R., 28
Sidman, M., 552
Siegel, W., 358
Sierra-Honigmann, M. R., 26
Siervogel, R. M., 190
Sievers, M. L., 85
Silberstein, L. R., 448
Siliquini, R., 345
Silla, R., 549
Silver, K., 59
Silverman, B. L., 173, 175
Silverman, W. K., 547
Silvers, W. K., 59
Silverstone, J. T., 147
Simansky, K. J., 30
Simkin-Silverman, L. R., 127, 571
Simonetti D'Arca, A., 559, 569
Simpson, M. A., 26
Simpson, W. S., 351
Sims, E. A. H., 19, 58, 177
Singh, R. B., 136, 137
Sinha, M. K., 56
Sismanis, A., 178
Sivitz, W. I., 25
Sjöström, C. D., 96, 134, 135
Sjöström, D., 188, 189, 190, 201, 351
Sjöström, L., 9, 12, 96, 135, 149, 160, 188, 201, 237, 243, 327, 328, 351
Skender, M. S., 303, 307
Skottova, N., 326
Slabber, M., 258
Slade, P. D., 453, 454
Slavens, G., 544
Slinkard, L. A., 534, 538, 545, 546
Smit, J. L., 329
Smith, C. K., 24, 30
Smith, C., 311, 313
Smith, D. E., 111, 158, 201, 371, 372, 427, 438, 456
Smith, D. K., 323
Smith, D., 310, 427, 438
Smith, E. O., 517
Smith, F. J., 27, 30, 59, 258, 383
Smith, F., 374
Smith, G. P., 326
Smith, I. G., 323
Smith, J. A., 544
Smith, J., 59
Smith, M., 112, 157, 293
Smith, N. J., 483
Smith, R. E., 173
Smith, T. P., 21
Smith, V., 201
Smoller, J. W., 155, 159

Snell, M. K., 358
Snitker, S., 45, 46, 49, 56, 425
Snook, J. T., 44, 401
Snyder, F. F., 175, 483, 507
Snyder, J., 308, 583
Snyder, M. P., 101, 583
Snyder, P., 583
Snyder, W. S., 50, 51
Sobal, J., 145, 147, 523, 558
Sobol, A. M., 12, 145, 525
Sokol, A., 264
Sokol, R. J., 522, 558
Soler, J. T., 8
Solow, C., 159
Sonne-Holm, S., 12
Sonuga-Barke, E. J. S., 448
Sorensen, T. I. A., 55, 77, 558
Sorensen, T. I., 12
Sorenson, T. I., 453
Soriano, E., 575, 581
Sorkin, J. D., 55, 125
Soveny, C., 258
Sowers, M., 4
Sox, H. C., 129
Sparling, P. B., 46
Specker, S., 152
Speckman, R. A., 23
Spector, T. D., 11
Spence, S. H., 534, 537, 538, 542, 543, 546, 547
Spiegelman, B. M., 76
Spinetta, M., 448
Spinnler, G., 43
Spitzer, R. L., 107, 108, 109, 110, 111, 151, 152, 156, 162, 193
Spraul, M., 46, 56
Spring, B., 145
Spurrell, E. B., 109, 110, 152, 157
Srebnik, D., 453
Srole, L., 146
Staelin, R., 581
Staffieri, J. R., 145, 480, 482
Stallings, V. A., 56, 110, 157, 518, 519, 521, 522, 525
Stalonas, P. M., 358, 359
Stamler, J., 125
Stampfer, M. J., 9, 11
Stanley, M., 518
Stanner, S. A., 173, 175
Stark, O., 516
Starkey, J. V., 342, 343, 344
States, 1995., 3, 7, 9, 10, 11, 12, 13
Statt, M., 330
Steen, S. N., 201
Steer, R. A., 151, 153, 156, 186, 450
Stefanick, M. L., 126, 571
Steffe, W. P., 388
Steffee, W. P., 367
Stehling, O., 24
Stein, Z. A., 522, 558
Steinberg, C. M., 202, 239, 240, 242, 449, 460
Steinhardt, M. A., 495
Stephen, A. M., 557
Steranchak, L., 543
Sterky, G., 544
Stern, J. S., 20, 287, 367
Stern, M. P., 46, 569
Sternberg, J. A., 161, 162, 237, 358

Stevens, J., 5, 96, 98, 173, 357, 420
Stevens, V. J., 420, 423, 424
Steward, H. L., 258, 259
Stewart, A. L., 147
Stewart-Brown, S. L., 149
Stice, E., 152
Stinnett, J. L., 159
Stock, M. J., 44, 47, 192, 243, 323, 360
Stoker, R. C., 572, 574
Stolley, M. R., 150
Stolmaker, L., 545
Stone, J. M., 467, 497
Story, M., 101, 145, 416, 558, 576, 581, 582
Strack, I., 27
Strain, G. W., 330
Stratment, F., 46
Strauss, R. S., 173, 175
Stricker-Krongrad, A., 28
Striegel-Moore, R. H., 428
Striegel-Moore, R. J., 147
Strobe, A., 189
Strobel, A., 59
Strobel, R. J., 127
Strodel, W. E., 351
Strosberg, A. D., 59, 189
Strupp, B. J., 263
Stuart, R. B., 233, 301
Stubbs, R. J., 263
Stunkard, A. J., 12, 43, 56, 57, 75, 76, 96, 107, 108,
    110, 111, 112, 113, 114, 115, 117, 144, 145,
    146, 147, 148, 150, 151, 152, 153, 155, 157,
    158, 159, 161, 162, 186, 189, 190, 192, 193,
    195, 197, 198, 230, 234, 237, 239, 241, 244,
    305, 358, 388, 398, 401, 405, 407, 447, 451,
    453, 454, 456, 457, 470, 480, 482, 483, 518,
    519, 520, 521, 522, 523, 525, 532, 545, 558, 583
Suchard, M. A., 236, 408
Sucher, K. P., 417, 426, 427, 438
Sugerman, H. J., 158, 178, 342, 343, 344, 347, 349,
    350, 391
Sugimori, H., 98
Sullivan, A. C., 329
Sullivan, J., 430
Sullivan, M., 149, 153, 160
Sullivan, S. P., 154
Summerbell, C. D., 177, 517
Sundquist, J., 55, 416
Suskind, R. M., 543
Susser, M. W., 522, 558
Svec, F., 330
Sveger, T., 543
Swain, R. M., 425
Swan, K. F., 26
Swanson, C. A., 439
Swap, W. C., 457
Swenson, W. M., 150
Swierczynki, J., 50
Swift, K., 159
Swinburn, B. A., 52, 55, 99, 101, 360, 426
Syngal, S., 127, 131
Szabo, G., 21
Szczypka, M. S., 30
Szmukler, G., 448

Tagliabue, J., 98
Takahashi, H., 190, 522

Talamini, G., 190
Tam, Y. K., 326
Tamir, D., 559, 564, 567, 568, 569
Tanaka, T., 23
Tanco, S., 477, 498, 499, 504, 505, 506
Tang-Christensen, M., 31
Tanner, J. M., 75
Tanofsky, M. B., 109, 110, 157
Tanrikut, C., 111, 112, 113
Tantleff-Dunn, S., 451, 452
Tapscott, E. B., 24
Taras, H. L., 99
Tartaglia, L. A., 26, 59, 325, 326
Tartara, A., 116
Tataranni, P. A., 46, 47, 56, 61, 74, 521
Tate, D. F., 312, 409
Tatemoto, K., 28
Tato, L., 190
Taussig, M. T., 429
Taylor, C. B., 100, 154, 155, 358, 569
Taylor, H. L., 46, 57, 154, 155
Taylor, M. J., 449
Taylor, W. C., 112, 437
Tecott, L. H., 30
Telch, C. F., 108, 111, 112, 151, 152, 155, 158, 193,
    483
Tell, G. S., 559, 566, 567, 568
Ten Have, T. R., 126, 435
Terry, B. E., 351
Terwilliger, J., 86
Theriault, G., 58
Thomas, D. B., 10
Thomas, F., 323
Thomas, L. N., 517
Thompson, D. B., 59
Thompson, D., 13
Thompson, H. R., 330
Thompson, J. K., 451, 452, 453, 454, 455, 456
Thompson, M. A., 453, 454
Thompson, M. P., 129
Thonney, P. F., 581
Thorburn, A. W., 259
Thorne, A., 47
Thorson, C., 244, 309, 368
Thorwart, M. L., 263, 323, 518
Thurlby, P. L., 24
Tijhuis, M. A. R., 269
Tindale, R. S., 145
Tirodhar, M. A., 427
Titze, S., 583, 585
Togerson, J. S., 237, 238
Tomarken, A. J., 545
Tonstad, S., 327, 328
Tontonoz, P., 23
Toppino, M., 345
Torjeson, P. A., 126
Tornberg, S. A., 3, 10
Toubro, S., 55, 192, 323, 332
Trayhurn, P., 24
Treiber, F., 544
Tremblay, A., 46, 58, 76, 284, 466
Tribole, E., 264, 494
Troendle, J. F., 517
Troiano, R. P., 42, 416, 515, 516, 519
Truett, G. E., 77
Truloff, C., 22

Truswell, A. S., 259
Tsukahara, S., 237
Tuck, M. L., 9
Tucker, L. A., 518
Tumer, N., 24
Tuomilehto, J., 136
Turton, M. D., 31
Twentyman, C. T., 364
Tzankoff, S. P., 46

Uchiyama, M., 190, 522
Udall, J. N., 522, 558
Ulbrecht, J. S., 323
Ulstrom, R., 558
Umesono, K., 23
Usiskin, K. S., 330

Vaisse, C., 26, 27, 28, 60
Valdez, R., 55
Valencia, M. E., 76, 97, 424
Valley, V., 198
Valoski, A. M., 194, 534, 535, 539, 540, 543, 544,
    545, 546, 547, 549, 557
Van Amelsvoort, J. M., 258
van Brummelen, P., 326
Van Den Berghe, G., 544
Van Es, A. J., 43
van Leer, E. M., 8
van Santen, E., 47
Vandenbergh, J. G., 26
Vanderschueren-Lodeweyckx, M., 544
Vandongen, R., 559, 563, 564, 567, 568
VanItallie, T. B., 4, 96, 97, 98, 127, 173, 251, 262,
    357
Vannotti, A., 43
Vara, L. S., 535, 540, 543, 544
Varady, A. N., 419, 427
Vartiainen, E., 559, 566, 568
Vastine, V. L., 350
Vaucher, Y., 558
Vaughan, L., 46
Vaughn, T. L., 10
Vazquez, I. M., 427, 428
Veith, R. C., 46
Vellar, O. D., 559, 566, 567, 568
Venditti, E. M., 126, 161, 162, 307, 361
Venes, A. M., 145
Venter, J. C., 73
Vernet, O., 47
Vernon-Roberts, J., 457, 497
Verschuren, W. M., 8
Vetrovec, G. W., 350
Vettor, R., 29
Vichitbandra, S., 236, 402
Vickers, S. P., 30
Viegener, B. J., 357, 361, 362
Vinckx, J., 544
Viteri, J. E., 571
Vito, D., 524
Vobecky, J. S., 558
Vogt, R. A., 126, 152, 155, 158, 159, 161, 201, 202,
    240, 306, 361, 373, 387, 425, 449, 450, 456,
    460
Voigt, L. F., 10

Volkmar, F. R., 234, 398
von Almen, T. K., 543
Vuori, I. M., 583, 585

Wadden, T. A., 12, 109, 111, 112, 126, 127, 144,
    146, 147, 148, 150, 151, 152, 154, 155, 156,
    157, 158, 159, 161, 162, 178, 186, 190, 193,
    195, 196, 197, 198, 199, 200, 201, 202, 203,
    229, 230, 231, 232, 234, 236, 237, 238, 239,
    240, 241, 242, 243, 244, 254, 255, 302, 304,
    305, 306, 307, 358, 359, 360, 361, 362, 363,
    366, 368, 372, 373, 374, 386, 387, 388, 392,
    396, 401, 402, 407, 411, 425, 449, 450, 451,
    456, 459, 460, 467, 469, 475, 477, 480, 482,
    483, 495, 507, 508, 525, 537, 542, 544, 546
Wade, T. J., 558
Wagner, J. L., 579, 581, 582
Waguespack, J., 77
Wahren, J., 47
Wainscott, D. B., 319
Walberg, J., 177
Wald, N. J., 557
Walder, K., 46, 60, 81
Wallace, J. P., 498
Wallentin, I., 135
Walsh, B. T., 111
Walsh, T., 151
Walson, P. D., 558
Walter, H. J., 559, 565, 568
Wand, J., 58
Wandel, M., 97
Wander, G. S., 98
Wang, H. J., 407
Wang, J., 25, 230
Wang, N. D., 23
Wang, T. C., 31
Ward Montague, N., 581
Ward, A., 257
Warden, C. H., 78
Wardlaw, S. L., 27, 28
Wardle, J., 466, 487, 497
Ware, J. E., 149, 161, 195
Warren, C. W., 523
Wassertheil-Smoller, S., 421
Waterlow, J., 45
Waters, G. S., 159
Watts, D. M., 343
Waxman, M., 518, 519, 520
Webb, P., 43, 45
Webber, E. M., 482, 483
Weber, C., 326
Weber, J. M., 524
Wedding, D., 103
Wedel, H., 12, 96, 135
Wehner, J. M., 30
Wei, M., 295, 297, 298
Wei, Y., 330
Weidner, G., 147, 148
Weigle, D. S., 44
Weinsier, R. L., 54, 95, 127, 193, 372, 425
Weinstock, P. H., 26
Weinstock, R. S., 126, 361, 363
Weintraub, M., 323, 332
Weisnagel, S. J., 61, 173

Weiss, N. S., 10
Weiss, W., 521
Weissfeld, L. A., 4
Weizman, A., 545
Welch, R., 109, 152
Welch, S. L., 109
Welle, S. L., 47, 330
Wells, J. C. K., 518, 521, 525
Wendt, S., 453
Wener, M. H., 340
Wengholt, H., 331
Wertheim, E. H., 448
West, D. B., 77
Westenhoefer, J., 110
Westerterp-Plantenga, M. S., 249, 258
Westlake, R. J., 407
Weststrate, J. A., 46, 47
Weyer, C., 45, 49, 50, 53, 57, 58, 425
Wharen, J., 47
Whelan, J., 312
Whelton, P. K., 135, 136, 358, 359, 420
Whitaker, L. A., 449
Whitaker, R. C., 102, 190, 516, 517, 521
Whitney, C., 257
White, A., 520
White, D. W., 26
White, E., 10
White, S. L., 421, 438
Whitehead, J. P., 25
Whitehead, R. G., 43
Whitehouse, R. H., 75
Whitikar, R. C., 558
Wichstrom, L., 448
Widdowson, E. M., 20
Wiederman, M. W., 198
Wilbur, C. S., 580, 581, 582
Wilbur, D. C., 483
Wilfley, D. E., 109, 110, 111, 152, 153, 157, 195, 428, 450
Wilk, J. E., 151, 193
Wilkens, L. R., 10
Wilkinson, J. E., 28
Will, J. C., 249
Willer, J. C., 177
Willett, W. C., 4, 7, 9, 11, 129, 177, 269
Willi, S. M., 189
Williams, G. S., 342, 344
Williams, J. H., 436
Williams, P. T., 100, 126, 569
Williams, R. C., 85
Williams, R. R., 78
Williams, S. B. W., 151
Williams, T. D., 27, 28
Williamson, D. A., 152, 453, 454
Williamson, D. F., 13, 125, 127, 128, 129, 130, 131, 132, 230, 232, 285, 428, 558
Williamson, J., 80
Wilson, B. D., 27, 28
Wilson, E. M., 243, 322
Wilson, G. T., 96, 109, 110, 111, 154, 157, 158, 357, 371, 372, 467, 469, 473, 474, 509
Wilson, J. F., 448, 487
Wilson, L. J., 127
Wilson, R. H., 436
Wilson, S., 333
Winett, R. A., 312, 409, 579, 581, 582

Wing, A. L., 193
Wing, R. R., 8, 96, 108, 109, 112, 126, 127, 129, 136, 137, 151, 155, 156, 157, 158, 162, 177, 193, 194, 200, 201, 202, 233, 234, 235, 236, 237, 238, 244, 269, 287, 288, 291, 301, 302, 304, 305, 306, 307, 309, 310, 311, 312, 313, 358, 361, 362, 363, 364, 366, 367, 368, 372, 373, 388, 401, 407, 409, 420, 423, 424, 466, 469, 475, 477, 534, 535, 539, 543, 544, 546, 547, 549, 557, 571
Wingard, D. L., 9
Wingate, B. J., 201
Winkelby, M. A., 416
Winkler, E., 22
Winters, C., 291, 361
Winther, E., 259
Wisser, M., 340
Witgrove, A. C., 346
Witteman, J. C. M., 4, 8
Wolever, T. M. S., 257, 258
Wolf, A. M., 42, 96, 126, 556
Wolff, G. L., 28
Wolff, H. G., 114, 193
Wolff, O. H., 516
Womble, L. G., 195, 230, 233, 242, 243, 244
Wong, W. W., 517
Wood, P. D., 126
Woodall, K., 535, 539, 543
Woods, M., 192
Woodward, E. R., 341
Wooley, S. C., 110, 154, 494, 495, 496
Woolston, J., 234, 398
Wootan, M. G., 572
Worsley, A., 559, 562, 567, 569
Woychik, R. P., 28
Wright, J. A., 102, 190, 516, 517
Wu-Peng, X. S., 26
Wurtman, J. J., 116
Wurtman, R. J., 116
Wyatt, H. R., 193
Wyatt, M., 264
Wylie, R. J., 420, 422
Wyshak, G., 405

Xia, J., 46
Xu, M., 30

Yaari, S., 130, 132
Yalom, I. D., 404, 507
Yang, M. U., 58, 251, 262
Yang, Q., 86
Yanovski, J. A., 152, 157, 158, 162
Yanovski, S. Z., 108, 109, 110, 129, 139, 152, 157, 158, 162, 193, 422
Yaswen, L., 28
Yawn, B. P., 145
Yen, S. S. C., 330
Yen, T. T., 28
Yeo, G. S. H., 28, 60
Yiengst, M. J., 46
Yokogoshi, H., 116
Yong, L. C., 8
York, B., 77
Yoshida, N., 23
Yost, T., 55
You, S., 20

Young, D. R., 437, 558, 571
Young, J. B., 56, 194
Yutrzenka, B. A., 438

Zanni, E., 46
Zansky, S. M., 523
Zarjevski, N., 28
Zavela, K., 147, 148
Zeanah, C. H., 520

Zelewski, M., 50
Zelitch, D. S., 405
Zemel, M. B., 557
Zhai, F., 557
Zhang, Q., 73
Zhang, Y., 24, 56, 59, 73
Zhi, J., 326, 328
Zhou, Q. Y., 29
Ziegler, E. E., 517
Ziegler, R. G., 97
Zifferblatt, S. M., 578, 581

Subject Index

Page numbers followed by "A" indicate appendix, "f" indicate figure, and "t" indicate table.

Adipose tissue
  brown (BAT), effects on body weight, 22
  energy, 250
  location, and Type 2 diabetes, 9
  white (WAT)
    development and proliferation, 23–24
    effects of lipolysis disruption, 25–26
    and lepetin secretion, 24–25
Adiposis dolorosa, 180–181
Age and obesity
  BMI index and elderly persons, 4
  children, 13
  of onset, 189–190
    and body image, 159, 482
  premenopausal/postmenopausal cancer risks, 10
Alcohol, 278A
Atkins diets, 261

Bariatric surgery, 351, 390–391
  complications
    late, 349–350
    nutritional, 350
    perioperative, 347–349
  considerations, 244, 340
  current procedures, 342
    gastric banding, 343, 391
    gastric bypass (RYGBP), 343, 344f, 355A–356A
    gastroplasty, 342–343
  and cytokines decrease, 340
  early procedures
    complications, 340–341
    gastric bypass (RYGBP), 341
    intestinal bypass (JIB), 340
    vertical banded gastroplasty (VBG), 341, 342f, 391
  and eating disorders, 158
  laparoscopic surgery, 344
    adjustable gastric banding (LASGB), 344–346, 345f

gastric bypass (LRYGBP), 346
  outcomes
    failed surgery/reoperation, 351
    positive, 350–351
  partial biliopancreatic diversion, 346–347, 346f
    distal gastric bypass, 347
    with duodenal switch, 347, 348f
BDD (balanced-deficit diet), 236, 256–257
  commercial programs, 257
  comparison with VLCDs, 238t
BDD (body dysmorphic disorder), 451
BDI-II (Beck Depression Inventory), 186
Behavioral assessment (of obese patient), 186, 203–204
  Beck Depression Inventory (BDI-II), 186
  interview initiation, 187
    and primary care physicians, 187–188
  summarization of assessment, 201
  treatment goals identification, 201–202
    and weight loss goals, 202
  treatment options, 202–203
    selected treatment overview, 203
  Weight and Lifestyle Inventory (WALI), 186–187
Behavioral assessment (of obese patient). See also
    BEST behavioral assessment model
Behavioral choice treatment, 467, 477n
Behavioral weight loss programs, 233, 388
  changing eating behavior, 302, 305
    structured meal plans, 305–306
  changing physical activity, 306–307
    improving exercise adherence, 308–310
    and long-term weight loss, 307–308
  components, 234
    frequent visits, 234
    group treatment, 234–235
    time-limited therapy, 234
    treatment flexibility, 235
    treatment limitations, 235
  effectiveness, 313–314

Behavioral weight loss programs *(continued)*
  historical overview, 301–302
  long-term effects, 357–358, 359t, 360
  posttreatment weight gain factors, 360
  relation of pharmacological treatment, 239–241, 240f
  studies, 303t–304t
  summary, 302f
Benign prostatic hyperplasia (BPH), and obesity, 11
BEST behavioral assessment model, 186
  Biological factors
    classification, 188, 189f
    discussion issues with patient, 190–191
    genetic factors, 189–190
  Environmental factors, 191
    discussion issues with patient, 194
    food intake, 191–193
    physical activity, 193–194
  Social/psychological factors, 194
    discussion issues with patient, 198–199
    mood disorder, 196–198, 196t, 197t
    psychosocial effects of obesity, 195
    social context of weight loss, 195
    substance abuse/physical or sexual abuse history, 198
  Temporal factors
    discussion issues with patient, 200–201
    favorable timing assessment, 199–200
    weight loss timing, 199
BIA (Bioelectric impedance analysis machines), 181
BMI (body mass index), 4, 5f, 179–180, 179f, 188
  and age, 4
  correlation with triglyceride levels, 8
  and overweight classification, 385t
  and risk–benefit evaluation of drug treatment, 333
  and treatment options, 229
Body image, 452t
  dissatisfaction, 152–153, 159
    clinical significance, 459–460
  dissatisfaction treatment, 456, 460
    with weight reduction, 457
    without weight reduction, 457–459
  as incentive for weight loss, 451
  therapy, 458
  weigh loss effects on, 158–159
Body image. *See also* Self-esteem issues and obesity
Body image disturbance (and obesity)
  and age at obesity onset, 159
  assessment, 451–452, 454t–455t
    general considerations, 455–456
    measures of appearance satisfaction, 453
    measures of size perception, 453, 455
    measures of weight satisfaction, 453
  etiology, 447
    clinical significance, 450–451
    prevalence, 447–448, 448t
    severity, 449–450
    specificity, 448–449
  future research directions, 459–460

Body weight regulation, 19, 31
  by the gut, 30–31
  by skeletal muscle metabolism, 21–22
  and early environmental factors, 20
Body weight regulation. *See also* Adipose tissue; Central nervous system; Hypothalamus
Bulimia. *See also* Eating disorders/binge eating, 107

Callipyge and muscle mass, 21–22
The Calloway Diet, 257
Cancer Prevention Study I, 132
Cancers and obesity as risk factor, 3, 9–10
Carbohydrates, 251, 276A–277A
  high-carbohydrate diets, 262–264
  low-carbohydrate diets, 261–262
  "poison," 259
Cardiovascular disease
  heart disease, 7–8
  hypertension, 8–9
  obesity as risk factor, 3, 5
Central nervous system
  control of ingestion
    dopaminergic pathways, 29–30
    serotonergic pathways, 30
Children and obesity, 525–526
  and advertising
    advocacy groups, 99
    limitations to combat toxic environment, 101
  energy expenditure
    metabolic rate, 521
    physical activity, 520
    television viewing, 520–521
  energy intake
    breast and bottle feeding, 517
    caloric consumption and dietary composition, 518–519
    feeding style, 519
    modern food environment, 519
  environmental and cultural change, 523
  fetal development issues, 522–523
  heredity, 521–522
  increase of, 57, 515–516
  metabolic risk factors, 56–57
  parents
    advice to, 490–492
    training, 545–546
  and prediction of obesity in adulthood, 516, 517f
  prejudices, 145
  prevention, 559
    changes in BMI vs. behavior, 567–568
    interventions/diverse settings, 568–569
    physical activity intervention, 567
    Planet Health intervention, 559, 567
  psychological factors, 525
  self-regulation vs. parental regulation of food intake, 524
  socioeconomic factors, 523–524
  syndromes, 525
Children and obesity. *See also* Treatment of pediatric obesity

Cognitive-behavioral treatment of obesity
  elements, 469
  evolution, 466–467
  phases, 472f
    addressing obstacles to maintenance (modules VI–VIII), 470–471, 473–474
    maintenance (module IX), 474–476
    weight loss (modules I–V), 469–470
  skills consolidation, 476–477
  theoretical foundation
    cognitive conceptualization, 465
    modification of maintaining mechanism, 466
    use of cognitive and behavioral procedures, 466
  weight regain issue, 467–468
    cognitive-behavioral analysis, 468
CT (computerized tomography), and visceral fat assessment, 182
Cultural changes and obesity, 98

De novo lipogenesis, 50, 277A–278A
Diabetes
  obesity as risk factor, 3
  Type 2, 9
    increase among children, 56
Diathesis–stress model of obesity, 97
Diet Center, 257
Dietitians
  and behavioral assessment, 186
  and dietary assessment, 176
Diets/dieting, 154, 254–255, 388–389
  books/regimens, 406
    "glycemic index" diets, 257–259
    high-carbohydrate diets, 262–264
    high-protein diets, 259–260
    LEARN program, 406–407
    lifestyle changes, 264–265, 388
    low-carbohydrate diets, 261–262
    low-protein diets, 260–261
    miscellaneous/inappropriate, 264, 407
  composition, 251, 253t
    carbohydrate, 251
    electrolytes and water, 252
    protein, 251–252
    vitamins and minerals, 252
  and depression, 154–155
  fasts, 255
  liquid meal replacement uses, 237, 306
  products, 256, 265–266, 407–409
    and consumer protection, 395
    low-fat/low-sugar/low-calorie products, 266, 267t–268t, 268
  programs
    nonmedical, 397–400
    proprietary/medically based, 401–413
    residential, 403–404
    self-help, 404–407
    supermarket self-help, 407–409
    Web-based, 409
  as risk factor for binge eating disorder, 110, 157–158
  structured meal plan, 191, 305–306
  "traffic-light diet" (for pediatric obesity), 543
  "unbalanced-deficit diets," 256
Diets/dieting. See also BDD; LCDs; Nondieting approaches; Psychosocial effects of dieting; VLCDs; Weight loss/criteria for strategy evaluation
Drug treatment of obesity, 389, 389t
  altered metabolism, 320
  drugs for other indication
    dehydroepiandrosterone (DHEA), 330
    testosterone/dihydrotestosterone, 330–331
  drugs that alter metabolism/postabsorptive drugs
    hydroxycitrate, 329–330
    metformin, 329
  drugs that alter metabolism/preabsorptive agents, orlistat, 326–329, 328f, 390
  drugs that increase energy expenditure
    ephedrine and caffeine, 331–333, 332f
    thyroid hormones, 331
  drugs that reduce food intake, 321t
    mazindol, 322–323
    noradrenergic drugs, 320, 322, 325
    phentermine and diethylpropion, 322, 322f
    phenylpropanolamine, 322
  negative issues, 317–318, 318t
  patient selection criteria, 333
  peptides that reduce food intake
    Cholecystokinin (CCK), 326
    leptin, 325–326
    neuropeptide Y (NPY), 326
    pancreatic hormones, 326
  reduction of food intake
    monoamine mechanisms, 319t
    noradrenergic receptors, 318–319
    serotonergic receptors, 319–320
  sympathomimetic drugs (long-term use)
    safety, 325
    sibutramine, 323–325, 324f, 389–390
Duke Diet and Fitness Center (DFC), 403

Eating disorders, 117
  binge-eating disorder, 151–152, 151f
    associated features, 108–109
    binge components, 109
    diagnostic criteria, 107–108, 108t
    and emotional distress, 192, 482
    placebo responsiveness, 112–113, 113t
    prevalence, 111
    risk factors, 109–110
    spontaneous remission study, 113–114
    and VLCDs, 157–158
    and weight cycling, 162
  binge-eating disorder treatments, 111, 112
    pharmacotherapy, 112
    psychological/cognitive-behavioral, 111
    psychological/interpersonal therapy, 111
    standard weight reduction programs, 112

Eating disorders *(continued)*
    night-eating syndrome, 114, 193
        differences from nocturnal sleep-related eating
            disorders, 116–117
        neuroendocrine study, 116, 117f
        provisional criteria, 114–115, 115t
Eating Inventory scale (Stunkard and Messick), 110
Energy balance
    animal models research, 59–60
    equations, 48
    equations (dynamic), dynamic energy balance
        equation, 50
    equations (static)
        equations during weight maintenance, 48–49,
            49f
        static energy balance equation, 49–50
        and fat oxidation, 52
        regulation, 21
Energy metabolism
    components, 44f, 45
        physical activity, 47–48
        resting metabolic rate (RMR), 45–46
        thermic effect of food, 46–47
    measurement methods, 43
        direct calorimetry, 43
        doubly labeled water technique, 45
        field methods (indirect), 44
        indirect calorimetry, 43–44
    metabolic adaptation, 57–58, 58f
    and obesity, 42
    risk factors for adult weight gain, 52–53
        insulin sensitivity, 55
        low metabolic rate, 53–54, 53f, 54f
        low physical activity, 54–55
        low plasma concentration of leptin, 56
        low rates of fat oxidation, 55
        low SNS activity, 56
    risk factors for weight gain/children, 56–57
Environmental determinants of obesity, 62, 76–77,
        175–176, 245, 558
    cultural impact on populations, 98
    lack of public health attention, 98–99
    toxic environment pervasiveness, 99–100
        intervention proposals, 100–103
    worldwide evidence, 97–98
Ethnicity/race and obesity, 3, 77, 175, 416, 441
    and cancer rates, 9
    community context, 418
    guidelines (theoretically based), 437–439, 438t
        adherence issues, 439–440, 440t
    health implications, 420
    population differences, 75–76, 97, 416–418
    prevalence, 418–420, 418t
    and program outcomes, 420, 421t–423t, 424
    studies, 429
        clinical settings, 429, 435
        community settings, 430t–434t, 435–437
    theoretical influences of race/ethnicity on weight
        management, 424–425, 425f, 426f, 426t,
        427–428

Evolution, and fat accumulation, 42
"Eye–mouth" gap, 48–49, 95, 408

Fast-food impact, 98, 99
    and limitations to combat toxic environment, 101
Fat
    high-fat diets, 261
    storage and oxidation, 277A
Fat. *See also* De novo lipogenesis
The Fat Attack Plan, 257
Fat balance equation, 52
FTC monitoring of weight loss programs, 396–397
    Voluntary Guidelines, 397

Gallstone formation and weight loss, 127
Gallstones and obesity, 10–11
Gender and obesity, 3, 75
    and cardiovascular disease, 7–8
    maternal vs. paternal obesity as risk factors, 190
    and nondieting approaches, 494
    and prejudice, 145
    and psychosocial consequences, 147–148, 149t
Genetics and body weight, 42, 73–74, 173
    gene–environment interaction, 77
    gene–gene interaction, 77
    genes affecting muscle mass, 21
    genes expressed in central nervous system, 20, 20t
    genes expressed in peripheral tissues, 21t
    methodological issues
        false-positives and false-negatives, 79–80
        genome scans for obesity-related phenotypes,
            80–83, 81t
        identifying genes for common obesities, 78–79
        multiple testing for multiple genes, 79–80
        other genomic regions with linkages, 83
    predisposition studies, 56
    research with animal models, 59–60
    and RMR, 46
    single-gene defects, 175
    "thrifty" genotype, 76
    variations within families, 74, 76
Genetics and body weight. *See also* Leptin
GI (glycemic index), 257
    concept shortcomings, 259
    diets, 257–258
    foods (high/low GI), 258–259

Health care professionals
    advise, 484–486
    impact on patient's self-esteem, 482–483
    preparations, 392
    resources available, 391–392
    terminology issues, 485t
Health Management Resources (HMR), 402–403
Hyperinsulinemia, 9
Hyperlipidemia, 8
Hyperphagia, 42
Hypothalamus and body mass regulation, 20, 21
    hypothalamic NYP and its receptors, 28–29
    MCH neurons of lateral hypothalamus, 29

mediation of lepitin by LEPR, 26–27
melanocortin system regulation and glycemic
control, 28

Insulin sensitivity, as risk factor for adult weight gain, 55
Internet and dieting/weight control industry
eDiets.com, 409
nutrisystems.com, 400
Iowa Women's Health Study, 132

Jenny Craig, Inc., 399
JIB procedures. *See* Bariatric surgery/early procedures

L.A. Weight Loss, 399–400
LCDs (low-calorie diets), 256
and carbohydrate levels, 261–262
LEARN program, 392, 406–407
Learning theory, contribution to behavioral treatment
of obesity, 301
Leptin (LEPR), 26, 76, 374
deficiency, 56
mechanisms producing obesity in mice, 25, 59
mediation by LEPR, 26–27
and plateau in weight loss trials, 383
Lifestyle physical activity interventions, 288, 290, 388
activity plus diet, 290–291
and *LEARN* program, 392
Project Active, 288, 289t–290t, 291f

Mc3r (melanocortin 3 receptor), 76
Medical evaluation (of obese patient), 182
body composition assessment, 181–182
complications of obesity assessment, 177–178, 178t
current weight control efforts/readiness, 176, 386
dietary assessment, 176–177
etiologies
endocrine dysfunction, 174–175
environmental contributors, 175–176
genetic background, 175
history, 174, 384–385
family history of obesity, 174
general, 178
onset/progression of obesity, 174
laboratory tests, 181
physical activity assessment, 177
physical examination, 181, 384–385
anthropometric measurements, 178–180, 179f
contraindications to weight reduction, 385–386, 385t
specific obesity-related complications, 180–181
previous weight loss efforts assessment, 176
Medical treatment (of obese patient)
by primary care physicians, 383–384
focus on medical benefits of weight loss, 387
monitoring, 387
preparations for, 392
resources available, 391–392
treatment complications assessment, 182

treatment selection, 173–174, 386–387, 386t
Metabolic adaptation, 57–58, 58f
Montignac Method, 261
Mortality, as consequence of overweight, 5, 6f, 7
MYO (myostatin) and muscle mass, 21–22

National Weight Control Registry, 269
Nondieting approaches, 494, 510
assumptions, 495
causes/consequences of overweight are not
understood, 496
benefits, 506–507
"dieting" definition questions, 508–509
empirical support, 499, 500t–504t, 506
controlled comparisons, 505–506
descriptive studies, 499
goals, 496–497
harmfulness of dieting, 495–496
ineffectiveness of dieting, 495
methods, 497–499
research issues, 509
weaknesses, 507–508
Nurses' Health Study, 128, 129
Nutrient balance, 50
alcohol balance, 52
carbohydrate balance, 51
diet composition, 251–252, 253t
fat balance, 52
-feedback model, 318, 319f
macronutrient storage in humans, 276t,
278A–279A
protein balance, 50–51, 51f
Nutrisystem.com, 400

OA (Overeaters Anonymous) program, 233, 257,
404–405
Obesity, 3,4
as chronic disease, 98, 173
as a "culture bound" syndrome, 428
and decreasing "health-related quality of life,"
149
determinants, 96
biological, 97
determinants. *See also* Environmental
determinants
discrimination and federal law, 146
disease risk factors, 3, 7f, 96, 97, 339
evolutionary factors, 42
and fat balance equation, 52
hyperplastic, 188, 189f
hypertrophic, 188, 189f
and infectious agents, 173
and intrauterine and early postnatal factors, 173,
175–176
and physical activity, 284
physical health problems, 3–4, 293
prevalence, 283, 392
causes of, 283–284
emphasis on dietary assessment, 284–285
paucity of focus on physical activity, 285

Obesity *(continued)*
  as public health problem, 3, 283
    economic costs, 12–13, 42, 96, 125
    global obesity epidemic, 95, 103
  and television viewing, 99
Obesity. *See also* Body image disturbance; Eating
    disorders; Medical evaluation
Obesity research
  with animal models, 59–60
  future studies, 87–88
    additional linkage studies, 83–84
    association studies/linkage disequilibrium, 84–85
  with humans, 74
    environmental determinants, 62
    family-based association methods, 86–87
    genetic linkage studies, 61
    longitudinal studies, 52–53
    molecular mechanisms, 60–61
    population-based association methods, 85–86
    special populations, 85
    twin studies, 75, 76
  methodological issues
    gene identification, 78–79
    genome scans, 80–83, 81t
    measurement, 77–78
    multiple testing for multiple genes, 79–80
    other genome regions, 83
    phenotype instability, 78
OPTIFAST 800, 237, 389, 401–402
Orlistat. *See* Pharmacological treatment of obesity
Ornish Program, 262
Osteoarthritis and obesity, 11
Overweight, 3, 4

Pharmacological treatment of obesity
  and behavioral treatment, 239–241, 240f
  facilitating medication adherence, 241–242
  long-term medication use, 242–243, 242f, 243f
  maintenance benefits, 237
  size of weight losses (sibutramine/orlistat), 239
Physical activity, 297–298
  as energy metabolism component, 47–48
  fitness/obesity/mortality study, 293–297, 294f, 295t,
    296f, 297f
  home-based exercise, 368
  importance of, 13, 306–307
  improving exercise adherence, 308–309
    personal trainer, 309–310
  lack of emphasis on, 285
  and long-term weight loss, 307–308, 388
  and measures to combat toxic environment, 101
  in nondieting approach, 498–499
  personal trainers, 368–369
  public health recommendations, 287–288
  relationship with weight change, 285–286
    and weight loss, 287–288
    and weight loss maintenance, 287, 369
  short bouts study, 291–293, 292f, 309, 369
Physical activity. *See also* Lifestyle physical activity
    interventions

Physicians' Weight Loss Centers, 257
Pima Indian population
  environmental studies, 97–98
  longitudinal studies, 52–53
  and obesity, 76, 85
Planet Health intervention, 559, 567
POMC/CART neuron, 28
Pound of Prevention study, 571–572
Prevention issues, 556
  adult studies
    community trials/multiple risk factors focus,
      569–570
    prevention trials, 570–572
    worksite interventions, 570
  early efforts, 100
  environmental studies, 572
    cafeteria-based interventions, 581–582
    mass media campaigns, 572, 573t, 574
    nutrition environmental interventions, 574,
      575t–580t, 581
    physical activity interventions, 583, 584t–585t
    restaurant-based interventions, 582
    vending machines, 582–583
  future directions, 583, 586–587
  predictors of obesity, 557
    risk factors, 557–558
  three-tiered "bull's-eye" approach, 558
  toxic environment interventions proposal, 100–103
  youth studies, 559, 560t–566t
    changes in BMI vs. behavior, 567–568
    interventions/diverse settings, 568–569
    physical activity intervention, 567
    Planet Health intervention, 559, 567
Primary care physicians, and treatment of obesity,
    232
Pritikin Program, 403–404
  diet, 263
Professional societies associated with weight control
    issues, 253
Protein, 251–252, 276A
  high-protein diets, 259–260
  low-protein diets, 260–261
PSMF (protein-sparing modified fast), 543
Psychosocial effects of dieting, 339
  effects on body image, 158–159
    weight loss threshold, 159
  effects on eating disorders, 157
    bariatric surgery, 158
    and VLCDs (very-low-calorie diets), 157–158
  effects on mood, 154–155
    clinical issues, 155–156, 156f
    self-directed weight loss, 156–157
Psychosocial effects of dieting. *See also* Psychosocial
    effects of weight loss/extremely obese
    individuals
Psychosocial effects of obesity, 4, 11–12, 144,
    162–163, 195
  discrimination, 145–146
  prejudice, 144–145
  psychosocial status of individuals (clinical

populations), psychological functioning. *See also* Body image dissatisfaction; Eating disorders
psychosocial status of individuals (extremely obese individuals), 153–154, 153t
psychosocial status of individuals (general population)
  psychological functioning, 146–148, 149t
  quality of life, 149–150
Psychosocial effects of obesity. *See also* Self-esteem issues and obesity
Psychosocial effects of weight loss/extremely obese individuals
  mood improvements, 159, 160f, 161
  quality of life improvements, 161

Respiratory chambers, 43–44
Restraint Scale (Herman and Polivy), 110
RMR (resting metabolic rate), 45–46
  use in calculation of energy needs, 249–250
Rolls, Barbara, 263
Ryanodine receptor 1 (RYR1) and muscle mass, 21–22
RYGBP procedures. *See* Bariatric surgery

Satiety, 258, 262
Self-esteem issues and obesity, 480–481
  consequences of low self-esteem, 483–484
  health care professionals
    advise, 484–486
    impact on patient's self-esteem, 482–483, 492
    terminology issues, 485t
  helping to improve self-esteem (by individual), 488–490
  helping to improve self-esteem (by parents), 490–492
  helping to improve self-esteem (research findings), 486–488
  impact on weight management, 484
  importance in nondieting approach, 498
  reasons for low self-esteem, 481–482
  variables
    age of obesity onset, 482
    binge-eating disorder, 482
Sibutramine. *See* Pharmacological treatment of obesity
SlimFast, 236, 265, 306, 407–408
SNS (sympathetic nervous system) impairment
  link with RMR, 46
  and obesity, 42, 56
Surgical interventions for obesity, 244

The T-Factor Diet, 257, 262, 263
TEF (thermic effect of food), 44, 46–47
"Thrifty" genotype, 76, 85
TOPS (Take Off Pounds Sensibly) program, 233, 257, 405
Treatment of obesity
  algorithms for selecting treatment, 230
  limitations, 96
  options for "extremely obese" category, 244

options for "obese" category, 235
  low-calorie/portion-controlled diet, 235–236
  pharmacological treatment, 237, 239–243
  structured meal plans/liquid replacements, 236
  VLCDs, 236–237, 238t
options for "overweight" category, 232
  behavioral weight loss programs, 233–235
  commercial programs, 233
  primary care physicians, 232
  self-help programs, 233
standard weight reduction programs, as binge-eating disorder treatment, 112
three-stage process for selecting treatment, 231f
treatment selections
  importance of history, 230
  individual preferences, 231–232
  safety/efficacy/cost considerations, 230–231
Treatment of obesity. *See also* Weight control issues; Weight loss
Treatment of pediatric obesity, 552
  behavior change, 545
    parent training, 545–546, 549
    problem solving, 546–547
    treatment frequency, 546
  common clinical problems, 550
    family treatment, 551
    motivation, 551
    positive reinforcement, 551–552
    self-monitoring, 550–551
  dietary interventions
    individualized dietary interventions, 533
    protein-sparing modified fast, 543
    "traffic-light diet," 543
  exercise interventions, 543–545, 548
  goals, 532
  length of treatment, 532
    and weight change, 547–548, 548f
  research questions, 549–550
  treatment outcome studies, 538t–542t
  treatment studies, 534t–537t
Trevose Behavior Modification Program, 405–406

VBG. *See* Bariatric surgery
VLCDs (very-low-calorie diets), 157–158, 236–237, 255–256
  comparison with BDDs, 238t
  diet composition, 251–252, 253t
  and medically based proprietary weight loss programs, 401
  problems, 305
  and protein needs, 255
  and water balance, 255–256
Volumetrics, 263

WALI (Weight and Lifestyle Inventory), 186–187, 209A–226A
Weight control issues, 269
  dieting/weight control industries, 95, 256, 395
    consumer protection issues, 395
    and FTC, 396–397

Weight control issues *(continued)*
  and the Internet, 400
  "eye–mouth" gap, 48–49, 95
  future directions
    clinical, 372
    research, 372–374
  maintenance, 244–245, 374–375
    and body image interventions, 460
    effective strategies, 371–372
    extended treatment strategy, 361, 362t–363t, 364, 371–372
    food provision/monetary incentives, 364, 367
    importance in cognitive-behavioral treatment, 474–475
    multicomponent posttreatment programs, 369–370
    peer support, 367
    and physical activity, 286, 367–369
    "problem," 357
    relapse prevention training (RPT), 364
    strategy overview, 365t–366t
    telephone prompts, 367
    of "weight loss" vs. "weight lost," 374, 468
  plateaus, 242, 371
    and leptin, 383
    success redefinition, 372
Weight control issues. *See also* Bariatric surgery; Behavioral weight loss programs; Cognitive-behavioral treatment; Diets/dieting; Drug treatment of obesity; Physical activity; Prevention issues; Treatment of obesity; Weight loss
Weight cycling, 127, 161
  and binge eating, 162
  harmful effects, 495
  posttreatment weight gain factors, 360
  psychosocial effects
    clinical implications, 162
    on mood, 161–162
  regain problem, 467–468
    cognitive-behavioral analysis, 468
Weight loss
  circumstances, 125
  criteria for strategy evaluation, 249, 250t
    calories, 249–251
    coexisting health risks/conditions, 254
    components of weight management, 254
    composition, 251–252, 253t
    consumer friendliness, 253–254
    cost, 253

  long-term maintenance provisions, 254
  effective approaches, 313–314
  epidemiological studies, 127–128, 138
    future research directions, 138–139
    methodological limitations, 128–129
  intentional
    physiological effects, 126f
      negative, 127
      positive, 126–127
  intentional (studies of), 129
    mortality, 132–133
    observational cohort studies, 129, 130t–131t
    osteoporotic fractures, 133
  media usage, 312–313
  motivational strategies, 310–311
    social support, 311
    weight loss satisfaction, 311
  nonrandomized controlled trials (NCTs) of interventions, 133, 134t
    diabetes, 133, 135
    mortality, 135
  and physical activity, 286–287
  physiological basis, 276A
    diet composition, 280A–281A
    energy density, 281A–282A
    energy-providing substrates, 276A–280A
  programs, 409–410
    and FTC, 396–397
    future research, 411–412
    nonmedical, 397–400
    proprietary/medically based, 401–403
    residential, 403–404
    selection, 410–411, 410t
    self-help, 404–407
    supermarket self-help, 407–409
    Voluntary Guidelines, 396, 397t
    Web-based, 409
  programs. *See also* individual programs
  randomized controlled trials (RCTs) of interventions, 135, 136t
    CVD and mortality, 137–138
    diabetes, 137
    hypertension, 135, 137
  social context, 195
Weight loss. *See also* Behavioral assessment; Weight control issues
Weight Watchers program, 233, 257, 397–398
  outcome data/interpretation, 398–399
Women's Healthy Lifestyle Project (WHLP), 571
Wyden, Congressman Ron, 396